Orthodontic Treatment of Class III Malocclusion

Editors

Peter W. Ngan

Department of Orthodontics
West Virginia University
USA

Toshio Deguchi

Department of Orthodontics
Matsumoto Dental University
Japan

&

Eugene W. Roberts

Indiana University School of Dentistry
USA

CONTENTS

PART III: DIAGNOSIS AND TREATMENT IN THE NON-GROWING PATIENTS

PART IV: CONTEMPORARY APPLIANCES IN TREATMENT OF CLASS III PATIENTS

PART V: TREATMENT OF CLASS III PATIENTS WITH CRANIOFACIAL ANOMALIES

FOREWORD

I was very flattered having received the invitation to preface this book. After reviewing its contents, I wish to take this opportunity to thank each of the authors who have contributed so magnificently to the orthodontic literature.

Orthodontic management of the Class III malocclusion has been a genuine challenge to the profession and remains a controversial issue among clinicians and researchers. Some support the dictum that growth and size of the craniofacial complex are genetically predetermined and cannot be altered. They assume that the great majority of Class III cases are "untreatable" by orthodontics alone, and that surgical management after growth has been completed is inevitable. Others agree that heredity plays a major role in this type of deviation, yet support the contention that the pattern and direction of growth can be modified and that forces generated in orthopedic and orthodontic treatments are able to minimize and even successfully correct some Class III malocclusions. The controversy is real and one question still to be answered: How much can orthodontics really do?

Orthodontic Treatment of Class III Malocclusions helps to answer many questions and leads to fascinating suggestions for more research. It is truly an indoctrination of the very basic issues of growth and development and the influence of heredity in the growing and non-growing patient. Skeletal anchorage devices, surgical protocols, lingual orthodontics and a very interesting chapter on cleft lip and palate patients can be found in the text. All the material presented is well anchored on scientific and clinical evidence.

As an academician who has devoted a great deal of time to Class III treatment, I would say that this text is a great addition to the literature, reinforcing and supporting the premise that appropriate interventions at the proper time, accompanied by a family growth study may very well minimize or camouflage the Class III to acceptable and stable results without surgical intervention. There is clinical and scientific evidence that selected procedures can change questionable prognoses.

And yet, with the introduction of the vast amount of new knowledge promulgated by the most recent research; the many authors, in their brilliant presentations offer evidence that the influence of skeletal anchorage, early intervention and heredity can certainly help the orthodontist make a more cogent decision in the ultimate treatment plan for the patient with the disfigured countenance.

Yes, indeed, this is a book packed with nuggets, and well worth reading.

Eustaquio Araújo, DDS, MDS

Masters and Certificate in Orthodontics, University of Pittsburgh, PA, USA
The Pete Sotiropoulos Professor of Orthodontics
Clinic Director, Center for Advanced Dental Education, Saint Louis University, St. Louis, Missouri
Adjunct Professor, Kunghee University, Seoul, South Korea
Diplomate of the American Board of Orthodontics
Diplomate of the Brazilian Board of Orthodontics
Former President of the Pontificia Universidade Católica de Minas Gerais (Pontifical Catholic University of Minas Gerais), PUCMinas, Belo Horizonte, Brazil
Member of the Angle Society of Orthodontics, Midwest Component
Member of the International College of Dentists
Member of the American College of Dentists

PREFACE

This new eBook is a clinical text with plentiful illustrations to highlight both research findings, as well as clinical treatment of patients with Class III malocclusions. In addition, the craniofacial biology behind the various treatment strategies will empower clinicians with a sound knowledge for treatment of Class III problems. Contemporary orthodontic appliances, using micro-implants as anchorage, provide new avenues in the treatment of Class III patients. This text has appeal for both academicians and clinicians, but the targeted readership involves all practicing professionals in the field of orthodontics globally. The prevalence of Class III malocclusion is higher in Southern Asia countries. The international expertise addressing this important clinical area will be particularly appealing to clinicians throughout the world where there is a high influx of Asians with Class III malocclusions.

This book is broadly divided into five parts. Part I of the book introduces the Class III skeletal growth pattern and the genetics of mandibular prognathism. Since chincaps, facemasks and Class III elastics are routinely used for modifying Class III growth patterns, it is appropriate to update the readers on the biologic response of the mandibular condyle to orthopedic/orthodontic forces. Part II focuses on the diagnosis and treatment of Class III malocclusions in the growing patients. There are three main treatment options for skeletal Class III malocclusion: growth modification, dentoalveolar compensation, and orthognathic surgery. The authors present guidelines for choosing among these treatment options. The emphasis is on the discriminative diagnosis and the characteristic procedures of each treatment option. A systematic review on the current literature on the stability of early treatment was included and a novel approach for using micro-implants for early orthopedic treatment was introduced. Part III focuses on the diagnosis and treatment of Class III malocclusion in non-growing patients. This part introduced the use of self-ligating bracket system and temporary anchorage devices (TAD) to camouflage adult patients with mild to moderate Class III malocclusion. The use of TAD facilitates the treatment for specific types of Class III malocclusion and expands the range of orthodontic camouflage treatment. Patients with severe Class III malocclusion will require orthognathic surgery to correct the deformity. A significant number of these patients have mandibular asymmetry. The authors will present a contemporary way to treat these patients with combined orthodontics and orthognathic surgery. Part IV provides plentiful illustrations to guide the readers on the treatment of non-growing Class III patients, with camouflage to lingual treatment. The last portion of the text provides clinical insight and concerns relative the treatment of dentoalveolar craniofacial anomalies. The emphasis is on the scar-associated physiological and developmental problems that plague the orthodontic treatment of cleft lip and palate orthodontic patients. We would like to thank Dr. Araujo Eustaquio for writing the foreword and Bentham Science Publishers, particularly Manager Publication Aniza Naveed, for their support and efforts.

Peter W. Ngan
Department of Orthodontics
West Virginia University
USA

Toshio Deguchi
Department of Orthodontics
Matsumoto Dental University
Japan

&

Eugene W. Roberts
Indiana University School of Dentistry
USA

List of Contributors

Peter, Ngan

Department of Orthodontics, West, Virginia University, School of Dentistry, 1073 Health Science Center North, P.O. Box 9480, Morgantown, WV, USA

Toshio, Deguchi

Indiana University School of Dentistry (IUSD), Jarabak, Scholar Award, Department of Orthodontics, Matsumoto Dental University, Nagano, Japan

Liliana M., Otero

University of Kentucky, College of Dentistry, 800 Rose, Street, Room D416, Lexington, Kentucky, USA

Lorri Ann, Morford

University of Kentucky, College of Dentistry, 800 Rose, Street, Room D416, Lexington, Kentucky, USA

James K, Hartsfield

University of Kentucky, College of Dentistry, 800 Rose, Street, Room D416, Lexington, Kentucky, USA

Koshio, Sato

Isahai Dental Clinic, Tohoku University Graduate School of, Dentistry, Sendai, Japan, Sendai, Japan

Ichiro, Takahashi

Section of Orthodontics and Dentofacial Orthopedics, Division of Oral Health, Growth and Development, Kyushu University, Faculty of Dental Science, 3-1-1, Maidashi, Higashi-ku Fukuoka, 812-8582, Japan

Hong, He

Department of Orthodontics, Wuhan University and Key Lab for Oral, Biomedical Engineering and Wuhan University, Ministry of Education, China

Benedict, Wilmes

Department of Orthodontics, University of Duesseldorf, Germany

Won, Moon

UCLA School of Dentistry, Section of Orthodontics, CHS 63-, 082, Box 951668, 10833 Le Conte Avenue, Los Angeles, CA 90095-1668, USA

Reena, Khullar

UCLA School of Dentistry, Section of Orthodontics, CHS 63-, 082, Box 951668, 10833 Le Conte Avenue, Los Angeles, CA 90095-1668, USA

Toru, Kageyama

Department of Orthodontics, Hard Tissue Research Institute, Graduate School, Matsumoto, Dental University, Nagano, Japan

Mohammad, Razavi

University of Alberta, Clinical Instructor, School of Dentistry, Dept. Of, Orthodontics, Edmonton Clinic Health Academy, 11405-87 Avenue NW, Edmonton, Alberta T6G1C9, Case Western Reserve University, School of Dental, Medicine, Dept. Of Orthodontics, 10900 Euclid Ave., Cleveland, OH 44106, Canada, USA

Teruko, Takano-Yamamoto

Division of Orthodontics and Dentofacial, Orthopedics, Tohoku University Graduate School of Dentistry, 4-1, Seiryo-machi, Aoba-ku, Sendai, 980-8575, Japan

Isao, Saito

Division of Orthodontics, Niigata University Graduate School of Medical and, Dental Sciences, Niigata, Japan

Naoko, Watanabe

Division of Orthodontics, Niigata University Graduate School of Medical and, Dental Sciences, Niigata, Japan

Hyoung-Seon, Baik

Department of Orthodontics, College of Dentistry, Yonsei University, 50 YONSEI-RO SEODAE MUN KU, Seoul, South Korea

Nobuyuki, Ishii

Kanomi Orthodontic Office, 30 Minamiekimae-cho, Himeji, 670-0962, Japan

Ryuzo, Kanomi

Kanomi Orthodontic Office, 30 Minamiekimae-cho, Himeji, 670-0962, Japan

Young-Chel, Park

Department of Orthodontics, The institute of craniofacial, deformity, Dental College and Dental Hospital, Yonsei University, SEO DAI MUN GU, SHIN, CHONDONG1234, Seoul, South Korea

Yoonjeong, Choi

Department of Orthodontics, The institute of craniofacial, deformity, Dental College and Dental Hospital, Yonsei University, SEO DAI MUN GU, SHIN, CHONDONG1234, Seoul, South Korea

Tohiyaki, Hiro

Hiro Orthodontic Clinic, Nagano, Japan

Takashi, Yamashiro

Department of Orthodontics and Dentofacial, Orthopedics, Graduate School of Dentistry, Osaka University, 1-8 Yamada-Oka, Suita, Osaka, Japan

Seiji, Iida

Department, of Oral and Maxillofacial Surgery, Graduate School of Medicine, Dentistry and Pharmaceutical Sciences Okayama University, Okayama, Japan

Eugene W. Roberts

Indiana University School of Dentistry, USA

PART I: DEVELOPMENT OF CLASS III MALOCCLUSION

Send Orders for Reprints to reprints@benthamscience.net
Orthodontic Treatment of Class III Malocclusion, 2014, 3-24

CHAPTER 1

Family History and Genetics of Mandibular Prognathism

Liliana M. Otero[1,3], Lorri Ann Morford[2,3], Gabriel Falcão-Alencar[2] and James K. Hartsfield, Jr.[2,3,*]

[1]Pontificia Universidad Javeriana, Bogotá, Colombia; [2]Hereditary Genetics/Genomics Laboratory, University of Kentucky, College of Dentistry, Lexington, Kentucky, USA; [3]Department of Oral Health Science, University of Kentucky, Lexington, Kentucky, USA

Abstract: Often referred to as mandibular prognathism, the Class III phenotype can be a result of mandibular prognathism, maxillary hypoplasia (also termed maxillary retrognathism), or a combination of the two. These terms reflect the anatomical heterogeneity of Class III, as either or both jaws may be affected in sagittal length, or in position relative to each other. Familial aggregation studies suggest that familial environmental factors and/or heredity can play a substantial role in the etiology of Class III phenotype. This is supported by the findings that prevalence and anatomical characteristics of Class III malocclusions vary largely according to ethnic background, and may represent the effects of cultural differences at least to some degree. Current genetic inheritance patterns proposed for the Class III malocclusion include autosomal-recessive, autosomal-dominant, autosomal-dominant with incomplete penetrance, and a polygenic threshold model. Studies will be presented showing that the familial distribution of mandibular prognathism could be explained by the presence of a dominant major gene with an autosomal Mendelian mode of transmission that is affected by other genes and environmental factors leading to incomplete penetrance and variable expressivity. Finally, findings from both genetic linkage and association analyses in humans will be presented implicating variation in chromosomal locations with the Class III phenotype, including 1p35, 1p36. 4p16.1, 6q25, 12q13, 14q24.3-31.2 and 19p13.2 in Asian populations; and 1p22.1, 3q26.2, 7p22, 11q22, 12q13.13, and 12q23 in families from South American; and 12q24.11 in primarily a Caucasian sample residing in the United States.

Keywords: Mandibular prognathism, Class III malocclusion, Craniofacial genetics, Genetics, Genetic linkage.

***Address correspondence to James K. Hartsfield:** University of Kentucky, College of Dentistry, 800 Rose Street, Room D416, Lexington, Kentucky, USA, 40536-0297; Tel: (859) 323-0296; Fax: (859) 257-8878; E-mail: James.Hartsfield@uky.edu

INTRODUCTION

Although all Angle occlusion types were initially based on the sagittal relationship of the permanent first molars, including the Class III malocclusion, it has generally been recognized that this dental relationship is often observed with a corresponding skeletal relationship as well. This is exemplified in Class III malocclusion cases, which characteristically result in the appearance of a prominent mandible. In its most severe form, the Class III malocclusion can be functionally and/or socially debilitating [1]. Affected individuals with a distinctive facial profile often seek orthodontic treatment, frequently combined with orthognathic surgery, to correct this malocclusion [2]. Often referred to as mandibular prognathism (taken from the Greek *pro* =forward and *gnathos* =jaw), skeletal aspects of this disorder can be a result of pure mandibular prognathism, maxillary hypoplasia/retrognathism, or a combination of the two. These phenotypic variations create a significant heterogeneity among Class III subjects and account for some of the difficulty encountered when scientifically investigating the condition [2].

Environmental factors that have been thought to influence Class III malocclusion as reviewed by El-Gheriani *et al.* [3] include enlarged tonsils [4], endocrine "imbalances"/hormonal disturbances [5, 6], posture, trauma and disease including premature loss of the first permanent molars [7]; nasal blockage [8], "congenital" anatomic defects [9], instrument deliveries [10], and trauma, infection or inflammation in the temporomandibular joint [11]. The roles these factors in Class III, however, are largely based on only a few observations. Clearly, different anatomical features of Class III can be classified into subgroups that appear to be influenced by ethnicity and may have a common environmental and/or genetic basis. While the relative contribution and interaction of genetic and/or environmental factors in the complex etiology of Class III is unclear, familial aggregation studies suggest that heredity plays a substantial role [2, 12, 13].

Prevalence of Class III Malocclusion

It has been demonstrated that both prevalence rates and anatomical characteristics of the Class III malocclusion vary largely according to ethnic background, with the highest prevalence observed in East Asian populations such as Korean, Chinese, and Japanese (8%-40%) [1, 4, 14-17]. By comparison, African populations exhibit a reduced Class III prevalence rate (3%-8%) compared to Asians and Class III is relatively rare in individuals of European-American descent (0.48%-4%) [4, 8, 16, 17]. Additional studies in the United States of America (US) have suggested that the prevalence of Class III malocclusion in Caucasians can be as high as (5.5%-9.5%) [18-20], while the prevalence in US Native American Indian populations is relatively low (2.6%-3.1%) [21]. North American Eskimos in Labrador, Canada have a Class III prevalence of approximately 16% [22].

Populations in South America are often a mixture of Caucasian/European, African and Amerindian decent. While the percentage of children in Bogotá, Colombia with Class III has been reported as 3.7%, Brazilian children exhibited a frequency between (4%-10%) [23-25]. The prevalence of Class III in Europe appears to vary based largely on geography with 2.9% reported in Britain [26], 4% in Sweden [27], 5% in Finland [28], (1.4%-4.3%) in Germany [29, 30] and 8% in Scotland [31]. In areas of the Middle East, the prevalence of Class III also displays geographic tendencies with the highest prevalence in Egypt at 10.6% [32], followed by 7.8% in Iran [33] and 5.1% in Lebanon [34].

Influence of Ethnicity on Class III-Related Facial Dimensions

When comparing craniofacial features of soft and skeletal tissue between ethnicities, a number of features may appear accentuated or diminished. These ethnicity-related features are most likely determined or at least strongly influenced by genetic factors [2]. For example, Singh and colleagues demonstrated differences in both horizontal and vertical craniofacial dimensions when comparing Korean and American-Caucasian patients with Class III malocclusions. Korean subjects with Class III malocclusion had shorter anterior cranial base and more pronounced midfacial retrusion compared with European Americans [35]. Additional studies by Ngan *et al.* (1997) have reported on the ethnic differences between Chinese and Caucasians with Class III malocclusion. Chinese subjects exhibited a shorter anterior cranial base, a larger posterior cranial base, a smaller gonial angle, and an increased mandibular length compared to Caucasians [36].

Several differences have also been reported between Japanese and Caucasians. Japanese subjects with severe Class III malocclusion exhibit an increased mandibular ramus and total mandibular length when compared to Caucasians. Japanese females showed a statistically significant reduction in the anterior cranial base, a reduced midfacial component, and increased lower anterior face height associated with a more obtuse gonial angle when compared to Caucasians. In addition, more proclined upper incisors were also noted in the Japanese females [15]. Finally, differences in the cephalometric measurements between Saudi and Japanese adult females have also been reported in the literature. Saudi females had an increased anterior cranial base length, decreased posterior cranial base length, smaller cranial base angle, smaller anterior and posterior facial heights, downward tipping of the maxilla, retruded chin, less steep mandibular plane, increased joint angle, smaller ramus, body and total mandibular length, and less retroclined mandibular incisors when compared to their Japanese counterparts [37].

Gender and Class III-Related Facial Dimensions

It should not be surprising that gender differences exist during normal craniofacial growth that are influenced, at least in part, by variations in sex hormone concentrations during the pubertal growth spurt [38]. The ratio of estrogen and testosterone is responsible for skeletal sexual dimorphisms like greater bone mass in adult males [39], and characteristics of the human face [40]. A high testosterone/estrogen (T/E) ratio in puberty facilitates facial characteristics such as the lateral growth of mandible and chin, and the lengthening of the lower face [40, 41].

Although preliminary indications suggest that Class III skeletal disharmony can become apparent as early as in the deciduous dentition phase, few papers have reported on gender differences specifically related to the Class III malocclusion [42]. In one study, a greater maxillary and mandibular protrusion with reduced facial convexity has been described for Chinese girls than observed for boys [43]. In a Slovenian population sample with mixed dentition, larger than average values for anterior and posterior face height were observed in males than in females [44]. In addition, studies have shown a significant degree of sexual dimorphism in craniofacial features especially after the age of 13 in Caucasian subjects with Class III malocclusion, with female subjects presenting smaller linear dimensions in the maxilla, mandible, and anterior facial heights than male subjects [45]. Miyajima and colleagues reported similar changes in Japanese females, with the retruded position of the maxilla maintained during growth, while the mandible became more protrusive [46].

Class III Anatomical Characteristics and Subphenotypes

Several studies have suggested the existence of multiple patterns or sub-phenotypes of the Class III malocclusion based on anatomical appearance. For example, Ellis and McNamara (1984) reported considerable variation among Class III malocclusion patients, where the most common combination of variables included a retrusive maxilla with protrusive incisors, a protrusive mandible with retrusive incisors, and a long lower facial height. Interestingly, they also found no significant gender differences [47]. Martone and colleagues have suggested the existence of three anatomical subgroupings of Class III in a study of craniofacial growth and head form including the brachycephalic, dolichocephalic and dinaric patterns [48]. In a cluster analysis of skull shapes among fifty British mandibular prognathism subjects, only 15% of them also presented with maxillary retrognathism, it was demonstrated that 58% of the subjects exhibited increased lower facial height, and five sub-grouping of Class III skull shapes could be defined [49]. Cluster analysis of 106 Korean patients with Class III malocclusion resulted in seven distinct clusters being identified [50]. Differences in the methods between these two cluster analyses make a clear comparison of the studies difficult.

Following along this same idea, with a view more towards genetic analysis, was a detailed phenotypic characterization of Class III malocclusions that resulted in five clusters representing distinct sub-phenotypes in a sample of 309 North Carolina subjects. Several ethnic groups were represented in the study, although 73% of the sample was Caucasian. The groupings of variables reflected anteroposterior and vertical dimensions rather than specific craniofacial structures, suggesting that different genes are involved in controlling dimension *vs.* structure. The five subgroupings or "*Prototype Clusters*" were described as follows: (1) prognathic mandible with long face, (2) maxillary deficiency with decreased vertical dimension (low angle), (3) maxillary deficiency with increased vertical dimension (high angle), (4) mild prognathic mandible with normal vertical dimension, and (5) a combination of prognathic mandible and maxillary deficiency with normal vertical dimension [51].

Inheritance Models of the Class III Malocclusion

Although the relative contribution and interaction of genetic and environmental factors in the etiology of the Class III malocclusion is unclear, familial aggregation studies suggests that heredity plays a substantial role. The familial nature of mandibular prognathism was first reported by Strohmayer in 1937 as noted by Wolff *et al.* (1993) in their analysis of the pedigree of the Hapsburg family [52]. Chudley presented examples of the Habsburg jaw printed on postage stamps of Spain and wrote that autosomal recessive and multifactorial inheritance were considered as possibilities by some geneticists, because of the incomplete penetrance in association with extensive consanguinity in the "Royal" Family [53]. It is also possible that portraits of the Hapsburg Family may have enhanced the prominence of the lower jaw as a feature of royalty, thereby making unbiased ascertainment of the affected in the family potentially problematic. Investigations of less inbred groups have resulted in a variety of modes of inheritance being proposed, with monogenic influences in some families (usually autosomal dominant with incomplete penetrance and variable expressivity) and multifactorial (polygenic complex) influences in others [3, 5, 12, 13, 52, 54-58]. Although the X chromosome does play a role in some syndromes with mandibular prognathism, the Class III phenotype is not X-linked since the numbers of affected males and females are similar [59].

Genetic Analyses of the Class III Phenotype

With the broad range of phenotypic heterogeneity observed among Class III cases, it is not surprising that genetic linkage studies have implicated multiple genetic loci, located on a number of different chromosomes in this malocclusion [60-68]. In this complex disorder, it has been hypothesized that the effects of one or more genes are modified (diminished, masked, enhanced, *etc...*) by another gene and/or its gene product, thereby leading to variable gene expressivity, incomplete gene penetrance, and ultimately large phenotypic variations. Statistically, this phenomenon is termed "*genetic epistasis*" and it describes a departure from the theoretical concept that a single genetic locus will act "independent" of another genetic allele. In addition to epistasis, variations in the incidence of Class III malocclusion by ethnicity may reflect a variation in the genes or gene sets contributing to the overall phenotype within a specific genetic background.

Genetics of Class III in Asians

Up until recently, the vast majority of Class III genetic research had been completed with Asian populations and has implicated genetic linkage to on multiple chromosomal regions including 1p35, 1p36, 4p16.1, 6q25, 12q13, 14q24.3 and 19p13.2 [60-64, 68] (Table **1A**). One of the most promising genetic regions connected to Class III malocclusion within this population appears to be on human chromosome 1. In a case-control genetic Linkage Disequilibrium (LD) association analysis of Korean individuals with mandibular prognathism, a haplotype of three single nucleotide polymorphisms (SNPs) within the Matrilin 1 (*MATN1) gene* (1p35) was identified as conferring an increased risk for mandibular prognathism (rs1149054 T>C, rs20566 G>A and rs1065755 C>T; $p<0.01$ and OR= 5.16) [61] In addition, the *MATN1* rs20566-AA genotype was shown to be protective against mandibular prognathism formation (OR = 0.16) while the rs1065755-TT genotype conferred an increased risk of mandibular prognathism (OR = 9.28) [61]. The *MATN1* gene encodes a cartilage matrix protein that belongs to the von Willebrand Factor type A (VWA) family of proteins and it appears to play a role in skeletal formation (reviewed in [69-71]). Since mandibular shape originates both from bone growth and/or surrounding muscle growth and function (reviewed in [72-74]), the *MATN1* gene is a reasonable gene candidate for Class III formation. At this time, however, there is no direct evidence that these particular SNPs are themselves causal, and may just be predictors of susceptibility to the phenotype. Thus, sequencing analysis of the *MATN1* gene in Asian Class III cases could be highly informative. It is also noteworthy that genetic variations in *MATN1* have been associated with osteochondrodysplasias (disorders of bone and cartilage development) and idiopathic scoliosis (which affects the musculoskeletal system) [75, 76]. Moreover, evidence for the role of *MATN1* in Class III malocclusion exists in a dental occlusion model in *Equus asinus*, the Zamorano-Leonés donkey [77]. In this model, Rodrigues *et al.,* identified a genetic variation within intron 7 (g503G > A) of the donkey *MATN1* gene that was significantly associated with donkeys exhibiting a prognatic lower jaw compared to the donkeys with normal occlusion. Both the GA and AA genotypes are associated with a decreased risk of prognathism formation , supporting the possible role of *MATN1* variation with mandibular prognathism [77]. No equivalent variation to the donkey g503G>A variation has yet been identified in human.

In addition to these findings with the *MATN1* gene loci, studies in Asians have implicated several additional loci which may influence the Class III phenotype. For example, a case-control genetic linkage disequilibrium association analysis of chromosome 1p36 in a presumably Hong Kong Chinese population said to have "mandibular prognathism" found four SNPs located within the *Erythrocyte Membrane Protein Band 4.1 (EPB4.1)* gene to be significant [62]. The implication(s) of this finding remains to be determined given the known roles/functions of *EPB4.1,* which appear to be restricted largely to red blood cells. In a genome wide linkage analysis of mandibular prognathism in 40 Korean sibling pairs and 50 Japanese sibling pairs encompassing a total of 42 families, researchers identified linkage at three chromosomal locations: 1p36 (D1S234; maximum Z(lr) = 2.51, p=0.0012), 6q25 (D6S305; maximum Z(lr) = 2.23, p=0.025) and 19p13.2 (D19S884; maximum Z(lr) = 1.93, p=0.0089) [60]. Microsatellite marker D1S234 resides within an intron of the *Chloride intracellular channel 4, (CLIC4)* gene and near the *Runt-related transcription factor 3 (RUNX3)* gene on human chromosome 1. D6S305 resides witin an intron of the *Parkin RBR E3 Ubiquitin Protein Ligase (PARK2)* gene, and D19S884 resides within an intron of the *fibrillin 3 (FBN3)* gene. The potential significance of these gene loci in Class III remains to be determined. Multipoint linkage analysis of a genome wide scan with 6,090 single nucleotide polymorphisms (SNP) in two Chinese families found significant (highest LOD 3.308) linkage to chromosome 4p16.1 for mandibular prognathism [63]. Suggestive linkage (LOD 2.03) of mandibular prognathism to chromosomal region 14q24.3-31.2 has also been found in one Han Chinese family [64]. Finally, an association has been identified between mandibular prognathism and rs1793953, which is associated with the *Collagen, type II, alpha 1 (COL2A1)* gene [68]. This is particularly noteworthy since the *COL2A1* gene is located at 12q13, which is a chromosomal region that has also been found to be significiant for Class III maloclussion in a South American sample [65].

Table 1A: Studies Examining the Genetics of Class III Malocclusions within Asian Populations

Chromosomal Location	Type of Study	Number of Subjects Studies	Phenotype	Markers	Findings / Significance Level	Refs.
1p35	Case Control	164 Korean subjects with Mandibular Prognathism 132 Controls	MP= Mandibular Prognathism	rs1149054 (-158T/C); rs20566 (+7987G/A); rs1065755 (+8572C/T)	rs1149054 rs20566 rs1065755 alleles together had a pronounced risk effect for MP	[61]
1p36	Case Control	Hong Kong Chinese	MP	rs2249138 rs2254241 rs2788890 rs2788888	p=0.018 p=0.015 p=0.028 p=0.023	[62]
1p36	GWAS	40 Korean Sibling Pairs (SPs) 50 Japanese SPs 42 Families Total	MP	D1S234	Maximum Z(Ir)=2.51 P=0.0012	[60]
4p16.1	Genome Wide Linkage Scan (GWLS); 6,090 SNP markers; Illumina Linkage-12 DNA Analysis Kit (average spacing 0.58 cM)	Two Unrelated Chinese Han Families (from different provinces) each comprised of 4 generations; 42 total individuals 18 affected individuals	MP	rs726111 rs875864 rs7658616 rs875579	NPL=2.71 LOD=3.308; NPL=3.65 LOD=3.166; NPL=3.63 LOD=3.156; NPL=3.54 LOD=3.106	[63]
6q25	GWAS	40 Korean SPs 50 Japanese SPs 42 Families Total	MP	D6S305	Maximum Z(Ir)=2.23 P=0.025	[60]
12q13	Association	211 cases and 224 controls of Hong Kong Chinese Han ethnicity However, MP was not associated with haplotypes that included rs1793953	MP	rs1793953	p=0.025	[68]

Table 1A: contd...

Chromosomal Location	Type of Study	Number of subjects studies	Phenotype	Markers	Findings / Significance Level	Refs.
14q24.3	GWLS; 6,090 SNP markers; Illumina Linkage-12 DNA Analysis Kit (average spacing 0.58 cM)	1 Han Chinese Family; 11 Affected 10 unaffected	MP	between rs1468507 and rs7141857	NPL=11.341 (empirical p = 0.020); LOD= 2.032 (empirical p = 0.008)	[64]
19p13.2	GWAS	40 Korean SPs 50 Japanese SPs 42 Families Total	MP	D19S884	Maximum Z(Ir)=1.93 P=0.0089	[60]

SPs = Sibling Pairs; GWAS=Genome wide association study; GWLS=Genome wide linkage scan; *NPL = Nonparametric Linkage; **PL = parametric Linkage; ***LOD= logarithm (base 10) of the odds score for parametric analysis; ****Zlr for nonparametric analysis.

Genetics of Class III in South Americans

These findings for the Asian subjects are in contrast to a recent study of four Hispanic families primarily with maxillary hypoplasia that were recruited at the Universidad de Antiouqia in Medellin, Colombia, South America [65] (Table **1B**). For this study, researchers performed a genome wide scan followed by a statistical linkage analysis. In this analysis, 10 of 500 microsatellite markers found on 5 different chromosomal locations segregated in an autosomal-dominant manner with the Class III phenotype [65]. These 5 locations included 1p22.1-22.2 (D1S2865 and D1S435), 3q26.2 (D3S3041), 11q22.2-q22.3 (D11S1886 and D11S4206), 12q13.13 (D12S1613, D12S1583, D12S354 and D12S369), and 12q23 (D12S368) [65].

In a separate genome wide linkage scan of one large Hispanic family from Bogotá, Colombia, South America, researchers have identified genetic linkage on chromosome 7 [78]. Further analysis of additional Hispanic families from Bogotá along with 10 families from Brasilia, Brazil, all primarily with mandibular prognathism in the presence or absence of maxillary hypoplasia, has confirmed this linkage to the Class III phenotype on chromosome 7 [78]. In studies of South

American families, Turner *et al.* (2011) was unable to confirm genetic linkage on chromosome 11 in the regions of D11S1886 and D11S4206 when examining cases of Class III with mandibular prognathism in the presence and absence of maxillary hypoplasia [79]. Recently Cruz *et al.* (2011) studied the genetic linkage with 6 microsatellite markers (D1S234, D4S3038, D6S1689, D7S503, D10S1483, and D19S56) for Class III malocclusion. They showed that there was no evidence

Table 1B: Studies Examining the Genetics of Class III Malocclusions within South American Populations

Chromosomal Location	Type of Study	Number of Subjects Studies	Phenotype	Markers	Findings / Significance Level	Refs.
1p22.1-22.2	4 cM Genome wide microsatellite scan (GWMS); 546 markers	4 Families from Medellín, Colombia; (Dichotomous classification) 28 affected 29 unaffected	primarily maxillary deficiency	D1S2865 D1S435	ZLR=2.92 (PL) LOD=1.8554 ZLR=2.54 (NPL) LOD=1.6382	[65]
1p36.11	Microsatellite Study	42 individuals from 10 Families in Brazil		D1S234	No Linkage Identified	[66]
3q26.2	4 cM GWMS; 546 markers	4 Families from Medellin, Colombia; (Dichotomous classification) 28 affected 29 unaffected	primarily maxillary deficiency	D3S3041	ZLR=2.97 (NPL) LOD=1.9136	[65]
4p16.3	Microsatellite Study	42 individuals from 10 Families in Brazil		D4S3038	No Linkage Identified	[66]
4p16 region		32 Colombian families	MP and maxilla retrognathia		No association to Class III identified for *MSX1* located on chromosome 4p16.3-p16.1	[67]
6p21	Microsatellite Study	42 individuals from 10 Families in Brazil		D6S1689	No Linkage Identified	[66]
7p22	*Illumina® Infinium Human Linkage*-y; 6,090 SNPs;	40 Individuals in 1 Family from Bogotá, Colombia; 25 Affected	MP +/- maxillary hypoplasia	rs1044701 rs1299548 rs1882600	LOD =2.3 LOD = 1.52 LOD = 1.9	[78]

Table 1B: contd…

Chromosomal Location	Type of Study	Number of Subjects Studies	Phenotype	Markers	Findings / Significance Level	Refs.
7p22	SNP Study	156 individuals in 21 families from Bogotá, Colombia and 77 individuals in 14 Families from Brasilia, Brazil	Mandibular Prognathism +/-maxillary hypoplasia	rs1044701 rs1299548 rs1882600 rs1294611 rs9640034 rs9640038 rs11526212 rs7800782	evidence of linkage(PL) at rs1882600 (LOD=2.36); Exclusion of linkage (PL) in the marker rs1044701	[78]
7p21.2	Microsatellite Study	42 individuals from 10 Families in Brazil		D7S503	No Linkage Identified	[66]
10q26	Microsatellite Study	42 individuals from 10 Families in Brazil		D10S1483	No Linkage Identified	[66]
11q22.2-q22.3	4 cM GWMS; 546 markers	4 Families from Medellín, Colombia; (Dichotomous classification) 28 affected 29 unaffected	primarily maxillary deficiency	D11S1886 D11S4206	ZLR=3.03 (PL) LOD=1.9960; ZLR=2.90 (PL) LOD=1.8377	[65]
11q22.2-q22.3	4 SNP markers in regions of D11S1886 and D11S4206	21 families from Bogotá, Colombia and 10 Families from Brasilia, Brazil	MP +/- maxillary hypoplasia	rs666723 rs578169 rs12416856 rs1386719	No Linkage Identified	[79]
12q13.13	4 cM GWMS; 546 markers	4 Families from Medellin, Colombia; (Dichotomous classification) 28 affected 29 unaffected	primarily maxillary deficiency	D12S1613 D12S1583 D12S354 D12S369	ZLR=2.79 (PL) LOD=1.6971; ZLR=2.93 (PL) LOD= 1.8730; ZLR=2.91 (PL) LOD=1.8412; ZLR=2.91 (PL) LOD=1.8355	[65]
12q23	4 cM GWMS; 546 markers	4 Families from Medellin, Colombia; (Dichotomous classification) 28 affected 29 unaffected	primarily maxillary deficiency	D12S368	ZLR=2.70 (NPL) LOD=1.7820	[65]
19p13.1	Microsatellite Study	42 individuals from 10 Families in Brazil		D19S56	No Linkage Identified	[66]

for linkage of any of the 6 microsatellite markers and excluded 5 of the 6 markers evaluated [66]. These findings emphasize the importance to ultimately study genetic factors of each sub-phenotype of Class III independently, since the genetic factors that influence maxillary hypoplasia may differ dramatically from those leading only to true mandibular prognathism.

Genetics of Class III in Other Ethnic Groups

Most of the Class III studies cited have been genetic linkage studies in families or linkage disequilibrium association studies in unrelated individuals. Another study of the later type was recently performed at the University of Pittsburgh [80, 81]. In this study, 40-44 mandibular prognathic cases were matched based on race, age and gender to 36-40 Class I/orthognathic control subjects in an association analysis examining 33-36 single nucleotide polymorphisms (SNPs) within 8 to10 previously reported candidate gene loci, including 1p22.1, 1p22.2, 1p36, 3q26.2, 5p13-p12, 6q25, 11q22.2-q22.3, 12q23, 12q13.13, and 19p13.2 (Table **1C**). They identified a significant (p=0.02) association of the Class III malocclusion with the marker rs10850110 located upstream of the Myosin 1H gene (*MYO1H*) on chromosome 12q24.11 [80, 81]. Four additional candidate genes within this region of human chromosome 12q24.11 were also noted that may play a role in the Class III phenotype including *ACACB* (acetyl-CoA carboxylase beta), *FOXN4* (forkhead box N4), *KCTD10* (potassium channel tetramerisation domain containing 10), and *UBE3B* (ubiquitin protein ligase E3B) [81].

Myosins, in general, are actin-based, ATPase driven motor molecules. MYO1H, however, is an unconventional myosin (Class I type), which has a role in intracellular movements in contrast with the conventional Class II myosins. Myosin-1H interacts with membranous compartments to move them relative to actin fibers and is involved in such processes as cell motility, phagocytosis and vesicle transport.

MYO1H is expressed in the musculoskeletal-craniofacial tissues [80], and in a preliminary examination, Class II Orthognathic surgery patients (n=4) expressed higher levels of MYO1H mRNA in their Masseter muscle than Class III orthognathic patients (n=2). Among Class III surgical patients examined, the trend of MYO1H mRNA expression was lowest in the single deep bite case examined and highest in the two Class III cases with normal bite. Overall, mRNA expression of MYO1H in Masseter muscle was ~0.4X of the levels observed in skeletal muscle of the limb [82]. Gene expression evaluation in masseter muscle from dentofacial deformity subjects undergoing orthoganathic surgery for skeleton-based malocclusions found a trend for increased MYO1H and MYO1C expression in class III malocclusion compared to class II malocclusion. There were significant correlations ($p < 0.05$) between MYO1C expression and fiber type percent occupancy in masseter muscle from subjects with normal and deep bite malocclusions. Significant correlations were also identified between MYO1C and MHC (myosin heavy chain) gene expression.The mechanism of how the *MYO1H* and *MYO1C* genes and their protein products influence the Class III phenotype, however, remains unknown. It has been postulated that altered glucose transport during condylar cartilage growth may be one of the cellular mechanisms that promotes mandibular prognathism, as well as development of open and deep bite skeletal malocclusions through masseter muscle fiber type differences [83].

It should be noted that the Pittsburgh group examined a small cohort size of 80 individuals including subjects with a variety of different ethnic backgrounds (26 Class I and 24 Class III cases of European descent, 6 Class I and 15 Class III cases of African descent and 3 Class I and 5 Class III cases were a combination of individuals of Hispanic, Asian and other descent) [81]. Since (1) the phenotypic expression of Class III can vary greatly between different ethnicities and may be influenced by a combination of genetics plus environmental factors, and (2) the Minor Allele Frequencies (MAFs) of the rs10850110 marker vary greatly between ethnicities (MAFs according to HapMap: 27% Caucasian, 1% African, 9% Chinese and 15% Japanese), it will remain to be determined how these findings will compare to future association studies.

Using whole exome sequencing techniques on the DNA from an Estonian family, scientists have recently uncovered a rare heterozygous missense mutation associated with Class III skeletal malocclusion in the Dual-Specificity Phosphatase 6 (*DUSP6*) gene (c.545C>T ; p.Ser182Phe; rs139318648). Affected individuals in this family were largely characterized as having a straight profile with maxillary deficiency. This rare variant co-segregated with the disease and followed an autosomal-dominant pattern of inheritance with incomplete penetrance. The *DUSP6* gene encodes is a cytoplasmic dual-specificity phosphatase that acts as a negative regulator of the MAP kinases, ERK1/2. This protein is involved in the some fundamental signaling processes that occur at the early stages of skeletal development, and can be transcriptionally upregulated *via* the fibroblast growth factor (FGF)/FGF receptor signaling pathway [84].

Table 1C: Studies Examining the Genetics of Class III Malocclusions within North American and European Populations

Chromosomal Location	Type of Study	Number of Subjects Studies	Phenotype	Markers	Findings / Significance Level	Refs.
12q24.11	Case Control	44 Class III cases of mixed ethnicity 36 Class I controls Pittsburgh, Pennsylvania USA		33 SNPs spanning all candidate regions; (1p22.1, 1p22.2, 1p36, 3q26.2, 5p13-p12, 6q25, 11q22.2-q22.3, 12q23, 12q13.13, and 19p13.2)	*MYO1H* (rs10850110) p=-0.03	[80, 81]
12q23-24	whole-exome sequencing	five siblings from an Estonian family affected by Class III malocclusion	Straight profile with maxillary hypoplasia	rs139318648	*DUSP6* *(c.545C>T ; p.Ser182Phe;*	[84]

In summary, there remains a great deal of work to be done to understand the genetic components of the Class III malocclusion. Studying the individual subgroupings of the Class III phenotype will be essential to define the genes with influence Class III heterogeneity. While linkage analysis within families will be valuable in defining ethnic contributions to the phenotype, large association analyses may help to better define genes, which influence the Class III phenotype independent of ethnicity. Clinically this reinforces the importance of a family history, including in regard to presence of, or treatment for, a "strong" lower jaw, "underbite" in lay term, or Class III malocclusion.

The patient who has a first degree relative (parent or full sibling) with a Class III malocclusion has up to a 50% likelihood of also developing a Class III malocclusion, although even in families with a clear multi-generation inheritance of Class III malocclusion, there can be unaffected "transmitting" member in which it "skipped a generation," termed non-penetrance in clinical genetics. The principle of variable expressivity is also illustrated in these families with their variation in the severity of the Class III malocclusion of affected members. These observations within families reinforce the understanding that even in autosomal dominant traits, other genetic and environmental factors may contribute to the variation in the phenotype (Fig. **1**) [85, 86].

DNA analysis in the future will likely determine the presence of genetic marker(s) present in the patient associated with the development of a Class III malocclusion. As the possible genetic factors that might be involved at this time appear likely to be several, the particular one(s) that are prognostic in a particular patient may depend on ethnic and family background. In addition, anatomical variation may contribute to Class III malocclusion. The most valuable contribution to clinical practice will be the next step. The study of how different patients respond based upon their genotypes to different treatments and the time of their utilization. These may or may not be the same genetic factors that influenced the development of the malocclusion [87, 88].

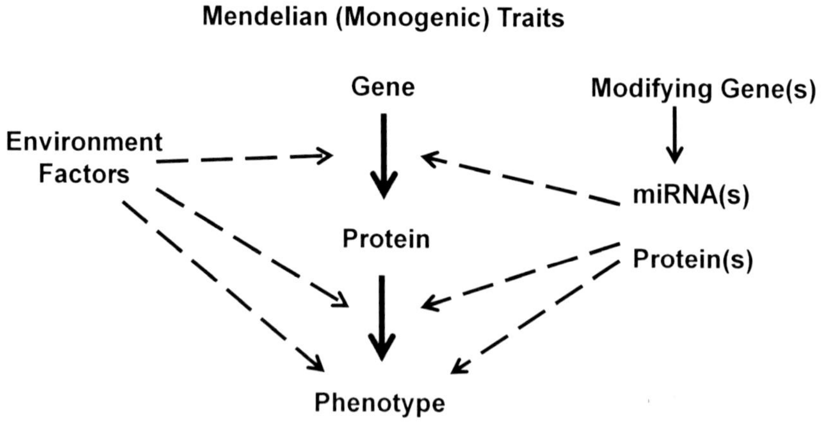

Figure 1: Genetic and environmental factors that contribute to the variation in the phenotype.

SUMMARY POINTS

- Mandibular prognathism (Class III malocclusion) can be a result of pure mandibular prognathism, maxillary hypoplasia/retrognathism, or a combination of the two.
- The prevalence of mandibular prognathism varies among different ethnic groups.
- Different anatomical features of Class III can be classified into subgroups that appear to be influenced by ethnicity and may have a common environmental and/or genetic basis.
- These phenotypic and ethnic variations indicate significant heterogeneity among Class III subjects and account for some of the difficulty encountered when scientifically investigating the condition.
- Familial aggregation and genetic linkage or association studies suggest that heredity plays a substantial role.
- It is probable that the mandibular prognathism in the Royal (Habsburg) Families of Europe was heavily influenced by inbreeding, autosomal recessive patterns, and other multifactorial inheritance possibilities. Analysis of less inbred groups usually indicate an autosomal dominant mode of inheritance with incomplete penetrance and variable expressivity) in some families and multifactorial (polygenic complex) influences in others.
- Genome wide scans indicate a number of genetic factors may be involved in different families, even within the same ethnic group.

ACKNOWLEDGEMENTS

Support for LAM and JKH from the NIH P20GM103538 Center for Biomedical Research Excellence II (COBRE II) Project, and for JKH by the E. Preston Hicks Endowed Chair at the University of Kentucky .

CONFLICT OF INTEREST

The authors confirm that this chapter contents have no conflict of interest.

REFERENCES

[1] Proffit WR, Fields HW, Jr., Moray LJ. Prevalence of malocclusion and orthodontic treatment need in the United States: estimates from the NHANES III survey. The International journal of adult orthodontics and orthognathic surgery. 1998;13(2):97-106.

[2] Singh GD. Morphologic determinants in the etiology of class III malocclusions: a review. Clinical anatomy. 1999;12(5):382-405.

[3] El-Gheriani AA, Maher BS, El-Gheriani AS, Sciote JJ, Abu-Shahba FA, Al-Azemi R, *et al.* Segregation analysis of mandibular prognathism in Libya. Journal of dental research. 2003 Jul;82(7):523-7.

[4] Angle E. Treatment of malocclusion of the teeth. 7th ed. Philadelphia: S.S. White Manufacturing Company; 1907.

[5] Downs WG. Studies in the Causes of Dental Anomalies. Genetics. 1927 Nov;12(6):570-80.

[6] Pascoe JJ, Hayward JR, Costich ER. Mandibular prognathism: its etiology and a classification. Journal of oral surgery, anesthesia, and hospital dental service. 1960 Jan;18:21-4.

[7] Gold JK. A new approach to the treatment of mandibular prognathism. American journal of orthodontics. 1949 Dec;35(12):893-912, illust.

[8] Davidov S, Geseva N, Donveca T, Dehova L. Incidence of prognathism in Bulgaria. Dental Abstracts. 1961;6:240-2.

[9] Monteleone L, Duvigneaud JD. Prognathism. Journal of Oral Surgery. 1963;21:190-5.

[10] Schoenwetter RF. A possible relationship between certain malocclusions and difficult or instrument deliveries. The Angle orthodontist. 1974 Oct;44(4):336-40.

[11] Haraguchi S, Takada K, Yasuda Y. Facial asymmetry in subjects with skeletal Class III deformity. The Angle orthodontist. 2002 Feb;72(1):28-35.

[12] Litton SF, Ackermann LV, Isaacson RJ, Shapiro BL. A genetic study of Class 3 malocclusion. American journal of orthodontics. 1970 Dec;58(6):565-77.

[13] Cruz RM, Krieger H, Ferreira R, Mah J, Hartsfield J, Jr., Oliveira S. Major gene and multifactorial inheritance of mandibular prognathism. Am J Med Genet Part A. 2008 Jan 1;146A(1):71-7.

[14] Allwright WC. A survey of handicapping dentofacial anomalies among Chinese in Hong Kong. Int Dent J. 1964;14:505-19.

[15] Ishii N, Deguchi T, Hunt NP. Craniofacial differences between Japanese and British Caucasian females with a skeletal Class III malocclusion. European journal of orthodontics. 2002 Oct;24(5):493-9.

[16] Emrich RE, Brodie AG, Blayney JR. Prevalence of Class 1, Class 2, and Class 3 malocclusions (Angle) in an urban population. An epidemiological study. Journal of dental research. 1965 Sep-Oct;44(5):947-53.

[17] Garner LD, Butt MH. Malocclusion in black Americans and Nyeri Kenyans. An epidemiologic study. The Angle orthodontist. 1985 Apr;55(2):139-46.

[18] Massler M, Frankel JM. Prevalence of malocclusion in children aged 14 to 18 years. American journal of orthodontics. 1951 Oct;37(10):751-68.

[19] Tipton RT, Rinchuse DJ. The relationship between static occlusion and functional occlusion in a dental school population. The Angle orthodontist. 1991 Spring;61(1):57-66.

[20] Horowitz HS. A study of occlusal relations in 10 to 12 year old Caucasian and Negro children--summary report. International dental journal. 1970 Dec;20(4):593-605.

[21] Grewe JM, Cervenka J, Shapiro BL, Witkop CJ, Jr. Prevalence o f malocclusion in Chippewa Indian children. Journal of dental research. 1968 Mar-Apr;47(2):302-5.

[22] Zammit MP, Hans MG, Broadbent BH, Johnsen DC, Latimer BM, Nelson S. Malocclusion in Labrador Inuit youth: a psychosocial, dental and cephalometric evaluation. Arctic medical research. 1995 Jan;54(1):32-44.

[23] Martins Mda G, Lima KC. Prevalence of malocclusions in 10-to 12-year-old schoolchildren in Ceara, Brazil. Oral health & preventive dentistry. 2009;7(3):217-23.

[24] Thilander B, Pena L, Infante C, Parada SS, de Mayorga C. Prevalence of malocclusion and orthodontic treatment need in children and adolescents in Bogota, Colombia. An epidemiological study related to different stages of dental development. European journal of orthodontics. 2001 Apr;23(2):153-67.

[25] Grando G, Young AA, Vedovello Filho M, Vedovello SA, Ramirez-Yanez GO. Prevalence of malocclusions in a young Brazilian population. International journal of orthodontics. 2008 Summer;19(2):13-6.

[26] Goose DH, Thomson DG, Winter FC. Malocclusion in schoolchildren of the west Midlands. British Dental Journal. 1957;102:174-8.

[27] Ingervall B. Prevalence of dental and occlusal anomalies in Swedish conscripts. Acta odontologica Scandinavica. 1974;32(2):83-92.

[28] Laine T, Hausen H. Occlusal anomalies in Finnish students related to age, sex, absent permanent teeth and orthodontic treatment. European journal of orthodontics. 1983 May;5(2):125-31.

[29] Helm S. Malocclusion in Danish children with adolescent dentition: an epidemiologic study. American journal of orthodontics. 1968 May;54(5):352-66.

[30] Solow B, Helm S. A method for tabulation and statistical evaluation of epidemiological malocclusion data. Acta odontologica Scandinavica. 1968 May;26(1):63-88.

[31] Luffingham JK, Campbell HM. The need for orthodontic treatment. A pilot survey of 14 year old school children in Paisley, Scotland. Transactions European Orthodontic Society. 1974:259-67.

[32] El-Mangoury NH, Mostafa YA. Epidemiologic panorama of dental occlusion. The Angle orthodontist. 1990 Fall;60(3):207-14.

[33] Borzabadi-Farahani A, Borzabadi-Farahani A, Eslamipour F. Malocclusion and occlusal traits in an urban Iranian population. An epidemiological study of 11-to 14-year-old children. European journal of orthodontics. 2009 Oct;31(5):477-84.

[34] Saleh FK. Prevalence of malocclusion in a sample of Lebanese schoolchildren: an epidemiological study. Eastern Mediterranean health journal = La revue de sante de la Mediterranee orientale = al-Majallah al-sihhiyah li-sharq al-mutawassit. 1999 Mar;5(2):337-43.

[35] Singh GD, McNamara JA, Jr., Lozanoff S. Comparison of mandibular morphology in Korean and European-American children with Class III malocclusions using finite-element morphometry. Journal of orthodontics. 2000 Jun;27(2):135-42.

[36] Ngan P, Hagg U, Yiu C, Merwin D, Wei SH. Cephalometric comparisons of Chinese and Caucasian surgical Class III patients. The International journal of adult orthodontics and orthognathic surgery. 1997;12(3):177-88.
[37] Bukhary MT. Comparative cephalometric study of Class III malocclusion in Saudi and Japanese adult females. Journal of oral science. 2005 Jun;47(2):83-90.
[38] Ursi WJ, Trotman CA, McNamara JA, Jr., Behrents RG. Sexual dimorphism in normal craniofacial growth. The Angle orthodontist. 1993 Spring;63(1):47-56.
[39] Vanderschueren D, Vandenput L, Boonen S, Lindberg MK, Bouillon R, Ohlsson C. Androgens and bone. Endocr Rev. 2004 Jun;25(3):389-425.
[40] Schaefer K, Fink B, Mitteroecker P, Neave N, Bookstein FL. Visualizing facial shape regression upon 2nd to 4th digit ratio and testosterone. Coll Antropol. 2005 Dec;29(2):415-9.
[41] Schaefer K. Female appearance: facial and bodily attractiveness as shape. Psychology Science. 2006;48(2):187-204.
[42] Tollaro I, Baccetti T, Bassarelli V, Franchi L. Class III malocclusion in the deciduous dentition: a morphological and correlation study. European journal of orthodontics. 1994 Oct;16(5):401-8.
[43] Yeong P, Huggare J. Morphology of Singapore chinese. European journal of orthodontics. 2004 Dec;26(6):605-12.
[44] Drevensek M, Farcnik F, Vidmar G. Cephalometric standards for Slovenians in the mixed dentition period. European journal of orthodontics. 2006 Feb;28(1):51-7.
[45] Baccetti T, Reyes BC, McNamara JA, Jr. Gender differences in Class III malocclusion. The Angle orthodontist. 2005 Jul;75(4):510-20.
[46] Miyajima K, McNamara JA, Jr., Sana M, Murata S. An estimation of craniofacial growth in the untreated Class III female with anterior crossbite. American journal of orthodontics and dentofacial orthopedics : official publication of the American Association of Orthodontists, its constituent societies, and the American Board of Orthodontics. 1997 Oct;112(4):425-34.
[47] Ellis E, 3rd, McNamara JA, Jr. Components of adult Class III malocclusion. J Oral Maxillofacial Surg. 1984 May;42(5):295-305.
[48] Martone VD, Enlow DH, Hans MG, Broadbent BH, Jr., Oyen O. Class I and Class III malocclusion sub-groupings related to headform type. The Angle orthodontist. 1992 Spring;62(1):35-42; discussion 3-4.
[49] Mackay F, Jones JA, Thompson R, Simpson W. Craniofacial form in class III cases. British journal of orthodontics. 1992 Feb;19(1):15-20.
[50] Hong SX, Yi CK. A classification and characterization of skeletal class III on etio-pathogenic basis. International Journal of Oral and Maxillofacial Surgery. 2001;30(4):264-71.
[51] Bui C, King T, Proffit W, Frazier-Bowers S. Phenotypic characterization of Class III patients. The Angle orthodontist. 2006 Jul;76(4):564-9.
[52] Wolff G, Wienker TF, Sander H. On the genetics of mandibular prognathism: analysis of large European noble families. Journal of medical genetics. 1993 Feb;30(2):112-6.
[53] Chudley AE. Genetic landmarks through philately--the Habsburg jaw. Clinical Genet. 1998 Oct;54(4):283-4.
[54] Niswander JD. Genetics of common dental disorders. Dental clinics of North America. 1975 Jan;19(1):197-206.

[55] Thompson EM, Winter RM. Another family with the 'Habsburg jaw'. Journal of medical genetics. 1988 Dec;25(12):838-42.
[56] Strohmayer W. Die Vererbung des Hapsburger Familientypus. Nova Acta Leopoldina. 1937;5:219-96.
[57] Rubbrecht O. Study of the heredity of the anomalies of the jaws. Am J Orthodont. 1939;25:751-79.
[58] Stiles KA, Luke JE. The inheritance of malocclusion due to mandibular prognathism. J Hered. 1953;44:241-5.
[59] Gorlin RJ, Redman RS, Shapiro BL. Effect of X-Chromosome Aneuploidy on Jaw Growth. Journal of dental research. 1965 Jan-Feb;44:SUPPL:269-82.
[60] Yamaguchi T, Park SB, Narita A, Maki K, Inoue I. Genome-wide linkage analysis of mandibular prognathism in Korean and Japanese patients. Journal of dental research. 2005 Mar;84(3):255-9.
[61] Jang JY, Park EK, Ryoo HM, Shin HI, Kim TH, Jang JS, *et al.* Polymorphisms in the Matrilin-1 gene and risk of mandibular prognathism in Koreans. Journal of dental research. 2010 Nov;89(11):1203-7.
[62] Xue F, Wong RW, Rabie AB. Genes, genetics, and Class III malocclusion. Orthodontics & craniofacial research. 2010 May;13(2):69-74.
[63] Li Q, Zhang F, Li X, Chen F. Genome scan for locus involved in mandibular prognathism in pedigrees from China. PloS one. 2010;5(9).
[64] Li Q, Li X, Zhang F, Chen F. The identification of a novel locus for mandibular prognathism in the Han Chinese population. Journal of dental research. 2011 Jan;90(1):53-7.
[65] Frazier-Bowers S, Rincon-Rodriguez R, Zhou J, Alexander K, Lange E. Evidence of linkage in a Hispanic cohort with a Class III dentofacial phenotype. Journal of dental research. 2009 Jan;88(1):56-60.
[66] Cruz RM, Hartsfield JK, Jr., Falcao-Alencar G, Koller DL, Pereira RW, Mah J, *et al.* Exclusion of Class III malocclusion candidate loci in Brazilian families. J Dent Res. 2011 Oct;90(10):1202-5.
[67] Otero LM. Factores genéticos asociados a la maloclusión clase III en un grupo de familias Colombianas: Pontificia Universidad Javeriana; 2008.
[68] Xue F, Rabie A, Luo G. Analysis of the association of COL2A1 and IGF-1 with mandibular prognathism in a Chinese population. Orthodontics & craniofacial research. 2014.
[69] Deák F, Wagener R, Kiss I, Paulsson M. The matrilins: a novel family of oligomeric extracellular matrix proteins. Matrix Biology. 1999;18(1):55-64.
[70] Wagener R, Ehlen HWA, Ko Y-P, Kobbe B, Mann HH, Sengle G, *et al.* The matrilins – adaptor proteins in the extracellular matrix. Febs Letters. 2005;579(15):3323-9.
[71] Klatt AR, Becker A-KA, Neacsu CD, Paulsson M, Wagener R. The matrilins: Modulators of extracellular matrix assembly. The International Journal of Biochemistry & Cell Biology. 2011;43(3):320-30.
[72] Pepicelli A, Woods M, Briggs C. The mandibular muscles and their importance in orthodontics: A contemporary review. American Journal of Orthodontics and Dentofacial Orthopedics. 2005;128(6):774-80.
[73] Sciote JJ, Horton MJ, Rowlerson AM, Ferri J, Close JM, Raoul G. Human Masseter Muscle Fiber Type Properties, Skeletal Malocclusions, and Muscle Growth Factor Expression. Journal of Oral and Maxillofacial Surgery. 2012;70(2):440-8.

[74] Mao JJ, Nah H-D. Growth and development: hereditary and mechanical modulations. American Journal of Orthodontics and Dentofacial Orthopedics. 2004;125(6):676-89.

[75] Montanaro L, Parisini P, Greggi T, Di Silvestre M, Campoccia D, Rizzi S, *et al.* Evidence of a linkage between matrilin-1 gene (MATN1) and idiopathic scoliosis. Scoliosis. 2006;1(1):21.

[76] Bae JW, Cho CH, Min WK, Kim UK. Associations between matrilin-1 gene polymorphisms and adolescent idiopathic scoliosis curve patterns in a Korean population. Mol Biol Rep. 2012 May;39(5):5561-7.

[77] Rodrigues JB, Araújo S, Guedes-Pinto H, San Roman F, Viegas C, Bastos E. Analysis of new Matrilin-1 gene variants in a case–control study related to dental malocclusions in Equus asinus. Gene. 2013 6/10/;522(1):70-4.

[78] Falcão-Alencar G, Ortero LM, Cruz RM, Foroud TM, Dongbing L, Koller D, *et al.* Evidence for Genetic Linkage of the Class III Craniofacial Phenotype With Human Chromosome 7 in 36 South American Families. 2012.

[79] Turner J, Falcão-Alencar G, Otero LM, Cruz RM, Morford LA, Ferrari I, *et al.* Genetic Analysis of Class III Malocclusion in Brazil and Colombia. J Dent Res 90(Spec Iss A): abstract #249; 2011.

[80] Tassopoulou-Fishell M, Deeley K, Harvey E, Sciote J, Vieira A. MYO1H Contributes to Class III Malocclusion. Journal of Dental Research. 2011(90 (Special Issue A), #248).

[81] Tassopoulou-Fishell M, Deeley K, Harvey EM, Sciote J, Vieira AR. Genetic variation in Myosin 1H contributes to mandibular prognathism. American Journal of Orthodontics and Dentofacial Orthopedics. 2012;141(1):51-9.

[82] Gray SL, Horton MJ, Vieira AR, Tassopoulou-Fishell M, Raoul G, Ferri J, *et al.* Myosin 1H Expression in Masseter Muscle of Orthognathic Surgery Subjects. J Dent Res. 2012;91((Spec Iss B)):2959.

[83] Raoul G, Desh H, Gray SL, Horton MJ, Nicot R, Rowlerson AM, *et al.* Expression of unconventional type-1 myosins (1H/1C) in masseter muscle influence the development of skeletal malocclusion in orthognathic surgery subjects. International journal of oral and maxillofacial surgery. 2013;42(10):1335.

[84] Nikopensius T, Saag M, Jagomägi T, Annilo T, Kals M, Kivistik P, *et al.* A missense mutation in DUSP6 is associated with class III malocclusion. Journal of dental research. 2013;92(10):893-8.

[85] Hartsfield JK, Jr. Genetics and Orthodontics. In: Graber LW, Vanarsdall RL, Vig KWL, editors. Orthodontics : current principles and techniques. 5th ed. St. Louis: Elsevier Mosby; 2011.

[86] Hartsfield JK, Jr., Bixler D. Clinical Genetics for the Dental Practitioner. In: Dean JA, Avery DR, McDonald RE, editors. McDonald's and Avery's dentistry for the child and adolescent. 9th ed. St. Louis, Mo.: Mosby/Elsevier; 2011. p. 64-84.

[87] Hartsfield JK, Jr., Zhou J, Chen S. The Importance of Analyzing Specific Genetic Factors in Facial Growth for Diagnosis and Treatment Planning. In: McNamara JA, Kapila SD, editors. Surgical Enhancement of Orthodontic Treatment, Craniofacial Growth Series, Department of Orthodontics and Pediatric Dentistry and Center for Human Growth and Development. Ann Arbor: The University of Michigan; 2010. p. 267-81.

[88] Hartsfield JK, Jr. Personalized Orthodontics, The Future of Genetics in Practice. Semin Orthod. 2008;14:166-71.

Send Orders for Reprints to reprints@benthamscience.net
Orthodontic Treatment of Class III Malocclusion, **2014, 25-36**

CHAPTER 2

Class III Skeletal Growth Pattern

Koshi Sato*

Isahai Dental Clinic, Takasaki, Japan; Tohoku University Graduate School of Dentistry, Sendai, Japan

Abstract: The relationship between body height increments and facial growth is well documented in the literature. Correlations are also found between body height and mandibular growth because both lower extremities and mandible are long bones with epiphyseal cartilage. The growth characteristics are similar for the mandible and long bones. On the average, body height tends to be greater in Class III than in Class I individuals. Furthermore, Class III individuals mature slower than Class I individuals during puberty. This may mean the growth period is much longer in Class III subjects, but that still needs to be substantiated. However, studies show there is no significant difference in facial growth increments between Class III and Class I subjects during the pubertal growth period. This means there is already differences in facial growth pattern between Class III and Class I subjects before the pubertal growth spurt. It is also important to note that patients with acromegaly also exhibited abnormal growth. This chapter suggested a few reasons why the occlusion tends to be unstable in Class III patients after treatment. In Class I subjects, stability can be explained by skeletal and dental compensation; cranial base growth compensates occlusal changes. However, the growth of the posterior cranial base is smaller in Class III individuals during puberty so that mandibular growth more directly affects the occlusion. Other factors in occlusal stability occur after treatment. The prediction of mandibular growth potential is possible using hand-wrist X-rays after the pubertal growth spurt. Clinically, there are limitations of orthopedic treatment with chincup and/or maxillary protraction appliance. These appliances may inhibit or at least mask mandibular growth. However, if there is excess mandibular growth after removal of the orthopedic appliance(s), Class III malocclusion may reoccur. The risk of orthodontic and orthopedic treatment can be minimized by a better understanding of the characteristics of facial growth in Class III patients.

Keywords: Craniofacial growth, Body height, Skeletal maturation, Class III skeletal growth.

RELATIONSHIP BETWEEN BODY HEIGHT AND CRANIOFACIAL SKELETON

In 1990, the author evaluated the growth timing for standing height, the mandible

***Address correspondence to Koshi Sato:** 25-1 Nakano-aza-yanagihara, Miyagino-ku, 983-0013 Sendai, Japan; Tel: +81-22-254-6704; Fax: +81-22-254-6704; E-mail: koshi.sato@orthodontist.jp

Peter W. Ngan, Toshi Deguchi and Eugene W. Roberts (Eds)

and the hand bones in skeletal Class III Japanese females. Table **1** shows the correlation between body height and craniofacial cephalometric linear measurements in 180 Class III Japanese females [1]. In general, correlations between the body height and mandibular length (Cd-Gn) were the highest and/or most significant on all age groups except for the 13y group. Correlation between body height and total facial height (N-Me) was next highest overall. A significant correlation between body height and maxillary length (A-Ptm) was found only with the 7y group. These results indicated that as body height, mandibular length and facial height are positively correlated.

Table 1: Correlation coefficients between body height (BH) and some cephalometric measurements for different age groups (n=20 for each group) of Class III Japanese females [1].

	6y	7y	8y	9y	10y	11y	12y	13y	adult
BH × S-N		0.507	0.508		0.517				
N-Me	0.680	0.539	0.525	0.476	0.760	0.651		0.533	0.449
N-ANS	0.578	0.560		0.472	0.632				0.460
ANS-Me	0.575		0.481		0.636	0.473		0.490	
A'-Ptm'		0.478							
Cd-Gn	0.646	0.646	0.613	0.617	0.643	0.585	0.471	0.457	0.482
Pog'-Go					0.537				
Cd-Go		0.659	0.511		0.462	0.447		0.537	0.477

Black= significant at $p<0.05$,
Red = significant at $p<0.01$, Blank= no significant difference.

Fig. **1** illustrates the relationship between the peak height velocity of growth (PHV) and the increase in mandibular length. Mandibular growth usually lags body height [2]. During puberty, increase in body height is mainly due to lengthening of lower

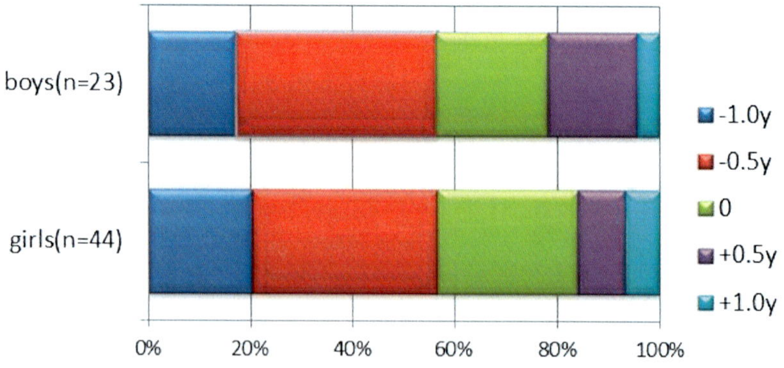

Figure 1: Time lag in pubertal growth peak between body height and mandibular length. (-) means body height is earlier, (+) means mandible is earlier [2].

extremities. Bones of lower extremities have epiphyseal cartilage and are classified as long bones. The mandible never has an epiphyseal cartilage like long bones, but the growth pattern and morphological characteristics are similar for the mandible and long bones (Fig. **2**). However, the growth process is much different for other facial bones associated with sutures, such as the maxilla.

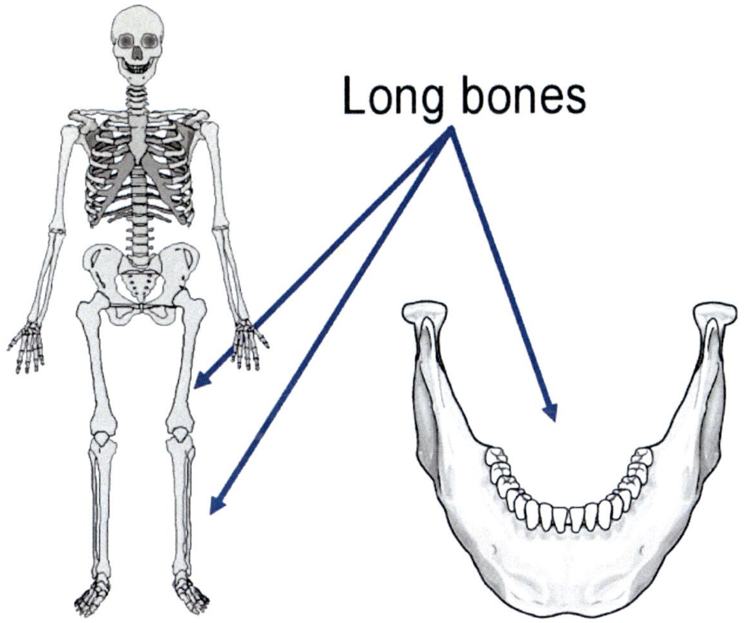

Figure 2: Based on overall morphology, bones of the lower extremities and mandible are classified as long bones.

RELATIONSHIP BETWEEN BODY HEIGHT AND CRANIOFACIAL SKELETON IN SKELETAL CLASS III SUBJECTS

If there is a strong correlation between body height and mandibular length, Class III subjects with a large mandible would have greater body height. Using longitudinal data during puberty [3], we found that the average body height in 30 Class III Japanese female was greater than that for Class I females of all age groups (Fig. **3**). The difference was about 2 cm during the pubertal growth period. The average body height of Class I females was about the same as the average body height of Japanese females. These results indicate that Class III subjects with larger mandible tend to be taller.

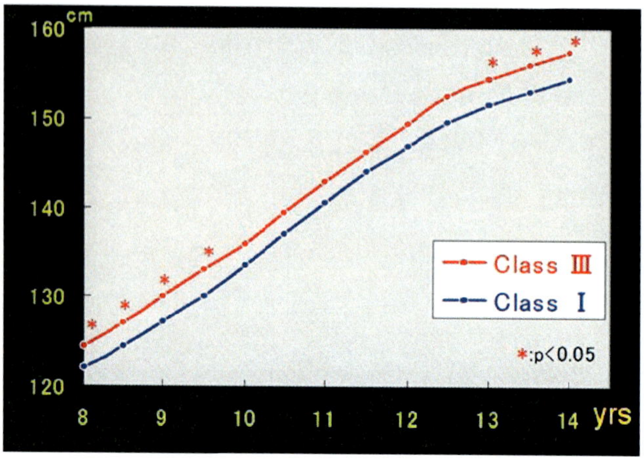

Figure 3: Average body height in Class III and Class I Japanese females (n=30) [3].

SKELETAL MATURATION TIMING IN CLASS III SUBJECTS

Using cross-sectional hand-wrist X-rays of Japanese females, the ratio of maturational stage was compared between Class I and Class III subjects during puberty [1]. There was no significant difference in the appearance of ulnar sesamoid bone (Figs. **4** and **5**). However, maturational stages of 3rd middle phalanx (Fig. **6**) and radius (Fig. **7**) were significantly different at ages 8 and 12y, indicating a tendency for earlier maturation than Class I subjects (Figs. **8** and **9**).

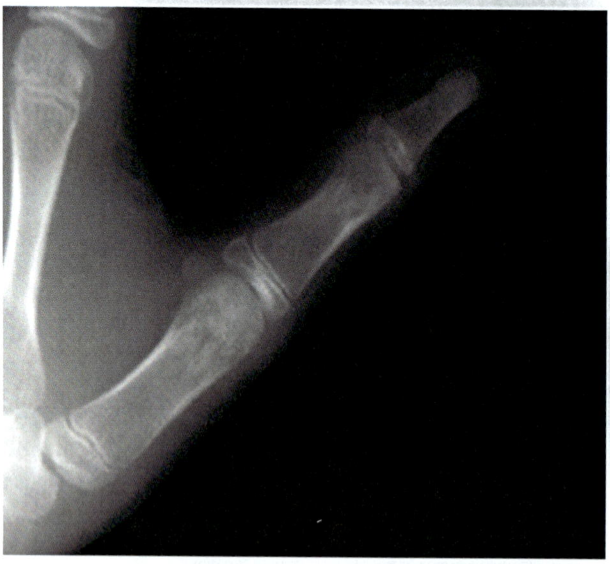

Figure 4: Appearance of the ulnar sesamoid bone.

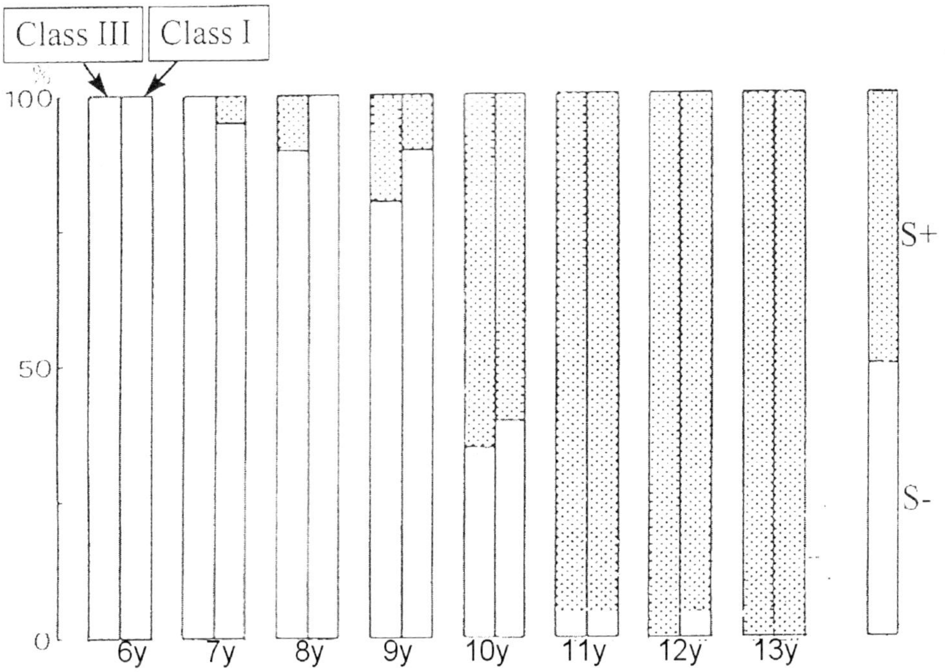

Figure 5: Appearance ratio of ulnar sesamoid bone in Class III and Class I subjects S+: appearance of sesamoid bone, S-: No appearance of sesamoid bone [1].

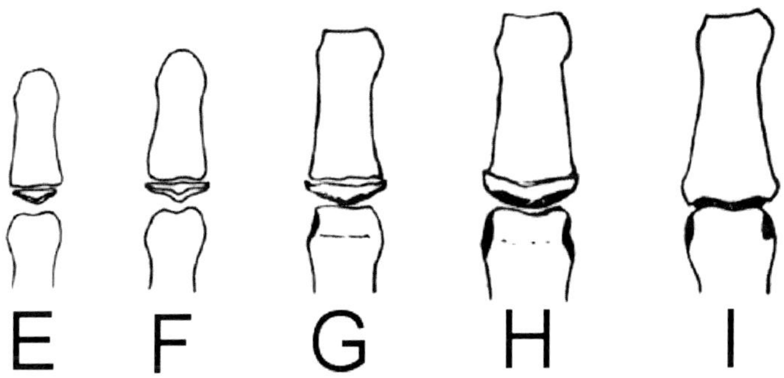

Figure 6: Maturational stages of 3rd middle phalanx [4].

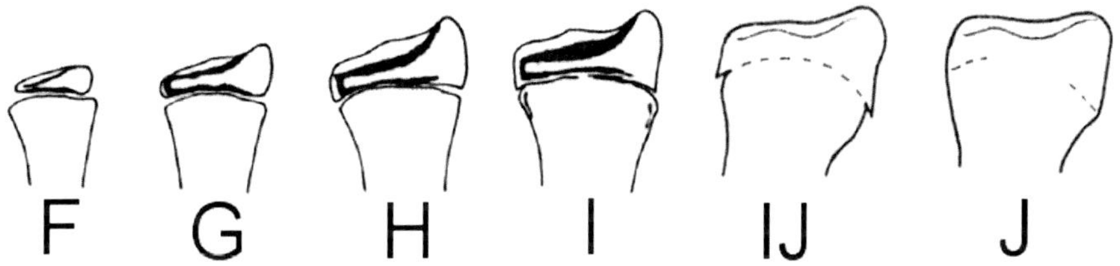

Figure 7: Maturational stages of the radius [4].

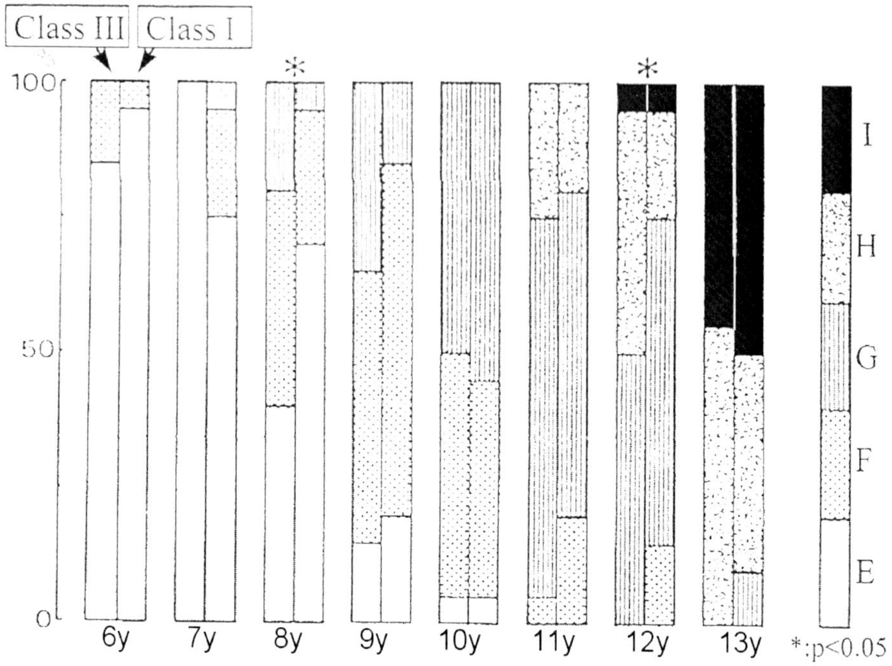

Figure 8: Maturational ratio of the 3rd middle phalanx in Class III and Class I subjects [1].

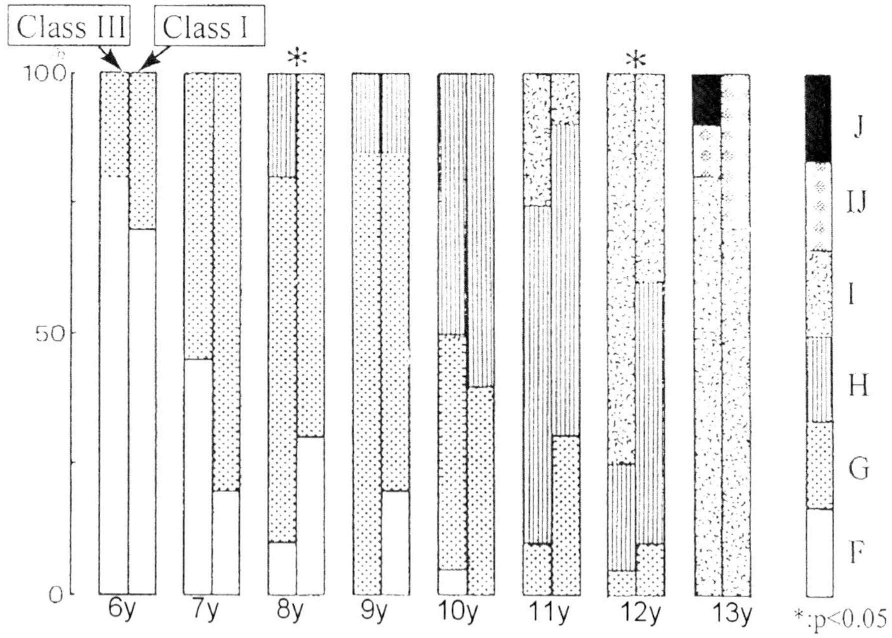

Figure 9: Maturational ratio of the radius in Class III and Class I subjects [1].

Using longitudinal hand-wrist X-rays, the exact maturational changes were investigated in Class I and Class III according to bone age by the Tanner-Whitehouse 2 (TW2) method [4]. Fig. **10** shows the maturational behavior of bone age in Class III and Class I Japanese boys. The maturation in Class III boys was slower than that of Class I boys before age 10. After 11 years of age, the maturation or bone age in Class III started to progress rapidly [3]. The acceleration of bone maturation gradually became slower, and eventually became the same as Class I boys after age 15. The difference of maturation was smaller in girls, but the tendency was almost same. These characteristics might mean that pubertal period is longer in Class III than in Class I adolescents.

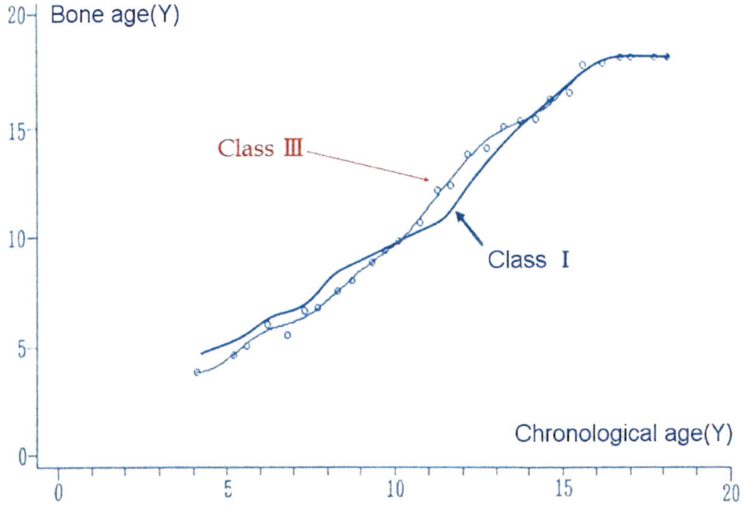

Figure 10: Maturational behavior of bone age (TW2 method) in Class III and Class I Japanese boys [3].

GROWTH INCREMENTS ON CLASS III SUBJECTS DURING PUBERTY

A few studies show that there are no significant difference in facial growth increments between Class III and Class I subjects during the pubertal growth period [5, 6]. Both from 9 to 14 years in girls and from 10 to 15 years in boys, the mean amount of maxillary and mandibular growth increments showed no significant difference between Class III and Class I groups. In late pubertal growth (from 14 to 17 years in females, and 15 to 18 years in males), similar results were recognized [7-9]. There was only a significant difference in the increment of anterior cranial base length (S-N) in girls between Class III and Class I groups (Figs. **11** and **12**). This means there is already a substantial difference in the facial pattern between Class III and Class I subjects before the pubertal growth spurt. It is important to note that patients with an over secretion of growth hormone (acromegaly) also exhibited an abnormal growth pattern like the Class III subjects.

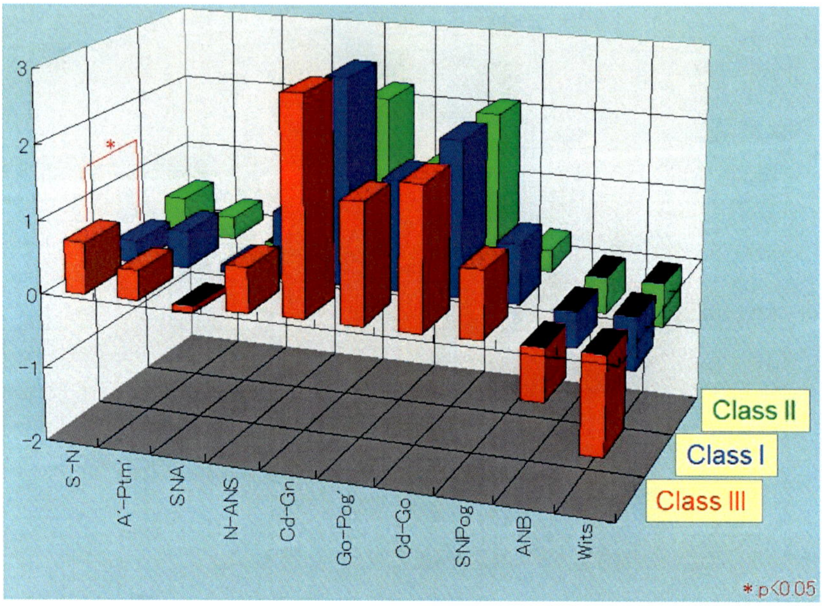

Figure 11: Facial growth increments in Japanese girls from 14 to 17 years [7, 9].

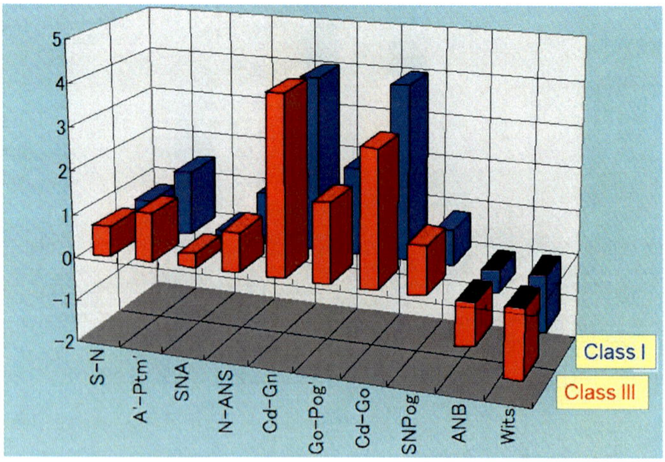

Figure 12: Facial growth increments in Japanese boys from 15 to 18 years [8,9].

MECHANISM FOR THE RELAPSE OF CROSSBITE IN CLASS III SUBJECTS

We often see the relapse of crossbite after 1st phase treatment in Class III subjects. However, the increment of mandibular growth is not different between Class I and Class III subjects during puberty. Why does the occlusion tend to be unstable in Class III patients after first phase treatment? The difference in craniofacial growth and skeletal profile between relapsed and nonrelapsed incisor reversed occlusion (anterior corssbite) in 35 treated Class III females, following maximum pubertal growth, was investigated [10]. Chincup therapy was applied from the beginning of treatment and was continued until a normal anterior bite was achieved. At 8 years of age, the skeletal profile showed significant differences in mandibular length, gonial angle and posterior cranial base length between the relapsed and nonrelapsed groups (Fig. **13**). The total incremental change in mandibular total length (Cd-Gn) and anterior facial height (N-Me) were significantly larger in the relapsed group, as compared to the nonrelapsed group, during pubertal growth period. The incremental change in mandibular total length and anterior facial height were significantly larger in the relapsed group. The total incremental change in posterior cranial base length (S-Ba) was significantly less in the relapsed group. Increments in the spheno-occipital synchondrosis might compensate for the differential growth between the maxilla and mandible. In conclusion, the reasons for the relapsed occlusion in treated skeletal class III patients after maximum pubertal growth were attributed to insufficient compensatory growth of the cranial base compared to an excessively growing mandible. Baccetti *et al.* [11] also reported that Class III disharmony showed a significant tendency to worsen with a long period of active mandibular growth, combined with the absence of any catchup growth in maxilla and/or compensation with more vertical facial growth.

Other factors in occlusal stability might be involved after treatment. There is clinical limitation of orthopedic force like chincup and maxillary protraction appliances. Orthopedic treatment certainly has an effect on maxillary and mandibular growth. However, significantly more growth of the mandible than in the maxilla, after removal of the orthopedic appliance, favors a relapse of Class III malocclusion. Eruptive force of lower third molars might effect on the labial inclination of the lower incisors if the anterior bite is not too deep. The prediction of mandibular growth potential is possible using hand-wrist X-rays during pubertal growth period [12]. The Tanner-Whitehouse 2 (TW2) method [13] is the most popular method. However, it is difficult to predict the individual occlusal changes accurately during puberty. One of the effective treatment options is to separate treatment timing into a first and second phase. The risk of orthodontic and orthopedic treatment can be minimized by a better understanding of the characteristics of facial growth in Class III patients.

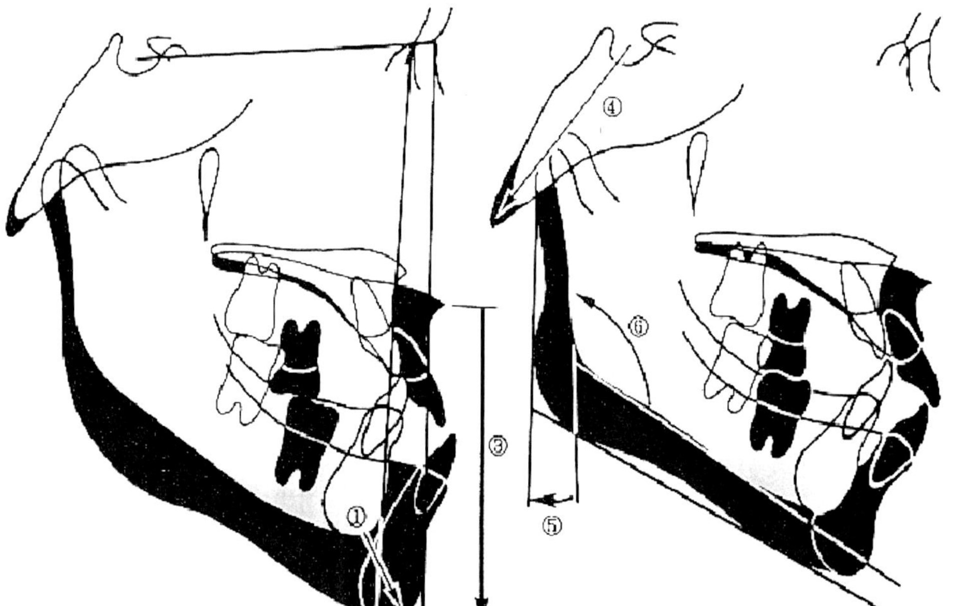

A B

Figure 13: Comparison of the facial change after first phase treatment between unstable (left) and stable (right) group [10]. For the unstable group (A), increments on mandible are large; the mandible indicates counter-clockwise rotation and the increments on lower facial height are large. For the stable group (B), the increments on posterior cranial base are large; the ramus indicates clockwise rotation; and the gonial angle becomes smaller.

SUMMARY

- Growth behavior of body height is synchronized with the mandibular growth pattern during puberty. However, the growth principle is much different between the mandible and other facial skeleton with sutures such as the maxilla.

- Skeletal Class III subjects with larger mandibles tend to have greater body height.
- Class III subjects tend to have earlier osseous maturation than Class I subjects, which is offset by a longer pubertal growth spurt.
- There is no significant difference in facial growth increments between Class III and Class I subjects during the pubertal growth period, suggesting the Class III skeletal pattern is established at a very young age.
- The principal reason for relapse of Class III occlusion in treated patients is attributed to insufficient compensatory growth of the cranial base to compensate for excessive growth of the mandible.
- The risk of orthodontic and orthopedic treatment can be minimized by a better understanding of the characteristics of facial growth in Class III patients.

ACKNOWLEDGEMENTS

Declared none.

CONFLICT OF INTEREST

The author confirms that this chapter contents have no conflicts of interest.

REFERENCES

[1] Sato K, Jinno K and Mitani H. Growth Timing of Standing Height, Mandible and Hand Bones in Skeletal Class III Females. Tohoku Univ Dent J 1990; 9: 65-72.

[2] Sato K. A study on growth timing of mandibular length, body height, hand bones and cervical vertebrae during puberty. J Jpn Orthod Soc 1987; 46: 517-33.

[3] Sato K. The latest results and a view of growth study. J Tohoku Orthod Soc 1996; 38-52.

[4] Tanner JM, Whitehouse RH, Cameron N, *et al.* Assessment of skeletal maturity and prediction of adult height (TW2 method). 2nd ed. Academic Press. London 1983.

[5] Bandai E, Sugawara J, Umemori M, *et al.* Craniofacial growth of mandibular prognathism in Japanese girls during pubertal growth period: Longitudinal study from 9 to 14 of age. Orthod Waves 2000; 59: 77-89.

[6] Sakamoto E, Sugawara J, Umemori M, *et al.* Craniofacial growth of mandibular prognathism during pubertal growth period in Japanese boys: Longitudinal study from 10 to 15 years of age. J Jpn Orthod Soc 1996; 55: 372-86.

[7] Sato K, Sugawara J and Mitani H. Longitudinal study on average craniofacial growth of Skeletal Cl. III girls in late adolescent period - Possibility of early orthognathic surgery-. J Jpn Orthod Soc 1989; 48: 21-8.

[8] Sato K, Sugawara J and Mitani H. Longitudinal study on average craniofacial growth of Skeletal Class III males in late adolescent period -Possibility of early orthognathic surgery-. J Jpn Orthod Soc 1992; 51: 25-30.

[9] Mitani H, Sato K and Sugawara J. Growth of mandibular prognathism after pubertal growth peak. Am J Orthod Dent Orthop 1993; 104: 330-6.

[10] Choi YH, Sato K and Mitani H. Growth characteristics of prognathic face with relapsed incisor reversed occlusion following chincap therapy. Orthod Waves 1999; 58: 1-14.

[11] Baccetti T, Franchi L, James A, *et al.* Growth in the untreated Class III subjects. Semin Orthod 2007; 13: 130-142.

[12] Sato K, Mito T and Mitani H. An accurate method of predicting mandibular growth potential based on bone maturity. Am J Orthod Dentofacial Orthop 2001; 120: 286-90.

[13] Tanner JM, Whitehouse RH, Cameron N, *et al.* Assessment of skeletal maturity and prediction of adult height (TW2 method). 2nd ed. London: Academic Press; 1983.

CHAPTER 3

Mechano-Reaction of Chondrocytes in the Mandibular Condyle During Orthopedic-Orthodontic Intervention

Ichiro Takahashi*

Section of Orthodontics and Dentofacial Orthopedics, Division of Oral Health, Growth and Development, Kyushu University, Faculty of Dental Science, Higashi-ku, Japan

Abstract: Early orthopedic treatment of skeletal malocclusions continues to challenge clinicians and the efficacy of mandibular growth modification by orthopedic appliances has long been a debate without conclusion. Several growth theories support the mandibular condyle as a growth site rather than a primary growth center. The response of cartilages and chondrocytes to mechanical stimulation is still considered a major parameter for controlling the growth of mandible. This chapter summarizes results of laboratory and clinical studies related to orthopedic interventions, focused on mandibular prognathism. The clinical problems with chincup therapy are discussed at the cellular level and with animal models. Based on the results from animal model studies, the magnitude and direction of the mechanical stress is analyzed relative to loading cells. Differentiating chondrocytes appear to be the effectors of the cellular physiologic and the pathologic reactions to mechanical stress. The possible mechano-transduction pathways in differentiating chondrocytes are discussed relative to cell-extracelluler matrix (ECM) adhesion and ion channels. A combined signal transduction mechanism is proposed for integrin based cell ECM adhesion, This mechanism, acting through a mitogen activated protein kinase (MAPK) pathway mediated by ion channels, is discussed as a possible mechanism for regulating mandibular growth. The promotion of endochondral bone formation in the mandibular condylar cartilage is proposed as an important example of this basic mechanism. Further horizons for craniofacial research in orthodontics and mechanobiology are proposed.

Keywords: Mandibular condylar cartilage, Mechanobiology, Cell-ECM adhesion, MAPK pathway, Orthopedic intervention.

INTRODUCTION

Orthodontic-orthopedic intervention for skeletal malocclusions has long been a

***Address correspondence to Ichiro Takahashi:** Section of Orthodontics and Dentofacial Orthopedics, Division of Oral Health, Growth and Development, Kyushu University, Faculty of Dental Science, 3-1-1, Maidashi, Higashi-ku Fukuoka, 812-8582, Japan; Tel: 011-81-92-642-6394; Fax: 011-81-92-642-6398; E-mail: takahashi@dent.kyushu-u.ac.jp

Peter W. Ngan, Toshi Deguchi and Eugene W. Roberts (Eds)

topic of discussion in orthodontics. Growth modification of the facial skeleton is largely dependent on the efficacy of orthopedic intervention in the maxilla and mandible. While this issue has long been debated, no clear consensus has been reached regarding the treatment modalities for skeletal malocclusion that are capable of modifying the growth of the maxillofacial complex. In the present chapter, mandibular growth, and especially the reaction of the mandibular condylar cartilages to orthopedic intervention, was addressed in the context of various aspects of orthodontic research and craniofacial biology.

Mandibular condylar cartilage is a secondary cartilage that differs substantially from the primary cartilage in long bone epiphyses [1]. Whether mechanical stress can affect the growth of bone formed by endochondral ossification is still debatable. Historical and regional craniofacial or maxillofacial deformation resulting from ethnic customs, such as foot binding in China, neck elongation by the Kayan people in Myanmar, and cranial deformation in Peru, led orthodontic researchers to believe that facial growth can be altered by mechanical stress. In general, endochondral bone formation in weight-bearing long bones, such as the femur and tibia, is believed to be a bone growth mechanism that can achieve longitudinal bone elongation under mechanical compressive force. As the epiphyseal growth plates of these bones are primary cartilage, this form of cartilage has generally been considered the active growth center of long bones. On the other hand, mandibular condylar cartilage, a secondary cartilage, was initially considered the growth center of the mandible, although this concept has gradually been revised such that it is now recognized as a passive growth site for the mandible [2]. Several leading scientists in the fields of orthodontics and dentofacial orthopedics have conceptualized the growth theory since about 1950. Up through the 1950s, it was commonly believed that growth of the facial skeleton was genetically regulated. Since the 1960s, the organ-specific roles of environmental factors have been emphasized. Nasal septal cartilage was shown to be a driving force of anterior growth in the maxilla [3]. Furthermore, nasal obstruction promoted an open bite in monkeys [4, 5], and the use of a mandibular protrusive appliance enhanced forward growth of the mandible in animal models [6, 7].

As described earlier, the growth plate cartilage is believed to be a growth center for long bones. However, the mandibular condylar cartilage is a secondary growth site in the mandible. According to the functional matrix hypothesis of Moss [8-12], the growth of skeletal tissues is largely affected by changes in nonskeletal tissue masses that compose the craniofacial complex, such as the eye, tongue, or any other organ that influences skeletal growth around it. This hypothesis proposed, that as the volume (mass) changes with the developing function of each matrix, predominant biomechanical factors regulate the growth of surrounding bone. After Petrovic [13,14] proposed the servo theory, development of the theoretical background to explain facial growth, at the macroscopic anatomical level, has stalled. Since the middle of the 1980s, molecular biology and genetics have focused on the subcellular level and gradually paved the way for the next generation of craniofacial research. Through the human genome project, information coded by the genome (coding sequences for proteins, regulatory elements for gene expression and suppression, and modifiers of expressed messages) has been explored. Interactions between genetic and epigenetic factors has focused on the molecular level [9-12].

In the present chapter, clinical research on orthopedic effects and growth of the temporomandibular joint (TMJ) were reviewed and summarized to clarify the discussion. Histologic studies were evaluated in the context of the molecular basis of the mechanobiology of cartilage. The roles of extracellular cell matrix (ECM) adhesion and ion channels in the mechanoreaction of chondrocytes are emphasized. Finally, promising research directions for clinical orthopedic intervention in orthodontic treatment during the growth stage are proposed.

Orthopedic Approaches to Mandibular Growth

Orthopedic force to retract the mandible of a Class III subject is delivered by a chincup. Functional appliances can produce protrusive force to modify growth to correct skeletal Class II problems. Most human studies are retrospective case control studies, demonstrating that retractive force to the mandible can redirect growth of the chin. In general, it was considered that when the chincup force was directed backward, the mandible would grow downward and rotate backward. When chincup force was directed upward, the mandible would grow forward. On the other hand, mandibular protrusive force is believed to accelerate growth at the posterior border of the mandible. When mandibular protrusion appliances are worn, forward growth of the mandible is stimulated and skeletal problems are corrected.

Cephalometric analyses of skeletal Class III patients show, in different studies, that orthopedic force directed at the TMJ (*via* chincup) either inhibited or failed to inhibit growth of the mandible [15-22]. Indeed, many previous studies have tried to clarify the effect of chincup therapy on skeletal Class III problems by varying parameters such as force magnitude, duration of application, and timing of application during the growth period. In a recent review, Barrett *et al.* [22] summarized the results of these previous human studies and concluded that a gentle force and a short duration of chincup force application had no effect on mandibular growth. Most of the studies described in their review used a chincup force of 200–350 g for 1 to 2 years.

On the other hand, Deguchi and McNamara [17] indicated that treatment with chin cup for two years could have some effects on mandibular growth, such as a reduction in mandibular length. The results of their subsequent study [19] indicated a decrease in the gonial angle, and a possible bending of the condylar neck has also been described [23, 24]. On the contrary, Sugawara *et al.* [16] insisted that the effect of chincup treatment was not maintained until the end of facial growth. However, none of these previous studies clearly showed an orthopedic effect for chincup treatment, because of a lack of control data, inadequate experimental design, or negative results. Therefore, the orthopedic inhibition of mandibular growth via chincup treatment remains controversial [25].

Orthopedic protrusion of the mandible with functional appliances has also been reported in the literature. The results of human studies have led to the suggestion that functional appliances achieve a limited enhancement of mandibular growth. Indeed, the results of a randomized controlled trial [26] indicated that the clinical outcome of two-phase treatment, with an orthopedic approach in the first phase, did not significantly benefit patients, compared to one-phase treatment. Herbst appliances have been shown to affect mandibular growth [27-29]. Although the mechanisms have not been clarified, condylar posterior growth and deformation, [30, 31] as well as relocation of the glenoid fossa seem to contribute to the orthopedic effects of mandibular protrusion [7].

Based on clinical studies, the orthopedic effects of various appliances remain unclear. Investigating the cellular and molecular mechanisms elicited by applying mechanical stress to chondrocytes may elucidate how tissues like the mandibular condylar cartilage react to orthopedic intervention.

Anatomy, Histology, and Development of Mandibular Condylar Cartilage

1) Structural Characteristics of the TMJ

Before discussing the molecular basis of orthopedic approaches to the TMJ, we need to discuss the anatomy, histology, and cellular biology of the mandibular condyle. Mandibular condylar cartilage is a secondary cartilage and thus differs from primary cartilage formed in the epiphyses of long bones, as described earlier. Whether mechanical stress can affect the growth of bone formed by endochondral ossification has been debated. In general, endochondral bone formation is induced by cyclic compression. The epiphyseal growth plates of long bones are primary cartilage, which produce bone in response to functional loading. On the other hand, secondary cartilage does not have the same capability for resisting mechanical stress which is the basis for orthopedic approach to inhibiting mandibular growth. However, historical and regional craniofacial or maxillofacial deformation resulting from ethnic customs, such as foot binding in China, neck elongation by the Kayan people in Myanmar, and cranial deformation in South America, led orthodontic researchers to believe that facial growth can be altered by mechanical stress, as described above. Interestingly, foot binding in China seemed to inhibit endochondral bone formation in primary cartilage.

Comparisons of the growth mechanisms of mandibular condylar cartilage with those of growth-plate or articular cartilage should focus on anatomical and histological differences in structure. The TMJ is phylogenetically classified as a secondary joint with a bony structure composed of the mandibular condyle facing the mandibular fossa of the temporal bone, mediated by a ligament-like TMJ disc in the articular capsule [1]. While most primary joints, such as the knee, elbow, and hip joints, demonstrate single- or multi-axial rotation in the adjacent fossa, TMJ movement occurs in combination with axial rotation and anteroposterior sliding of the mandibular condyle against the articular surface of the temporal fossa. Therefore, the mechanical environment around the mandibular condylar cartilage differs from those around articular and growth-plate cartilages in primary joints, which may differentiate the mechanical properties of mandibular condylar cartilage from those of primary joints.

2) Histological and Molecular Characteristics of Mandibular Condylar Cartilage

Initial Differentiation of Chondrocytes

Fig. **1** shows mandibular condylar cartilage, growth-plate cartilage, and articular cartilage. Mandibular condylar cartilage has a five-layer structure composed of a fibrous layer, a proliferative cell layer, a transitional cell layer, a mature cell layer, and a hypertrophic cell layer beyond the articular surface. Articular and growth-plate cartilages are composed of four layers of well-differentiated chondrocytes (the resting, proliferating, prehypertrophic (or mature), and hypertrophic cell layers) [32-34]. In previous studies, many researchers have demonstrated differences between growth-plate cartilage and mandibular condylar cartilage based on the localization and expression of various ECM macromolecules [34-38]. The most apparent difference is the existence of less differentiated cells in the upper three layers of mandibular condylar cartilage. The fibrous, proliferative, and transient cell layers in mandibular condylar cartilage are composed of fibroblasts and undifferentiated mesenchymal cells with proliferative activity. These cells are surrounded by ECM composed of type I and III collagens and/or fibronectin, which are found in the ECM of fibrous connective tissue, but not in mature cartilage [39, 40]. In addition, these cells express messenger RNAs (mRNAs) encoding type I collagen [35]. Cells in all cell layers of articular and growth-plate cartilages are surrounded by ECM of mature cartilage which is composed of type II collagen and aggrecan. They also express mRNAs for these two cartilage-specific ECM macromolecules.

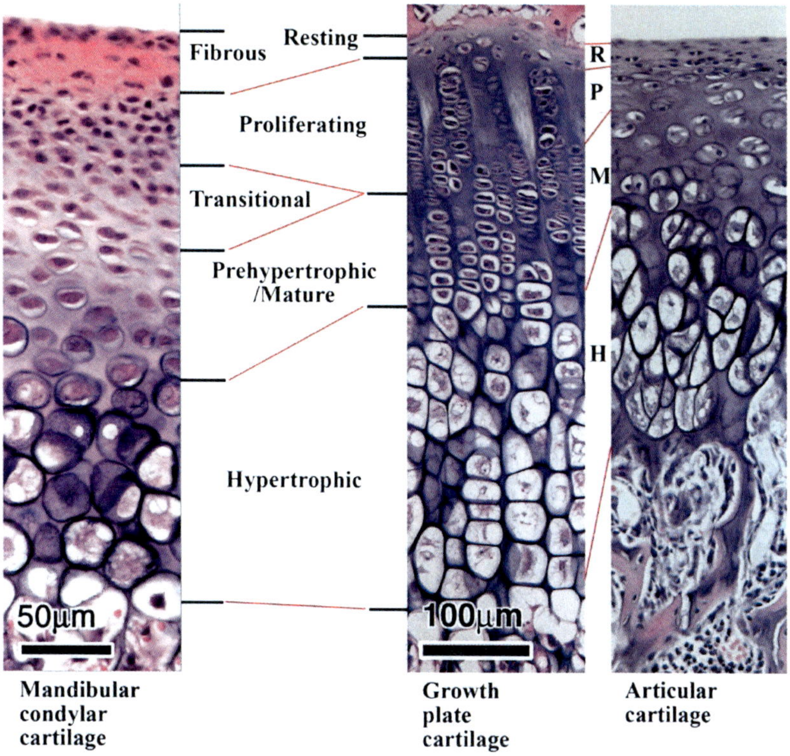

Figure 1: Illustrating the histological differences of three different types of hyaline cartilages. Left column shows a growing mandibular condylar cartilage in rat with five layered structures as indicated. Center column is a growth plate cartilage and the right column is an articular cartilage of rat tibia at 4 weeks of age. R: Resting cell layer, P: Proliferative cell layer, M: Mature (Prehypertrophic) cell layer and H: Hypertrophic cell layer.

These histological differences are established during chondrogenesis from the embryonic to fetal period. As described above, growth-plate cartilage is a primary cartilage, whereas mandibular condylar cartilage is a secondary cartilage. Primary cartilage is formed during an earlier embryonic stage than mandibular condylar cartilage. The latter is formed early in the fetal stage when embryonic development is largely complete. Generally, primary cartilage is formed from mesenchymal stem cells after cellular condensation, but before any organ is formed among the skeletal elements. This condensation occurs in the embryonic ECM, composed of type I and III collagens and fibronectin, which provides anchorage to the cells expressing α5β1 and α2β1 integrins on their surfaces. The cells that condense as cartilage anlage are also known to express the cell–cell adhesion molecules N-cadherin and neural cell adhesion molecule [41-44]. When cell aggregation begins, expression of the transcription factor SRY-box containing gene 9 (Sox-9) becomes apparent before expressing cartilage-specific ECM molecules [45-48]. Expression of Sox-9 and the related genes Sox-5 and Sox-6 in the condensing cells promotes expression of the genes encoding for type II collagen and aggrecan, and serves to enhance transcription at the very beginning of the phenotypic differentiation of chondrocytes [49]. Indeed, Sox-9 binds to the first intron of the type II collagen gene and enhances type II collagen gene expression [50]. Thereafter, the chondrocyte phenotype becomes more apparent. Cells become rounded as chondrocytes mature and cartilage-specific ECM proteins, such as type II collagen, aggrecan, and hyaluronic acid, occupy the intercellular space by replacing type I and III collagens and fibronectin, which are present at undifferentiated stages. Alteration of the cell–ECM adhesion status is known to contribute to chondrogenic differentiation. Inhibition of integrin-mediated cell–ECM adhesion by an RGD (Arg-Gly-Asp)-containing peptide promoted the chondrogenic differentiation of chondrocytes derived from costal cartilage [51]. Thus, release from cell–cell and cell–ECM adhesion appears to be a critical cellular event for further differentiation of chondrocytes. Thereafter, a complex three-dimensional network of these macromolecules may confer specific mechanical properties and characteristics to the cartilage ECM.

As described above, initial differentiation of primary cartilage occurs in the cranial base and Meckel's cartilage. Secondary cartilage is then produced in the TMJ when mesenchymal cells derived from cranial neural crest cells condense in a triangular zone bordered by the cranial base, Meckel's cartilage, and anlages of the masseter and internal pterygoid muscles. The anlage of mandibular condylar cartilage appears different from primary cartilage; it is surrounded by thick layers of fibrous and undifferentiated mesenchymal cells, instead of the thin perichondrium that covers primary cartilage. Thus, the structural differences in the cell layers between primary cartilage and mandibular condylar cartilage are established during early chondrogenic differentiation. Interestingly, whereas Sox-9 gene expression peaks after cell condensation and then decreases in primary cartilage, this expression has a patchy pattern in chondrocytes of other cartilage. Sox-9 is strongly expressed in differentiating chondrocytes of the proliferating cell layer, but it is only very weakly expressed in mature chondrocytes of the mandibular condylar cartilage [38, 39]. In addition, the expression and localization of type I collagen in the fibrous, proliferative, and transient cell layers has been related to the expression of connective tissue growth factor (CTGF) [52]. CTGF is generally known as the downstream effector of transforming growth factor β (TGF-β), which regulates the enhancement of type I collagen gene expression. In mandibular condylar cartilage, CTGF and type I collagen are co-expressed in the upper three cell layers and seem to contribute to the formation of the specific structure characteristic of this cartilage. No similar relationship has been observed in growth-plate cartilage.

Maturation and Terminal Differentiation of Chondrocytes

Matrix remodeling continues in the zone of differentiation from mature to hypertrophic chondrocytes,. Apparently as a result of chondrocytc differentiation, the amount of ECM increases, and cells also increase in size [33]. It is easy to speculate that the increase in cell size requires degradation of the matrix around the chondrocytes. Indeed, chondrocytes in both primary cartilage and mandibular condylar cartilage express genes encoding matrix metalloproteinases (MMPs) and aggrecanases. These enzymes are known to degrade ECM. As well as producing these proteinases, the cells regulate matrix degradation by producing proteinase inhibitors, namely tissue inhibitors of metalloproteinases. In our previous studies [36, 37], we showed that the patterns of MMP-9 and aggrecanase-1expression differed between growth-plate cartilage and mandibular condylar cartilage. Thus, metabolism of the ECM and tissue growth may be differentially controlled in the two different types of cartilage. Besides these metabolic changes during chondrogenesis, parathyroid hormone–related peptide and its receptor regulate the terminal differentiation of chondrocytes by regulating Indian hedgehog (IHH) [53], which could be a gatekeeper for the transition from mature (prehypertrophic) to hypertrophic chondrocytes. IHH is known to regulate the hypertrophy of chondrocytes in mandibular condylar cartilage [54]. Once chondrocytes terminally differentiate, they begin to: 1). secrete type X collagen [55] and chondromodulin [56, 57], 2). induce calcification of the surrounding ECM, and 3. promote angiogenesis in calcified cartilage and chondroclastic resorption of the matrix. The terminal differentiation of chondrocytes has shown no clear difference between growth-plate cartilage and mandibular condylar cartilage, except in matrix calcification. The cartilaginous matrix in the perpendicular septa of the hypertrophic cell layer in primary cartilage calcifies, whereas the cartilaginous matrix in the transverse septa does not. Hypertrophic chondrocytes in mandibular condylar cartilage are arranged randomly compared with those in growth-plate cartilage. Thus, calcification occurs all around the hypertrophic chondrocytes in an irregular pattern.

Histologic Effects of Orthopedic Intervention at the TMJ

1) Mandibular Advancement in Animal Models

Animal model studies of orthopedic intervention at the TMJ have described the effects of mandibular advancement on condylar remodeling and glenoid fossa relocation [6, 7, 58-60]. These animal experiments showed condylar remodeling and bone formation at the posterior border of the mandibular ramus and backward bending of the condylar neck after protrusive orthopedic functional intervention [6]. Forward relocation of the glenoid fossa was shown to occur in combination with condylar remodeling in monkeys [7]. In addition, a transient increase in the thickness of condylar cartilage was observed in monkeys [6] and in sheep [59]. As mentioned earlier, growth theories advocate that orofacial function is related to the skeletal morphology and growth of maxillofacial skeletal components. In this context, animal experiments indicate that electrical stimulation of the lateral pterygoid or masseter muscle induce transient histological changes in mandibular condylar cartilage [61-63]. Indeed, electrical stimulation of masseter muscle redirects condylar growth to a more forward direction, and increases the thickness of mandibular condylar cartilage in its anterior region [62]. Similarly, electrical stimulation of the lateral pterygoid muscle redirects condylar growth superiorly and causes transient thickening of the central mandibular condylar cartilage in growing rats [63]. Mandibular advancement using functional appliances transiently stimulates the lateral pterygoid, masseter, and digastric muscles in monkeys [64]. Transient thickening of the cartilage occurs, and growth is redirected, regardless of the method used to protrude the mandible. Although the mechanical environment may vary with specific experimental conditions, increased compressive stress usually induces the transient thickening of cartilage. Functional appliances produce forward displacement and upward movement of the condyles; masseter muscle activation and/or squeezing of the articular capsule, as a result of lateral pterygoid muscle activation, induces compressive stress and cartilage thickening is observed. One can also speculate that thickening of the cartilage would induce endochondral bone growth and redirect the growth of the mandibular condyle. Because the mechanical environment among experiments is variable, further studies will be needed to understand the relationship between the tissue response and mechanical conditions.

2) Application of Mandibular Retractive Force in Animal Models

A limited number of studies have established animal models of chincup therapy. Previous studies [65, 66] have tried to analyze the effect of mandibular retractive force on mandibular growth and the diurnal regulation of chondrogenic differentiation and cell proliferation using the same orthopedic approach. Asano [65] demonstrated that the application of retractive force to the mandible for 4 weeks inhibited mandibular growth in growing rats, a response that was maintained for a further 8 weeks without catchup growth of the mandible after the application of orthopedic force. Immediately after force application, mandibular condylar cartilage of the experimental rats showed reduced thickness, especially in the hypertrophic cell layer, and degenerative changes. The number and size of hypertrophic chondrocytes decreased and primary spongy bone levels were reduced during the force application and throughout the experimental period. Yamada *et al.* [66] demonstrated that the histological effect shown in the previous study was related to cell proliferation and the cartilage-specific ECM molecules of type II and X collagens. Apparently, levels of both of these collagens diminished in mandibular condylar cartilage when mandibular retraction force was applied. Specifically, in an experimental group to which orthopedic force was applied throughout the day, type X collagen completely disappeared from the matrix, while type II collagen was still weakly detected. Because type X collagen is a marker of hypertrophic chondrocytes, the application of mandibular retraction force can be assumed to completely inhibit the terminal differentiation of chondrocytes, which may consequently reduce endochondral bone formation. Diurnal variation was found in the cell proliferation of experimental animals, which was reduced when mandibular retraction force was applied during the resting period (the light period in the case of rats) compared with the active (dark) period (Fig. **2**). Although orthopedic intervention at the mandibular condyle using a mandibular retraction appliance could be effective, the degenerative response of the cartilaginous tissue could risk loss of the physiological function of the TMJ. Additionally, the anatomic structure of the TMJ in rats differs from that in humans, and the distribution of mechanical stress could differ when chincup force is applied to the human TMJ.

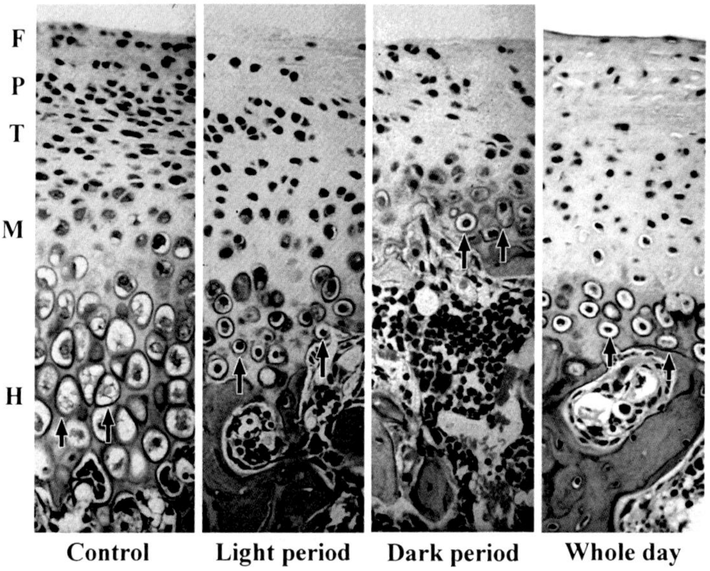

Figure 2: Effect of mandibular retractive force (MRF) on histological architecture of mandibular condylar cartilage in 5-week-old rats. MRF was applied for two weeks. Light and dark periods are controlled as 12/12-h light/dark illumination program. Light period: MRF applied during light period, Dark period: MRF applied during dark period and Whole day: MRF was applied for all day long. Note the cell size difference in the hypertrophic cell layer (arrows). F: fibrous layer, P: proliferative cell layer, T: transitional cell layer, M: mature (prehypertrophic) cell layer and H: hypertrophic cell layer.

3) Other Animal Models and In Vitro Tissue Culture Analysis of Tissue Responses to Applied Mechanical Stress

The distribution of mechanical stress in the TMJ is not uniform. Animal models and *in vitro* models have been established to simplify the experimental conditions. Midpalatal suture cartilage, which is classified as a secondary cartilage, is a simple model for observing the effects of expansive and compressive forces on the differentiation of chondrocytes. Orthodontic wires have been used to load compressive and expansive forces to this type of cartilage. Interestingly, expansive stress caused cartilaginous tissue between the right and left palatal bones to be replaced with fibrous suture tissue, whereas compressive stress promoted the hypertrophic differentiation of chondrocytes [67-69]. Organ culture systems were also tested using mandibular condyles from 4- or 5-day-old mice [70, 71]. Loading of an organ culture system with intermittent compressive stress induced matrix synthesis, but not cell proliferation [70]. Use of another organ culture system using the TMJ and the masseter muscle showed that electrical stimulation of the masseter muscle at 0.7 Hz contributed to the maintenance of the chondrocytic phenotype of mandibular condylar cartilage cells [71]. Without electrical stimulation, condylar cartilage lost its cartilaginous structure. In addition, intermittent stress had positive effects on the chondrogenic phenotype, but continuous stress did not.

The molecular basis of tissue reactions to mechanical stress loading on cartilage has been discussed. IHH is a key molecule during mechanical stress responses because, as described above, alterations in the terminal differentiation of prehypertrophic chondrocytes into hypertrophic chondrocytes are a prominent phenomenon during tissue responses. Indeed, mandibular advancement in rats induced the synthesis of IHH protein in the proliferative cell layer, a response that was related to the up-regulation of proliferative activity [72]. In a knee joint contracture model, joint immobilization induced the expression of TGF-β and CTGF in the articular capsule. Moreover, the ECM of the articular cartilage was partially composed of type I collagen at positions where the physiological loading pattern had been altered [73, 74]. In general, CTGF promotes type I collagen expression under the control of TGF-β. Thus, the mechanical stress response of chondrocytes may be regulated by mechanical stress–induced CTGF. In our previous study using midpalatal suture cartilage as a model [75], we found that extracellular signal–regulated kinase (ERK)-1/2 was phosphorylated by stretch stimulation. As a result of this phosphorylation, ERK-1/2 showed nuclear translocation after stimulation for 3 to 6 hours, as well as increased expression of α5β1-integrin. At the same time, stress fibers formed in differentiating chondrocytes, focal adhesion kinase (FAK) was upregulated, and focal adhesion contacts formed in midpalatal suture cartilage. Thus, cell–ECM adhesion may play crucial roles in the mechanical stress response.

In vitro tissue culture studies [76-79] have tested the influence of dynamic/cyclic or static compressive forces on chondrogenesis, chondrocyte differentiation, the chondrocytic phenotype, and chondrocyte metabolism. Many other studies have investigated the effects of dynamic/cyclic and static compressive stresses on cartilage differentiation and metabolism. The use of various experimental systems has led to two different conclusions: 1) cyclic/dynamic compressive stress can enhance chondrocytic metabolism and/or maturation by up-regulating the expression of genes encoding cartilage-specific macromolecules, whereas static compressive force inhibits chondrocyte metabolism [70, 71, 77, 78] and 2) both cyclic/dynamic and static compressive forces can induce the chondrogenic differentiation of undifferentiated mesenchymal cells and maintain the chondrocytic phenotype [76, 79]. Again, the mechanical stress applied differed among experimental systems and the mechanical properties of the tissues prepared varied widely. Whereas our study [76] utilized combined agarose/collagen gel culture, which swells by 40% under 1 kPa compressive stress during the 4-day loading period, cartilage explants with different stress relaxation properties may swell in different time courses. In addition, the source of the cells used also differed among studies, with some using cells derived from mature or growing articular cartilage and others using embryonic or mesenchymal stem cells. Thus, it appears that a certain level of compressive stress is needed to maintain the cartilage phenotype and induce chondrogenesis. As most of these previous investigations were performed using primary cartilage, the effects of mechanical stress on the metabolism, phenotype, and differentiation of mandibular condylar cartilage cells remain unclear.

Molecular Response of Chondrocytes to Mechanical Stress

Mechano-transduction is the mechanism by which changes in the extracellular mechanical environment are translated into intracellular biochemical reactions. Intracellular responses to mechanical stress have largely been discussed in the context of the phosphorylation of signaling molecules and the import of ions by cells.

Previous studies found that FAK, ERKs, and p38 mitogen-activated protein kinase (p38 MAPK) were activated because of the mechanical stimulation of chondrocytes. In our previous study [80, 81], stepwise stretch stimulation of differentiating chondrocytes inhibited chondrogenic differentiation of embryonic limb bud–derived mesenchymal stem cells through cell–ECM adhesion mediated by integrins. Inhibition of chondrogenesis through integrin-mediated ERK activation can be rescued by inhibiting mitogen-activated protein kinase kinase (MEK)-1/2, signaling molecules that act upstream of ERK-1/2. Since activation of ERK, as a result of fibroblast growth factor (FGF) signaling, is known to inhibit chondrogenesis [82], the crosstalk between integrin and receptor tyrosine kinase pathways may be a key mechanism of mechano-signal transduction. Thus, stretch-induced inhibition of chondrogenesis may result from crosstalk between mechano-transduction and tyrosine receptor kinase pathways. However, ERK was also activated as the result of dynamic/static and shear stress/compression, and p38 MAPK was activated due to the exposure of cartilage explant cultures to static compression [83]. Interestingly, FGF1 and FGF2 have been reported to enhance Sox-9 protein expression during limb chondrogenesis by activating an ERK-1/2 pathway [84]. Our data suggested that stretch stimulation; however, did not activate p38 MAPK during the inhibition of chondrogenesis. Therefore, multiple MAPK pathways appear to play crucial roles in the mechano-transduction pathway in combination with one another. Based on the molecular biological theory, mechanical stress is now considered one of those factors, like cytokines and growth factors.

The Ca^{2+} ion channel transient receptor potential vanilloids (TRPVs) are activated by osmotic stimulation. Targeted disruption of TRPV4 caused osteoarthritic joint degeneration in a mouse model, and TRPV4 promoted prostaglandin E_2 production under hypo-osmotic conditions [85, 86]. Large calcium-activated potassium channels (BK channels) have been shown in patch-clamp experiments to be involved in K^+ ion incorporation [87]. Interestingly, stretch-activated channels together induce activation of FAK under cyclical pressure–induced strain [88].

Although the molecular basis for mechano-transduction has been demonstrated in a variety of research fields, as described above, further investigations are necessary to clarify the mechanisms underlying the mechanical stress responses of cells and tissues. Recently, tissue engineering of cartilage has been attempted.

Cartilage can be engineered by loading dynamic mechanical stress through cell–ECM adhesion mediated by integrins, which may enhance cartilage maturation and improve the mechanical properties of tissue-engineered cartilage [89, 90]. Thus, the results of research into the molecular basis of chondrogenesis and mechano-transduction pathways have been translated into the development of technologies for tissue reconstruction.

SUMMARY AND FUTURE DIRECTIONS

The present chapter has reviewed the anatomy, histology, growth mechanisms, development, and differentiation of mandibular condylar cartilage, through comparison with other cartilages. Also discussed were the orthopedic effects on the mandibular condyle and the molecular basis of mechano-transduction in chondrocytes, as determined using various experimental models. Although extensive studies have been performed in the molecular and clinical fields, treatment modalities for skeletal class III problems are not generalized. Based on the results of the animal model studies, the complexity of tissue reactions were discussed to orthopedic approaches focused on the condyle relative to the complexity of the surrounding mechanical environment. Even at the cellular or tissue level (as explored in *in vitro* studies), the distribution of mechanical stress in experimental models is complex. In addition, we lack precise data on the distribution of stress in the TMJ during function and under orthopedic intervention. As the calculation capacity of computers increases, it may be possible to simulate stress distribution in the TMJ in the near future. Analysis of the relationships between stress distribution and tissue, cellular, and molecular responses may lead to an understanding of the mechanisms of orthopedic effects on the mandible. One hypothesis (Fig. **3**) that can be raised is that mechanical compressive stress at the physiological level could enhance chondrogenic differentiation and, consequently, endochondral bone formation. Whereas stress above a certain level, or shared stress under stretch stimulation (pathological stress), could inhibit the chondrocyte differentiation or induce the degeneration of cartilage and inhibit bone formation. Both of these pathologic processes are regulated by a molecular mechano-transduction pathway through tyrosine phosphorylation and ion channel activation (Fig. **4**).

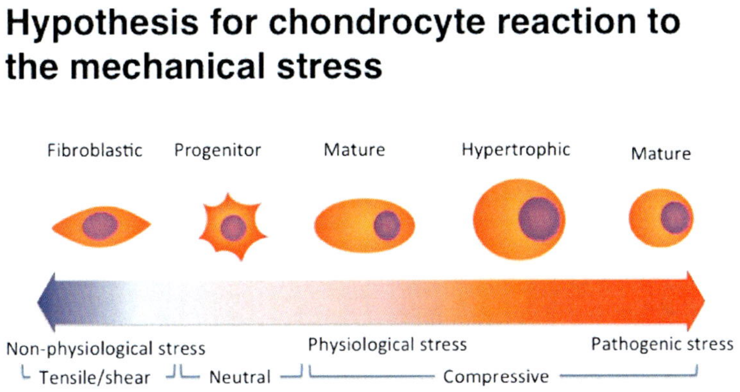

Figure 3: Illustration of the hypothesis cited in the present chapter. Mechanical compressive stress at the physiological level could enhance chondrogenic differentiation and, consequently, endochondral bone formation. On the other hand, stress above a certain level or shared stress under stretch stimulation (pathological stress) could inhibit chondrocyte differentiation, induce the degeneration of cartilage, and/or inhibit bone formation.

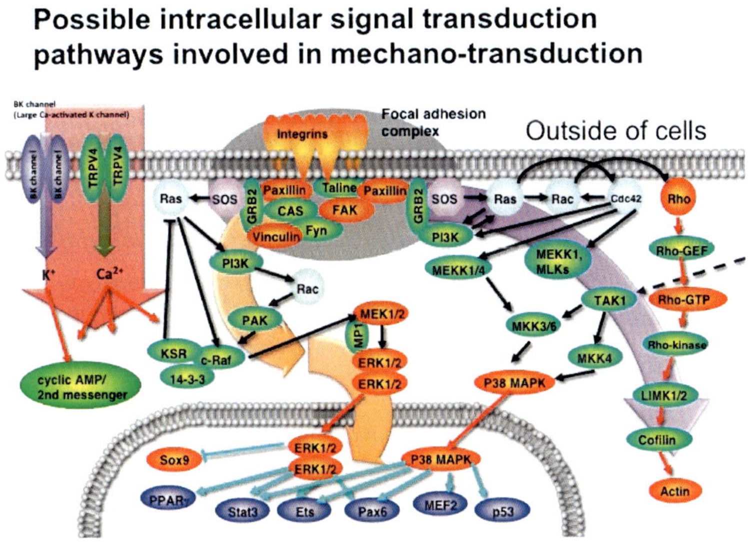

Figure 4: Illustration of mechano-transduction signaling pathway in the chondrocytes. Ion channels, MAPK pathway and cytoskeletal elements are affected by stretch or shear stress stimulation. Mechanical stress is conveyed *via* an array of chemical signals initially propagated near the cell wall.

Through the human genome project, information coded by the genome (coding sequences for proteins, regulatory elements for gene expression and suppression, and modifiers of expressed messages) have been explored. The interactions between genetic and epigenetic factors have been focused at the molecular level. In addition, individual-level variation in genomic sequences, such as single nucleotide polymorphisms (SNPs) and other types of variation, can be considered determinants of individual variation in mechanical responses and susceptibility to diseases. An important aspect of molecular studies is to understand the molecular mechanisms that regulate mechanical stress responses at the individual level. Recently, modalities of bioinformatics, involving various biological agents, have been developed that may enhance the further development of research and diagnostic modalities. If individual differences in mechanical stress responses based on individual variation in genomic sequences are clarified, diagnostic criteria for facial growth and response to orthopedic interventions could be established. An improved knowledge base could lead to a paradigm shift in orthodontic diagnosis, as well as the development of advanced treatment modalities, that focus long-term management on specific stages of growth.

SUMMARY POINTS

- So far, the orthopedic effects of various appliances remain unclear, but clinically relevant research has produced definitive evidence.
- The mechanical environment around the mandibular condylar cartilage differs from articular and growth-plate cartilages in primary joints, which may help explain the specific mechanical properties of mandibular condylar cartilage, compared to the joints of long bones.
- The process of differentiation and maturation of mandibular condylar cartilage is different from that of primary cartilage, relative to ECM production and regulation of cell differentiation.
- Animal studies indicate that retraction force on the mandible is effective, but the degenerative response of the cartilaginous tissue may compromise physiological function of the TMJ.
- It is hypothesized that physiologic compressive stress enhances chondrogenic differentiation and endochondral bone formation, but pathological stress inhibits chondrocyte differentiation, induces cartilage and/or inhibits bone formation.

- The molecular mechano-transduction pathway for condylar cartilage is *via* tyrosine phosphorylation and ion channel activation.

ACKNOWLEDGEMENTS

Declared none.

CONFLICT OF INTEREST

The author confirms that this chapter contents have no conflict of interest.

REFERENCES

[1] Ten Cate AR. (1994) Temporomandibular joint. In: Ten Cate AR (ed) Oral histology: development, structure, and function, 4th edn. Mosby, St. Louis, pp 432-455.
[2] Hall BK. From condensation to differentiation and temporomandibular joint and synchondrosis. In: Hall BK (ed) Bone and cartilage: Developmental and evolutionary skeletal biology, chapters 20 and 33. Elsevier 2005;272-281.
[3] Sarnat BG and Wexler MR. Growth of the face and jaws after resection of the septal cartilage in the rabbit. Am J Anat 1966;118:755-768.
[4] Harvold EP, Tomer BS, Vargervik K, *et al.* Primate experiments on oral respiration. Am J Orthod 1981;79:359-372.
[5] Yamada T, Tanne K, Miyamoto K, *et al.* Influences of nasal respiratory obstruction on craniofacial growth in young Macaca fuscata monkeys. Am J Orthod Dentofac Orthop 1997;111:38-43.
[6] McNamara JA Jr, Hinton RJ and Hoffman DL. Histologic analysis of temporomandibular joint adaptation to protrusive function in young adult rhesus monkeys (Macaca mulatta). Am J Orthod 1982;82:288-298.
[7] Woodside DG, Metaxas A and Altuna G. The influence of functional appliance therapy on glenoid fossa remodeling. Am J Orthod Dentofacial Orthop 1987;92:181-198.
[8] Moss ML. A theoretical analysis of the functional matrix. Acta Biotheor 1968;18:195-202.
[9] Moss ML. The functional matrix hypothesis revisited. 1. The role of mechanotransduction. Am J Orthod Dentofacial Orthop 1997;112:8-11.
[10] Moss ML. The functional matrix hypothesis revisited. 2. The role of an osseous connected cellular network. Am J Orthod Dentofacial Orthop 1997;112:221-216.
[11] Moss ML. The functional matrix hypothesis revisited. 3. The genomic thesis. Am J Orthod Dentofacial Orthop 1997;112:338-342.
[12] Moss ML. The functional matrix hypothesis revisited. 4. The epigenetic antithesis and the resolving synthesis. Am J Orthod Dentofacial Orthop 1997;112:410-417.
[13] Petrovic AG. Research methodology in craniofacial growth In: Graber TM, Rakosi T and Petrovic AG (eds) Dentofacial orthopedics with functional appliances, chapter 1. Mosby, St. Louis, 1985;5-18.
[14] Petrovic AG. Research methodology in craniofacial growth In: Graber TM, Rakosi T and Petrovic AG (eds) Dentofacial orthopedics with functional appliances, chapter 2. Mosby, St. Louis, 1985;19-67.

[15] Mitani H and Fukazawa H. Effects of chincap force on the timing and amount of mandibular growth associated with anterior reversed occlusion (Class III malocclusion) during puberty. Am J Orthod Dentofacial Orthop 1986;90:454-463.
[16] Sugawara J, Asano T, Endo N, *et al.* Long-term effects of chincap therapy on skeletal profile in mandibular prognathism. Am J Orthod Dentofacial Orthop 1990;98:127-133.
[17] Deguchi T and McNamara JA. Craniofacial adaptations induced by chincup therapy in Class III patients. Am J Orthod Dentofacial Orthop. 1999;115:175-182.
[18] Deguchi T, Kuroda T, Hunt NP, *et al.* Long-term application of chincup force alters the morphology of the dolichofacial Class III mandible. Am J Orthod Dentofacial Orthop 1999;116:610-615.
[19] Deguchi T, Kuroda T, Minoshima Y *et al.* Craniofacial features of patients with Class III abnormalities: growth-related changes and effects of short-term and long-term chincup therapy. Am J Orthod Dentofacial Orthop 2002;121:84-92.
[20] Tahmina K, Tanaka E and Tanne K. Craniofacial morphology in orthodontically treated patients of class III malocclusion with stable and unstable treatment outcomes. Am J Orthod Dentofacial Orthop 2000;117:681-690.
[21] Ko YI, Baek SH, Mah J *et al.* Determinants of successful chincup therapy in skeletal class III malocclusion. Am J Orthod Dentofacial Orthop 2004;126:33-41.
[22] Barrett AA, Baccetti T and McNamara JA Jr. Treatment effects of the light-force chincup. Am J Orthod Dentofacial Orthop 2010;138:468-476.
[23] Deguchi T. Force distribution of the temporomandibular joint and temporal bone surface subjected to the head-chincup force. Am J Orthod Dentofacial Orthop. 1998;114:277-282.
[24] Gökalp H and Kurt G. Magnetic resonance imaging of the condylar growth pattern and disk position after chin cup therapy: a preliminary study. Angle Orthod 2005;75:568-575.
[25] Liu ZP, Li CJ, Hu HK, *et al.* Efficacy of short-term chincup therapy for mandibular growth retardation in Class III malocclusion. Angle Orthod 2011;81:162-168.
[26] Tulloch JF, Proffit WR and Phillips C. Outcomes in a 2-phase randomized clinical trial of early Class II treatment. Am J Orthod Dentofacial Orthop 2004;125:657-667.
[27] Wieslander L. Long-term effect of treatment with the headgear-Herbst appliance in the early mixed dentition. Stability or relapse? Am J Orthod Dentofacial Orthop 1993;104:319-329.
[28] Hägg U, Du X and Rabie AB. Initial and late treatment effects of headgear-Herbst appliance with mandibular step-by-step advancement. Am J Orthod Dentofacial Orthop 2002;122:477-485.
[29] Serbesis-Tsarudis C and Pancherz H. "Effective" TMJ and chin position changes in Class II treatment. Angle Orthod 2008;78:813-818.
[30] Croft RS, Buschang PH, English JD, *et al.* A cephalometric and tomographic evaluation of Herbst treatment in the mixed dentition. Am J Orthod Dentofacial Orthop 1999;116:435-443.
[31] Güner DD, Oztürk Y and Sayman HB. Evaluation of the effects of functional orthopaedic treatment on temporomandibular joints with single-photon emission computerized tomography. Eur J Orthod 2003;25:9-12.
[32] Silbermann M, Reddi AH, Hand AR, *et al.* Further characterisation of the extracellular matrix in the mandibular condyle in neonatal mice. J Anat 1987;151:169-188.
[33] Luder HU, Leblond CP, and Von der Mark K. Cellular stages in cartilage formation as revealed by morphometry, radioautography and type II collagen immunostaining of the mandibular condyle from weanling rats. Am J Anat 1988;182:197-214.

[34] Mizoguchi I, Nakamura M, Takahashi I, *et al.* An immunohistochemical study of localization of type I and type II collagens in mandibular condylar cartilage compared with tibial growth plate. Histochemistry 1990;93:593-599.

[35] Bae JW, Takahashi I, Sasano Y, *et al.* Age-related changes in gene expression patterns of matrix metalloproteinases and their collagenous substrates in mandibular condylar cartilage in rats. J Anat 2003;203:235-241.

[36] Takahashi I, Onodera K, Bae JW, *et al.* Age-related changes in the expression of gelatinase and tissue inhibitor of metalloproteinase genes in mandibular condylar, growth plate, and articular cartilage in rats. J Mol Histol 2005;36:355-366.

[37] Mitani H, Takahashi I, Onodera K, *et al.* Comparison of age-dependent expression of aggrecan and ADAMTSs in mandibular condylar cartilage, tibial growth plate, and articular cartilage in rats. Histochem Cell Biol 2006;126:371-380.

[38] Shibata S, Suda N, Suzuki S, *et al.* An *in situ* hybridization study of Runx2, Osterix, and Sox9 at the onset of condylar cartilage formation in fetal mouse mandible. J Anat 2006;208:169-177.

[39] Ben Ami Y, Von der Mark K, Franzen A, *et al.* Immunohistochemical studies of the extracellular matrix in the condylar cartilage of the human fetal mandible: collagens and noncollagenous proteins. Am J Anat 1991;190:157-166.

[40] Mizoguchi I, Takahashi I, Sasano Y, *et al.* Localization of types I, II and III collagen and glycosaminoglycans in the mandibular condyle of growing monkeys: an immunohistochemical study. Anat Embryol (Berl) 1997;195:127-135.

[41] Oberlender SA and Tuan RS. Spatiotemporal profile of N-cadherin expression in the developing limb mesenchyme. Cell Adhes Commun 1994;2:521-537.

[42] Tavella S, Raffo P, Tacchetti C, *et al.* N-CAM and N-cadherin expression during *in vitro* chondrogenesis. Exp Cell Res 1994;215:354-362.

[43] Tsonis PA, Del Rio-Tsonis K, Millan JL, *et al.* Expression of N-cadherin and alkaline phosphatase in chick limb bud mesenchymal cells: regulation by 1, 25-dihydroxyvitamin D3 or TGF-beta1. Exp Cell Res 1994;213:433-437.

[44] Fang J and Hall BK. Differential expression of neural cell adhesion molecule (NCAM) during osteogenesis and secondary chondrogenesis in the embryonic chick. Int J Dev Biol 1995;39:519-528.

[45] Wright E, Hargrave MR, Christiansen J, *et al.* The Sry-related gene Sox9 is expressed during chondrogenesis in mouse embryos. Nat Genet 1995;9:15-20.

[46] Lefebvre V, Zhou G, Mukhopadhyay K, *et al.* An 18-base-pair sequence in the mouse proalpha1(II) collagen gene is sufficient for expression in cartilage and binds nuclear proteins that are selectively expressed in chondrocytes. Mol Cell Biol 196;16:4512-4523.

[47] Ng LJ, Wheatley S, Muscat GE, *et al.* SOX9 binds DNA, activates transcription, and coexpresses with type II collagen during chondrogenesis in the mouse. Dev Biol 1997;183:108-121.

[48] Zhao Q, Eberspaecher H and De Crombrugghe B. Parallel expression of Sox9 and Col2a1 in cells undergoing chondrogenesis. Dev Dynam 1997;209:377-386.

[49] Lefebvre V, Li P and Crombrugghe B. A new long form of Sox5 (L-Sox5), Sox6 and Sox9 are coexpressed in chondrogenesis and cooperatively activate the type II collagen gene. EMBO J 1998;17:5718-5733.

[50] Bell DM, Leung KK, Wheatley SC, *et al.* SOX9 directly regulates the type-II collagen gene. Nat Genet 1997;16:174-178.

[51] Yasuda T, Shimizu K, Nakagawa Y, *et al.* Possible involvement of RGD (Arg-Gly-Asp)-containing extracellular matrix proteins in rat growth plate chondrocyte differentiation in culture. J Bone Miner Res 1996;11:1430-1437.
[52] Fukunaga T, Yamashiro T, Oya S, *et al.* Connective tissue growth factor mRNA expression pattern in cartilages is associated with their type I collagen expression. Bone 2003;33:911-918.
[53] Vortkamp A, Lee K, Lanske B, *et al.* Regulation of rate of cartilage differentiation by Indian hedgehog and PTH-related protein. Science 1996;273:613-622.
[54] Shibukawa Y, Young B, Wu C, *et al.* Temporomandibular joint formation and condyle growth require Indian hedgehog signaling. Dev Dyn 2007;236:426-434.
[55] Ohashi N, Ejiri S, Hanada K, *et al.* Changes in type I, II, and X collagen immunoreactivity of the mandibular condylar cartilage in a naturally aging rat model. J Bone Miner Metab 1997;15:77-83.
[56] Hiraki Y and Shukunami C. Chondromodulin-I as a novel cartilage-specific growth-modulating factor. Pediatr Nephrol 2000;14:602-605.
[57] Shukunami C and Hiraki Y. Role of cartilage-derived anti-angiogenic factor, chondromodulin-I, during endochondral bone formation. Osteoarthritis Cartilage 9 Suppl A 2001:S91-101.
[58] McNamara JA Jr and Carlson DS. Quantitative analysis of temporomandibular joint adaptations to protrusive function. Am J Orthod 1979;76:593-611.
[59] Ma B, Sampson W, Fazzalari N, *et al.* Experimental forward mandibular displacement in sheep. Arch Oral Biol 2002;47:75-84.
[60] Tagliaro ML, Rassi Guimarães ML, Pereira Padilha DM, *et al.* Mandibular advancement and morphological changes in the mandibles of female mice of different ages. Exp Gerontol 2006;41:1157-1164.
[61] Kantomaa T and Rönning O. The effect of electrical stimulation of the lateral pterygoid muscle on the growth of the mandible in the rat. Proc Finn Dent Soc 1984;78:215-219.
[62] Watanabe Y. An experimental study on the effects of overactivity of the masseter muscle by electrical stimulation on the mandibular morphogenesis in rats. J Hiroshima Univ Dent Soc 1990;22:65-85.
[63] Takahashi I, Mizoguchi I, Nakamura M, *et al.* Effects of lateral pterygoid muscle hyperactivity on differentiation of mandibular condyles in rats. Anat Rec 1995;241:328-336.
[64] Sessle BJ, Woodside DG, Bourque P, *et al.* Effect of functional appliances on jaw muscle activity. Am J Orthod Dentofacial Orthop 1990;98:222-230.
[65] Asano T. The effects of mandibular retractive force on the growing rat mandible. Am J Orthod Dentofacial Orthop 1986;90:464-474.
[66] Yamada S, Saeki S, Takahashi I, *et al.* Diurnal variation in the response of the mandible to orthopedic force. J Dent Res 2002;81:711-715.
[67] Takahashi I, Mizoguchi I, Nakamura M, *et al.* Effects of expansive force on the differentiation of midpalatal suture cartilage in rats. Bone 1996;18:341-348.
[68] Saitoh S, Takahashi I, Mizoguchi I, *et al.* Compressive force promotes chondrogenic differentiation and hypertrophy in midpalatal suture cartilage in growing rats. Anat Rec 2000;260:392-401.
[69] Hou B, Fukai N and Olsen BR. Mechanical force-induced midpalatal suture remodeling in mice. Bone 2007;40:1483-1493.

[70] Copray JC, Jansen HW and Duterloo HS. Effects of compressive forces on proliferation and matrix synthesis in mandibular condylar cartilage of the rat *in vitro*. Arch Oral Biol 1985;30:299-304.

[71] Pirttiniemi P and Kantomaa T. Electrical stimulation of masseter muscles maintains condylar cartilage in long-term organ culture. J Dent Res 1996;75:1365-1371.

[72] Tang GH, Rabie AB and Hägg U. Indian hedgehog: a mechanotransduction mediator in condylar cartilage. J Dent Res 2004;83:434-438.

[73] Hagiwara Y, Chimoto E, Takahashi I, *et al.* Expression of transforming growth factor-beta1 and connective tissue growth factor in the capsule in a rat immobilized knee model. Ups J Med Sci 2008;113:221-234.

[74] Hagiwara Y, Ando A, Chimoto E, *et al.* Expression of collagen types I and II on articular cartilage in a rat knee contracture model. Connect Tissue Res 2010;51:22-30.

[75] Takahashi I, Onodera K, Sasano Y, *et al.* Effect of stretching on gene expression of beta1 integrin and focal adhesion kinase and on chondrogenesis through cell-extracellular matrix interactions. Eur J Cell Biol 2003;82:182-192.

[76] Takahashi I, Nuckolls GH, Takahashi K, *et al.* Compressive force promotes sox9, type II collagen and aggrecan and inhibits IL-1beta expression resulting in chondrogenesis in mouse embryonic limb bud mesenchymal cells. J Cell Sci 1998;111:2067-2076.

[77] Othman H, Thonar EJ and Mao JJ. Modulation of neonatal growth plate development by *ex vivo* intermittent mechanical stress. J Biomech 2007;40:2686-2693.

[78] Sergerie K, Parent S, Beauchemin PF, *et al.* Growth plate explants respond differently to *in vitro* static and dynamic loadings. J Orthop Res 2011;29:473-480.

[79] Tran SC, Cooley AJ and Elder SH. Effect of a mechanical stimulation bioreactor on tissue engineered, scaffold-free cartilage. Biotechnol Bioeng 2011;108:1421-1429.

[80] Onodera K, Takahashi I, Sasano Y, *et al.* Stepwise mechanical stretching inhibits chondrogenesis through cell-matrix adhesion mediated by integrins in embryonic rat limb-bud mesenchymal cells. Eur J Cell Biol 2005;84:45-58.

[81] Takahashi I, Masuda T, Arai F, *et al.* Mechanobiological Signal Transduction in Differentiating Chondrocyte and New Configuration for Mechanical Stress Culture. Proceedings of the 2nd IEEE International Conference on Nano/Micro Engineered and Molecular Systems 2007;1061-1064.

[82] Bobick BE and Kulyk WM. The MEK-ERK signaling pathway is a negative regulator of cartilage-specific gene expression in embryonic limb mesenchyme. J Biol Chem 2004;279:4588-4595.

[83] Fitzgerald JB, Jin M, Chai DH, *et al.* Shear- and compression-induced chondrocyte transcription requires MAPK activation in cartilage explants. J Biol Chem 2008;283:6735-6743.

[84] Murakami S, Kan M, McKeehan WL, *et al.* Up-regulation of the chondrogenic Sox9 gene by fibroblast growth factors is mediated by the mitogen-activated protein kinase pathway. Proc Natl Acad Sci U S A 2000;97:1113-1118.

[85] Phan MN, Leddy HA, Votta BJ, *et al.* Functional characterization of TRPV4 as an osmotically sensitive ion channel in porcine articular chondrocytes. Arthritis Rheum 2009;60:3028-3037.

[86] Clark AL, Votta BJ, Kumar S, *et al.* Chondroprotective role of the osmotically sensitive ion channel transient receptor potential vanilloid 4: age- and sex-dependent progression of osteoarthritis in Trpv4-deficient mice. Arthritis Rheum 2010;62:2973-2983.

[87] Mobasheri A, Lewis R, Maxwell JE, *et al.* Characterization of a stretch-activated potassium channel in chondrocytes. J Cell Physiol 2010;223:511-518.

[88] Lee HS, Millward-Sadler SJ, Wright MO, *et al.* Integrin and mechanosensitive ion channel-dependent tyrosine phosphorylation of focal adhesion proteins and beta-catenin in human articular chondrocytes after mechanical stimulation. J Bone Miner Res 2000;15:1501-1509.

[89] Chen R, Curran SJ, Curran JM, *et al.* The use of poly(l-lactide) and RGD modified microspheres as cell carriers in a flow intermittency bioreactor for tissue engineering cartilage. Biomaterials 2006;27:4453-4460.

[90] Villanueva I, Weigel CA and Bryant SJ. Cell-matrix interactions and dynamic mechanical loading influence chondrocyte gene expression and bioactivity in PEG-RGD hydrogels. Acta Biomater 2009;5:2832-2846.

PART II: DIAGNOSIS AND TREATMENT IN THE GROWING PATIENTS

CHAPTER 4

Treatment of Class III Malocclusions in the Growing Patients

Peter Ngan[1,*], Hong He[2] and Benedict Wilmes[3]

[1]Department of Orthodontics, West Virginia University School of Dentistry, USA; [2]Department of Orthodontics, Wuhan University and Key Lab for Oral Biomedical Engineering and Wuhan University, Ministry of Education, China and [3]Department of Orthodontics, University of Duesseldorf, Germany

Abstract: Class III malocclusion and anterior crossbite are common clinical problems, especially in patients of Asian ancestry. Management of the developing Class III malocclusion continues to challenge practicing clinicians. This chapter focuses on the treatment of Class III malocclusions in growing patients. The question arises as to what type of Class III malocclusion will benefit from early treatment; when is a good time to start an early phase of orthodontic or orthopedic treatment; how successful are these treatments long-term; and do we have evidence in the literature to support early treatment? Protraction facemask is used in the treatment of Class III malocclusions with maxillary deficiencies. The question is whether side effects such as proclination of maxillary incisors and loss of arch length can be resolved using a bone anchored protraction device. These questions will be addressed and illustrated with clinical cases.

Keywords: Class III malocclusion, Frequency, Etiology, Diagnosis, Growth Prediction, Early treatment, Chin cap therapy, Maxillary protraction, Bone anchored protraction.

INTRODUCTION

Prevalence of Class III Malocclusion

The prevalence of Class III malocclusion varies among different ethnic groups. The prevalence in Caucasians ranges between 1% and 4% depending on the method in studying the malocclusion and the age group evaluated [1-4]. A high prevalence of Class III malocclusion has been observed in the Asian populations such as Chinese (4% - 12%) [5-8], Japanese (2.3% - 13%) [9-10] and Koreans

***Address correspondence to Peter Ngan:** Professor and Chairman, Department of Orthodontics, West Virginia University, School of Dentistry, 1073 Health Science Center North, P.O. Box 9480, Morgantown, WV 26506, USA; Tel: 304-293-3222; Fax: 304-293-2327; Email: pngan@hsc.wvu.edu

(9% - 19%) [11]. A relatively high prevalence of Class III malocclusion was also reported in other countries such as Saudi Arabia (9.4%) [12] and Sweden (6%) [13]. This was in contrast with people of Northern European ancestry with estimates ranging from 0.8% to 4.2% [14-16], European Americans (0.8%) [17-18] and African Americans (0.6% - 1.2%) [17-18].

Components of Class III Malocclusion

Individuals with Class III malocclusion and anterior crossbites may have combinations of skeletal and dentoalveolar components (Fig. **1**). Consideration of the various components is essential so that the underlying cause of the discrepancy can be treated appropriately. This is particularly relevant to the treatment of Class III malocclusion because the components vary among different ethnic groups [19-22]. Guyer *et al.* [19] conducted a cephalometric study to identify the various types of skeletal Class III patterns between 13 and 15 years old Caucasian children. Approximately 57% of the patients with either a normal or prognathic mandible showed a deficiency in the maxilla. Masaki [20], in a comparative study of native Japanese and of Americans of Northern European ancestry, reported that maxillary skeletal retrusion occurred more often in the Asian face. The author reported that the posterior cranial base length and lower anterior facial height were significantly larger and the anterior cranial base length and facial depth were smaller in Japanese children. Masaki [20] stressed that a backward rotation of the mandible in the Japanese appeared to be necessary to coordinate occlusion because of a small maxilla. Ishii *et al.* [21] compared the major craniofacial differences between Japanese and Caucasians with Class III malocclusion and found that Japanese patients had a significantly reduced anterior cranial base; a significantly more obtuse gonial angle; a high angle facial pattern with a significantly increased lower anterior face height; and significantly more proclined upper incisors. Ngan *et al.* [22] compared the adult Chinese and Caucasian Class III craniofacial differences and found that the Chinese adults had a shorter anterior cranial base length, a larger posterior cranial base length and an increase mandibular length that contributed to the increase in mandibular prognathism.

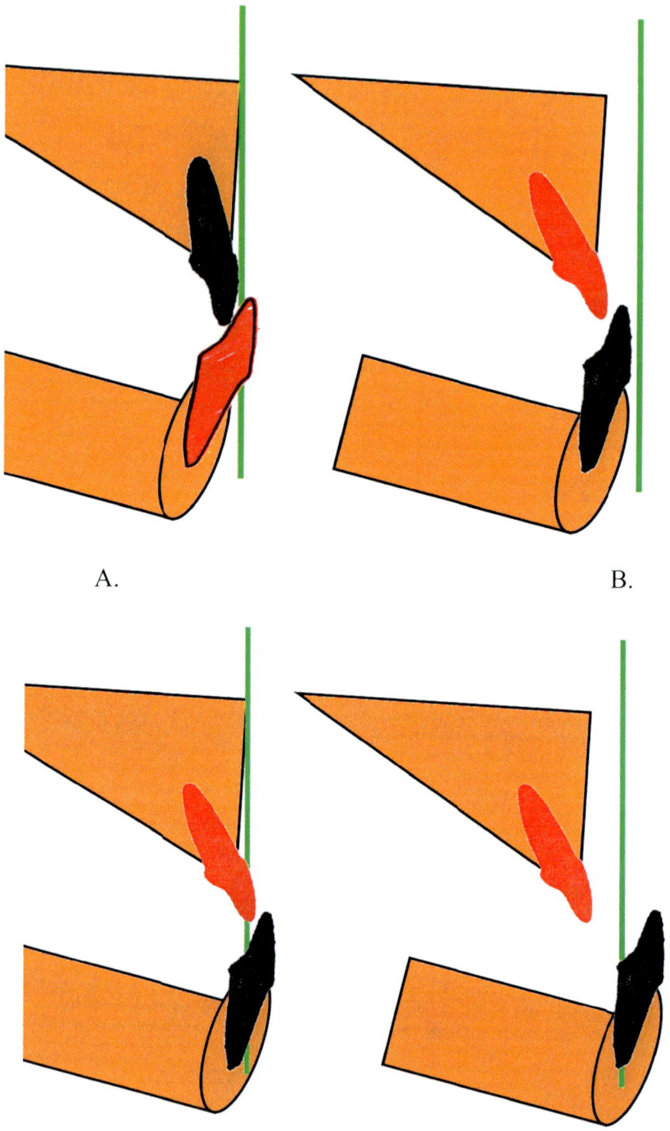

A. B. C. D.

Figure 1: (A to D) Schematic diagrams of four different types of Class III facial skeletal profiles with reference to a line (green) dropped down from the forehead. A. Anterior crossbite resulted from a normal maxilla, normal mandible, retroclined maxillary incisors and proclined mandibular incisors. B. Anterior crossbite resulted from a retrognathic maxilla, normal mandible, proclined maxillary incisors and retroclined mandibular incisors. C. Anterior crossbite resulted from a normal maxilla, prognathic mandible, proclined maxillary incisors and retroclined mandibular incisors. D. Anterior crossbite resulted from a retrognathic maxilla, prognathic mandible, proclined maxillary incisors and retroclined mandibular incisors.

Differential Diagnosis of Class III Malocclusion

Class III patients may present with symptoms such as multiple teeth in anterior crossbite, minimal overjet or lingually inclined mandibular incisors. Anterior crossbites may be due to the improper inclination of the maxillary and mandibular incisors (dentoalveolar mal-relationship), occlusal interferences (pseudo Class III malocclusion), or true skeletal discrepancies of the maxilla and/or mandible (Fig. **2**).

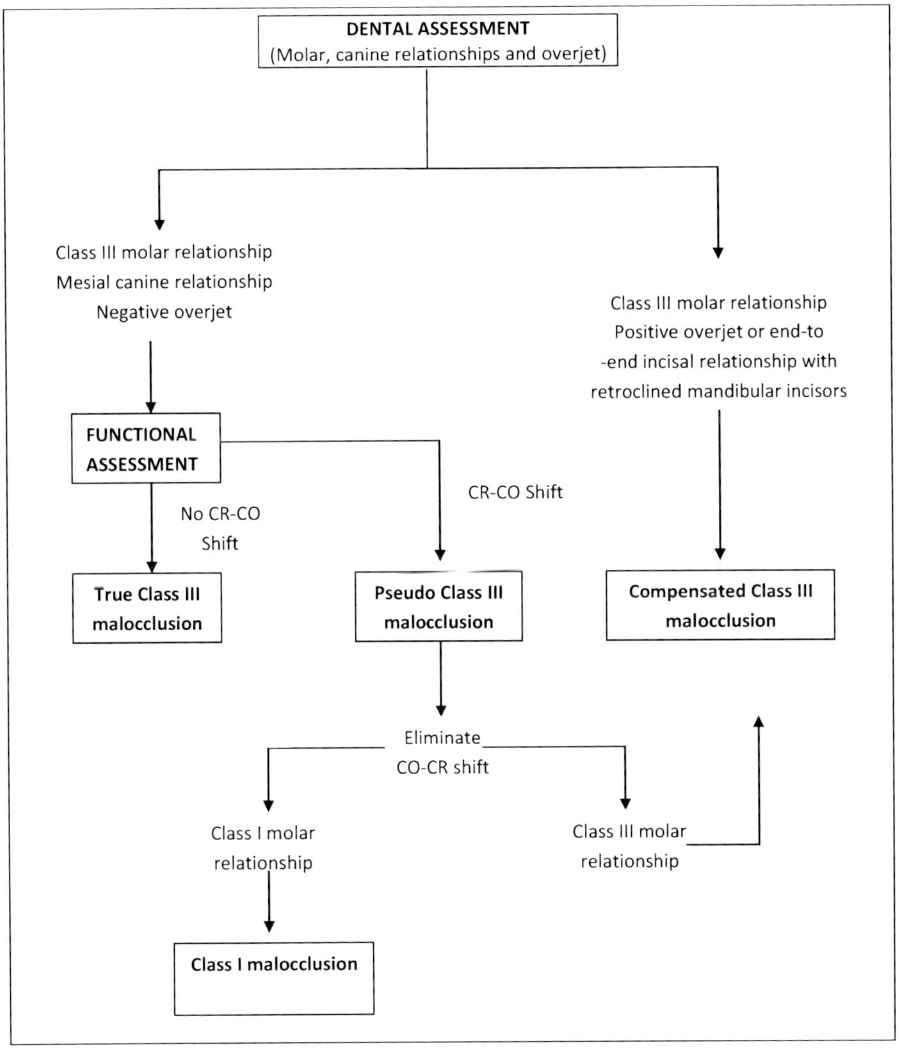

Figure 2: Diagnostic scheme for dental and skeletal anterior crossbites. (From Ngan P, Hu AM, Fields HW: Pediatr Dent 19:386-395.1997).

i. *Dental Assessment:* Check if Class III molar relationship is associated with a negative overjet. If a positive overjet or end to end incisal relationship is found, together with retroclined mandibular incisors, a compensated Class III malocclusion is suspected, meaing that upper incisors are proclined and lower incisors are retroclined to compensate for the skeletal discrepancy. If a negative overjet is found, proceed to functional assessment.

ii. *Functional Assessment:* Assess the relationship of the mandible to the maxilla in order to determine if a centric relation (C_r) to centric occlusion (C_o) discrepancy exists. Anterior positioning of the mandible may result from a premature tooth contact(s) that deflects the mandible anteriorly to achieve full intercuspation (centric occlusion). Patients who present with a forward shift of the mandible on closure may have a normal facial profile and Class I molar relationship in C_r, but a prognathic profile and Class III molar relationship in C_o. This situation is referred to as "pseudo Class III malocclusion." Elimination of C_o-C_r shift reveals whether it is a simple Class I malocclusion or a compensated Class III malocclusion. On the other hand, a patient presenting with no shift on closure, a full-step Class III molar relationship, and a mesial occlusion of the lower to upper canines is diagnostic of a true Class III malocclusion.

iii. *Clinical Assessment:* A profile evaluation involves an analysis of facial proportions, chin position, midface prominence, and vertical proportion [23]. Patients with maxillary deficiency usually have a concave profile, evidenced by a flattening of the infraorbital rim and the area adjacent to the nose. The chin should not be positioned anterior to a vertical line extending down from soft tissue Glabella. However, it is important to remember that facial convexity decreases as the patient matures. A degree of chin prominence that would be normal for an adult may suggest a Class III skeletal pattern in a young child. The vertical proportion should be checked in C_o and C_r. The normal ratio of lower to total facial height (LFH/TFH) is approximately 0.55. This ratio is decreased in patients with functional shift and overclosure of the mandible.

iv. *Cephalometric Assessment*: Intermaxillary cephalometric measurements can be used to confirm the contributions of the maxilla and mandible as well as the maxillary and mandibular incisors to the Class III skeletal and dental relationships (Table **1**).

Table 1: Cephalometric measurements for Class III evaluations

Intermaxillary Measurements	Standard (age 6-18 years)
WITS	0mm (female), -1mm (male)
Maxillo-mandibular differences	23mm (12 years old)
ANB	2 degrees
Point A to Nasion perpendicular	0-1mm
Pogonion to Nasion perpendicular	-4 to 0mm

Classification of Class III Malocclusions

Class III malocclusion can be categorized into dentoalveolar mal-relationship, pseudo Class III malocclusion, and true skeletal malocclusion. In patients with dentoalveolar mal-relationship (Fig. **1A**), there is no apparent sagittal skeletal discrepancy. The ANB angle is within normal limits. The problem is primarily due to lingual tipping of the maxillary incisors and labial tipping of the mandibular incisors. In true skeletal Class III malocclusion with mandibular protrusion/retrusive maxilla, or a combination of both (Figs. **1B** to **1D**), the ANB angle in the skeletal Class III patients is generally negative with a smaller than normal SNA angle and/or greater than normal SNB angle. Unfortunately, individual variations in cranial base flexure and anterior/posterior displacement of Nasion alter the ANB angle [24]. Alternative cephalometric values can be used to assess the anterior/posterior relationship of the maxilla and mandible (Table **1**). These measurements include Nasion perpendicular to "A" point, Wits appraisal, and effective maxillary and mandibular length. Vertically, patients with a long mandibular base usually have a large gonial angle. The incisal inclination in this type of Class III patients is the opposite to the dentoalveolar Class III problem, *i.e.*, the upper incisors are tipped labially, and the lower incisors are tipped lingually.

In patients with pseudo Class III malocclusion, Kwong and Lin [25] conducted a cephalometric study comparing the characteristics of Class I, pseudo Class III and skeletal Class III patients (Table **2**). Most of the cephalometric measurements suggested that pseudo Class III malocclusion is an intermediate form between Class I and skeletal Class III malocclusion. The only exception was the gonial angle, which was generally more obtuse in the skeletal Class III sample. Measurement of the gonial angle in the pseudo Class III sample was found to be similar to the Class I sample, making this measurement a key diagnostic feature in the differential diagnosis between pseudo and true skeletal Class III individuals.

Table 2: Cephalometric characteristics (°) of patients with Class I, pseudo Class III and true Class III malocclusions

		SNA	SNB	SN - MP	Gonial Angle	U1 - SN	L1 - MP
Class I	Mean	83.2	80.5	30.6	121.6	107.2	94.3
	S.D	3.2	3.0	4.3	5.4	6.1	5.5
Pseudo Class III	Mean	81.4	81.1	33.0	120.4	109.4	91.7
	S.D	3.9	3.5	4.8	5.6	5.8	6.8
True Class III	Mean	80.3	81.7	36.0	124.2	111.0	87.6
	S.D	3.6	3.2	4.2	14.3	5.4	6.7

(Data reproduced from Lin JJ. Creative Orthodontics: Blending the Damon System & TADs to manage difficult malocclusions, Yong Chieh Company, Taipei, Taiwan, ROC, 2007 pp. 34, Fig. **16**).

Class III Skeletal Growth Pattern

Cranial Base: Battagel [26] found the linear and angular measurements of the cranial base were decreased in patients with Class III malocclusion. Class III patients exhibited a cranial base angle (Ba-S-N) that was more acute and also exhibited a more anteriorly positioned articulare compared to Class I patients. In addition, the middle cranial fossa in the Class III individual had a posterior and superior alignment. This alignment positions the nasomaxillary complex in a more retrusive relationship in the Class III patient and contributes to a forward rotation of the mandible.

Maxilla: Class III patients commonly exhibits a decreased horizontal maxillary growth when compared to the Class I patients. The horizontal "A Point" movement is approximately 0.4 mm/yr compared to 1.0 mm/yr in Class I individuals [27].

Mandible: The Class III individual exhibits an increased length of the mandible while the mandibular articulation is more vertically oriented; resulting in a more prominent lower jaw [28]. The ascending ramus tends to be shorter with a steeper mandibular plane angle. The gonial angle is more obtuse than Class I patients. The mandibular prominence along with the decreased length of the maxillary complex may accentuate the typical straight to concave profile in these cases. Typically, Class III patients display dentoalveolar compensation in the form of proclination of the maxillary incisors accompanied with retroclination of the mandibular incisors.

Growth Increments: Sugawara and Mitani [29] reported similar mandibular growth increments between Class III and Class I patients during the pre-pubertal, pubertal and post-pubertal growth periods. The authors concluded that Class III skeletal pattern was established at a very young age. Facial growth in male and female Class III patients was different. Battagel [26] found the largest increment of facial growth for males occurred between the ages of 14 and 17. In female Class III patients, the maximum increment of facial growth occurred between the ages of 9.5 to 12 years, although active growth continued in the nasal area and both jaws after the age of 15. In contrast to the male Class III patients, Class III female patients possessed a more prominent mandible and an increased proclination of the maxillary incisors. For Class III patients, the mandible was growing almost twice as much as the maxilla in both the vertical and horizontal direction during the growth period. However, the anterior-posterior growth change of the mandible was similar to the Class I patients [29, 30].

Class III Growth Predictions

Treatment of children with a Class III malocclusion represents a challenge in orthodontics because an unsuccessful outcome of orthodontic/orthopedic therapy is frequent [31, 32] Despite elimination of the reverse overjet and achievement of an acceptable dental arch relationship during early intervention, relapse is observed irrespective of the treatment modality [33-34] and at different ages [26,33]. Deterioration of occlusion was found in Class III patients of different ethnicity [31,35] and the incidence of relapse has been reported to be almost 50 per cent [33]. The uncertainty regarding the long-term results of Class III treatment was a stimulus to identify potential predictors of therapeutic success or failure. If an unfavorable outcome of therapy could be anticipated prior to treatment, then the type and timing of orthodontic/orthopedic treatment could be modified.

Battagel recognized a need for a model to predict long-term outcome for orthodontics treatment of Class III malocclusions [26]. The author employed discriminant function analysis to identify predictors for relapse in a group of children treated with cervical headgear applied to the mandibular dentition. The author developed a four-variable discriminant model, capable of predicting relapse with high accuracy (U1/PP angle, Labrale superior to soft tissue Nasion, Labrale inferior to Sella vertical, and the number of anterior teeth in crossbite). Franchi *et al.* [33] reported a three-variable predictive model (Axis of condylar process to SBL angle, mandibular plane to palatal plane, and the mandibular intermolar width) that was quite different from Battagel. Tahmina *et al.* [34] examined a sample of Asians treated with a chincup and identified three predictive variables (Gonial angle, N-A-Pog angle, and RP/SN angle). Ghiz *et al.* [36] performed a retrospective study to select a model of cephalometric variables to predict future Class III growth patterns based on the results of early orthopedic treatment on 64 patients using a protraction facemask. According to the outcome of treatment at least 3 years after orthopedic treatment, all subjects were divided into 2 groups: a successful group with acceptable treatment outcome and an unsuccessful group with relapse in anterior overjet. Cephalometric measurements subjected to discriminant analysis identified 4 variables to be significant in predicting successful treatment outcomes: 1. position of condyle to cranial base, 2. ramal length, 3. mandibular length, and 4. gonial angle (Fig. **3**). A logistic equation was established that is accurate in predicting successfully treated Class III cases 95.5% of the time and unsuccessfully treated cases 70% of the time.

$$P = \frac{1}{1 + \text{Exp}(-L)}$$

Where $L = 30.557 + 0.196\,(\text{Co-GD}) - 0.129\,(\text{Co-Pg}) + 0.162\,(\text{Co-Goi}) - 0.206\,(\text{Ar-Goi-Me})$

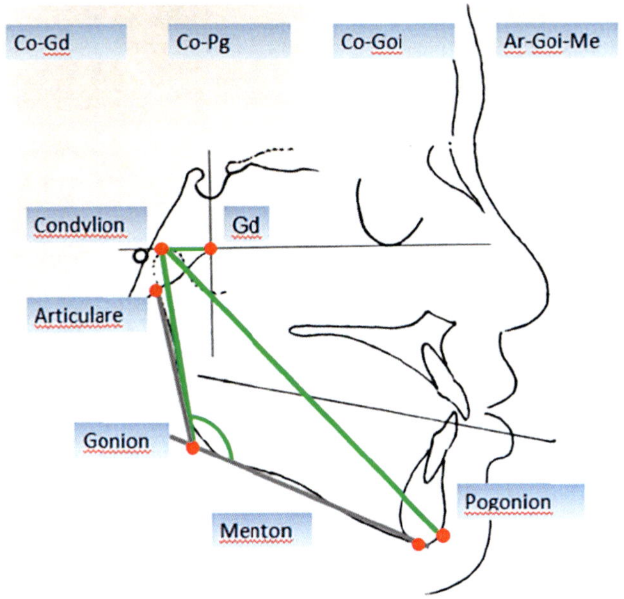

Figure 3: Significant predictors for successful Class III treatment outcomes: The position of the condyle with reference to the cranial base (Co-Gd); the ramal length (Co-Goi); the mandibular length (Co-Pg); and the gonial angle (An-Goi-Me).

Ngan *et al.* [37] evaluated the cephalometric radiographs taken after first phase treatment with rapid maxillary expansion and facemask (RME+FM) and at the follow-up visit. On the basis of post-treatment and follow-up cephalometric records, the authors developed a Growth Treatment Response Vector analysis or (GTRV) which consisted of a ratio of horizontal growth changes of the maxilla and mandible determined along the occlusal plane and a vector showing the direction of maxillary and mandibular growth.

$$\text{GTRV ratio} = \frac{\text{Horizontal growth changes of the maxilla}}{\text{Horizontal growth changes of the mandible}}$$

The ratio for a group of subjects from the Bolton Growth Study with good skeletal growth was 0.77. Table **3** shows the ratio of two groups of Class III patients treated successfully and unsuccessfully with protraction facemask. When the GTRV ratio fell below a certain value, it was reported to be suggestive of an unsuccessful second phase of treatment with fixed appliances. In such cases comprehensive edgewise treatment should be postponed.

Table 3: Growth Treatment Response Vector (GTRV) ratios of horizontal maxillary growth to mandibular growth in successful and unsuccessful groups

		Successful Group	Unsuccessful Group
GTRV Ratio	Mean	0.49	0.22
	SD	0.14	0.10
	Range	0.33 to 0.88	0.06 to 0.38

To perform the GTRV analysis, the horizontal growth changes of the maxilla and the mandible between the post-treatment radiograph and the follow-up radiograph were determined by locating the A point and B point on the post-treatment radiograph (Fig. **4**). The occlusal plane (O) was constructed by using the mesial buccal cusp of the maxillary molars and the incisal tip of the maxillary incisors as landmarks. The lines AO and BO were then constructed by connecting point A and B, perpendicular to the occlusal plane.

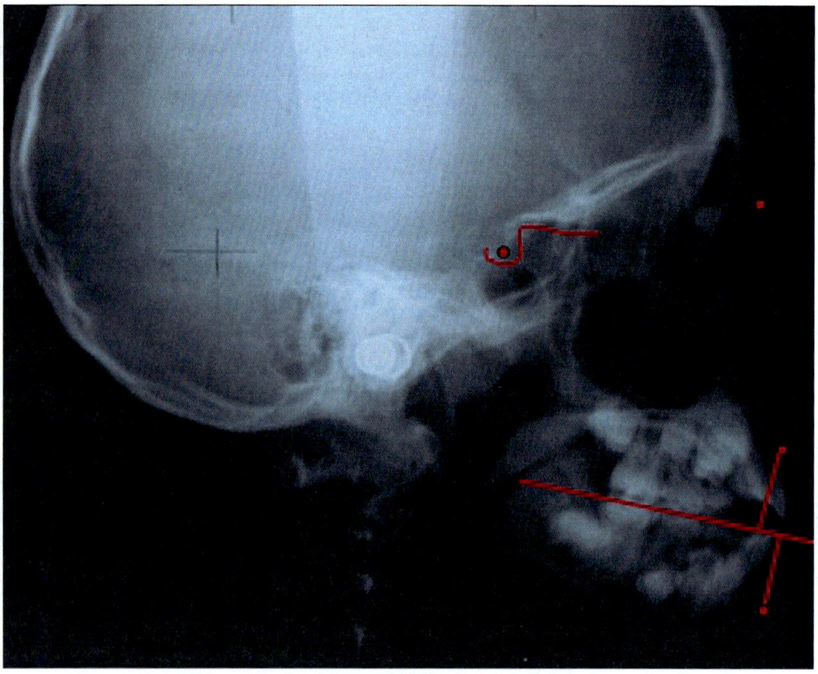

Figure 4: The occlusal plane (O) was constructed by using the mesial buccal cusp of the maxillary molars and the incisal tip of the maxillary incisors as landmarks. The line AO and BO were constructed by connecting A and B points perpendicular to the occlusal plane.

The first tracing was superimposed on the follow-up radiograph using the stable landmarks on the mid-sagittal cranial structure (Fig. **5**). The A point and B point on the follow-up radiograph was located and the lines AO and BO were then constructed by connecting point A and B of the follow-up radiograph to the occlusal plane of the first tracing. The distance between the A point of the two tracings along the occlusal plane represented the growth changes of the maxilla and the distance on the occlusal plane of the B point represented the growth changes of the mandible.

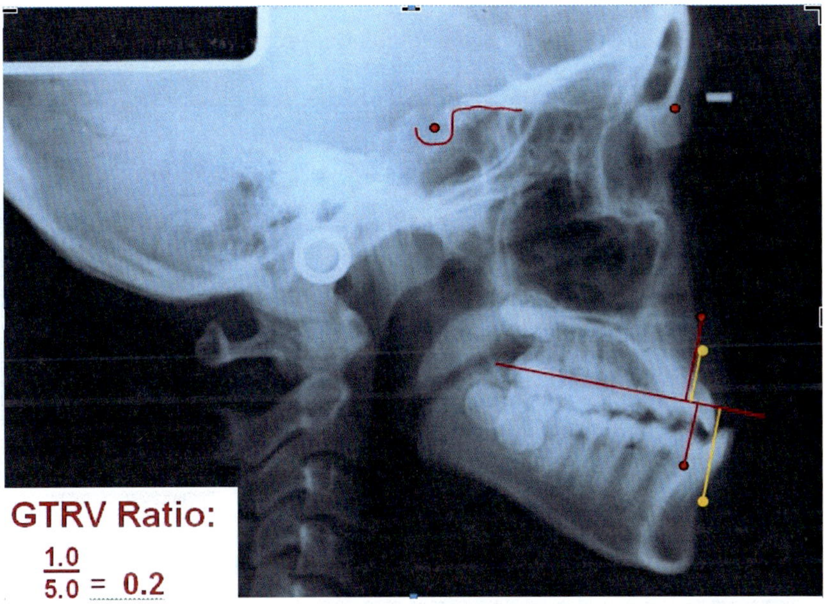

Figure 5: The first tracing was superimposed on the follow-up radiograph using the stable landmarks on the mid-sagittal cranial structure. The distance between the A point of the two tracing along the occlusal plane represented the growth changes of the maxilla and the distance on the occlusal plane of the B point represented the growth changes of the mandible. GTRV ratio was then calculated using the formula as depicted in the text.

Fudalej *et al.* [38] performed a systematic review on the various models used to predict outcome of orthodontic treatment of Class III malocclusion. The authors concluded that the possibility of accurate prediction of outcome of orthodontic/orthopedic treatment of Class III malocclusion was still questionable. Validation testing of the prediction model on the cases, which were not used to develop it, was needed in order to evaluate an actual discriminative power of the prediction model.

Indications and Contraindications for Early Class III Treatment

The objective of early orthodontic treatment is to create an environment in which a more favorable dentofacial development can exist. The goals of early interceptive Class III treatment may include 1. preventing progressive irreversible soft tissue or bony changes related to teeth in anterior crossbite, 2. improving skeletal discrepancies and minimizing dental compensation to skeletal discrepancies, 3. improving occlusal function, 4. minimizing the need for orthognathic surgery, and 5. providing a more pleasing facial esthetics thus improving the psychosocial development of a child (Fig. **6**).

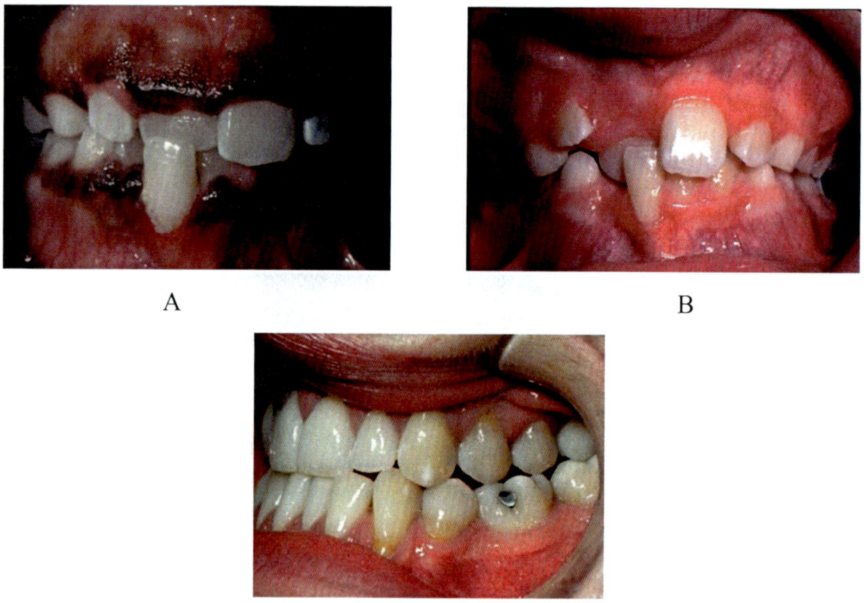

A B

C

Figure 6: (A to B) Progressive irreversible soft tissue and bony damage due to an anterior crossbite. (C) Dental compensation to skeletal Class III discrepancies.

Turpin [39] developed a list of positive and negative factors to aid in deciding when to intercept a developing Class III malocclusion. The positive factors include good facial esthetics, mild skeletal disharmony, no familial prognathism, A-P functional shift, convergent facial type, symmetrical condyle growth, growing patients with expected good cooperation. The negative factors include poor facial esthetics, severe skeletal disharmony, familial pattern established, no A-P shift, divergent facial type, asymmetrical growth, growth complete, and poor cooperation expected. The author recommends that early treatment should be considered for a patient that presents with characteristics listed in the positive column. For individuals who present with characteristics in the negative column, treatment can be delayed until growth is completed. Patients should be aware of the fact that surgery may be necessary at a later date, even when an initial phase of treatment may be successful.

Treatment of Pseudo Class III Malocclusion

Patients with pseudo Class III malocclusion often present with anterior crossbites that are due to a premature tooth contact or improper positioning of the maxillary and mandibular incisors [40]. Elimination of the C_o-C_r discrepancy may 1. avoid abnormal wear and traumatic occlusal forces to the affected teeth, 2. avoid potential adverse growth influences in the maxilla and mandible, 3. improve maxillary lip posture and facial appearance, and 4. avoid abnormal posterior occlusion which may develop as a result of habitual posturing of the mandible to accommodate the abnormal anterior occlusal contacts.

Correction of single tooth in anterior crossbite can be corrected using a fixed or removable appliance. A maxillary lingual arch with finger springs can be fabricated using an indirect technique. In the mixed dentition, bands are fitted on the maxillary second primary molars or the permanent first molars. An impression is made of the maxillary arch with the bands in place. Bands are transferred to the impression before pouring. A lingual arch is fabricated and soldered to the molar bands. Finger springs with helices are soldered to the lingual arch (Fig. **7**).

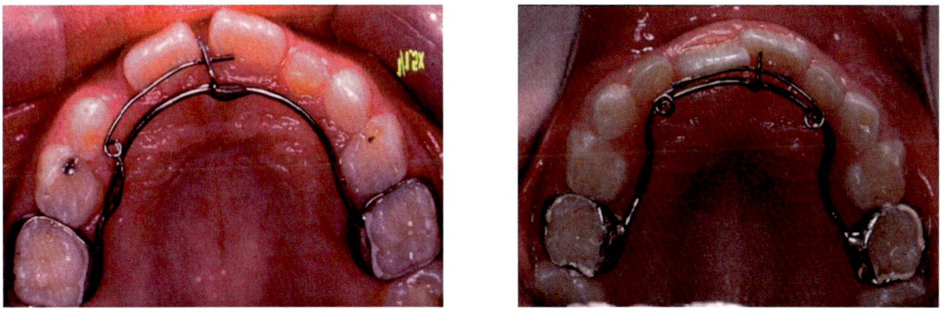

A B

Figure 7: (A to B) Maxillary arch with finger springs to correct single tooth in anterior crossbite.

Correction of multiple teeth in anterior crossbite is best accomplished with a fixed appliance. An expansion appliance or maxillary lingual arch can be used as anchorage to correct the anterior crossbite. Fig. **8** shows an 8-year-old patient presented with multiple teeth in anterior crossbite. A Hyrax maxillary expansion appliance was fabricated to create arch length for the alignment of the maxillary incisors (Fig. **8**). After expansion, a sequence of three archwires (0.012" NiTi, 0.018 NiTi and 0.018 SS) were used to align the maxillary incisors (Fig. **10**). A coil spring can be inserted between the maxillary lateral incisors and the first primary molars to provide an anterior force to correct the crossbite. The correction is usually accomplished within 6 months and retainers are usually not necessary if an adequate overbite is achieved after crossbite correction. If retention is indicated, a removable retainer (Fig. **8** N-O) with acrylic removed for the eruption of permanent premolars can be worn night time for about a year.

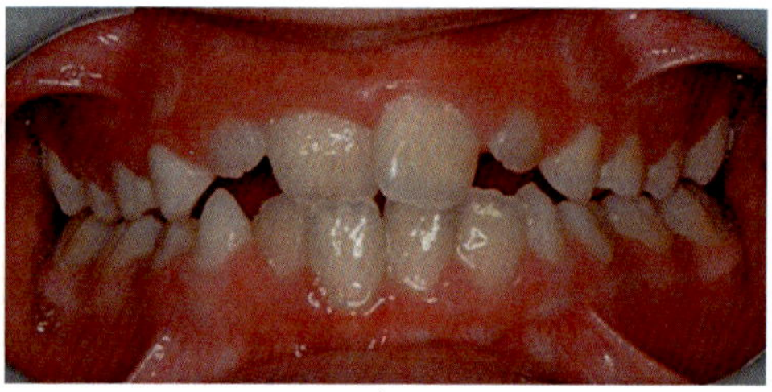

A

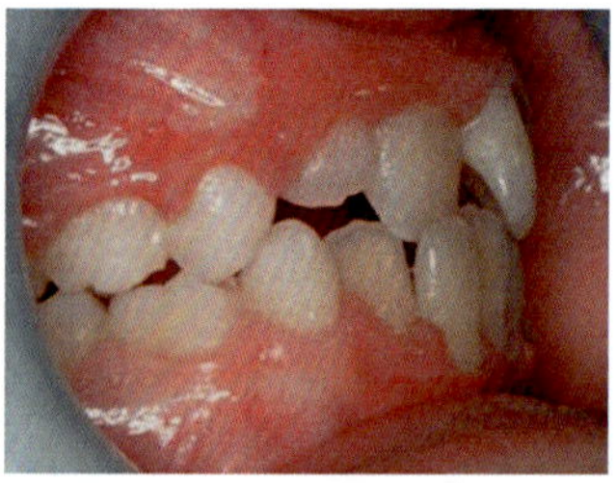

B

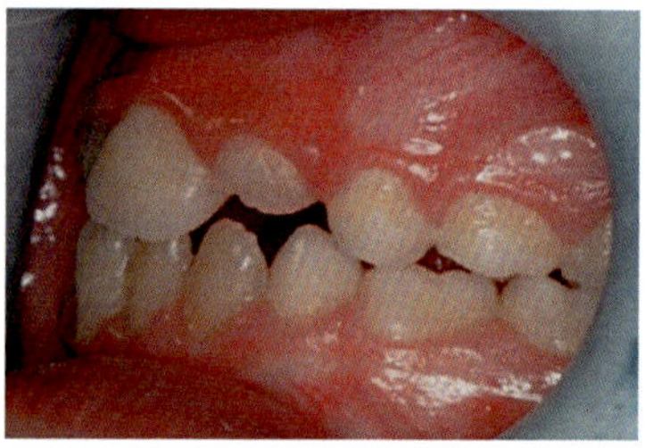

C

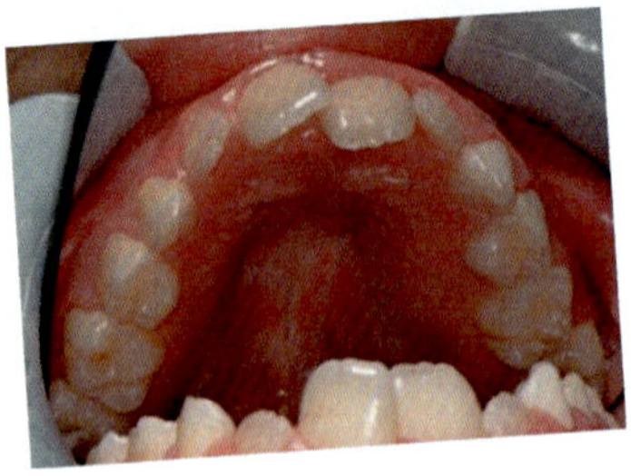

D

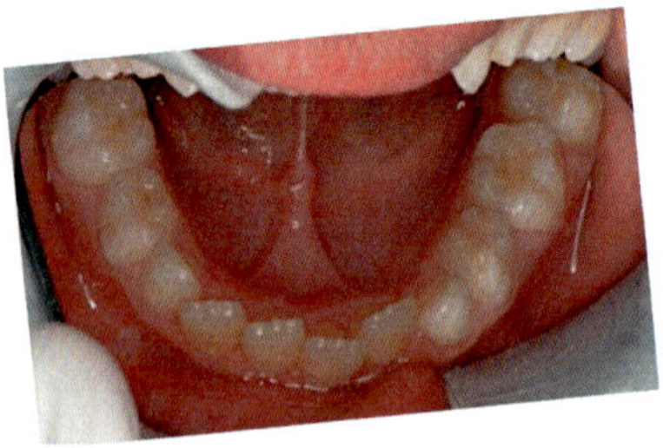

E

Fig. 8: contd....

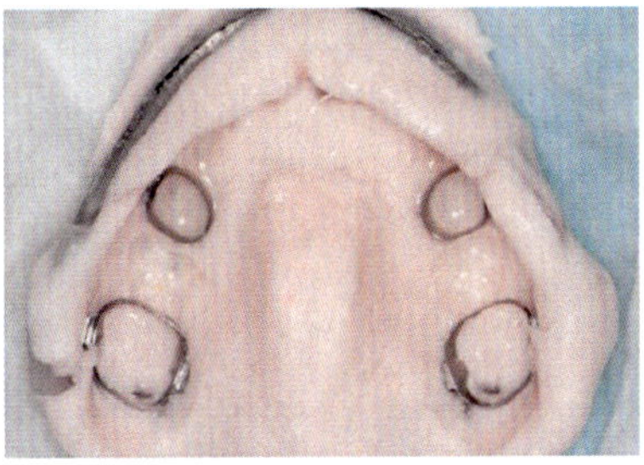

F

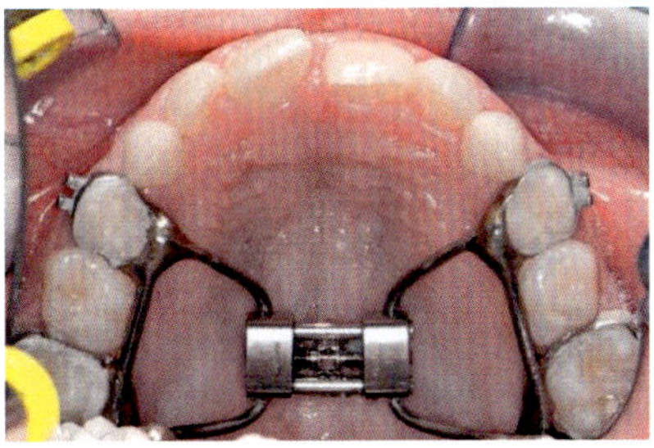

G

Figure 8: (A to E) The maxillary arch of an 8-year-old patient is shown with multiple teeth in anterior crossbite. (F to G) A rapid palatal expansion appliance is fabricated to serve as anchorage for the crossbite correction.

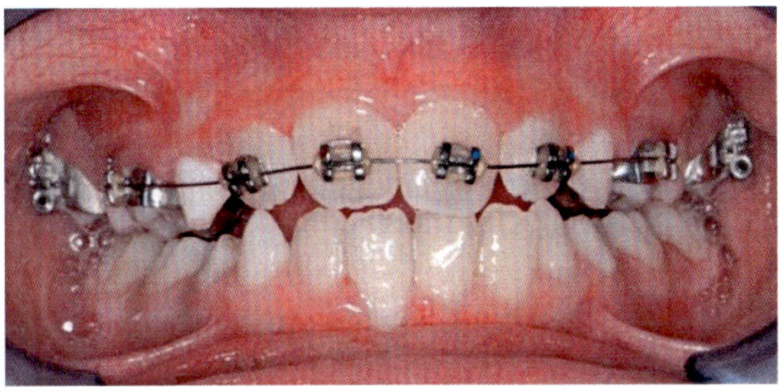

H

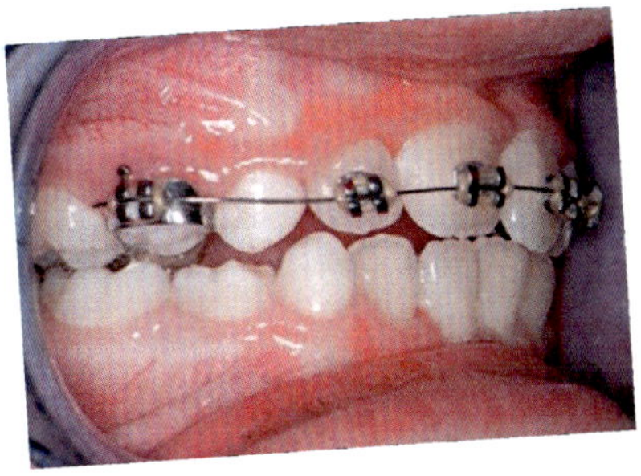

I

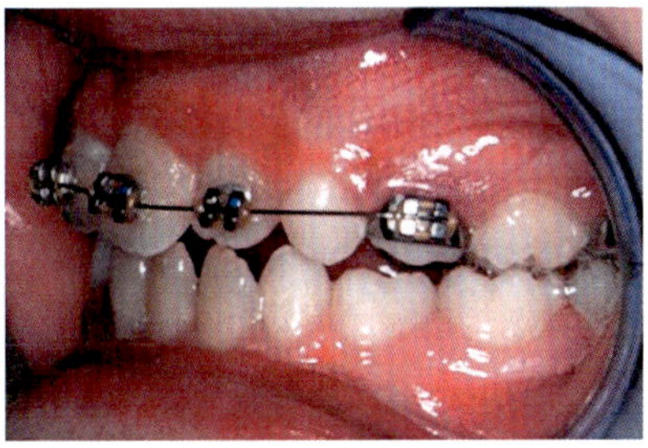

J

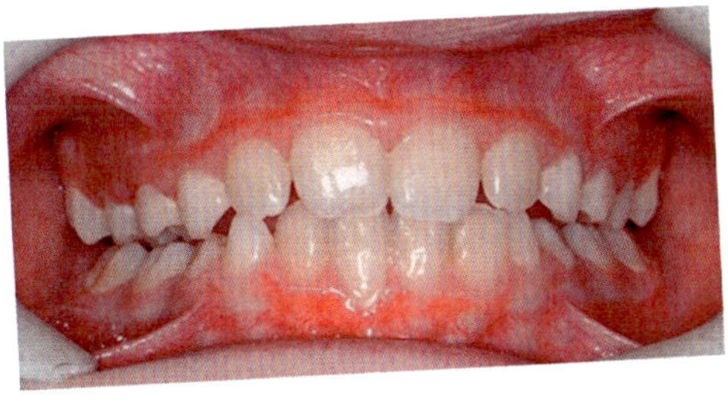

K

Fig. 8: contd....

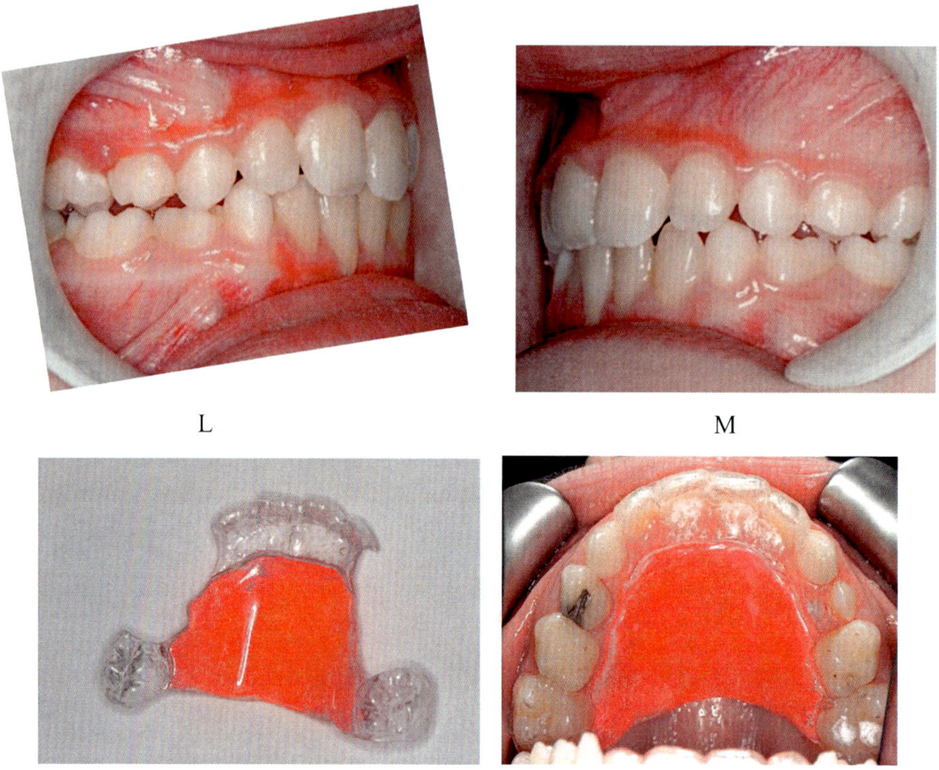

L M

N O

Figure 8: (H to J) Brackets are placed to align of maxillary incisors after maxillary expansion. (K to M) Post-treatment photographs show the corrected anterior crossbite. (N to O) Removable retainer for mixed dentittion treatment showing acrylic removed for eruption of permanent premolars.

Treatment of Skeletal Class III Malocclusion

Functional Appliance Therapy

The Frankel III Regulator (FRIII) is a functional appliance designed to counteract the muscle forces acting on the maxillary complex. According to Frankel [41], the vestibular shields in the depths of the sulcus were placed away from the alveolar buccal plates of the maxilla to stretch the periosteum and allow for forward development of the maxilla. The shields were fitted closely to the alveolar process of the mandible to hold or redirect growth posteriorly. Treatment of Class III malocclusions with a FR III Regulators or other types of functional appliances is more successful when patients presenting with a functional shift on closure. In two separate studies [42, 43], the FR III Regulators appeared to effect occlusal changes by proclination of the upper incisors and retroclination of the lower incisors. The mandible was repositioned downward and backward, decreasing the prognathism of the mandible and increasing the lower facial height. There were minimal changes in the position of the maxilla. The best response to treatment with FR III Regulator was reported in Class III patients with an increased overbite of 4-5mm in the early mixed dentition. Fig. **9** shows a 6 year old patient who presented with a mild Class III skeletal malocclusion and an anterior crossbite. The patient was treated with a FR III Regulator, and was instructed to wear the appliance full time. A positive overjet was obtained after 10 months of treatment. The patient was placed on observation until all permanent teeth in the buccal segments erupted.

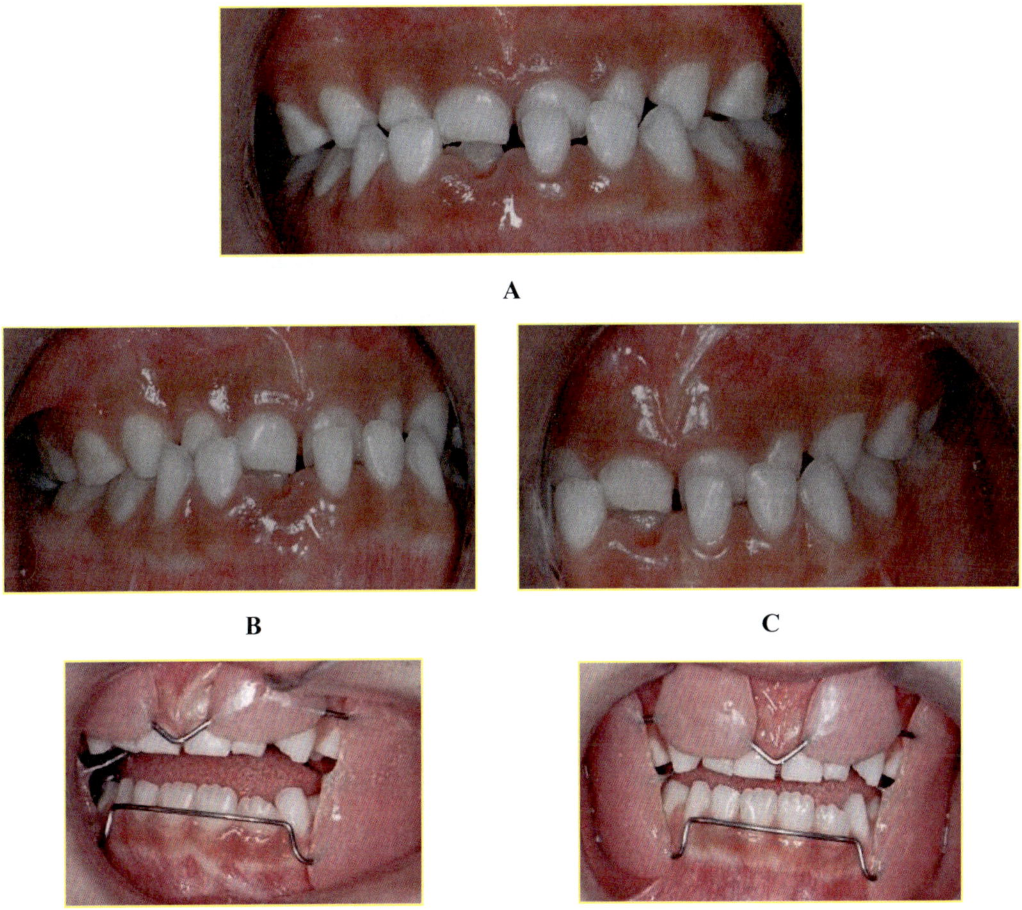

A B C D E

Figure 9: (A to C) A 6-year-old patient presented with a Class III malocclusion and an anterior crossbite. (D to E) A Frankel III regulator was used to correct the anterior crossbite.

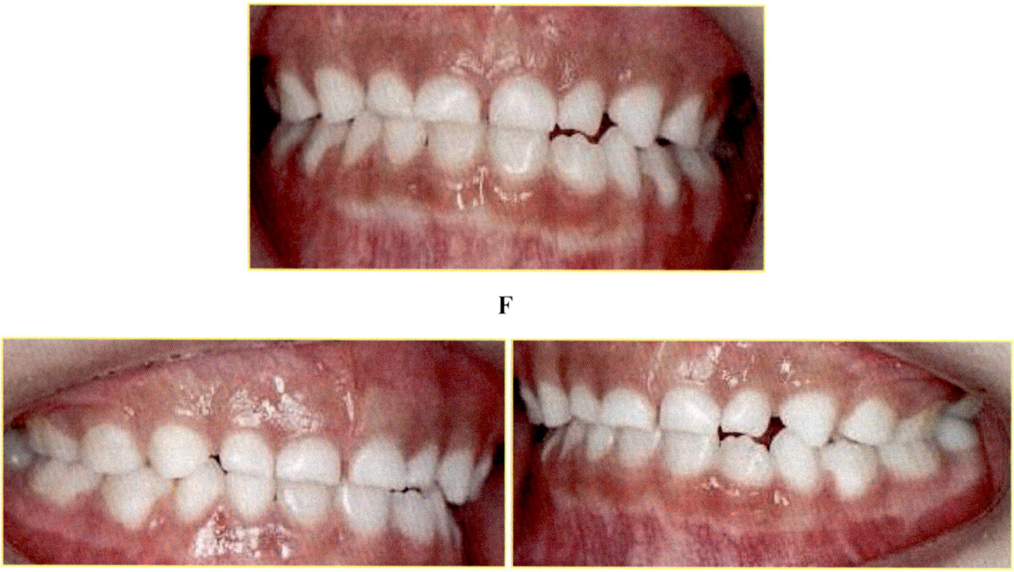

F

G H

Figure 9: (F to H) Correction of anterior crossbite was achieved after 8 months of treatment.

Chin Cup Therapy

Skeletal Class III malocclusion with a relatively normal maxilla and a moderately protrusive mandible can be treated using a chin cup. This treatment modality is popular among the Asian populations due to its favorable effects on the sagittal as well as vertical dimension. The objective of early treatment with chin cup is to provide growth inhibition or redirection with posterior positioning of the mandible.

Effects on Mandibular Growth

The orthopedic effects of chin cup on the mandible include: 1. redirection of mandibular growth vertically, 2. backward rotation of the mandible, 3. retardation of mandibular growth, and 4. remodeling of the mandible. To date, there is no agreement in the literature as to whether chin cup therapy may [44, 45] or may not [46] inhibit the growth of the mandible. However, chin cup therapy has been shown to produce a change in the mandible that is associated with a downward and backward rotation as well as a decrease in the angle of the mandible [47-49]. Treatment effects reported include a decrease in the gonial angle, less incremental increase in mandibular length and posterior movement of Point B and Pogonion. Control of vertical growth during chin cup treatment is difficult to manage.

Effects on Maxillary Growth

Some studies [46-48] have indicated that a chin cup appliance has no effect on the anteroposterior growth of the maxilla. However, Uner *et al.* [49] showed that early correction of anterior crossbite with chin cup appliance prevents retarded anteroposterior maxillary growth. Sugawara *et al.* [50] compared the growth changes of patients after chin cup treatment with control subjects and reported that at age 17, the midface is more deficient in patients of the control groups than in those of the treatment groups.

Force Magnitude and Direction

Chin cups are divided into two types: the occipital-pull chin cup that is used for patients with mandibular protrusion and the vertical-pull chin cup that is used in patients presenting with a steep mandibular plane angle and excessive anterior facial height. Most of the reported studies [49, 51, 52] recommended an orthopedic force of 300-500 grams per side. Patients are instructed to wear the appliance for 14 hrs/day. The orthopedic force is usually directed either through the condyle or below it.

Treatment Timing and Duration

Patients with mandibular excess can usually be recognized in the primary dentition despite the fact that the mandible appears retrognathic in the early years for most children. There is evidence that treatment to reduce mandibular protrusion is more successful when it is started in the primary or early mixed dentition [47-49]. The treatment time varies from one year to as long as 4 years depending on the severity of the original malocclusion.

Stability of Treatment

The stability of chin cup treatment remains unclear. Several investigators reported stability in horizontal maxillary and mandibular changes associated with chin cup treatment [52, 53]. However, a few studies reported a tendency to return to the original growth pattern after the chin cup is discontinued [44, 46, 49]. Sugarwara and colleagues [50] published a report on the long-term effects of chin cup therapy on three groups of Japanese girls who started chin cup treatment at 7, 9, and 11 years. All 63 patients were followed with serial lateral headfilms taken at the ages of 7, 9, 11, 14, and 17 years. The authors found that the skeletal profile was greatly improved during the initial stages of chin cup therapy, but these changes were not usually maintained. Patients who started treatment at an earlier age had a catch-up growth of the mandible in a forward and downward direction before the growth of the face was completed. The authors concluded that chin cup therapy did not necessarily guarantee a positive correction of the skeletal profile after completion of growth.

Effects on Temporomandibular Joint

There is some concern on the adverse effect of chin cup appliance on the temporomandibular joint (TMJ). In a study by Deguchi and Kitsugi [52], several patients complained of temporary soreness of the TMJ during the retention period. Two out of 40 patients continued to have TMJ pain and some degree of difficulty in opening the mouth after the end of active treatment. Several studies indicated that the chin cup not only affects the growth of the mandible, but cranial base structures as well [48]. However, a recent study failed to support the hypothesis that chin cup appliances induce the posterior displacement of the glenoid fossa [54].

Fig. **10** shows a 5-year-old female with a Class III malocclusion and a combination of maxillary deficiency and mandibular prognathism. In addition, she presented with a posterior crossbite and an anterior open bite with a steep mandibular plane angle. Treatment was started with maxillary expansion and protraction with a facemask (Fig. **10**). The patient was instructed to wear the facemask for 10 to 12 hours at night. A positive overjet was obtained after 8 months of facemask treatment. A maxillary transpalatal bar, a mandibular tongue crib and a chin cup were used to correct the remaining open bite problem.

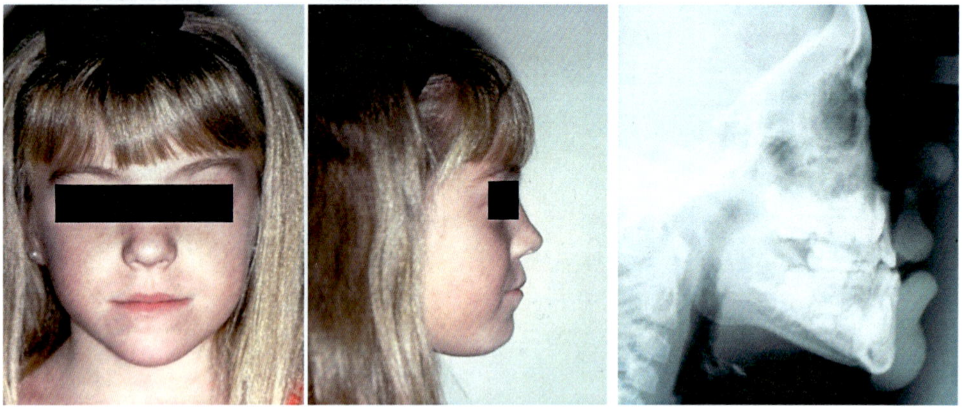

A **B** **C**

Fig. 10: contd....

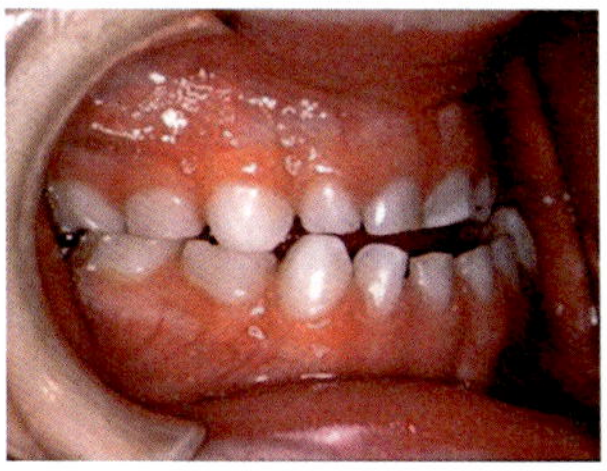

D

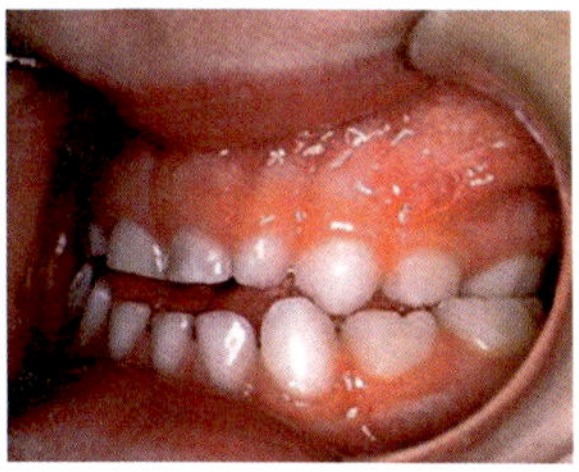

E

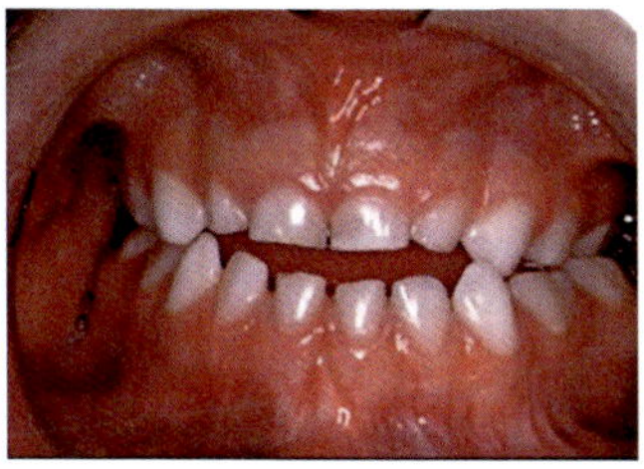

F

Figure 10: (A to F) 5-year-old female presented with a Class III malocclusion, anterior crossbite, posterior crossbite and an anterior open bite.

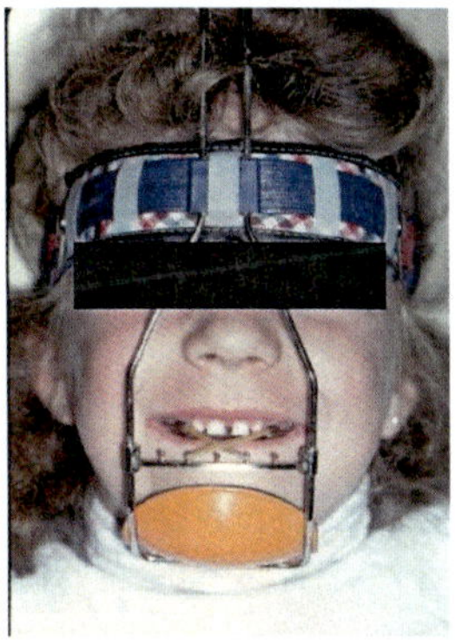

G

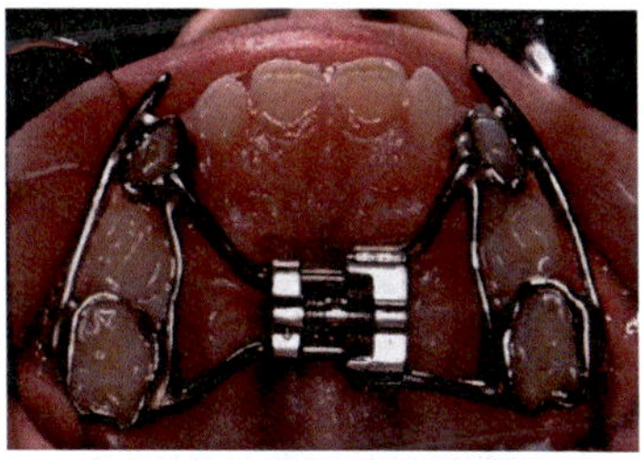

H

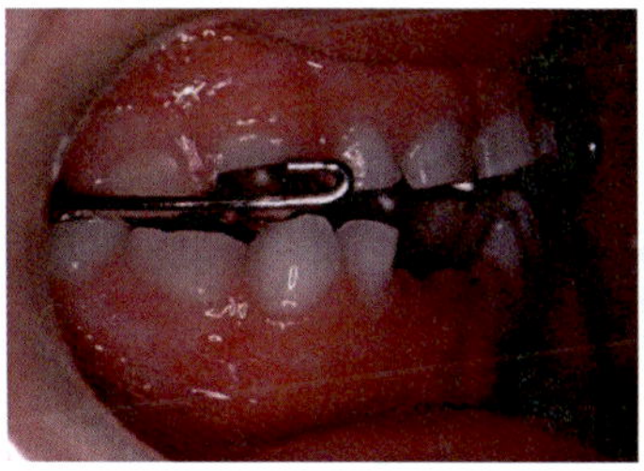

I

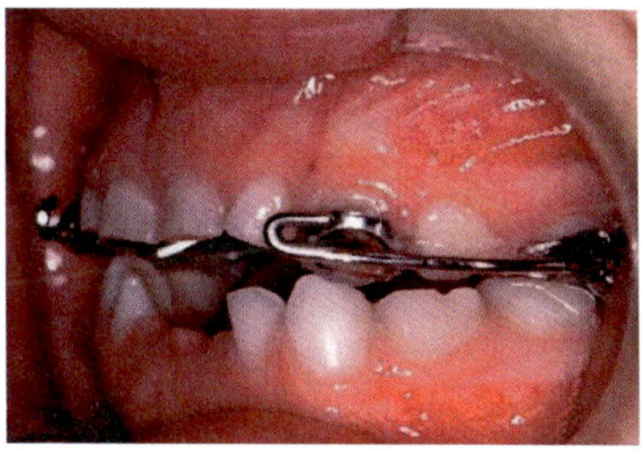

J

Figure 10: (G to J) Maxillary expansion and protraction was achieved with a Hyrax expansion appliance and a facemask.

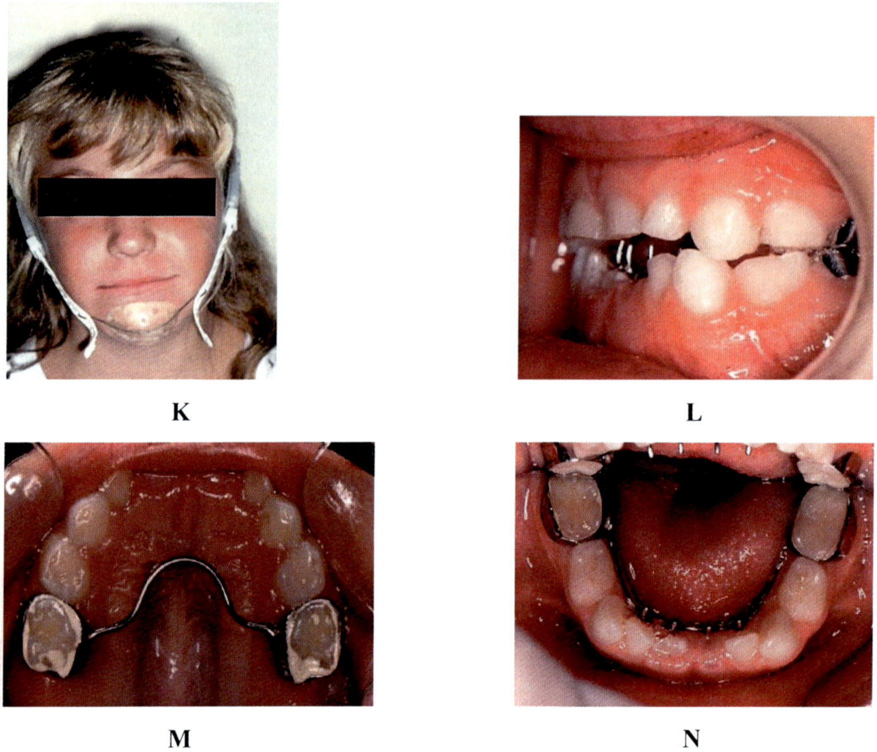

Figure 10: (K to N) A maxillary transpalatal bar, mandibular tongue crib and a chin cup were used to correct the remaining open bite problem.

Protraction Facemask Therapy

The protraction facemask has a long history for treatment of Class III patients with maxillary deficiency. In 1944, Oppenheim [55] felt that a clinician cannot control the growth or anterior displacement of the mandible so he suggested moving the maxilla forward in hope of counterbalancing mandibular protrusion. In the 1960's, Delaire [56] revived the interest in using a facemask for maxillary protraction. Petit [57] later modified Delaire's basic concept by increasing the amount of force generated by the appliance, thus decreasing the overall treatment time. In 1987, McNamara [58] introduced the use of a bonded expansion appliance with acrylic occlusal coverage for maxillary protraction. Turley [23] improved patient cooperation in wearing the appliance by fabricating customized facemasks. To date, short-term results show promising skeletal, dental and profile improvements with treatment [27,31,35]. The use of skeletal anchorage devices, such as mini-implants and miniplates, minimizes the side effects of maxillary protraction [59-61]. The long-term benefits of early facemask treatment need further substantiation awaiting results from prospective clinical trials.

Treatment Indications for Facemask Therapy

The facemask is most effective in the treatment of mild to moderate skeletal Class III malocclusions with a retrusive maxilla and a hypodivergent growth pattern. Several randomized clinical trials and meta-analyses have demonstrated the effectiveness of this appliance in treating Class III patients with maxillary deficiency [62-65]. Patients presenting with some degree of anterior functional shift and a moderate overbite have an improved treatment prognosis. In these cases, correction of the anterior crossbite and the mandibular shift result in a downward and backward rotation of the mandible, which diminishes its prognathism. The presence of an adequate overbite helps maintain the immediate dental correction after treatment. For patients presenting with a hyperdivergent growth pattern and a minimal overbite, a bonded acrylic palatal expansion appliance to control vertical eruption of molars has been recommended. However, a study comparing the use of banded or bonded expansion appliances as anchorage devices for maxillary expansion and protraction showed little differences in the skeletal and dental changes following the use of either appliance [66]. Specifically, vertical eruption of the posterior molars and an increase in lower facial height were observed in both groups.

The Protraction Facemask

The protraction facemask has two pads that contact the soft tissue in the forehead and chin region. The pads are connected by a midline framework and are adjustable through the loosening and tightening of a set-screw. An adjustable anterior wire with hooks is also connected to the midline framework to accommodate a downward and forward pull on the maxilla with elastics (Fig. **11**). To minimize the opening of the bite as the maxilla is repositioned; the protraction elastics are attached near the maxillary canines with a downward and forward pull of 30° to the occlusal plane. Maxillary protraction generally requires 300 to 600 grams of force per side, depending on the age of the patient. Tension of the elastics can be estimated using a tension stress gauge. A 3/8" 14 oz elastic will provide around 400 gm or 12 oz of force per side. Patients are instructed to wear the facemask for 12-14 hours a day.

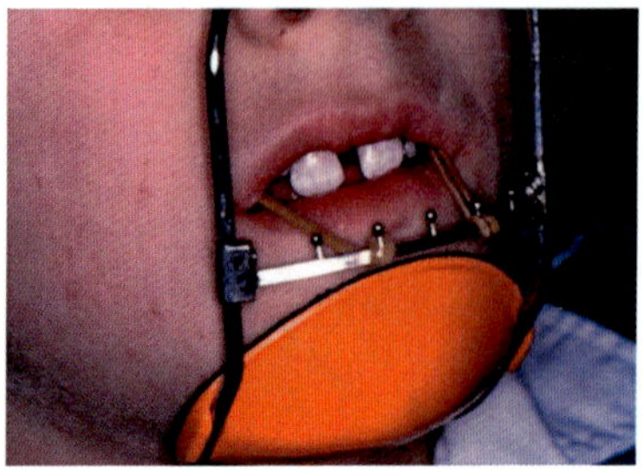

A

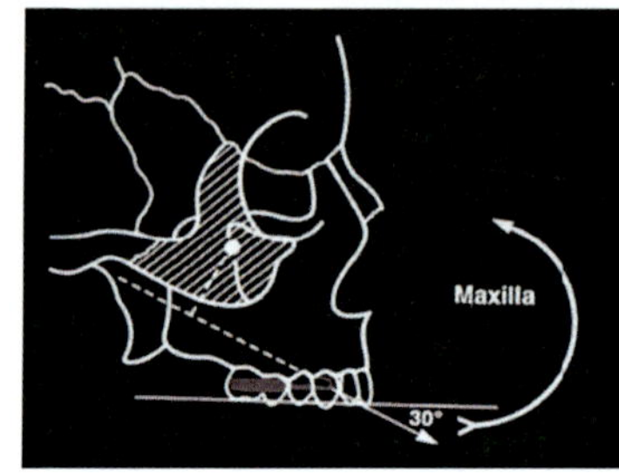

B

Figure 11: (A to B) A facemask is designed with an adjustable anterior wire to accommodate a downward and forward pull on the maxilla. To minimize the opening of the bite as the maxilla is repositioned, the protraction elastics are attached near the maxillary canines with a downward and forward pull of 30° to the occlusal plane.

Design and Construction of the Anchorage Appliance

1. Metallic Banded Palatal Expansion Appliance

In the mixed dentition, the banded palatal expansion appliance is constructed by fitting bands on the maxillary primary second molars and permanent first molars (Fig. **12**). In the primary dentition, bands are fitted on the primary first and second molars. Taking a compound impression of the bands and maxillary teeth is recommended to improve the accuracy of transferring the bands to the impression. The impression is then poured up. Molar bands are joined by soldering a heavy wire (0.043-inch) to the palatal plate, which has a Hyrax-type screw (Palex^{TM} expansion screw, Great Lakes Orthodontic Products, Tonawanda, NY) in the midline. A 0.045-inch wire is soldered bilaterally to the buccal aspects of the molar bands, and extended anteriorly to the canine area, wherea hook is formed for protraction of the maxilla with elastics. The appliance is activated twice daily (0.25 mm per turn) for 1 week by the patient or parent. In patients with a more constricted maxilla, activation of the expansion screw is carried out for 2 weeks.

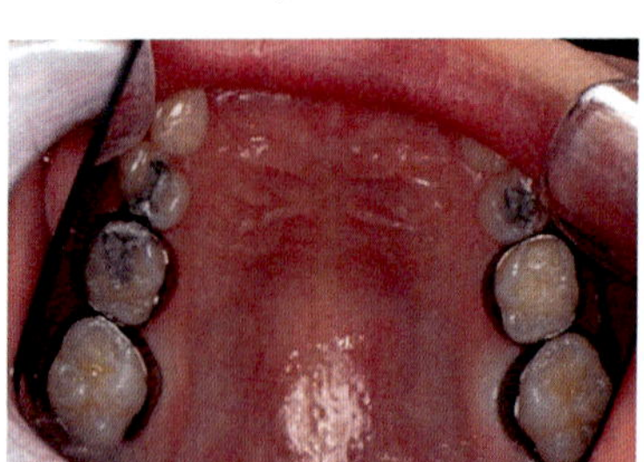

A

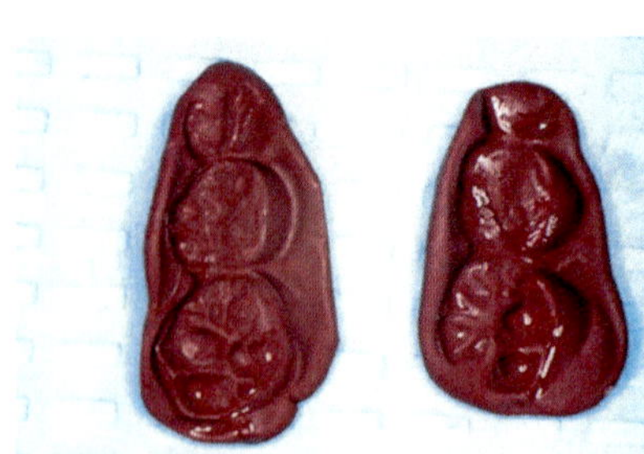

B

Fig. 12: contd....

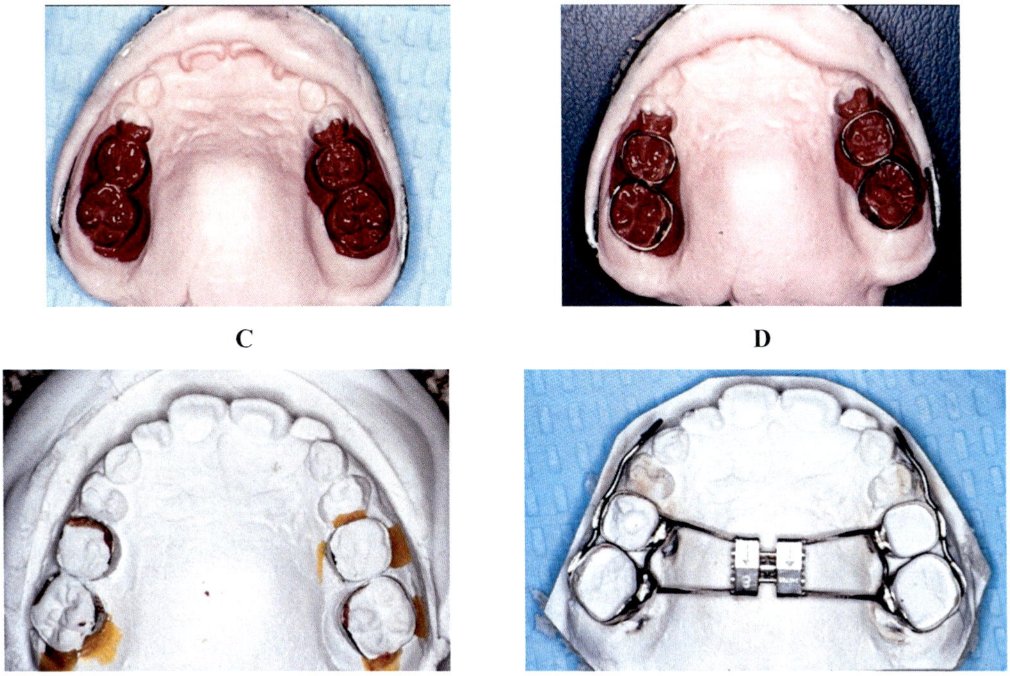

C D E F

Figure 12: (A to F) Fabrication of a banded expansion appliance for maxillary protraction: a. bands are fitted on maxillary second primary molars and permanent first molars, b. compound impression material is used to record the band positions relative the maxillary arch, c. an alginate impression is taken on top of the compound molding, d. molar bands are transferred to the impression, e. the composite impression is poured up in stone, and f. expansion appliance was fabricated with 0.045" stainless steel wires soldered to the molar bands both on the lingual and buccal aspects .

2. Acrylic Bonded Palatal Expansion Appliance

The acrylic bonded palatal expansion appliance incorporates a Hyrax-type screw into a wire framework made from 0.040-inch stainless steel (Fig. **13**). The framework extends around the buccal and lingual surfaces of the dentition. A separate 0.040-inch stainless steel wire is bent to cross the occlusion between the canine and the primary first molars and terminates with a hook for protraction with elastics. Acrylic is then added on all the occlusal surfaces of the primary molars and permanent first molars using a "salt and pepper" application of methyl methacrylate monomer and polymer. The appliance is bonded to the teeth using a chemical-cure adhesive (Excel™, Reliance Orthodontic Products, Itasca, IL) that is specially formulated for the bonding of large acrylic appliances.

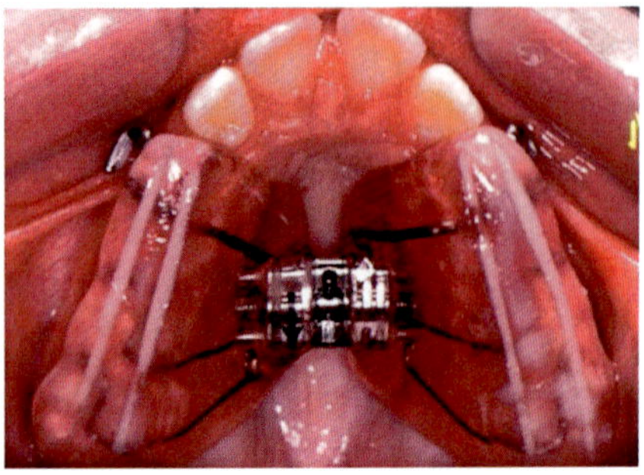

A

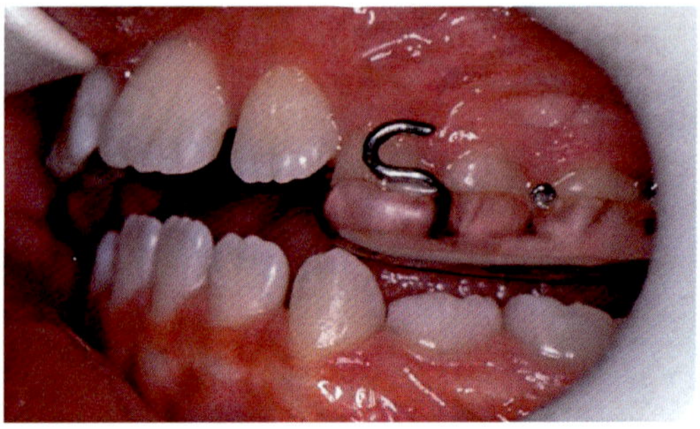

B

Figure 13: (A to B) A bonded expansion appliance for maxillary protraction is shown in the occlusal view. An 0.040-inch stainless steel wire is bent to cross the occlusion between the canine and the primary first molars and ends with a hook for protraction with elastics.

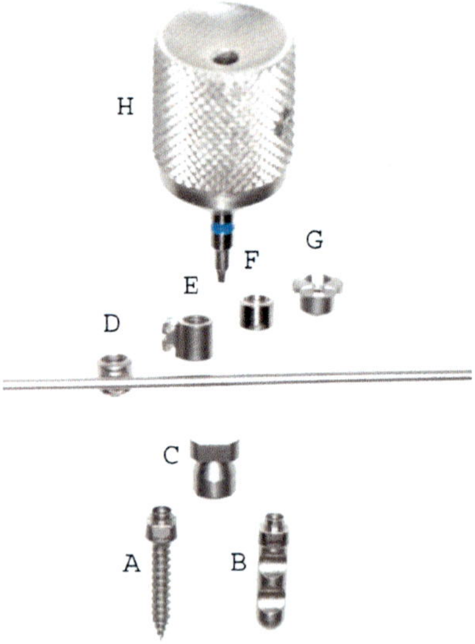

A

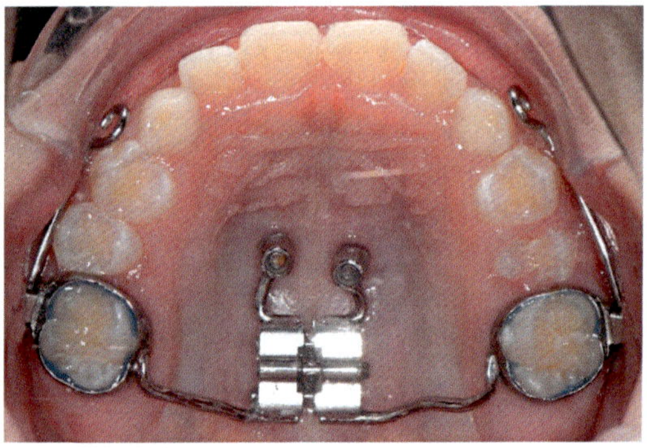

B

Figure 14: (A to B) Mini-implant is shown with the interchangeable abutments (Benefit System). Insertion of two mini-implants on the palate nearby the third palatal rugae was used as anchorage for rapid palatal expansion.

3. Mini-Implants Supported Metallic Banded Palatal Expansion Appliance (Hybrid Hyrax Appliance)

Fig. **14** shows the Benefit System utilizing mini-implants as anchorage for maxillary expansion and protraction. After administration of topical anesthesia, two mini-implants with interchangeable abutments (2mmx9mm) are inserted with a contra-angle screwdriver next to the mid-palatal suture, near the second and third palatal rugae. Pre-drilling is not needed in young patients because of the relatively low bone density. At the same appointment, bands are fitted on the upper first molars. After transfer caps are placed over the miniscrews, a silicon impression is taken. Following the impression, the laboratory analogs are placed over the transfer caps. Two standard Benefit system abutments are then screwed over the laboratory analogs. A standard Hyrax palatal split screw is connected to the device by laser-welding it anterior to the two abutments and posteriorly to the molar bands. The Hybrid Hyrax appliance is inserted by pressing it gently over the mini-implants and alternately screwing the two abutments onto the mini-implants.

Skeletal Effects of Maxillary Protraction

Several circum-maxillary sutures play an important role in the development of the nasomaxillary complex (Fig. **15**): frontomaxillary, nasomaxillary, zygomatico-temporal, zygomaticomaxillary, pterygopalatine, intermaxillary, ethmoidalmaxillary and the lacrymomaxillary sutures. Animal studies have shown that the maxillary complex can be displaced anteriorly with significant changes in the circum-maxillary sutures and the maxillary tuberosity [67]. Maxillary protraction, however, does not always result in forward movement of the maxilla. Nanda [68] showed that with the same line of force, different midfacial bones displaced in different directions depending on the moments of force generated at the sutures. Jackson, Kokich and Shapiro [69] found that anterior positioning of the maxillary complex was accompanied with a small amount of counterclockwise rotation during the treatment period. The center of resistance of the maxilla was found to be located at the distal contacts of the maxillary first molars one half the distances from the functional occlusal plane to the inferior border of the orbit [70]. Protraction of the maxilla below the center of resistance produces counterclockwise rotation of the maxilla. Using human skulls, Hata and colleagues [71] also found that protraction forces at the level of the maxillary arch produced forward with counterclockwise rotation of the maxilla unless a heavy downward vector of force was applied.

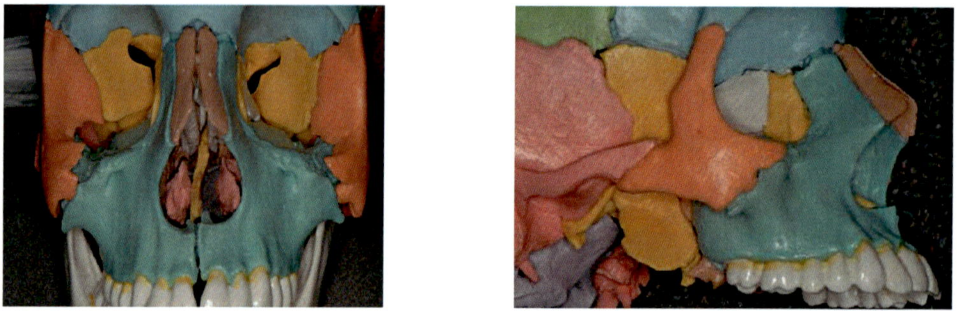

A B

Figure 15: (A to B) Circummaxillary sutures connecting the maxilla to the rest of the skull.

Clinical Response to Maxillary Protraction

Clinically, anterior crossbites can be corrected with 3-4 months of maxillary expansion and protraction depending on the severity of the malocclusion. Improvement in overbite and molar relationship can be expected with an additional 4-6 months of maxillary protraction. In a prospective clinical trial [35], overjet correction was found to be the result of forward maxillary movement (31%), backward movement of the mandible (21%), labial movement of the maxillary incisors (28%), and lingual movement of the mandibular incisors (20%). The molar relationship was corrected to a Class I or Class II dental relationship by a combination of skeletal movements and differential movement of the maxillary and mandibular molars. Anchorage loss was observed during maxillary protraction with mesial movement of the maxillary molars. Overbite was improved by eruption of the maxillary and mandibular molars. The total facial height was increased by inferior movement of the maxilla, downward and backward rotation of the mandible, as well as a concomitant increase in the mandibular plane angle.

Patients with skeletal Class III malocclusion often present with a concave facial profile, a retrusive nasomaxillary area, and a prominent lower third of the face. The lower lip is often protruded relative to the upper lip. Treatment with maxillary expansion and protraction can straighten the skeletal and soft tissue facial profiles and improve the posture of the lips. It is important to note that the profile and occlusion of Class III patients usually becomes worse with no treatment because the lack of horizontal maxillary growth and excess mandibular growth often lead to compensated incisal changes and overclosure of the mandible. In a prospective clinical trial, patients treated with 8 months of maxillary protraction, the maxilla came forward an average of 2.1 mm. In control patients without treatment, the maxilla came forward only 0.5 mm. On average, the mandible was positioned about 1.0 mm posteriorly with treatment. With no treatment, the mandible came forward 1.7 mm. In addition, without treatment, the incisors compensated to the skeletal discrepancy by proclination of the maxillary incisors and retroclination of the mandibular incisors. In general, the direction of these changes is similar to those occurring with treatment. With the advent of 3-D imaging, the forward movement of the maxilla, upper incisors and upper lip and the backward movement of the mandible, lower incisors and lower lip can be seen graphically with color changes (Fig. **16**).

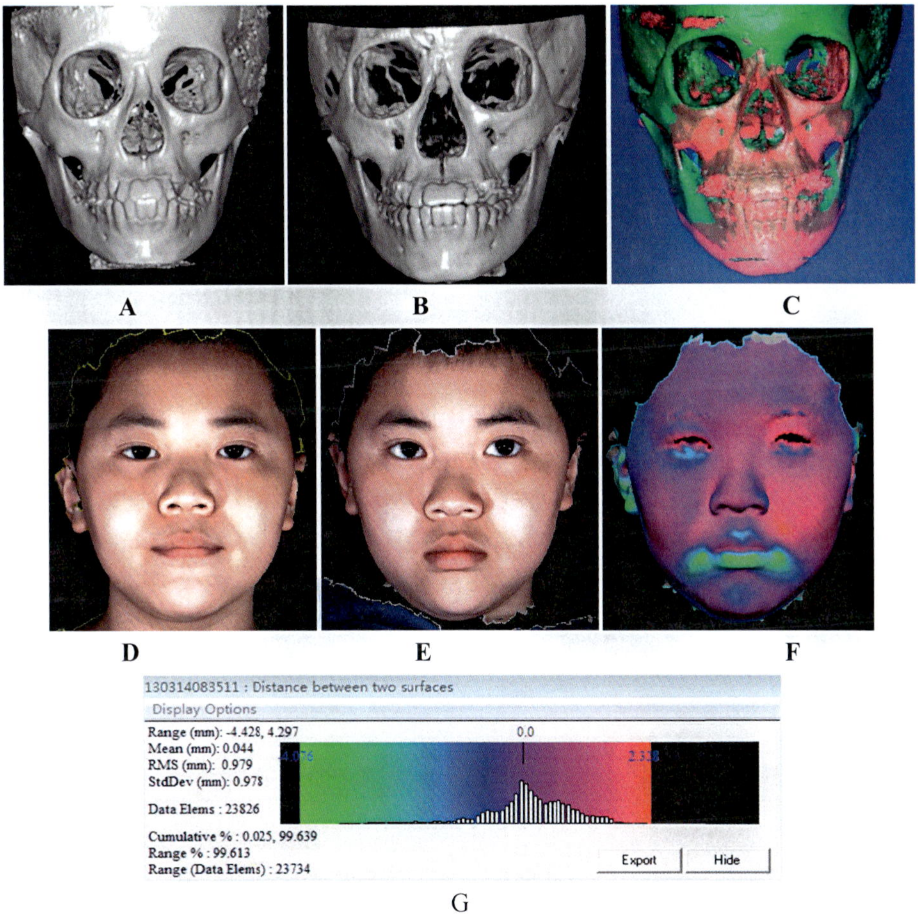

Figure 16: 3-D PA radiographs and stereophotometric photographs of a 12-year-old patient treated 8 months with protraction facemask. (A-C) Pre-, post- and superimposed radiographs showing forward movement of the maxilla and maxillary incisors. (D-F) Pre-, post- and superimposed soft tissue data showing forward movement of the mid-face and backward movement of the lower lip. G. Color spectrum showing data of soft tissue movement.

Variability in Clinical Response

Clinically, the maxilla can be advanced 2 to 4 mm over an 8 to 12 months period of maxillary protraction. The amount of forward maxillary movement is influenced by a number of factors including: age of the patient, expansion prior to protraction, tooth-borne *vs.* skeletal anchorage system, the force level, as well as its direction and point of application, and treatment time (Table **4**) [31,51,72-86].

Table 4: Factors influencing the forward movement of the maxilla (A Point) with protraction facemask

Author	**Year**	**Expansion**	**Force Level (per side)**	**Treatment Time**	**"A" Point Movement**
Nanda [76]	'80	Haas	500g	4m	1.5mm
Ishii [51]	'87	No expansion	250g	11-24m	2.7mm
Tindlund [77]	'89	Quadhelix	700g	12m	3.0mm
Merwin [73]	'97	Hyrax	400g	6m	2.0mm
Nartallo-Turley [80]	'97	Hyrax	200-450g	11m	3.3mm
da Silva [78]	'98	Haas	350g	12m	1.5mm
Gallagher [79]	'98	Slow Expansion	300-400g	8-9m	1.6mm/yr
Baik [72]	'98	Hyrax	300-400g	6-8m	2.1mm
Pangrezio-Kulbersh [81]	'98	Bonded RME	400-600g	7-8m	1.8mm
Kapust [74]	'98	Hyrax	300-400g	9-10m	2.8mm
Baccetti [75]	'98	Bonded RME	400g	11m	2.1mm
Ngan [83]	'98	Hyrax	400g	8-9m	2.1mm
Sung [82]	'98	Hyrax	300-400g	8-9m	2.1mm
Westwood [31]	'03	Bonded RME	400g	10m	1.8mm
Kajiyama [84]	'04	None	400g	12m	1.9mm
Vaughan [85]	'05	Hyrax	400g	12m	2.0mm
Cha [86]	'11	Bonded RME	400g	12m	2.1mm

1. Age of Patient

The optimal time to intervene in an early Class III patient is at the time of eruption of the upper central incisors. The erupted maxillary first molars provide better anchorage for maxillary protraction. A positive overjet and overbite at the end of facemask treatment appears to maintain the anterior occlusion after treatment. However, there is some evidence that one can obtain a better skeletal and dental response in the primary and early mixed dentition [85]. More recent clinical studies indicate that maxillary protraction is effective through puberty with diminishing skeletal response as the sutures mature [82-85]. Fig. **17** shows a 10-year-old boy presenting with a Class III malocclusion and an anterior crossbite. A phase I treatment was initiated using a maxillary expansion appliance in conjunction with a facemask. After 12 months of maxillary protraction treatment to correct the anterior crossbite, the patient was placed on growth observation until the eruption of all permanent dentition. Subsequently the patient was treated with a fixed orthodontic appliance for 14 months and stable results were achieved (Fig. **17**).

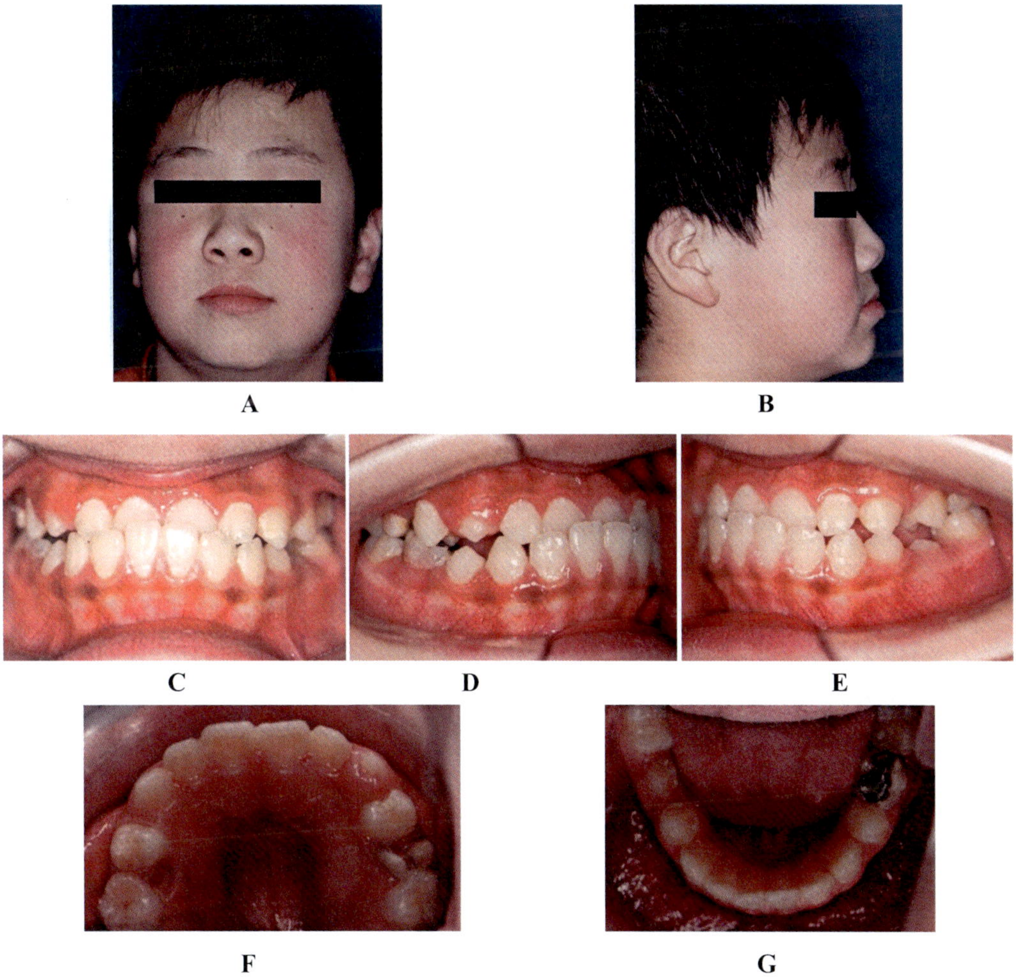

Figure 17: (A to G) A 10-year-old boy presented with a Class III malocclusion and an anterior crossbite.

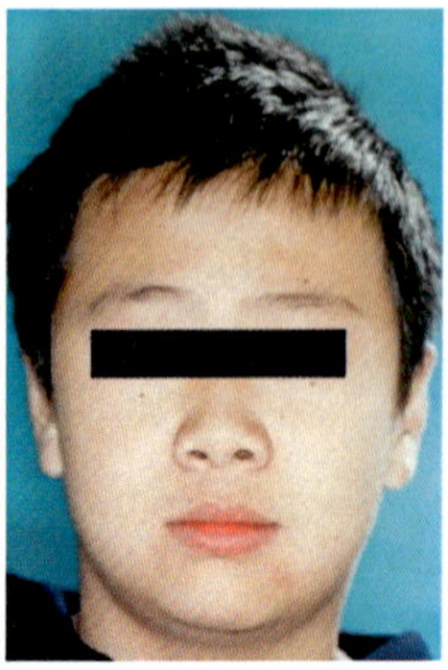

H

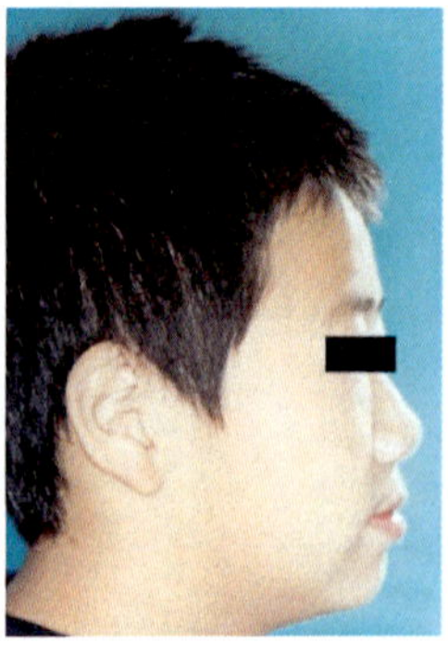

I

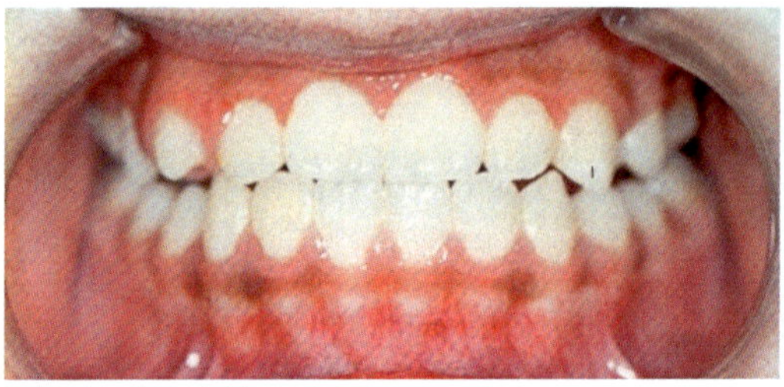

J

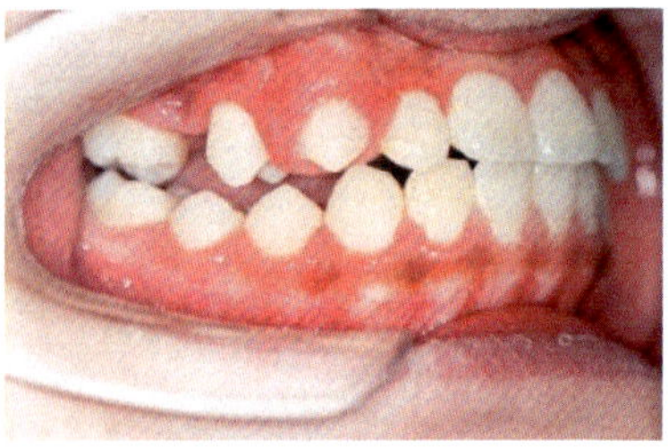

K

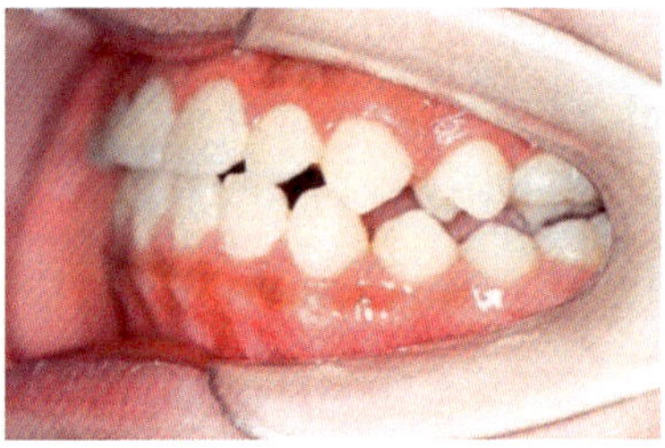

L

Figure 17: (H to L) Progress photographs after 12 months of facemask treatment.

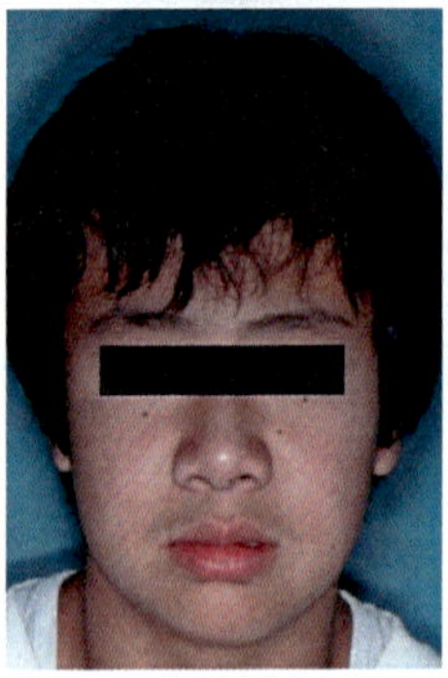

M

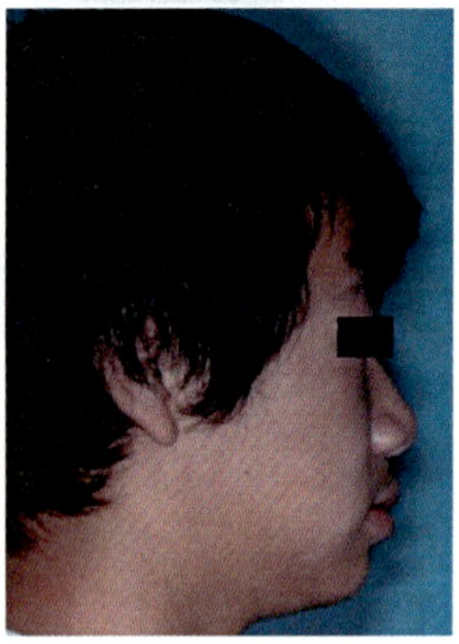

N

Fig. 17: contd…

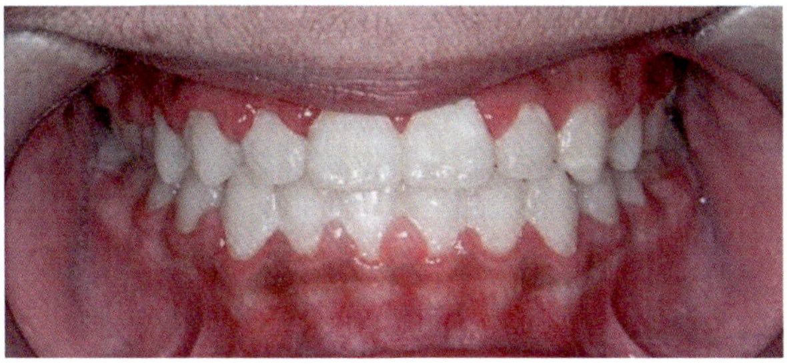

O

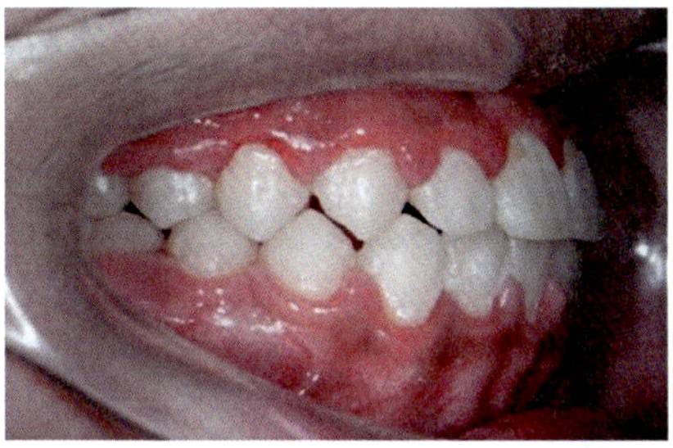

P

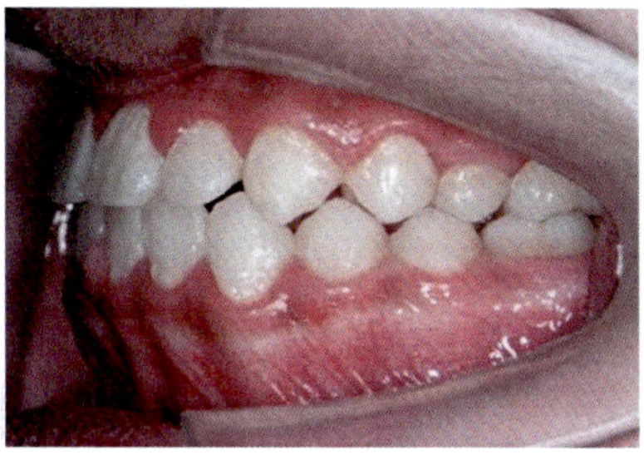

Q

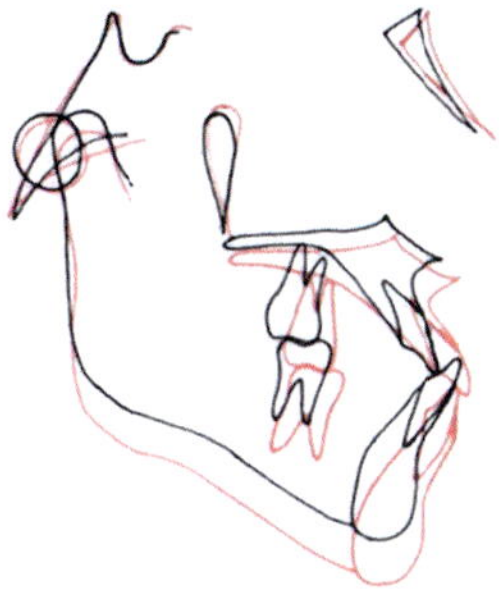

R

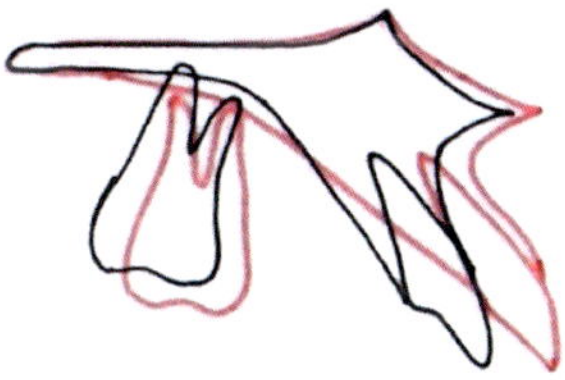

S

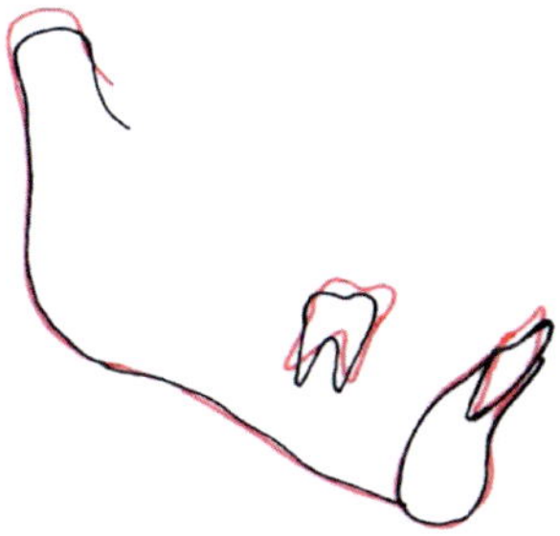

T

Figure 17: (M to Q) Post-treatment photographs after 14 months of fixed appliance treatment document the change. (R to T) Superimposition of the pre- and post-treatment cephalometric tracings show the skeletal and dentoalveolar responses.

2. Expansion Prior to Maxillary Protraction

The need to expand the maxilla prior to protraction is not entirely clear. Sutural expansion and/or protraction induce new bone growth by mechanically stretching the sutures [87-89]. The response to mechanical traction includes a widening of the sutures, changes in the orientation of fiber bundles, an increase in the number of osteoblasts, and deposition of osteoid on both sutural bone surfaces [89]. Clinically, it has been shown that maxillary expansion can disarticulate the maxilla to allow a more favorable forward movement of the maxilla [31,35,72-86]. However, when using tooth-borne devices for orthopedic effects, a well-disarticulated maxilla seems to be critical. In a study by Baik [72], 60 patients treated with protraction facemask were divided into 2 groups with or without RME.

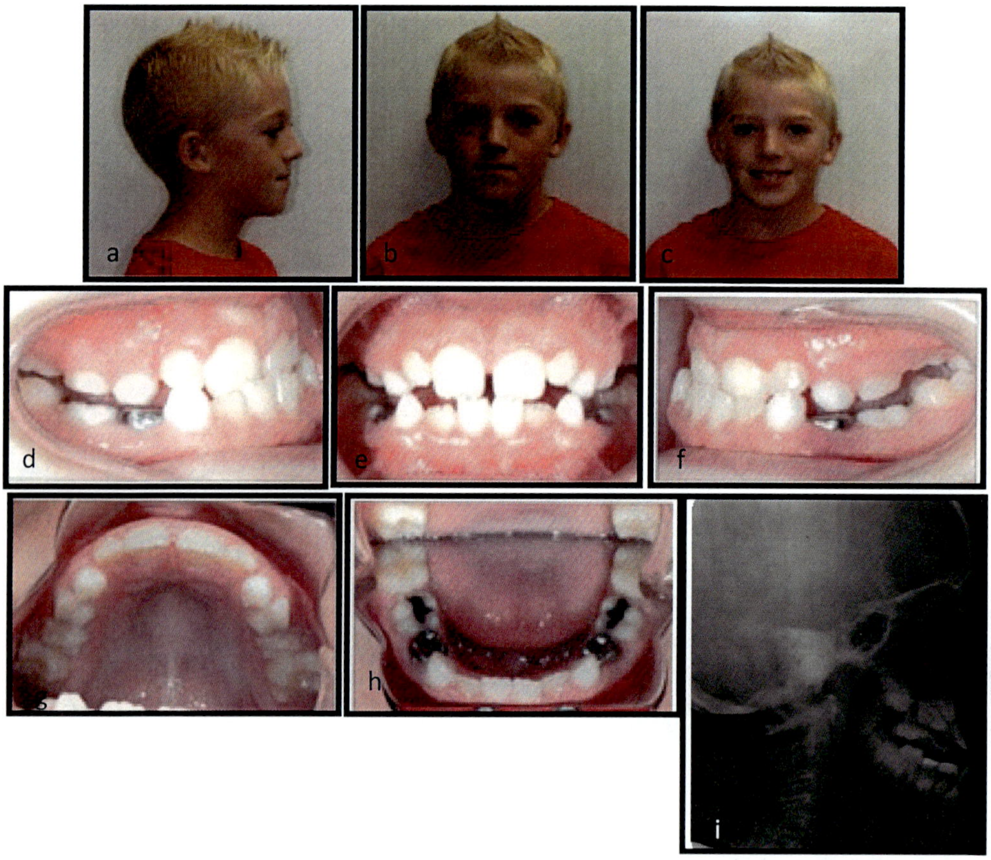

Figure 18: (A to I) A 9-year-old male presents with a Class III malocclusion and a deficient maxilla.

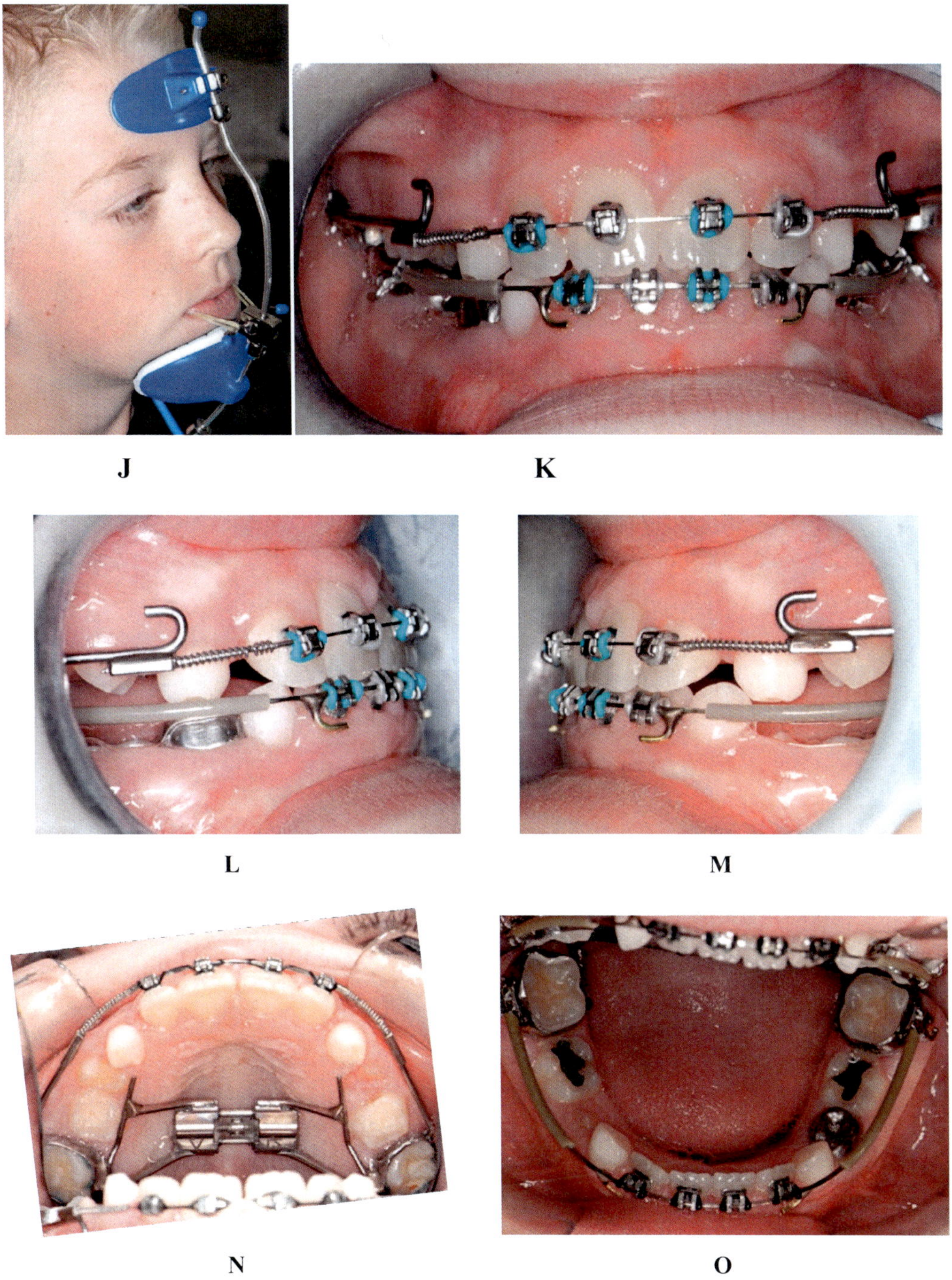

Figure 18: (J to O) Treatment was with a facemask using the maxillary expansion and constriction protocol. The patient was instructed to wear the facemask at night and Class III elastics during the day time, from the maxillary first molars to the post on the mandibular.018X.025 ss arch wire.

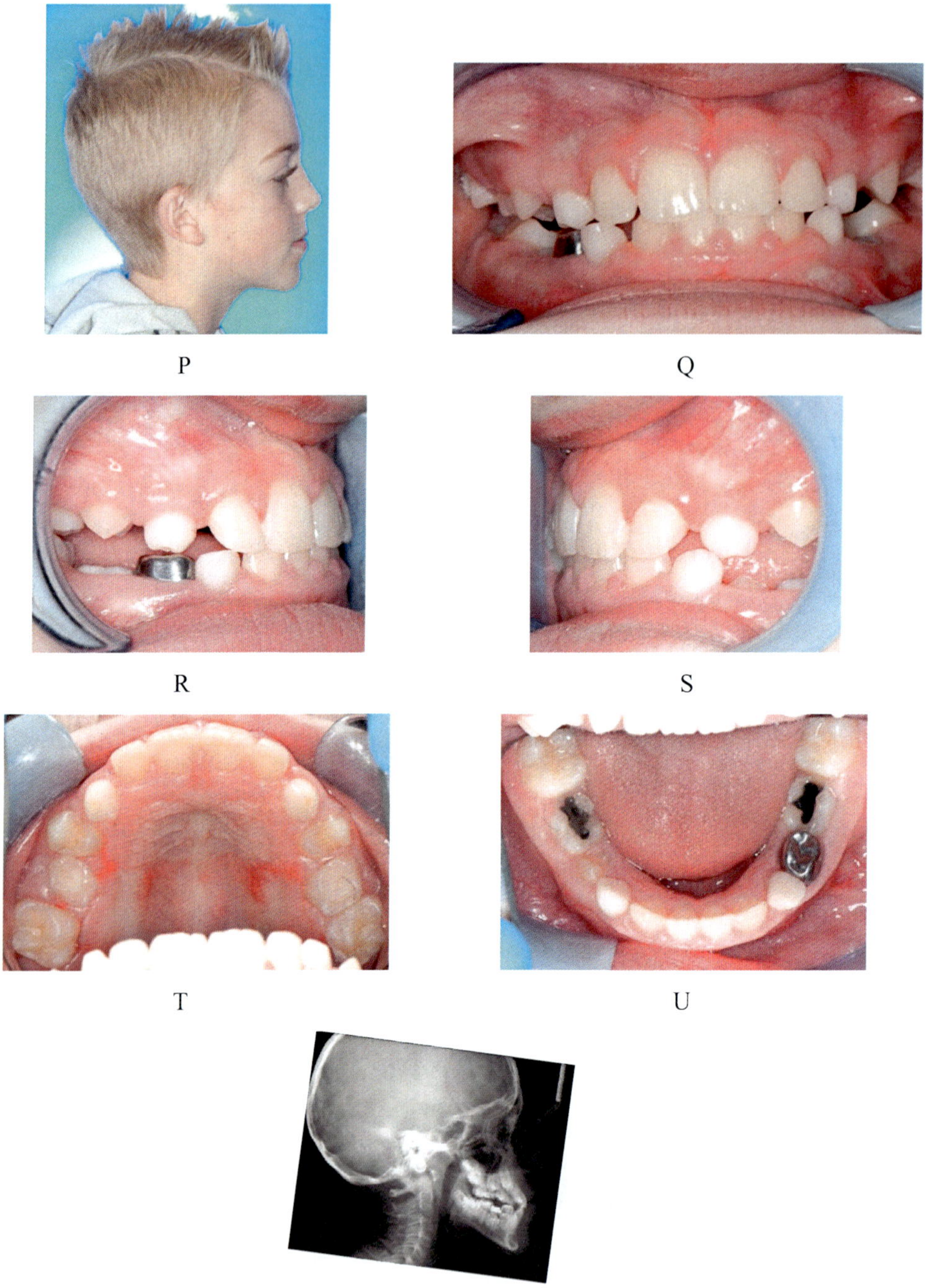

Figure 18: (P to V) Post-treatment photographs and radiograph show changes after 6 months of maxillary protraction.

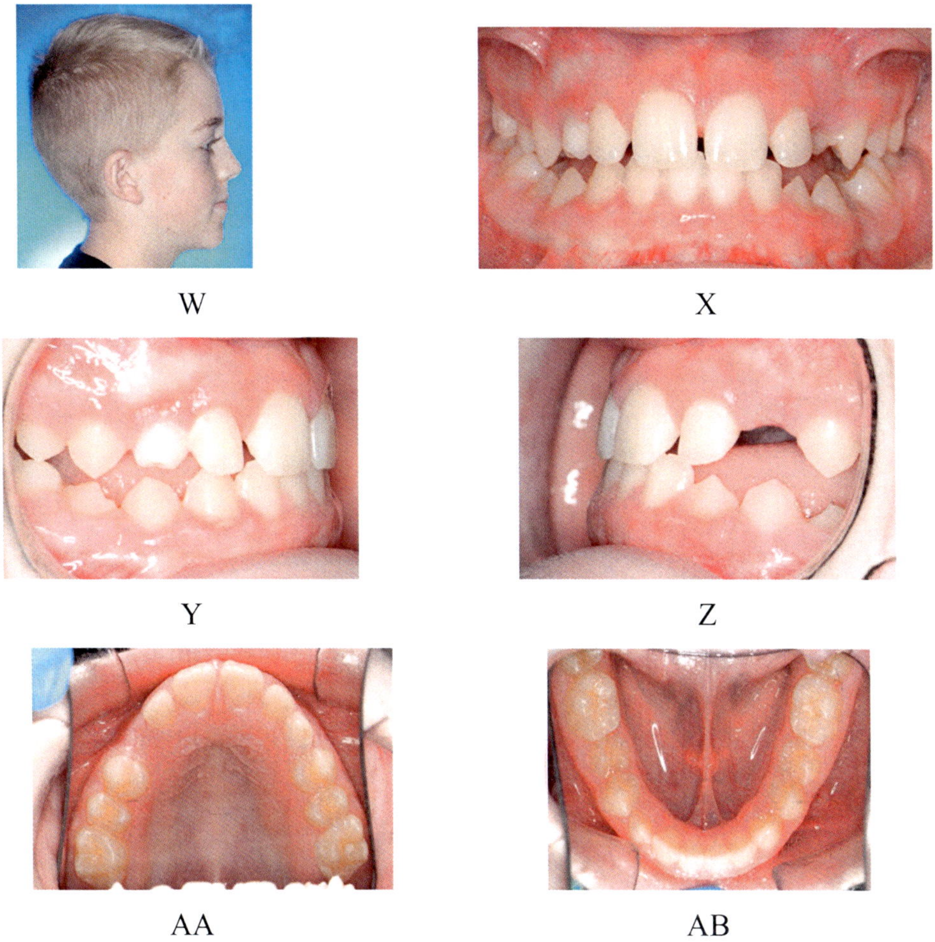

Figure 18: (W to AB) One year post-treatment photographs document stability of the overbite and overjet after maxillary protraction.

The author found significantly greater forward movement of the maxilla (+2.0 mm) when protraction was used in conjunction with RME compared with protraction without RME (+0.9 mm). In the same study, greater forward movement of the maxilla (+2.8mm) was found when protraction was initiated during maxillary expansion compared with protraction after expansion (1.85mm). Liou [90, 91] suggested a protocol of repetitive weekly alternate rapid maxillary expansion and constriction of the maxilla to disarticulate the maxilla without over-expanding. Usually, it requires 7-9 weeks to loosen the maxilla. Liou reported an average of 5.8 mm of forward movement of the maxilla at A point using this method [91]. Fig. **18** shows a 9-year-old male presented with a Class III malocclusion and maxillary deficiency. A phase I treatment was initiated with facemask in conjunction with rapid palatal expansion appliance. A protocol of repeated expansion and constriction of the maxilla was employed to loosen the maxillary sutures prior to maxillary protraction. The expansion appliance was turned twice (0.5mm) in the morning and twice in the evening for the first week for expansion. The appliance was turned backwards with the same rate the second week for constriction. This protocol was repeated for 6 weeks. Patient was then instructed to wear the facemask for 12 to 14 hours at night to "protract" the maxilla. In addition, a 2x4 appliance was placed in the mandibular arch together with a posted .018x.025 stainless steel wire. Patient was instructed to wear Class III elastics (3/8" 6 oz) during day time for no more than 8 hours to "hold" the maxilla in a forward position. The anterior crossbite was corrected after 6 months of maxillary protraction.

3. Tooth-Borne *vs.* Skeletal Anchorage for Maxillary Protraction

Conventional tooth-borne appliances rely on an almost complete dentition to transmit the relatively high level of forces to the bony structure of the maxilla and midface. In most situations, tooth-borne protraction appliances produce adverse effects such as buccal tipping of the first molars, proclination of the maxillary incisors as well as loss of arch length as a result of mesial migration of the maxillary first molars. To overcome these drawbacks, a bone anchored maxillary protraction device was developed [92-96]. Wilmes *et al.* reported a rapid palatal expansion appliance that utilizes mini-implants, placed anteriorly in the palate for skeletal anchorage [94-96]. Fig. **19** shows a 9-year-old female presented with a Class III skeletal malocclusion and a deficient maxilla (Wits: -8.3mm). Treatment was initiated with a Hybrid Hyrax rapid palatal expansion appliance together with a Mentoplate (bone plate place in the mental region of the mandible) as anchorage for Class III elastics. Two micro-implants were placed in the palate and an impression was taken to fabricate the Hybrid Hyrax expansion appliance using the Benefit System. The oral surgeon places the titanium Mentoplate in the mandible under local anesthesia. After preparation of a mucoperiosteal flap, the two extensions are shortened and adapted. The Mentoplate is fixed with four screws; the flap is repositioned and sutured. Class III elastics (3.5 oz, 3/16") are used to protract the maxilla after maxillary expansion. After one week of maxillary expansion, Class III elastics are applied. After nine months of treatment, the patient's occlusion and profile showed marked improvement. The soft tissues appeared healthy throughout treatment. The pre- and post-treatment lateral cephalograms show an improvement in the anteroposterior jaw position (Wits = -2.8mm).

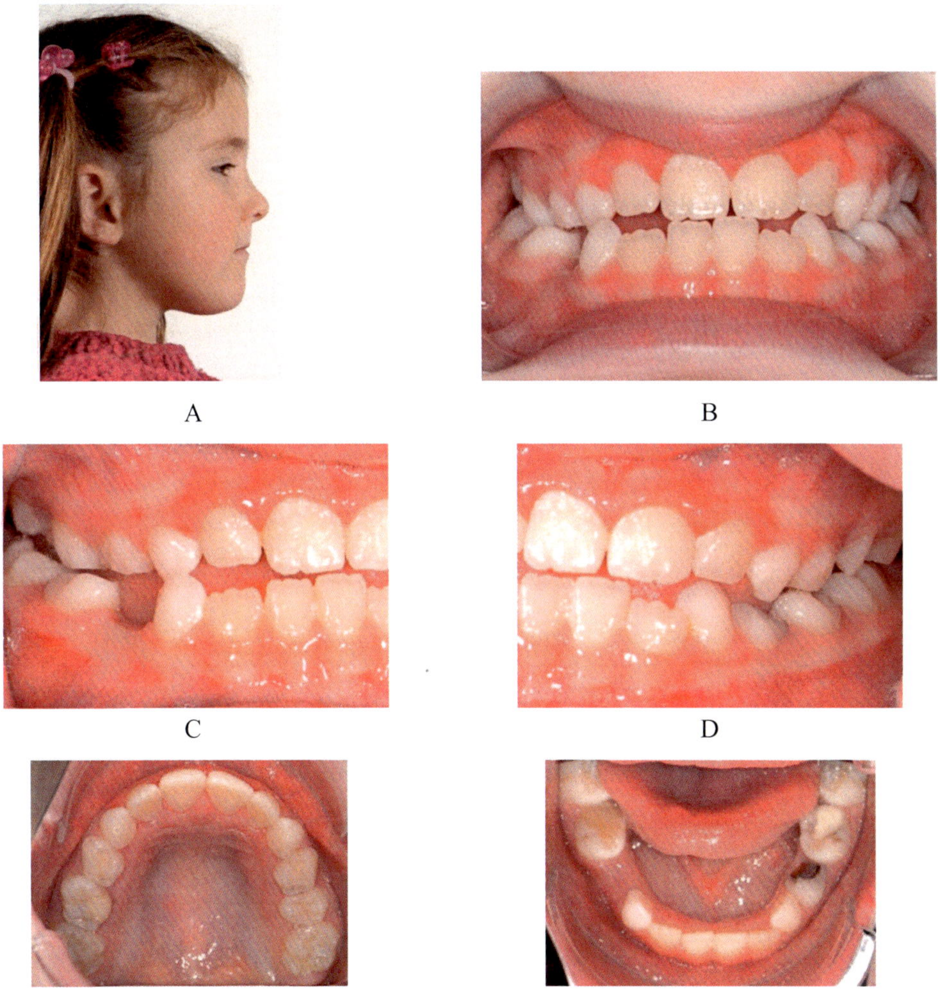

A B C D E F

Fig. 19: contd...

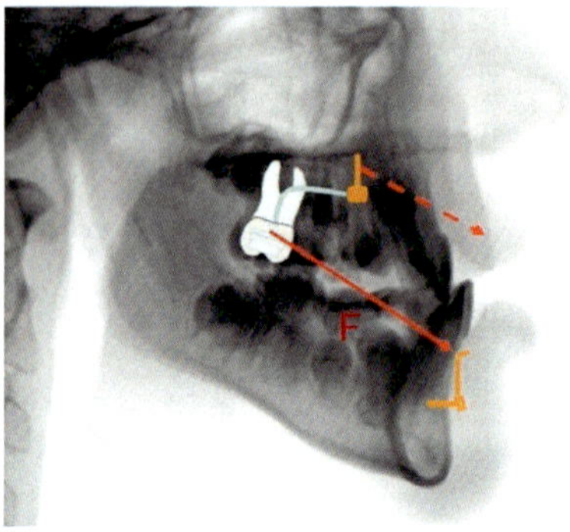

G

Figure 19: (A to G) 9-year-old female presented with Class III malocclusion and a deficient maxilla. A schematic diagram shows the treatment protocol with a Hybrid Hyrax rapid palatal expansion appliance, together with a Mentoplate, as anchorage for Class III elastics.

The use of Hybrid Hyrax and Mentoplate appliances as anchorage and Class III elastics for maxillary protraction requires minimal compliance by the patient. However, the placement of a Mentoplate is a surgical procedure and could be quite invasive. If patient is very cooperative, one can use a combination of a Hybrid Hyrax appliance as anchorage and a facemask for maxillary protraction. Fig. **20** shows a 10-year old girl with maxillary deficiency (Wits 8.3mm). Treatment was initiated with a Hybrid Hyrax expansion appliance and a facemask. After 2 weeks of expansion, the facemask was worn 4 hours during day time and 8 hours at night. After 9 months of treatment, the patient profile and occlusion show impressive improvement. The pre- and post-treatment lateral cephalograms showed a dramatic improvement in the anteroposterior jaw relationship (Wits 0mm).

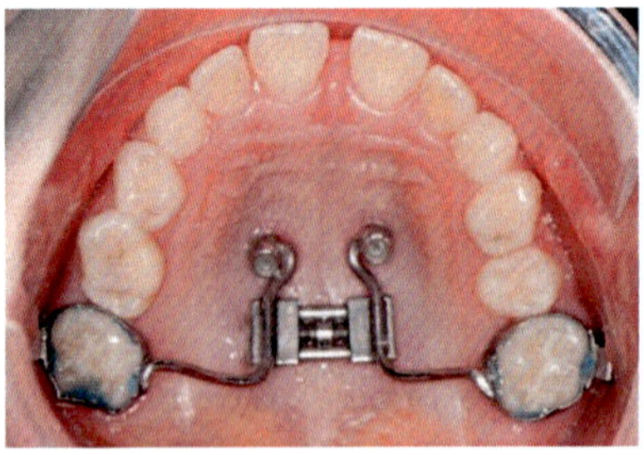

H

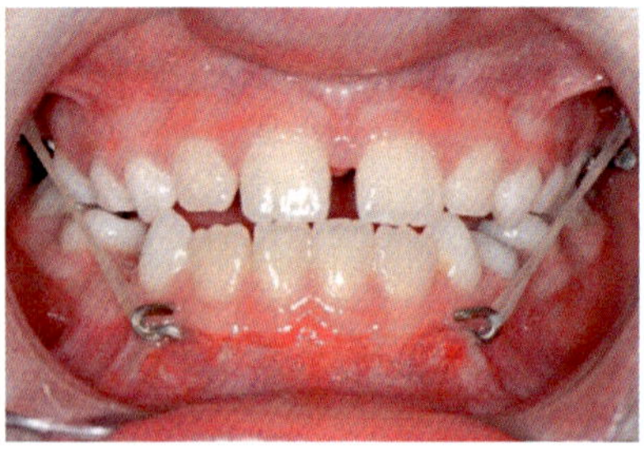

I

Fig. 19: contd...

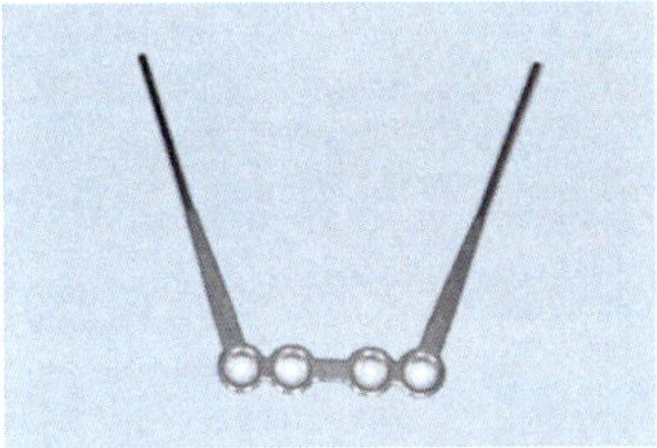

J

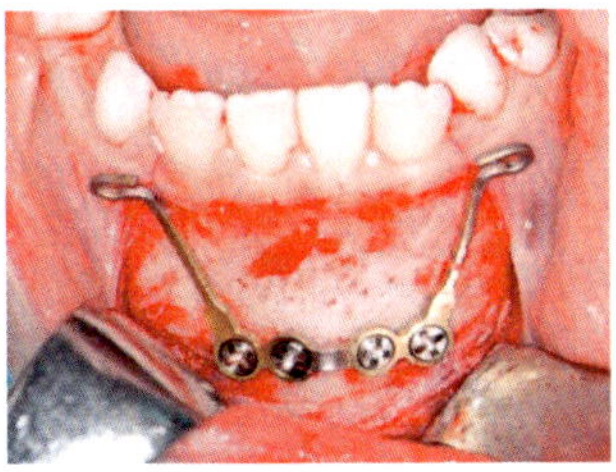

K

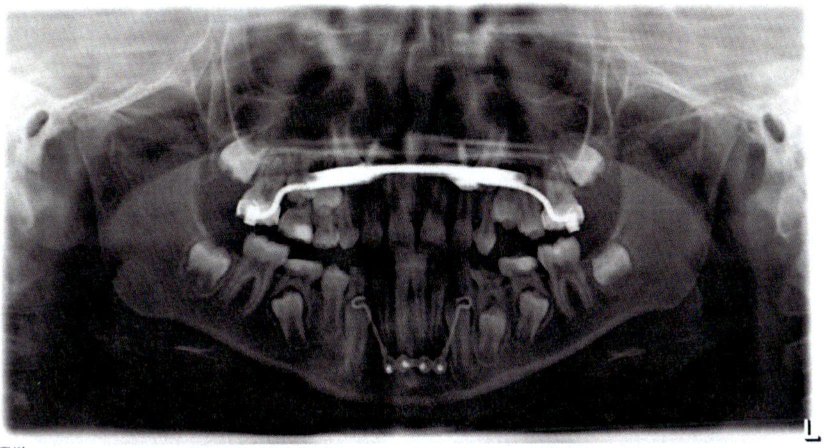

L

Figure 19: (H to L) Placement of Hybrid Hyrax rapid palatal expansion appliance in the palate is used along with a Mentoplate as anchorage for Class III elastics to achieve maxillary protraction.

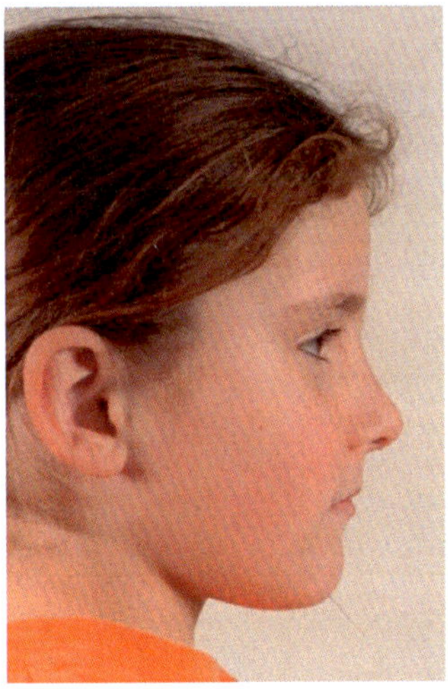

M

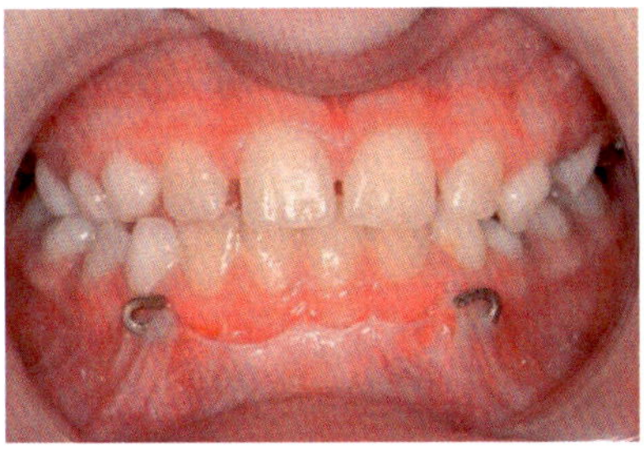

N

Fig. 19: contd...

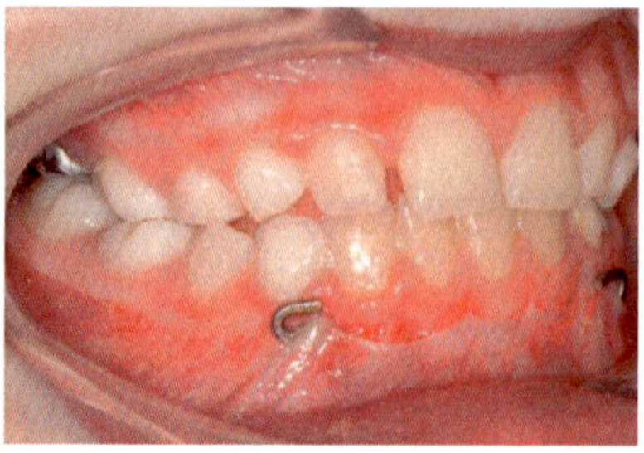

O

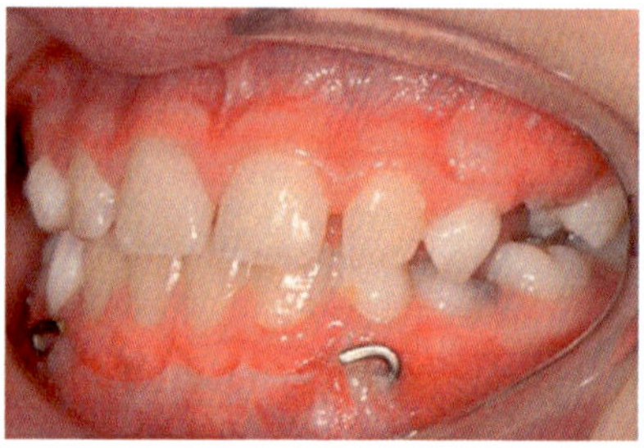

P

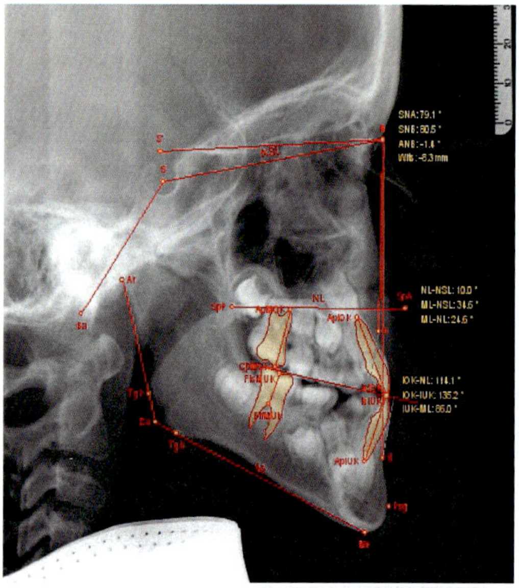

Q

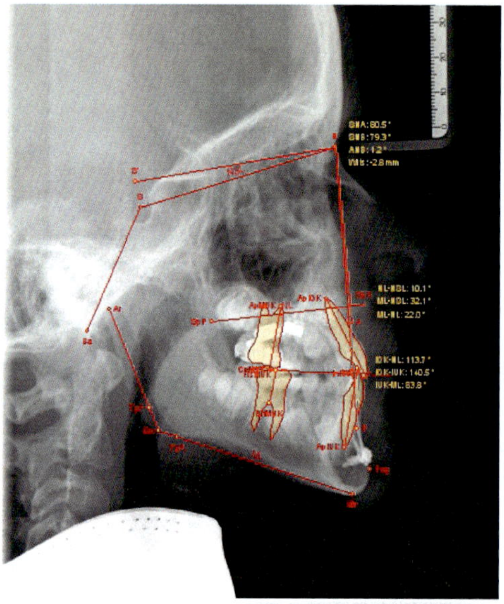

R

Figure 19: (M to R) Post-treatment extraoral and intraoral photographs show improvement in profile and occlusion with healthy soft tissue throughout the treatment. q. Pre-treatment and r. post-treatment lateral cephalograms document the improvement in anteroposterior jaw position.

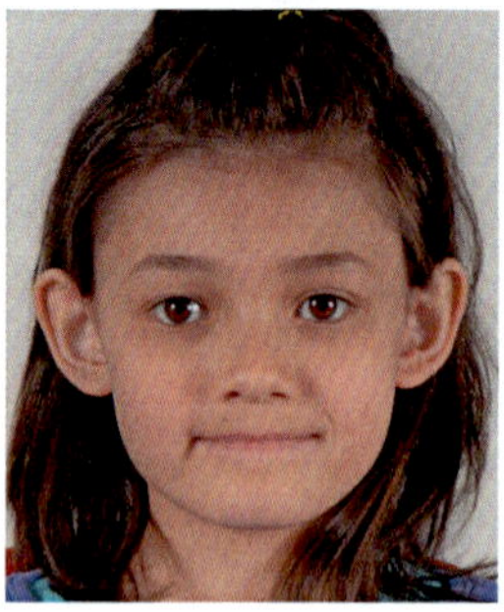

A

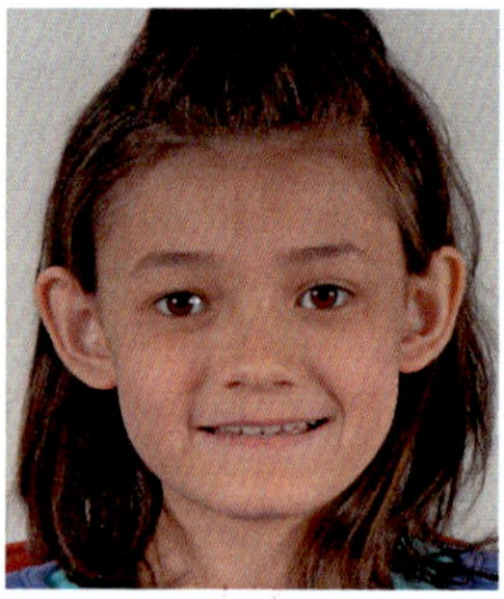

B

Fig. 20: contd...

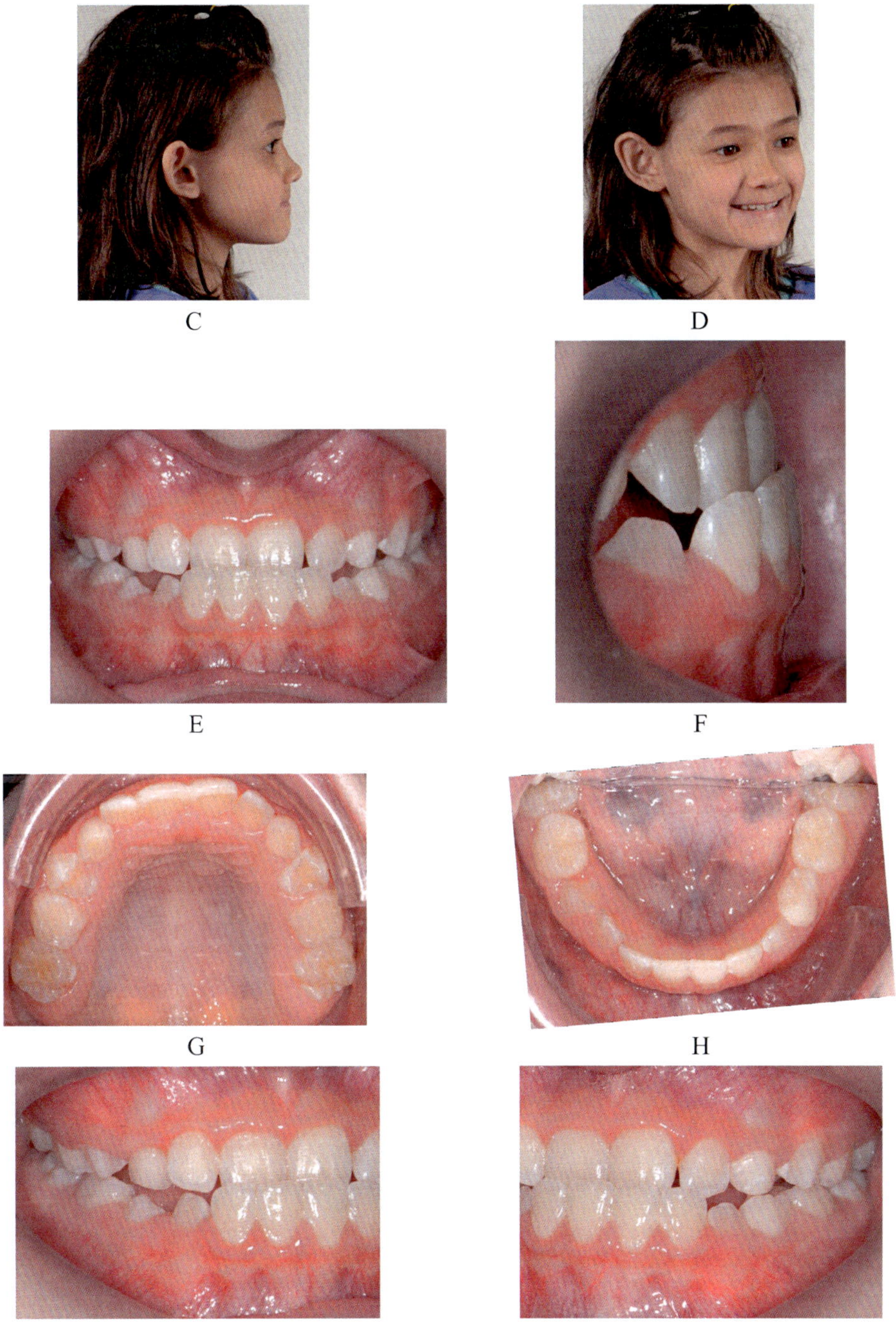

C D E F G H I J

Fig. 20: contd...

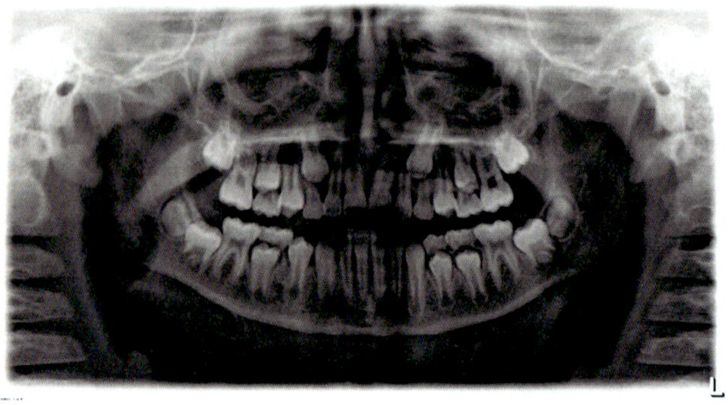

K

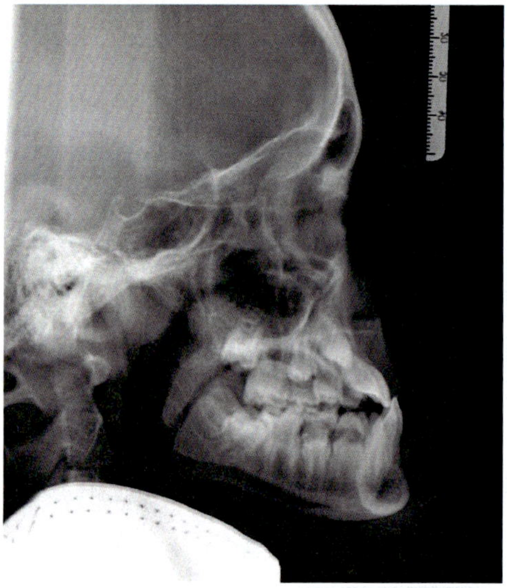

L

Figure 20: (A to L) 10 year old female with Class III malloclusion and maxillary deficiency.

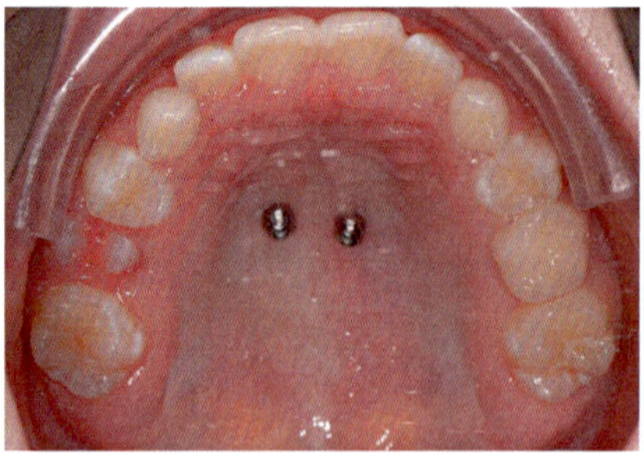

M

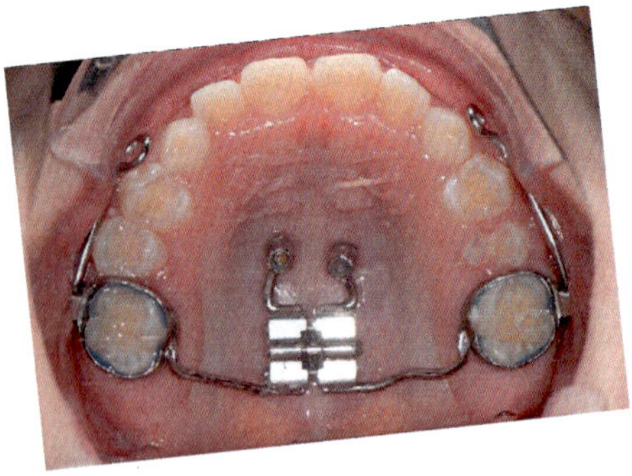

N

Fig. 20: contd...

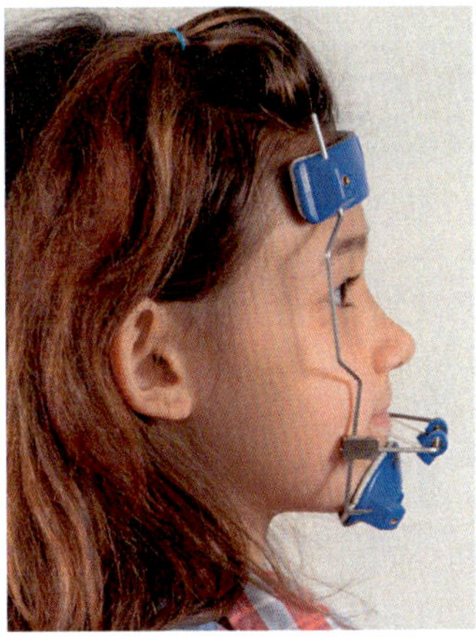

O

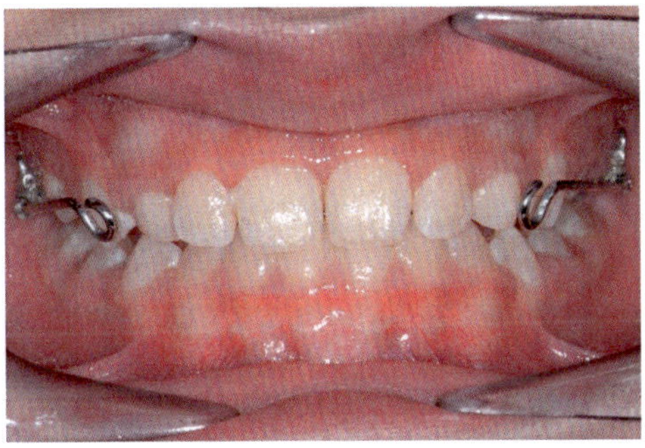

P

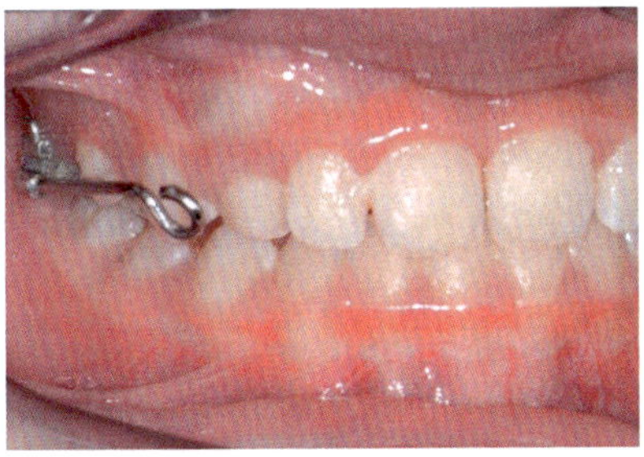

Q

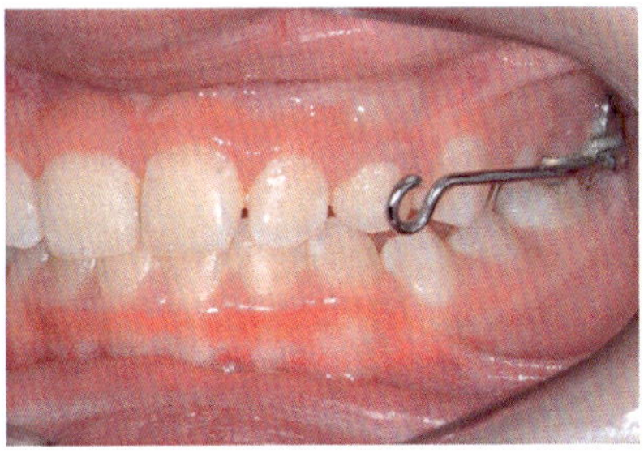

R

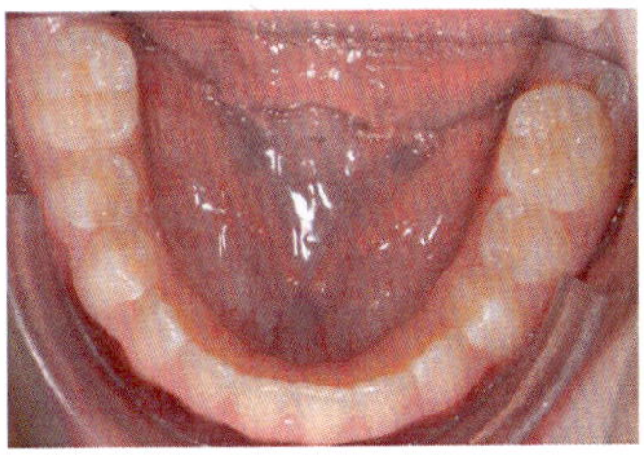

S

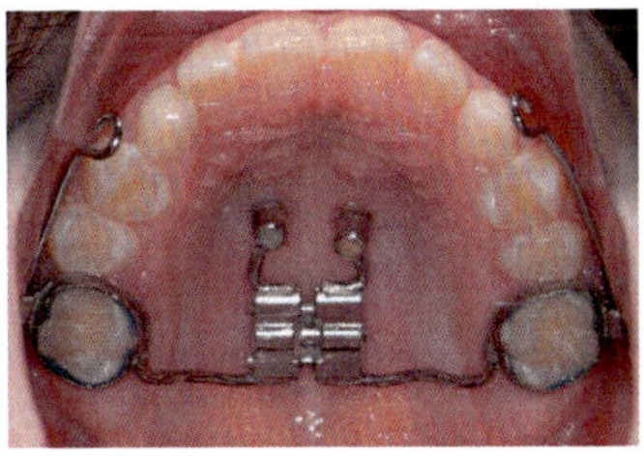

T

Fig. 20: contd...

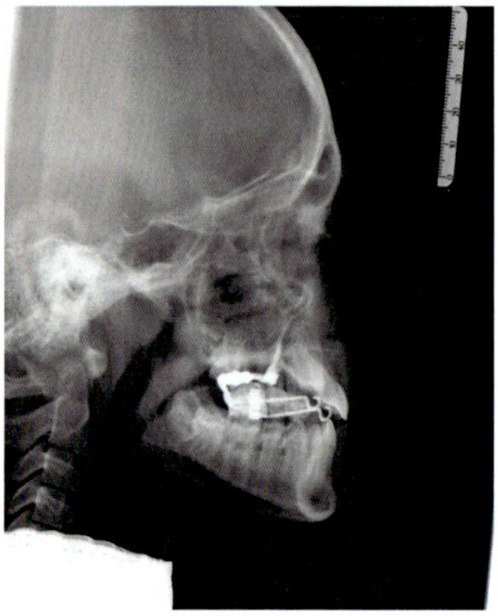

U

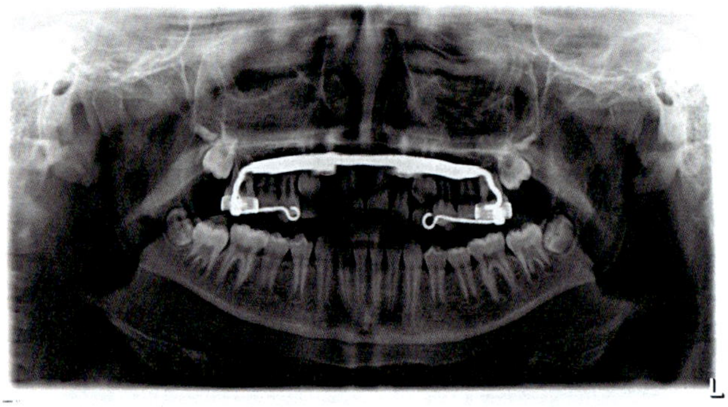

V

Figure 20: (M to V) Hybrid Hyrax rapid palatal expansion appliance in conjunction with a facemask was used to correct the anterior crossbite.

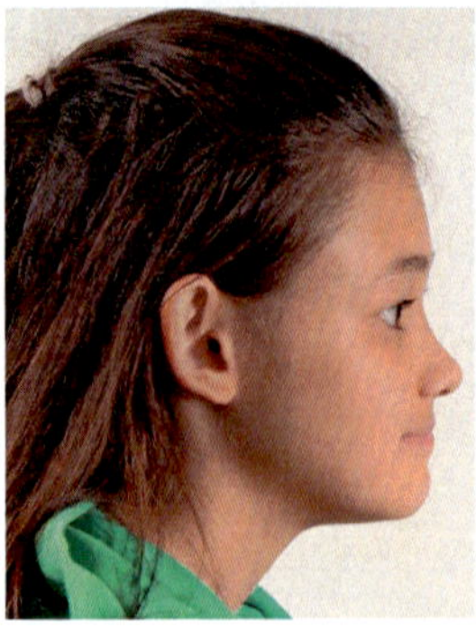

W

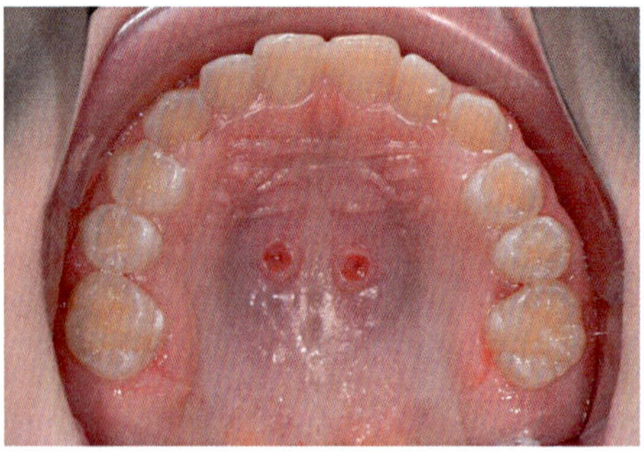

X

Figure 20: (W to X) Post treatment extraoral photograph showing improvement in profile and intraoral photograph showing removal of the mini-implants.

4. Force Level, Direction and Point of Application

Orthopedic effects require greater forces than do orthodontic movements. Successful maxillary protraction has been reported using 300 to 500 g of force per side in the primary and mixed dentitions (Table **4**). Most of these studies recommended a 10 to 12 hours/day of headgear wear.

Hata *et al.* [71] suggested that an effective forward displacement of the maxilla can be obtained clinically from a force applied 5 mm above the palatal plane. In deep overbite cases in which an opening of the bite is desired, a forward pull from the level of the maxillary arch with a concomitant anterior rotation of the maxilla will aid in the treatment of these malocclusions. In several clinical studies, a 30° to 45° forward and downward protraction force applied at the canine region produced an acceptable clinical response with one degree of counterclockwise rotation of the palatal plane [35].

5. Length of Treatment Time

There is no consensus on the length of treatment with protraction headgear. A review of the literature shows the treatment time varies from 4 to 12 months (Table **3**). Most of the orthopedic changes are observed within the first 3-6 months after maxillary expansion. Prolonged use of protraction force results in dentoalveolar changes including mesial movement of maxillary molars and proclination of maxillary incisors. The benefit of repeated maxillary expansion and protraction has not been reported in the literature. Increased treatment time may compromise patient oral hygiene and cooperation.

Post-Treatment Stability

Animal and human studies have shown that the effects on the maxilla remained stable for 1 to 2 years after treatment. In a few studies [27, 31, 35] where patients were followed after maxillary expansion and protraction, the anterior position of the maxilla was maintained post-treatment. During this growth period the maxilla and mandible reverted back to the original growth pattern. In some cases, Class III correction was lost due to excess mandibular growth. Few studies followed the early treatment patients through the pubertal growth period. In a prospective clinical trial

[27, 35], a group of Chinese patients were over-treated to a Class I or II relationship with maxillary expansion and protraction and then retained with a Class III functional appliance for one year. When these patients were followed after the pubertal growth period, 67% of the patients maintained a positive overjet. In patients that relapsed back to a negative overjet, the mandible outgrew the maxilla in the horizontal direction. The overjet reverted back to an anterior crossbite due to excessive forward mandibular growth. As a result, the authors recommend overcorrection of the overjet and molar relationships to anticipate subsequent horizontal mandibular growth. It is also advisable to use a retention device such as a mandibular retractor or a functional appliance following maxillary protraction.

Camouflage Class III Treatment and its Limitations

Skeletal discrepancies that cannot be resolved during mixed dentition by growth modification may require comprehensive appliance therapy and/or surgical correction. Patients treated during childhood may have the malocclusion recur during adolescence. Treatment of Class III malocclusion in adolescence is indicated in many instances to alleviate the potential psychosocial problems [97] and perhaps reduce the need for surgery [98]. Malocclusions with a mild mandibular prognathism and a moderate overbite can be corrected with dentoalveolar movements. Class III elastics with/without extraction of teeth have been used to camouflage the skeletal discrepancy resulting in an acceptable facial profile. Studies have shown that a wide range of tooth movement to compensate for the skeletal changes in Class III patients. The upper and lower limits for incisal movement to compensate for Class III skeletal changes were 120° to SN and 80 ° to MP, respectfully [99].

SUMMARY POINTS

- To differentiate a dental anterior crossbite from a true skeletal discrepancy, one must take into account the molar relationship, functional shift, and profile evaluation in addition to supplementing the diagnosis with intermaxillary cephalometric measurements.

- Class III skeletal growth pattern is established at a very young age. Even though mandibular growth increments are similar between Class I and Class III individuals during the pre-pubertal, pubertal and post-pubertal periods, the mandible typically grows for a longer period of time.

- The uncertainty regarding the long-term results of Class III treatment necessitates the identification of potential predictors of therapeutic success or failure.

- Protraction facemask therapy can be used in the treatment of Class III malocclusions with maxillary deficiencies in both the sagittal and vertical dimensions. The optimal time to address a Class III malocclusion is during primary and early mixed dentitions.

- The use of a tooth-borne appliance as anchorage for maxillary protraction produces adverse effects such as buccal tipping of the posterior molars, proclination of the maxillary incisors and loss of arch length, as a result of mesial migration of the maxillary first molars.

- An expansion and constriction protocol can be used to "disarticulate" the circummaxillary sutures connecting the maxilla to the skull. This process is thought to lower the level of force for orthopedic protraction as well as the length of time needed for maxillary protraction.

- Bone anchored protraction devices using mini-implants can also be used to minimize the side effects associated with maxillary expansion and protraction.

ACKNOWLEDGEMENTS

Declared none.

CONFLICT OF INTEREST

The authors confirm that this chapter contents have no conflict of interest.

REFERENCES

[1] Emrich RE, Brodie AG and Blayney JR. Prevalence of Class I, Class II, and Class III malocclusions (Angle) in an urban population: an epidemiological study. J Dent Res 1965;44:947-1014.

[2] Thilander B and Myrberg N. The prevalence of malocclusion in Swedish school children. Scan J Dent Res 1973;81:12-20.

[3] Magnusson TE. An epidemiologic study of occlusal anomalies in relation to the development of the dentition in Icelandic children. Community Dent Oral Epidemiol 1976;4:121-128.

[4] Tschill P, Bacon W and Sonko A. Malocclusion in the deciduous dentition of Caucasian children. Eur J Orthod 1997;19:361-367.

[5] Chan GK. Class III malocclusion in Chinese: Etiology and treatment. Am J Orthod 1974;65:152-156.

[6] Lew KKK, Foong WC and Loh E. Malocclusion status in Singapore school children. Cited in: Lew KKK, Foong, WC. Horizontal skeletal typing in an ethnic Chinese population with true Class III malocclusion. Br J Orthod 1993;20:19-23.

[7] Allwright WC and Burndred WH. A survey of handicapping dentofacial anomalies among Chinese in Hong Kong. Int Dent J 1964; 14: 505-519.

[8] Lin JJ. Prevalence of malocclusion in Chinese children age 9-15. Clinical Dentistry (Chinese) 1985; 5: 57-65.

[9] Endo T. An epidemiological study of reversed occlusion. Part 1. Incidence of reversed occlusion in children 6 to 14 years old. J Jpn Orthod Soc 1971;30:73-77.

[10] Susami R, Asai Y, Hirose K, *et al.* The prevalence of malocclusion in Japanese school children. J Jpn Orthod Soc 1972;31:319-324.

[11] Baik HS, Han HK, Kim DJ, *et al.* Cephalometric characteristics of Korean Class III surgical patients and their relationship to plans for surgical treatment. Int J Adult Orthod Orthognath Surg 2000;15:119-128.

[12] Toms AP. Class IIII malocclusion: a cephalometric study of Saudi Arabians. Br J Orthod 1989;16:201-206.

[13] Ingervall B, Mohlin B and Thilander B. Prevalence and awareness of malocclusion in Swedish men. Community Dent Oral Epidemiol 1979;6:308-314.

[14] Altemus LA. Frequency of the incidence of malocclusion in American Negro children aged 12-16. Angle Orthod 1959;29:189-200.

[15] Foster TD and Day AJW. A survey of malocclusion and the need for treatment in a Shropshire school population. Br J Orthod 1974;1:73-78.

[16] Hannuksela A. The prevalence of malocclusion and the need for orthodontic treatment in 9-year Finnish school children. Proc Finn Dent Soc 1977;73:21-26.

[17] Kelly JE, Sanchez M and Van Kirk LE. An assessment of the occlusion of the teeth of children. DHEW Publication No (HRA) 74-1612, Washington, DC: National Center for Health Statistics, 1973.

[18] Kelly JE and Harvey C. An assessment of the teeth of youths 12-17 years. DHEW Publication No (HRA) 77-1644, Washington DC: National Center for Health Statistics, 1977.

[19] Guyer EC, Ellis EE, McNamara JA, *et al.* Components of Class III malocclusions in juveniles and adolescents. Angle Orthod 1986; 56: 7-30.

[20] Masaki F. Longitudinal study of morphological differences in the cranial base and facial structure between Japanese and American white. J Jpn Orthod Soc 1980; 39: 436-56.

[21] Ishii N, Deguchi T and Hunt NP. Craniofacial differences between Japanese and British Caucasian female with a skeletal Class III malocclusion. Eur J Orthod 2002;24:493-499.

[22] Ngan P, Hagg U, Yiu C, *et al.* Cephalometric comparisons of Chinese and Caucasian surgical Class III patients. Int J Adult Orthod Orthognath Surg 1997;12:177-188.

[23] Turley P. Orthopedic correction of Class III malocclusion with palatal expansion and custom protraction headgear. J Clin Orthod 1988; May: 314-325.

[24] Latham RA. The sella point and postnatal growth of the human cranial base. Am J Orthod 1972; 61: 156-62.

[25] Kwong WL and Lin JJ. Comparison between pseudo and true Class III malocclusion byVeterans' General Hospital cephalometric analysis. Clin Dent 1987; 69-78.

[26] Battagel J. The aetiological factors in Class III malocclusion. Eur J Orthod 1993; 15: 347-370.

[27] Hagg U, Tse A, Bendeus M, *et al.* Long-term follow-up of early treatment with reverse headgear. Eur J Orthod 2003;25:95-102.

[28] Miyajima K, McNamara JA Jr, Sana M, *et al.* An estimation of craniofacial growth in the untreated Class III female with anterior crossbite. Am J Orthod Dentofac Orthop 1997;112:425-434.

[29] Sugawara J and Mitani H. Facial growth of skeletal Class III malocclusion and the effects, limitations, and long-term dentofacial adaptations to chin cap therapy. Sem in Orthod 1997; 3: 244-254.

[30] Reyes BC, Baccetti T and McNamara JA Jr. An estimate of craniofacial growth in Class III malocclusion. Angle Orthod 2006;76:577-584.

[31] Westwood PV, McNamara JA Jr, Baccetti T, *et al.* Long-term effects of Class III treatment with rapid maxillary expansion and facemask therapy followed by fixed appliances. Am J Orthod Dentofac Orthop 2003;123;306-320.

[32] Baik HS. Limitations in orthopedic and camouflage treatment for Class III malocclusion. Sem in Orthod 2007;13:158-174.

[33] Franchi L, Baccetti T and Tollaro I. Predictive variables for the outcome of early functional treatment of Class III malocclusion. Am J Orthod Dentofac Orthop 1997;112:80-86.

[34] Tahmina K, Tanaka E and Tanne K. Craniofacial morphology in orthodontically treated patients of Class III malocclusion with stable and unstable treatment outcomes. Am J Orthod Dentofac Orthop 2000;117:681-690.

[35] Ngan PW, Hagg U, Yiu C, *et al.* Treatment response and long-term dentofacial adaptations to maxillary expansion and protraction. Sem in Orthod 1997;3:255-264.

[36] Ghiz MA, Ngan P and Gunel E. Cephalometric variables to predict future success of early orthopedic Class III treatment. American Journal of Orthodontics and Dentofacial Orthopedics 2005;127:301-306.

[37] Ngan PW and Wei SHY. Early treatment of Class III patients to improve facial esthetics and predict future growth. Hong Kong Dental Journal 2004;1:28-34.

[38] Piotr Fudalej, Magdalena Dragan and Barbara Wedrychowska-Szulc. Prediction of the outcome of orthodontic treatment of Class III malocclusions—a systematic review. Eur J Orthod 2011;33:190-197.

[39] Turpin DL. Early Class III treatment. Unpublished thesis presented at 81st session, Am Assoc Orthod, San Francisco, 1981.

[40] Rabie ABM and Wong RWK. Early treatment of pseudo Class III malocclusion: A 10-year follow up study. J Clin Orthod 2009;43:692-698.

[41] Frankel R. Maxillary retrusion in Class III and treatment with the functional corrector III. Trans Eur Orthod Soc 1970; 46: 249-259.
[42] Loh MK and Kerr WJS. The function regulator III: Effects and indications for use. Brit J Orthod 1985; 12: 153-157.
[43] Ulgen M and Firatli S. The effects of Frankel's function regulator on the Class III malocclusion. Am J Orthod 1994; 105: 561-567.
[44] Sakamoto T, Iwase I, Uka A, *et al.* A roentgenocephalometric study of skeletal changes during and after chin cup treatment. Am J Orthod 1984; 85: 341-50.
[45] Wendell P, Nanda R, Sakamoto T, *et al.* The effects of chin cup therapy on the mandible: A longitudinal study. Am J Orthod 1985; 87: 265-274.
[46] Mitani H and FuKazawa. Effects of chin cup force on the timing and amount of mandibular growth associated with anterior reverse occlusion. (Class III malocclusion) during puberty. Am J Orthod Dentofac Orthop 1986; 9: 454-6.
[47] Graber LW. Chin cup therapy for mandibular prognathism. Am J Orthod 1977; 72: 23-41.
[48] Ritucci R and Nanda R. The effect of chin cup therapy on the growth and development of the cranial base and midface. Am J Orthod Dentofac Orthop 1984; 85: 341-50.
[49] Uner O, YuKsel S and Ucuncu N. Long-term evaluation after chin cup treatment. Eur J Orthod 1995; 17: 135-141.
[50] Sugawara J, Asano T, Endo N, *et al.* Long-term effects of chin cu p therapy on skeletal profile in mandibular prognathism. Am J Orthod Dentofac Orthop 1990; 98: 127-133.
[51] Ishii H, Morita S, Takeuchi Y, *et al.* Treatment effect of combined maxillary protraction and chincap appliance in severe skeletal Class III cases. Am J Orthod Dentofac Orthop 1987; 92: 304-312.
[52] Deguchi T and Kitsugi A. Stability of changes associated with chin cup treatment. Angle Orthod 1996; 66: 193-146.
[53] Ohyama Y. A longitudinal cephalometric study on craniofacial growth of the orthodontically treated patient with mandibular prognathism. J Osaka Univ Dental School, 1981, 26: 270-94.
[54] Deguchi T and McNamara JA. Craniofacial adaptations induced by chin cup therapy in Class III patients. Am J Orthod Dentofac Orthop 1999; 115: 175-182.
[55] Oppenheim A. A possibility for physiologic orthodontic movement. Am J Orthodont Oral Surgery 1944; 30: 277-328, 345-68.
[56] Delaire VJ, Verdon P and Floor J. Ziele und ergebnisse extraoraler Zuge in postero- anteriore Richtung in anwendung einer orthopadischen Maske bei der Behandlung von Fallen der Klasse III. Fortschr Kiefer Orthop 1976; 37: 246-262.
[57] Petit H. Adaptations following accelerated facial mask therapy in clinical alteration of the growing face. JA McNamara, Jr., KA Ribbens and RP Howe, eds, Monograph 14, Craniofacial Growth Series, Center for Human Growth and Development, University of Michigan, Ann Arbor, 1983.
[58] McNamara JA, Jr. An orthopedic approach to the treatment of Class III malocclusion in growing children. J Clin Orthod 1987; 21: 598-608.
[59] Wilmes B, Nienkemper M, Ludwig B, *et al.* Early Class III treatment with a Hybrid hyrax-Mentoplate combination. J Clin Orthod 2011;55:1-7.
[60] Cha BK and Ngan PW. Skeletal anchorage for orthopedic correction of growing Class III patients. Sem in Orthod 2011;17:124-137.
[61] Hong H, Ngan P, Hang GL, *et al.* Use of onplant as stable anchorage for facemask treatment: A case report. Angle Orthod 2005;75:453-460.

[62] Mandall N, Dibiase A, Littlewood S *et al.* Is early Class III protraction facemask treatment effective? A multicenter, randomized, controlled trial: 15-month follow-up. J Orthod 2010;37:149-161.
[63] Kim JH, Viana MA, Graber TM, Omerza FF, Begole EA. The effectiveness of protraction facemask therapy: a meta-analysis. Am J Orthod Dentofac Orthop 1999;115:675-685.
[64] Jager A, Braumann B, Kim C, Wahner S. Skeletal and dental effects of maxillary protraction in patients with class III malocclusion. A meta analysis. J Orofac Orthop 2001; 62:275-284.
[65] Toffol LD, Pavoni C, Baccetti T, Franchi L, Cozza P. Orthopedic treatment outcome in Class III malocclusion. Angle Orthod 2008; 78:561-573.
[66] Ngan P, Cheung E and Wei SHY. Comparison of protraction facemask response using banded and bonded expansion appliances as anchorage. Sem in Orthod 2007;13:175-184.
[67] Kambara T. Dentofacial changes produced by extraoral forward force in Macaca Irus. Am J Orthod 1977; 71: 249-277.
[68] Nanda R. Protraction of maxilla in rhesus monkeys by controlled extraoral forces. Am J Orthod 1978; 74: 121-141.
[69] Jackson GW, Kokich VG and Shapiro PA. Experimental and postexperimental response to anteriorly directed extraoral force in young Macaca nemestrina. Am J Orthod 1979; 75: 318-333.
[70] Lee K, Ryu Y, Park Y, *et al.*. A study of holographic inferometry on the initial reaction of the maxillofacial complex during protraction. Am J Orthod Dentofac Orthop 1997; 111: 623-32.
[71] Hata S, Itoh T, Nakagawa M, *et al.* Biomechanical effects of maxillary protraction on the craniofacial complex. Am J Orthod Dentofac Orthop 1987; 91: 305-311.
[72] Baik HS. Clinical results of the maxillary protraction in Korean children. Am J Orthod Dentofac Orthop 1995; 108: 583-592.
[73] Merwin D, Ngan P, Hagg U, *et al.* Timing for effective application of anteriorly directed orthopedic force to the maxilla. Am J Orthod Dentofac Orthop 1997; 112: 292-9.
[74] Kapust AJ, Sinclair PM and Turley PK. Cephalometric effects of facemask expansion therapy in Class III children: A comparison of three age groups. Am J Orthod Dentofac Orthop 1998; 113: 204-12.
[75] Baccetti T, McGill JS, Franchi L, *et al.* Skeletal effects of early treatment of Class III malocclusion with maxillary expansion and face-mask therapy. Am J Orthod Dentofac Orthop 1998; 113: 333-43.
[76] Nanda R. Biomechanical and clinical considerations of a protraction headgear. Am J Orthod 1980; 78: 125-139.
[77] Tindlund RS. Orthopaedic protraction of the midface in the deciduous dentition. J Cranio Maxillofac Surg 1989; 17: 17-19.
[78] da Silva Filho OG and Boas MCV, Capelozza Filho L. Rapid maxillary expansion in the primary and mixed dentitions: a cephalometric evaluation. Am J Orthod Dentofac Orthop 1991; 100: 171-179.
[79] Gallagher RW, Miranda F and Buschang PH. Maxillary protraction - Treatment and posttreatment effects. Am J Orthod Dentofac Orthop 1998; 113: 612-9.
[80] Nartallo-Turley P and Turley, P. Cephalometric effects of combined palatal Expansion and facemask therapy on Class III malocclusion. Angle Orthod 1998; 68: 217-223.
[81] Pangrazio-Kulbersh V, Berger J and Kersten G. Effects of protraction mechanics on the midface. Am J Orthod Dentofac Orthop 1998; 114: 484-91.

[82] Sung SJ and Baik HS. Assessment of skeletal and dental changes by maxillary protraction. Am J Orthod Dentofac Orthop 1998; 114: 492-502.

[83] Ngan P, Yiu C, Hagg U, *et al.* Cephalometric and occlusal changes in Class III patients after maxillary expansion and protraction. Eur J Orthod 20:237-45, 1998.

[84] Kajiyama K, Murakami T and Suzuki A. A comparison of orthodontic and Orthopaedic effects of a modified maxillary protractor between deciduous and early mixed dentitions. Am J Orthod Dentofac Orthop 2004; 126:23-32.

[85] Vaughan GA, Mason B, Moon HB *et al.* The effects of maxillary protraction therapy with and without rapid palatal expansion: a prospective randomized clinical trial. Am J Orthod Dentofac Orthop 2005;128:299-309.

[86] Cha BK and Ngan P. Skeletal anchorage for orthopaedic correction of growing Class III patients. Sem in Orthod 2011.

[87] Droshl H. The effect of heavy orthopedic forces on the sutures of the facial bones. Angle Orthod 1975;45:26-33.

[88] Engstrom C and Thilander B. Premature facial synostosis: the influence of biomechanical factors in normal and hypocalcemia young rats. Eur J Orthod 1985;78:35-47.

[89] Linge L. Tissue reactions incident to widening of facial sutures. An experimental study in Macaca mulatta. Trans Eur Orthod Soc 1972;48:481-497.

[90] Liou EJW. Effective maxillary orthopedic protraction for growing Class III patients: a clinical application simulates distraction osteogenesis. Prog Orthod 2005;6:36-53.

[91] Liou EJW. Toothborne orthopedic maxillary protraction in Class III patients. J Clin Orthod 2005;39:68-75.

[92] Ngugen T, Cevidanes L, Cornelis MA, *et al.* Three dimensional assessment of maxillary changes associated with bone anchored maxillary protraction. Am J Orthod Dentofac Orthop 2011;140:790-798.

[93] Cevidanes L, Baccetti T, Franchi L, *et al.* Comparison of two protocols for maxillary protraction: bone anchors *vs.* facemask with rapid maxillary expansion. Angle Orthod 2010;80:799-806.

[94] Wilmes B and Drescher D. A miniscrew system with interchangeable abutments. J Clin Orthod 2008;42:575-580.

[95] Wilmes B, Drescher D and Nienkemper M. A miniplate system for improved stability of skeletal anchorage. J Clin Orthod 2009;43:494-501.

[96] Wilmes B, Nienkemper M and Drescher D. Application and effectiveness of a mini-implant and tooth-borne rapid palatal expansion device: The Hybrid Hyrax. World J Orthod 2010;11:323-330.

[97] Phillips C and Edwards Beal KN. Self-concept and the perception of facial appearance on children. Am J Orthod Dentofac Orthop 1985;87:110-118.

[98] Proffit WR, White RP. The need for surgical-orthodontic treatment. In Proffit WR, White RP ed. Surgical Orthodontic Treatment, Mosby Year Book, St. Louis, 1991; pp 2-4.

[99] Burns NR, Musich DR, Martin CA, *et al.* Class III camouflage treatment: What are the limits? Am J Orthod Dentofac Orthop 2010;137:9.e1-9.e13.

116 *Orthodontic Treatment of Class III Malocclusion*, 2014, 116-150

CHAPTER 5

Class III Orthopedic Treatment with Skeletal Anchorage

Won Moon* and Reena Khullar

Section of Orthodontics, UCLA School of Dentistry, Los Angeles, CA, USA

Abstract: Class III malocclusion has been treated in the past using several different approaches. In growing patients, appliances such as the chin cup and facemask, with or without palatal expansion, have been used for orthopedic correction. Whereas the chin cup has been used to restrain or change the direction of mandibular growth, the facemask has been used to protract the maxilla. The traditional approach of facemask treatment with expansion involves using the maxillary dentition as an anchorage unit. This invariably results in an increase in the vertical dimension of occlusion, due to the buccal tipping and extrusion of the maxillary dentition as well as an increase in incisor inclination, due to the forward movement of maxillary dentition. In Class III high angle cases, both the transverse and anterior movements can cause tipping of the dentition which tends to open the bite; thus, controlling the vertical dimension is of utmost importance during the treatment phase. The aim of this chapter is to introduce a novel approach, using a combination of micro-implants with a rapid palatal expander, and a facemask. This approach skeletally expands and protracts the maxilla, leading to an almost negligible change in vertical dimension, an elimination of adverse dental movements, and a significantly positive change in the patient's facial profile.

Keywords: Class III, Orthopedic Correction, Micro-implants, Rapid Palatal Expansion, Facemask, Maxillary Deficiency, Dental Compensation, MARPE.

INTRODUCTION

A Class III malocclusion is a description of a particular dental relationship, but the underlying cause is frequently skeletal disharmony. Common findings of Class III malocclusion are listed in Table **1**.

An example of such a malocclusion is illustrated in Fig. **1**. It may be accompanied by a functional shift, which, if left untreated, will worsen the skeletal imbalance over time, as shown in Fig. **2**.

***Address correspondence to Won Moon:** UCLA School of Dentistry, Section of Orthodontics, CHS 63-082, Box 951668, 10833 Le Conte Avenue, Los Angeles, CA 90095-1668, USA; Tel: 310-825-4705; Fax: 310-206-5349; Email: wmoon@dentistry.ucla.edu

Peter W. Ngan, Toshi Deguchi and Eugene W. Roberts (Eds)

Table 1: Common findings of Class III malocclusion

Facial Profile	**Concave**
Maxilla	Underdeveloped/Retrognathic
Mandible	Prognathic
Maxillary arch	Narrow
Mandibular arch	Relatively wider than maxillary arch
Dentition	Posterior and/or anterior crossbite Anterior and/or lateral openbite Buccally flared maxillary posterior teeth Lingually tipped mandibular posterior teeth Proclined maxillary incisors Retroclined mandibular incisors

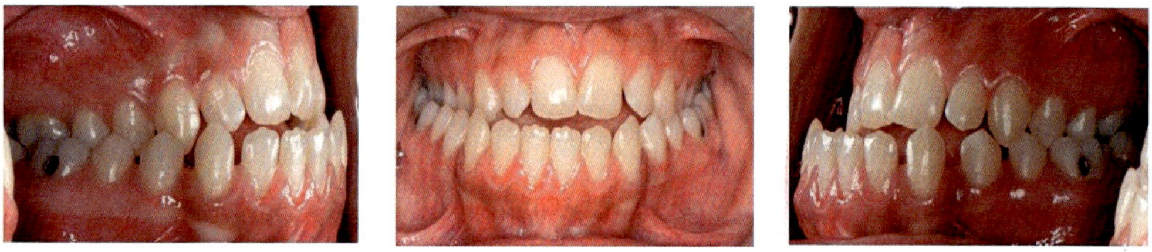

Figure 1: Typical dental compensation are seen in Class III malocclusions: proclined maxillary incisors, retroclined mandibular incisors, buccally tipped maxillary posterior dentition, and lingually tipped mandibular posterior dentition.

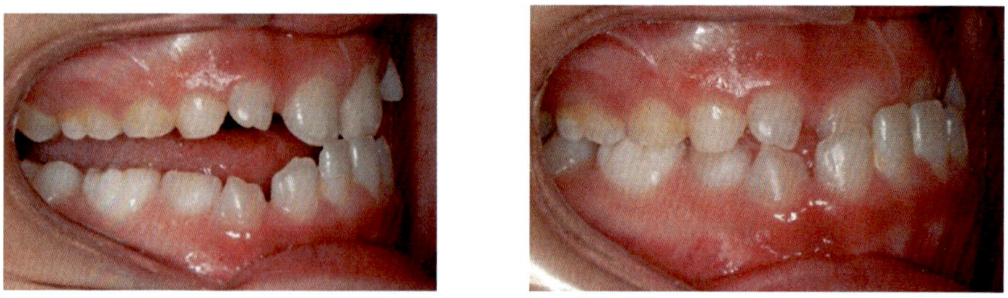

Figure 2: A functional shift due to interference of maxillary central incisors, results in worsening the Class III malocclusion.

In growing patients, attempts were made to reverse the growth pattern of these individuals utilizing various types of orthopedic/orthodontic appliances. In the past, a chin cup has been used to retard or change the direction of the growth of the mandible [1, 2] (Fig. **3**).

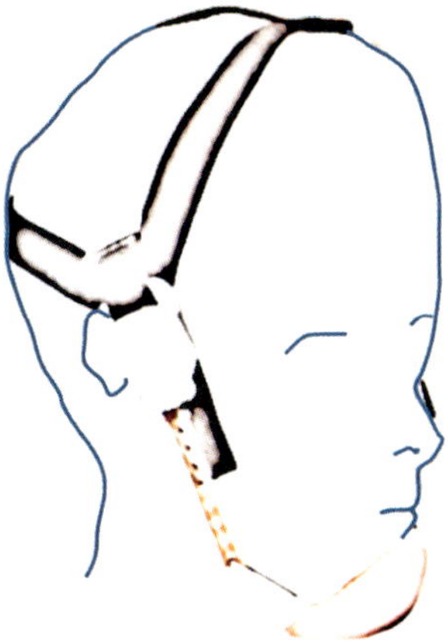

Figure 3: Chin cup is used to restrain and redirect mandibular growth.

Such a restraining effect of a chin cup on mandibular growth has not been found to be stable in the long term [1, 2]. Once the chin cup appliance is removed, condylar regrowth occurs [3] and forward displacement of the mandible takes place during the first year [4]. Furthermore, it is difficult to achieve complete inhibition of mandibular growth [5]. A study found that long-term use of the chin cup appliance for more than 5 years showed effective results in improving the Class III skeletal malocclusion [6]. Due to the unpredictable long-term effect of chin cup therapy and the potential disruption of the temporo-mandibular joint complex, maxillary protraction using a facemask is usually more favorable for treating Class III malocclusion [7] (Fig. **4**).

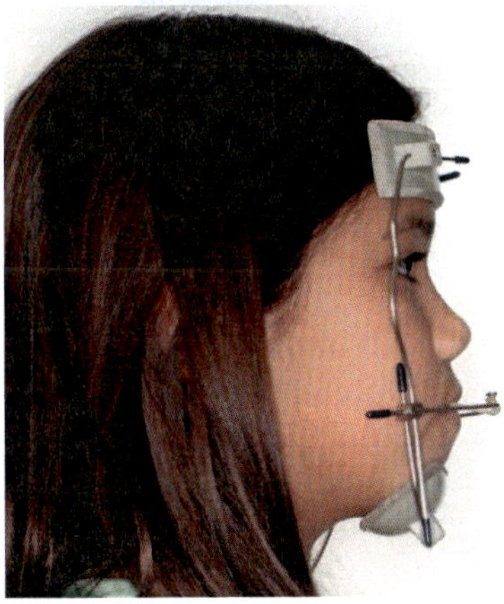

Figure 4: A facemask is used to correct Class III skeletal malocclusion.

CONVENTIONAL FACEMASK IN CLASS III TREATMENT

The facemask enhances the growth of the maxilla by force application to the circummaxillary sutures in an anterior direction. It has been used in combination with or without a maxillary rapid palatal expander (RPE) [8] to disarticulate the circummaxillary sutures, and aid in the forward movement of maxilla, as well as expand the narrow maxilla (Fig. **5**).

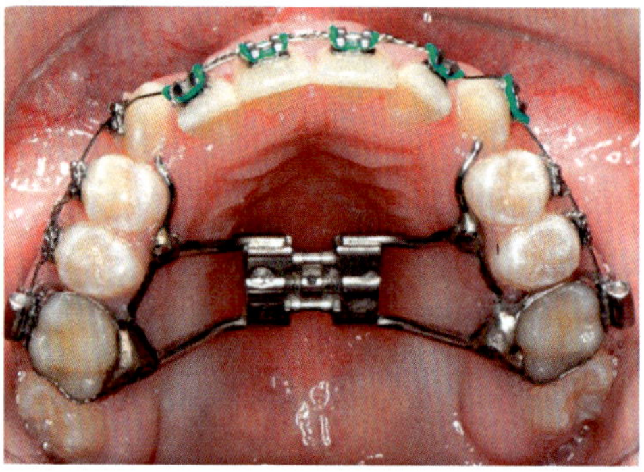

Figure 5: Rapid Palatal Expander (RPE) has bands on first molars for anchorage.

Maxillary expansion has been considered important during maxillary protraction with a facemask by some investigators [9]. A finite element model (FEM), comparing the displacement of craniofacial sutures with maxillary protraction alone and in combination with maxillary expansion, found that upward and forward rotation of the maxilla occurred with maxillary protraction alone [10]. When the maxillary protraction was combined with 4 mm of transverse expansion, there was no rotational movement of the maxilla. The study also indicated that displacement of the maxilla in all three planes of space was greater, when maxillary protraction was combined with maxillary expansion. Significant skeletal and dental changes have been reported with the simultaneous use of facemask and fixed palatal expansion [11-13].

In traditional maxillary expansion and protraction, the force application is tooth-borne. This resulted in undesirable side effects, such as excessive buccal tipping the maxillary posterior teeth and flaring of the already proclined maxillary incisors [14, 15] (Figs. **6** and **7**). A study was performed to evaluate the skeletal effects on the maxilla after rapid palatal expansion, using cone beam computed tomography [16]. The study concluded that the total amount of expansion resulted from a combination of orthopedic expansion, alveolar bone bending and orthodontic tipping. Often, treatment with traditional maxillary expansion combined with facemask therapy reduces the magnitude of Class III malocclusion in an A-P plane, but produces undesired dental movements: 1. increase in the vertical dimension, and 2. clockwise rotation of the mandible [17, 18]. The Class III correction is largely achieved from the clockwise rotation of the mandible, rather than from the forward movement of maxilla. In high-angle cases, the bite force is not adequate to overcome the dental tipping caused by the treatment, thereby leading to irreversible consequences such as anterior open-bite (Fig. 7).

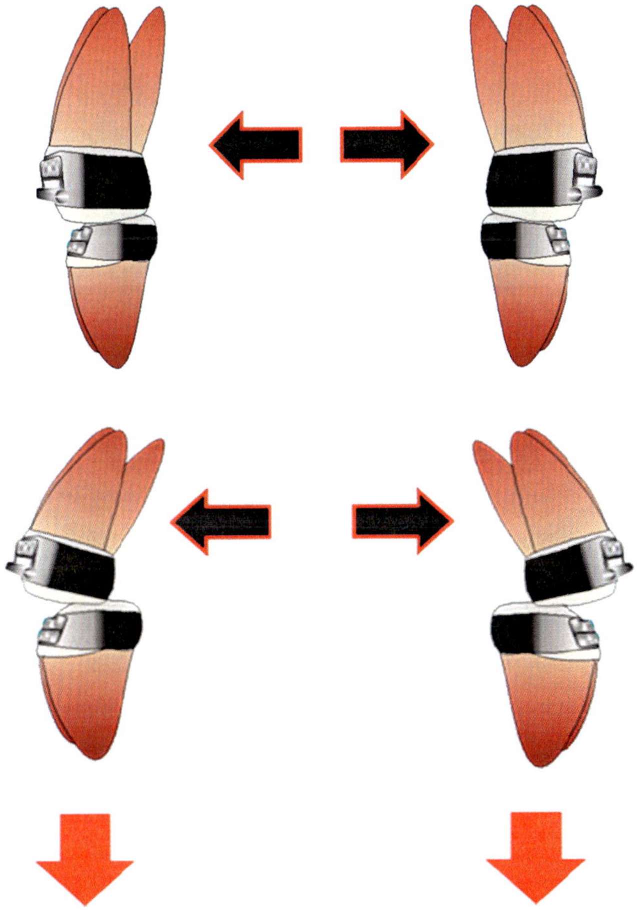

Figure 6: The above illustration shows the effect of traditional rapid palatal expansion, causing buccal tipping of maxillary molars, resulting in increased vertical dimensions.

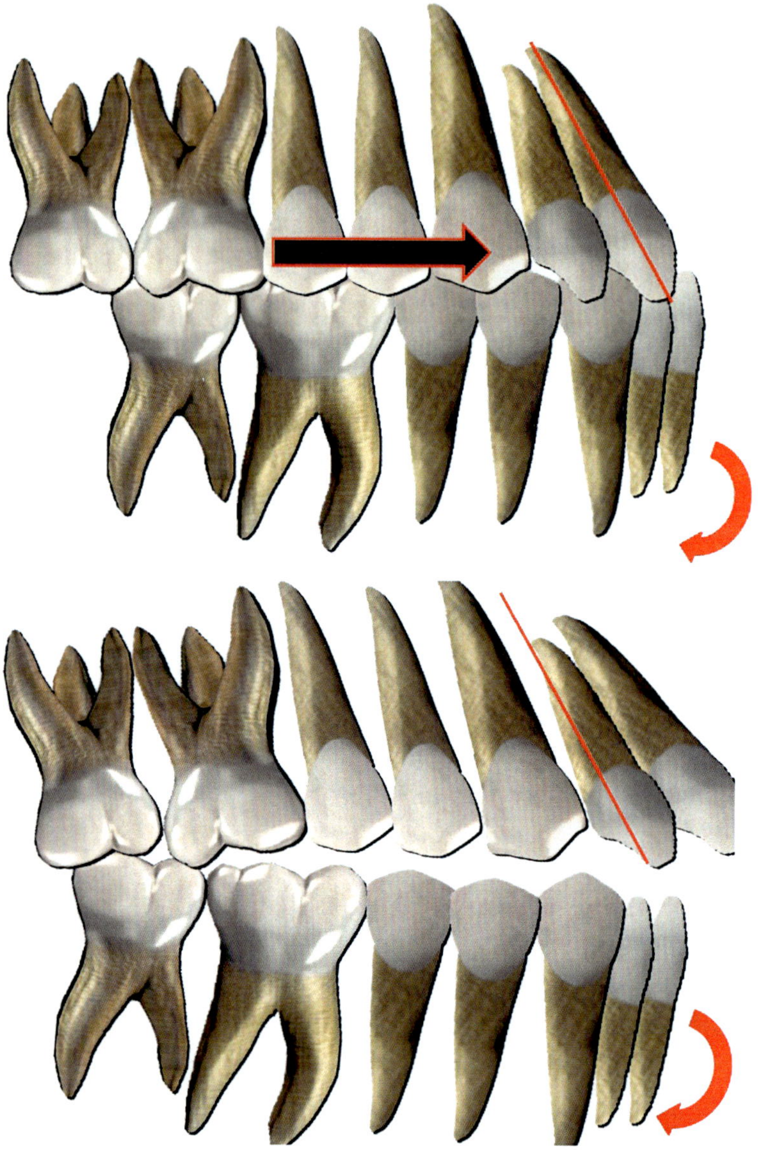

Figure 7: The line of force (above) and the resulting moment tips the maxillary dention mesially resulting in the bite opening (below), due to the clockwise rotation of the mandible in a high angle case.

Hence, it becomes difficult to assess the magnitude of the actual skeletal expansion and protraction due to the dentoalveolar changes in a 3-dimensional space. Furthermore, skeletal correction is largely limited by the increase in dental compensation during the treatment. Continuation of such a treatment until skeletal harmony is achieved will result in an undesirable dental relationship (*i.e.* Class II malocclusion).

NOVEL TREATMENT MODALITY UTILIZING MICRO-IMPLANTS

The previously mentioned problems can be controlled when the micro-implants are utilized [19] in combination with the traditional treatment protocol. The RPE can be modified as illustrated. The body of the device is fitted closely to the palatal vault, and it is fixated to the palatal bone using four micro-implants. Four cylinders with 1.5 mm internal diameter and 2 mm in length are soldered to the main frame of the RPE. These cylinders are used as jigs for implant placement, and they also provide support and prevent tipping of these implants during the RPE activation. After cementing the appliance securely, four micro-implants, 1.5 mm in diameters and 11 mm in length, are placed through the tubes. By using 11 mm implants, they provide 5-6 mm of palatal bone engagement. Two micro-implants, one on each side, are adequate; however, the entire apparatus has to be remade when one of the two micro-implants fails. Using four implants is advantageous when such a failure occurs; as long as each side has at least one intact implant, this appliance is fully functional. This micro-implant assisted RPE (MARPE) also has facemask hooks attached to the molar bands (Fig. **8**).

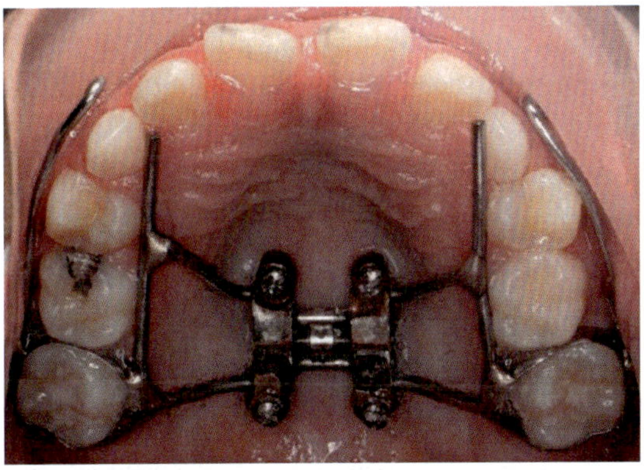

Figure 8: MARPE with facemask hooks.

The whole apparatus is attached to the palatal bone near the mid-palatal suture, and as this appliance is activated, expansion force is applied directly to the mid-palatal suture and subsequently to the circummaxillary sutures. The expansion and protraction forces are applied directly to the maxillary complex rather than the dentition. A recent FEM study at UCLA School of Dentistry by MacGinnis and Moon demonstrated the significantly favorable skeletal force distribution when the MARPE is used.

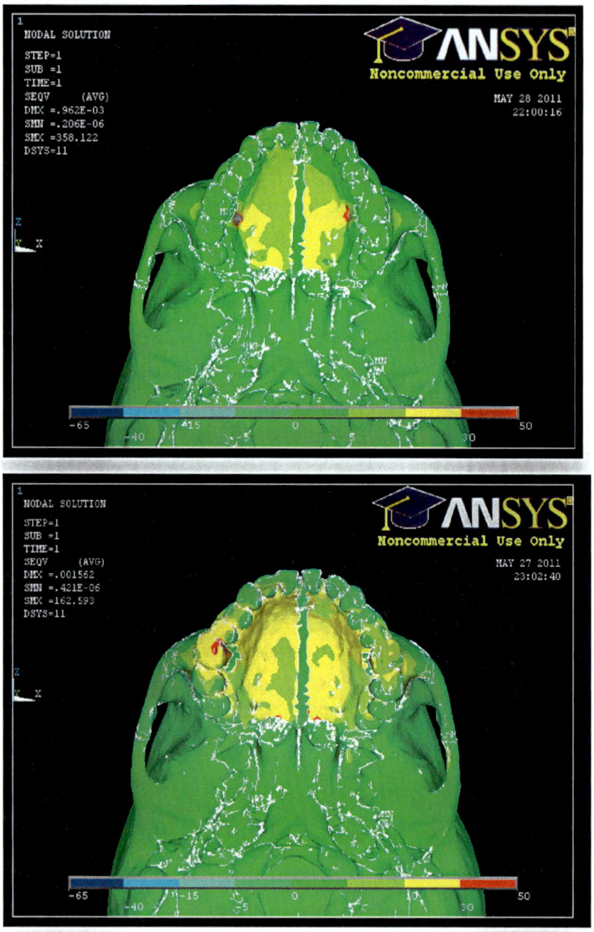

Figure 9: FEM study showing skeletal force level distribution for RPE (image above) *vs.* MARPE (image below).

The above illustration shows the expansion force is isolated to the palate with MARPE, whereas the significant amount of force was distributed to dentition with RPE. This implies that MARPE ensures skeletal expansion and less dental tipping (Fig. **9**).

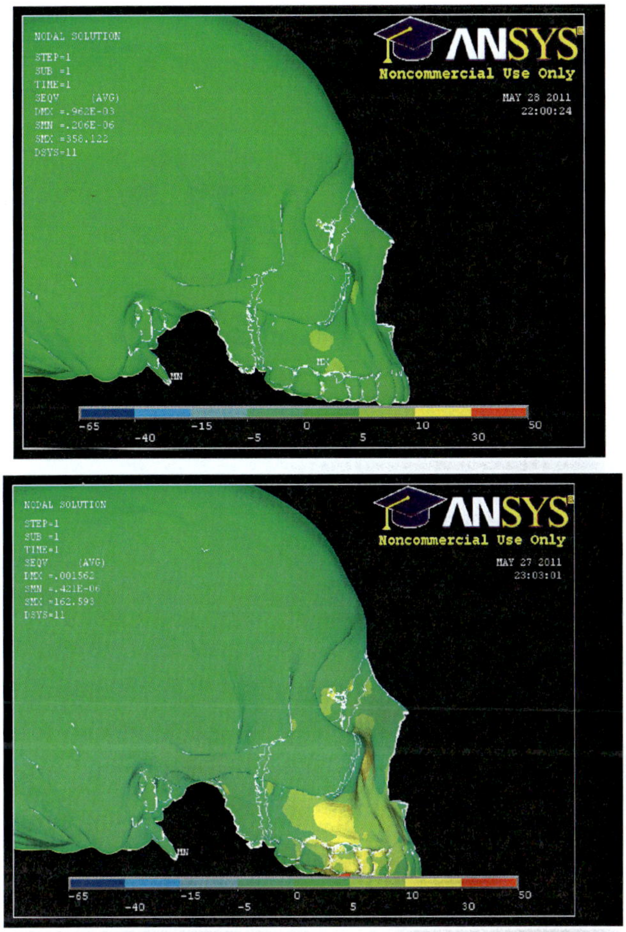

Figure 10: FEM study showing skeletal force level distribution for RPE (image on the right) *vs.* MARPE (image on the left).

The lateral views also show that a significantly higher force level is exerted around the buttress area with RPE compared to MARPE which implies that the rotational movements of the buccal segments is limited with the MARPE (Fig. **10**). The preliminary FEM study by Wu and Moon also demonstrates that pure skeletal protraction is possible when a facemask is used with MARPE.

Sutural loosening has been reported by several authors using a combination of a two-hinge rapid maxillary expander, intraoral maxillary protraction springs and/or a regular alternate maxillary expansion and constriction protocol [20]. This protocol mimicked distraction osteogenesis, resulting in effective disarticulation of maxilla without over expanding the maxilla. In another study, alternate rapid expansion and constriction of maxilla was compared with only rapid expansion of maxilla, both involving the use of using a two-hinge maxillary expander and maxillary protraction springs [21]. The study concluded that alternate rapid maxillary expansion and constriction resulted in more anterior displacement of the maxilla, which was found stable over a period of two years. In another study involving unilateral cleft lip and palate patients, conventional maxillary protraction with reverse pull headgear and Class III elastics was compared with an untreated control group [22]. Statistically significant changes in the amount of maxillary protraction, as well as in the maxillo-mandibular skeletal relationship were found in the treatment group.

The novel approach using micro-implants was used on over 60 patients in the last 8 years by Moon, the results of which are convincingly superior to the conventional approach. Adverse side effects (buccal tipping of the molars and proclination of the incisors) of the traditional RPE protocol can be completely eliminated. In addition, some of the existing dental compensations can also be reversed as the skeletal relationship improves. Most importantly, this novel approach is also effective in patients with extremely severe high angles. The Class III malocclusion patients with high mandibular plane angles are classified as a very difficult problem in orthodontics [23, 24], because control of the vertical dimensions is of utmost importance. This new treatment protocol can provide a critically needed solution to this problem. In this chapter, three clinical cases will be presented to illustrate utility of the MIRPE method.

CASE STUDY 1

An 11 year old female patient was presented with a skeletal and dental Class III malocclusion (SNA: 80.4, SNB: 83.2, ANB: -2.8°, Wits: -15.4 mm). The patient presented a concave facial profile, with bimaxillary protrusion, proclined maxillary incisors, incompetent lips, slight mentalis strain, and Class III malocclusion (Figs. **11** and **12**).

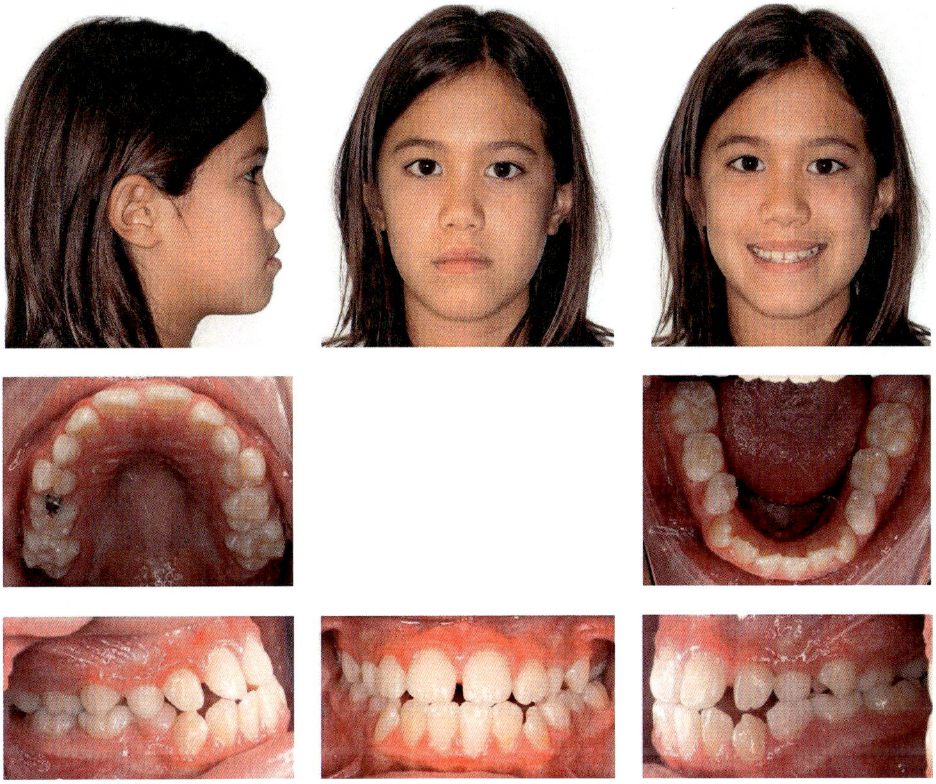

Figure 11: Composite of Patient 1, before starting orthopedic treatment.

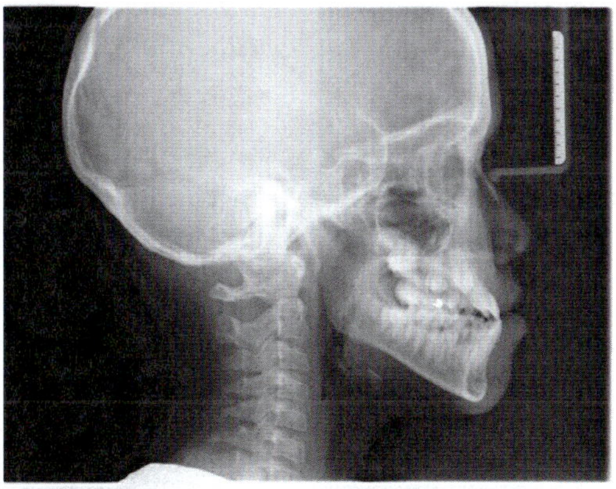

Figure 12: Lateral cephalogram of Patient 1, pre-treatment.

Treatment Plan

The treatment plan consisted of Phase I treatment using MARPE with a facemask, followed by a Phase II treatment.

Phase I Treatment (Orthopedic Treatment):

A MARPE was fabricated with bands on first molars, and extension arms with facemask hooks bilaterally. This MARPE also had four soldered tubes (2 mm in length and 1.5 mm of internal diameter) for micro-implant placement. After cementing the MARPE, four micro-implants (1.5 mm in diameter and 11 mm in length) were securely placed in the palate, two on each side of the mid-palatal suture (Fig. **13**).

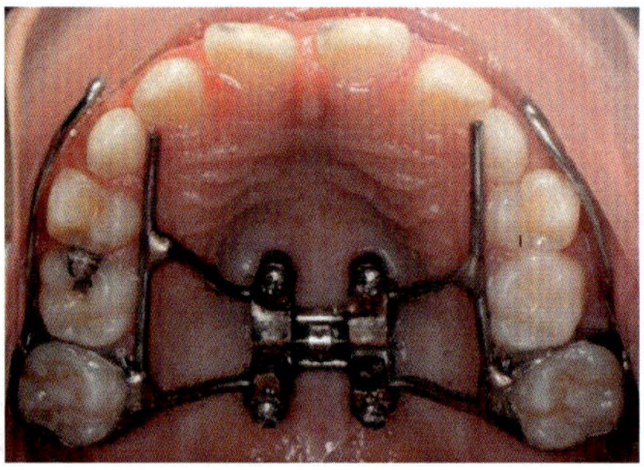

Figure 13: Micro-Implant assisted Rapid Palatal Expander (MARPE), used in Patient 1.

The molar bands were used merely as a guide to position the appliance against the palate until the micro-implants were inserted. After the implant placement, the bands play a minimal role in retention; they serve more as attachment points for the facemask hooks. The entire appliance is secured to the palate by the micro-implants, ensuring that both expansion and protraction forces will be delivered to the maxillary skeletal complex. The patient and her parents were instructed to turn the expansion screw three times a week and to wear a facemask for 12-14 hours per day. The expansion was stopped after 6 weeks.

Results

After 10 months of treatment, significant facial changes were noted (Figs. **14** and **15**). The previous concave facial profile was transformed into a convex facial profile with bimaxillary protrusion, and the soft tissue superimposition demonstrates the striking facial changes (Fig. **15**). The lateral cephalogram also shows significant orthopedic correction; the maxillary position has changed drastically only within a 10-month period (Fig. **16**). Considerable skeletal

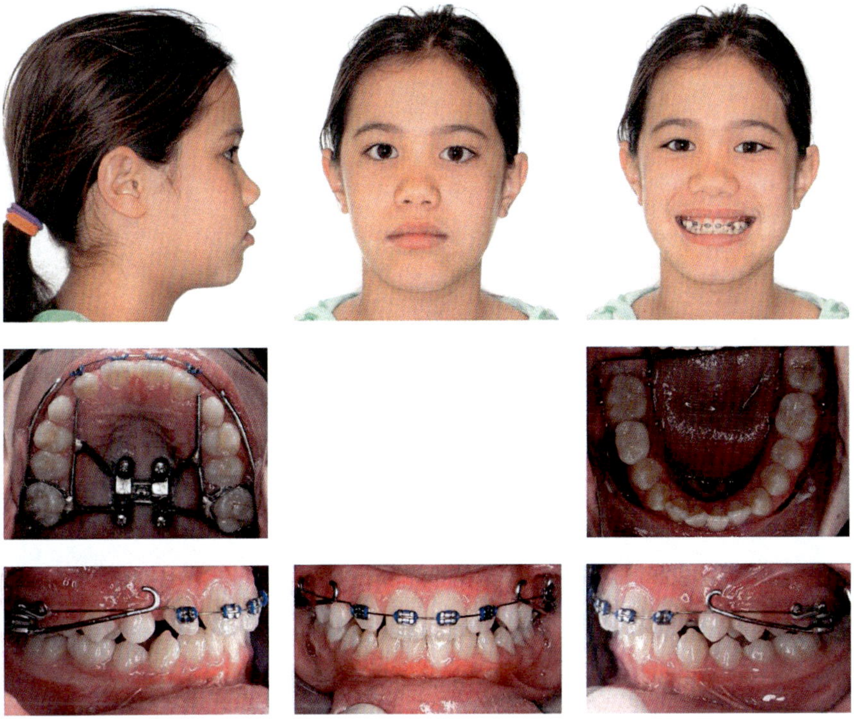

Figure 14: Composite of Patient 1, after 10 months of orthopedic treatment.

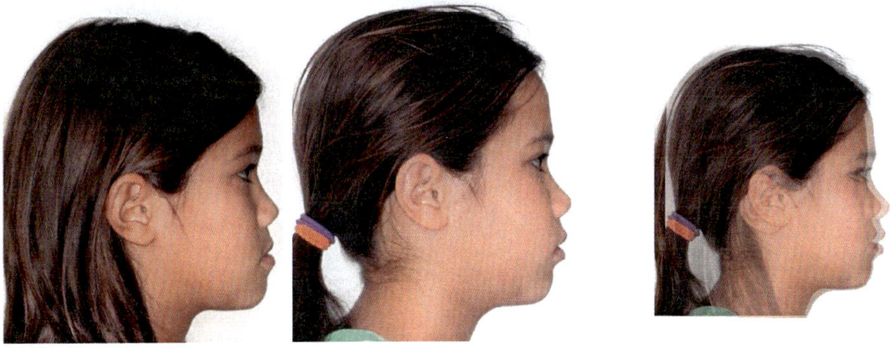

Figure 15: A comparison of the facial profiles shows a marked change from a pretreatment concave profile (image on the left) to a slightly convex profile (image on the right) after 10 months of treatment with facemask and MARPE. Superimposition of the two profiles (the bottom image) shows a significant facial change.

movement occurred: SNA angle increased by 7 degrees, ANB angle also increased by 7 degrees, and Wits measurement decreased by 14 mm. As the skeletal relationship improved, the U1-SN angle decreased from 119 to 109 degrees. Contrasted with the forward tipping of the incisors as seen with the conventional facemask therapy [25, 26], the dental compensation decompensated as skeletal harmony was achieved (Fig. **17**). This clearly demonstrates the functional matrix theory [27] in action. At this point, this patient no longer had skeletal disharmony, and she now became a Class I bimaxillary protrusive patient. Facemask treatment was discontinued at this time.

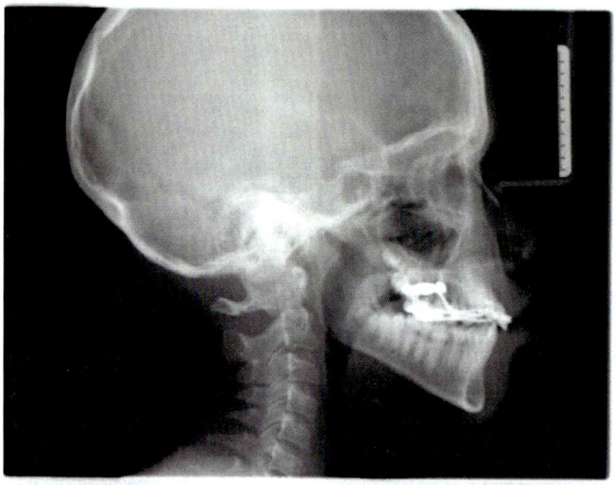

Figure 16: Lateral cephalogram for Patient 1 after 6 weeks of MARPE activation and 10 months of facemask wear.

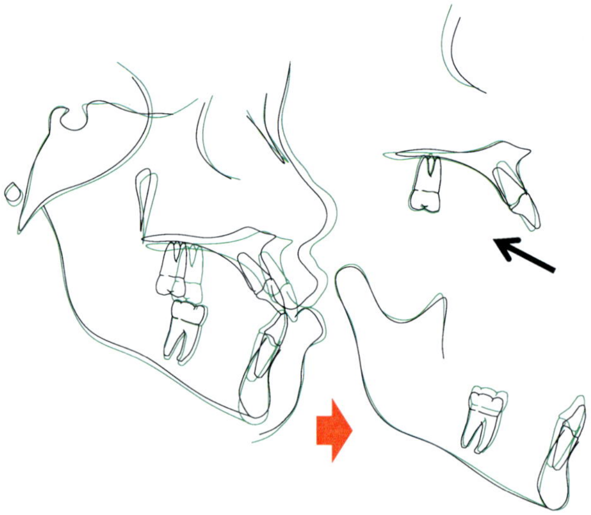

Figure 17: Superimposition showing significant skeletal change in maxilla and dental decompensation of upper and lower dentition; pretreatment (black) and 10 months post-orthopedic-treatment (green) The red arrow represents the direction of maxillary protraction and the black arrow shows the line of force, due to lip pressure, that tips the incisors distally.

Phase II Treatment (Orthodontic Treatment):

Mandibular dentition was banded and bonded. Micro-implants (1.5 mm in diameter and 6 mm in length) were placed between second bicuspids and first molars bilaterally. En-Masse retraction of mandibular dentition was performed until the ideal mandibular incisor position was achieved. The maxillary dentition was subsequently banded and bonded, and micro-implants (1.5 mm in diameter and 6 mm in length) were placed between second bicuspids and first molars bilaterally for En-Masse retraction of the maxillary dentition.

Results

After 28 months of treatment without a facemask, a significant change in profile was achieved. A straight facial profile with relaxed lips was observed, and the mentalis strain was eliminated (Fig. **18**). Fig. **19** illustrates facial profile changes during the two phases of the treatment. During the orthopedic phase of the treatment, facial convexity was achieved; however, the patient exhibited lip

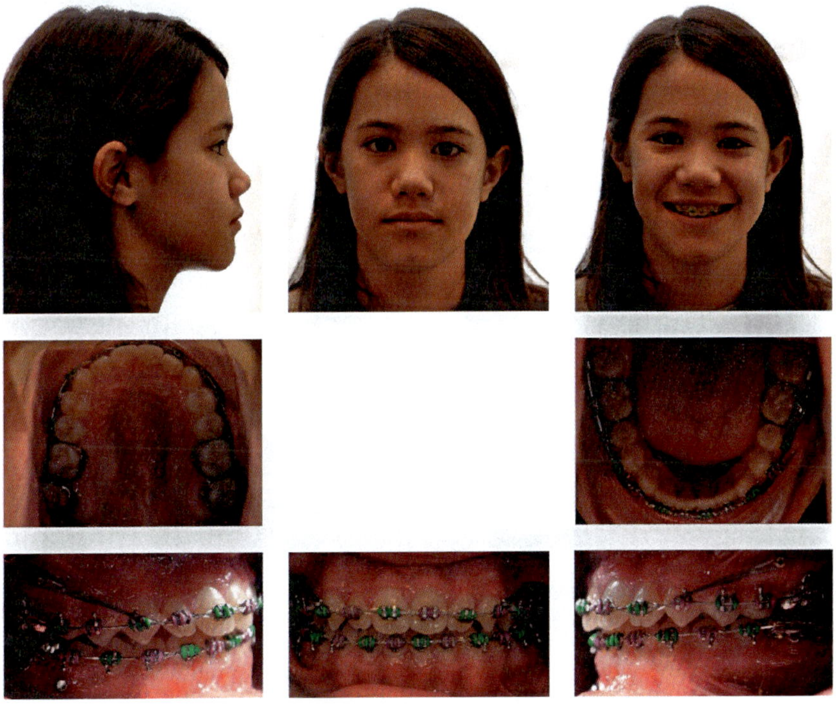

Figure 18: Composite after 28 months of orthodontic treatment without a facemask.

protrusion. During the orthodontic phase of the treatment, the lip protrusion was eliminated by distally driving the upper and lower dentition. During this phase of the treatment the SNA and ANB angles did not change illustrating the skeletal correction achieved during the phase I treatment was stable. Both maxilla and mandible grew significantly with an equal magnitude. The upper and lower incisor inclinations also changed, obviously from the retraction of upper and lower dentition (Figs. **20, 21** and **22**).

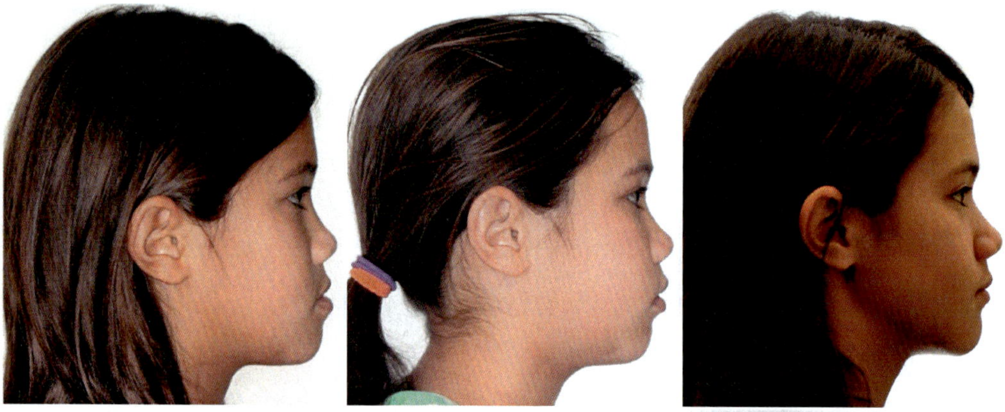

Figure 19: A comparison of facial profiles shows a change from being concave with lip protrusion (pretreatment) to slightly convex with lip protrusion (after 10 months of orthopedic treatment with MARPE and facemask) to slightly convex without lip protrusion (after 28 months of orthodontic treatment: En-Masse retraction), in order from left to right respectively.

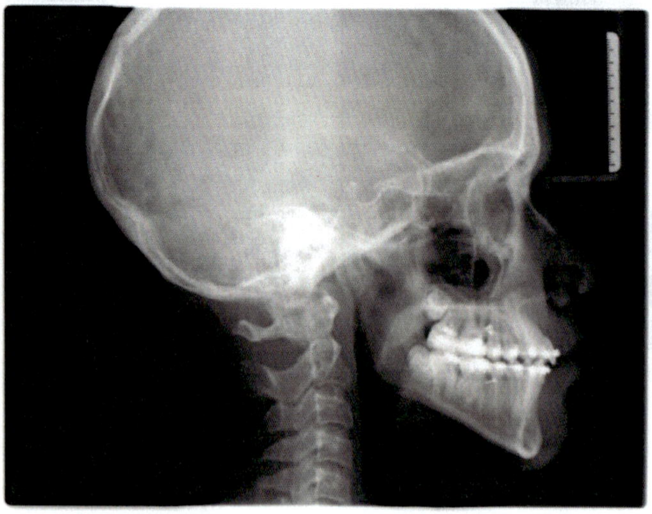

Figure 20: Lateral cephalogram after 28 months of orthodontic treatment.

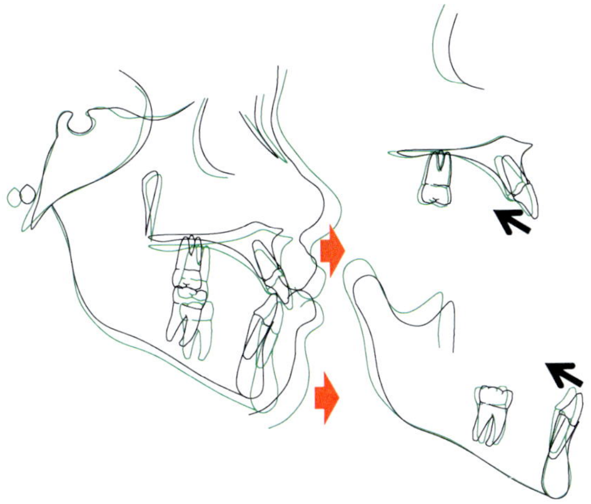

Figure 21: Superimposition showing significant growth in the maxilla and mandible together (red arrows), after 28 months of treatment without facemask (green), when compared with the timepoint of completion of Phase 1 treatment (black). Retraction of upper and lower incisors is also noted by the direction of the black arrows.

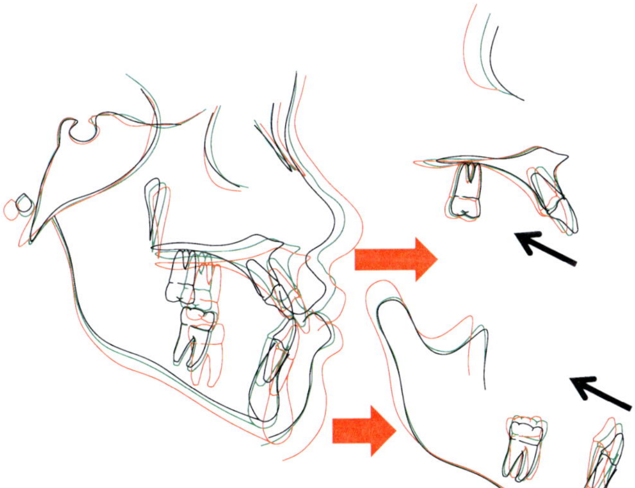

Figure 22: Superimposition: preorthopedic (black), post-orthopedic, preorthodontic (green) and post-orthodontic (red).

Throughout both phases of the treatment, the FMA and SN-GoGn angles were stable indicating that this treatment provided a good control of the vertical dimension. The cephalometric measurements are shown in Table **2**.

Table 2: Comparison of cephalometric measurements for Patient 1.

Measurement	Initial	Phase I (10 months with facemask)	Phase II (28 months without facemask)
SNA (°)	80.4	87.4	87.6
SNB (°)	83.2	82.8	83.5
ANB (°)	-2.8	4.6	4.2
Wits (mm)	-15.4	-1.3	2.2
U1-SN (°)	119.0	108.6	111.9
L1-GoGn (°)	87.0	88.1	81.7
FMA (°)	28.1	29.2	28.5
SN-GoGn (°)	32.3	32.5	31.1

Conclusions

With combining MARPE and facemask, it is possible to enhance the growth of the maxilla in antero-posterior (AP) direction without dental side effects, and the existing dental compensations can be corrected.

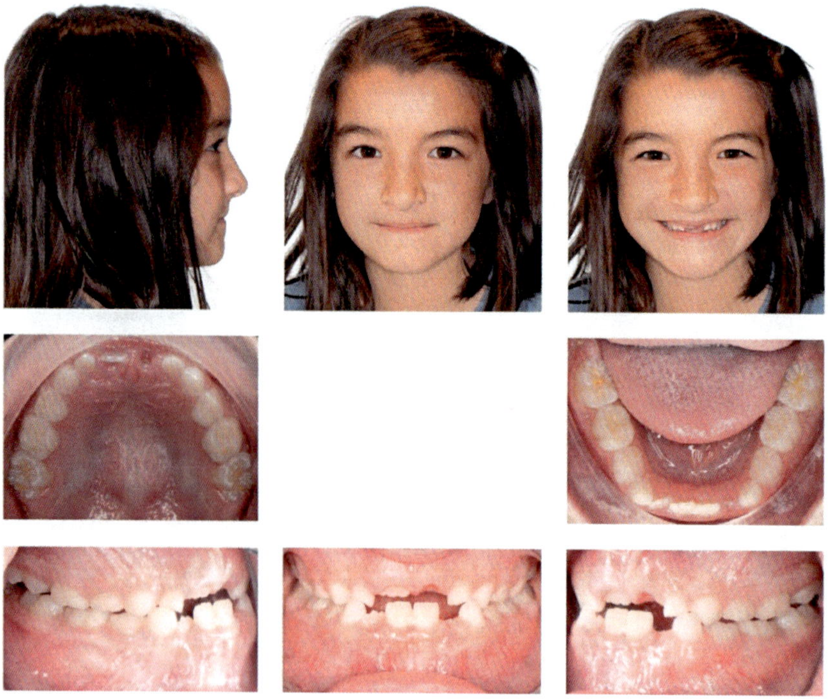

Figure 23: Composite of Patient 2, before initiation of orthopedic treatment.

CASE STUDY 2

An 8-year-old female patient was presented with a multiple family history of skeletal Class III. She had a concave facial profile in early mixed dentition with retroclined lower incisors, and compensated class I dental relationship (Fig. **23**). Her ANB measurement was -2.1° (Fig. **24**).

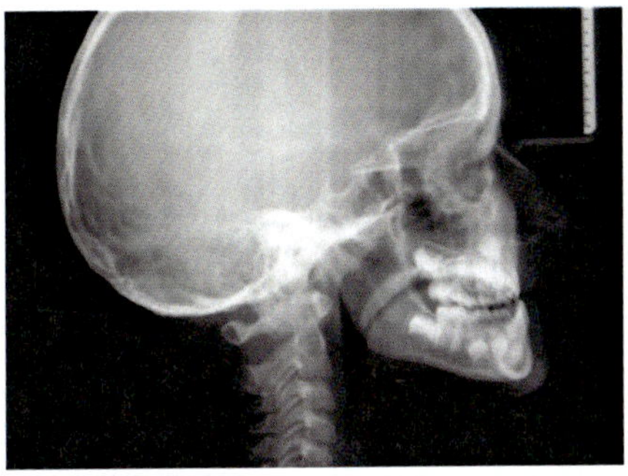

Figure 24: Lateral cephalogram of Patient 2, pretreatment.

Treatment Plan

The treatment plan consisted of Phase I treatment using MARPE with a facemask and monitoring the growth and development.

Phase I Treatment (Orthopedic Treatment):

The same treatment protocol was used as in the Case Study 1.

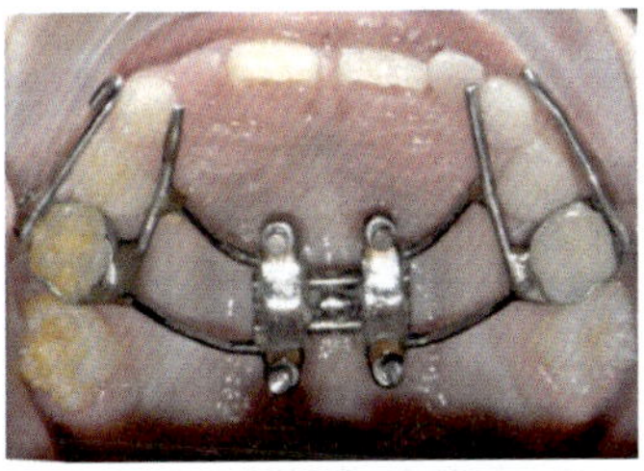

Figure 25: Micro-Implant assisted Rapid Palatal Expander with facemask hooks was used in Patient 2.

Results

After 14 months of treatment with MARPE and facemask therapy, significant facial changes were evident (Figs. **26** and **27**). A straight facial profile became more convex, and Fig. **27** clearly demonstrates the magnitude of this change.

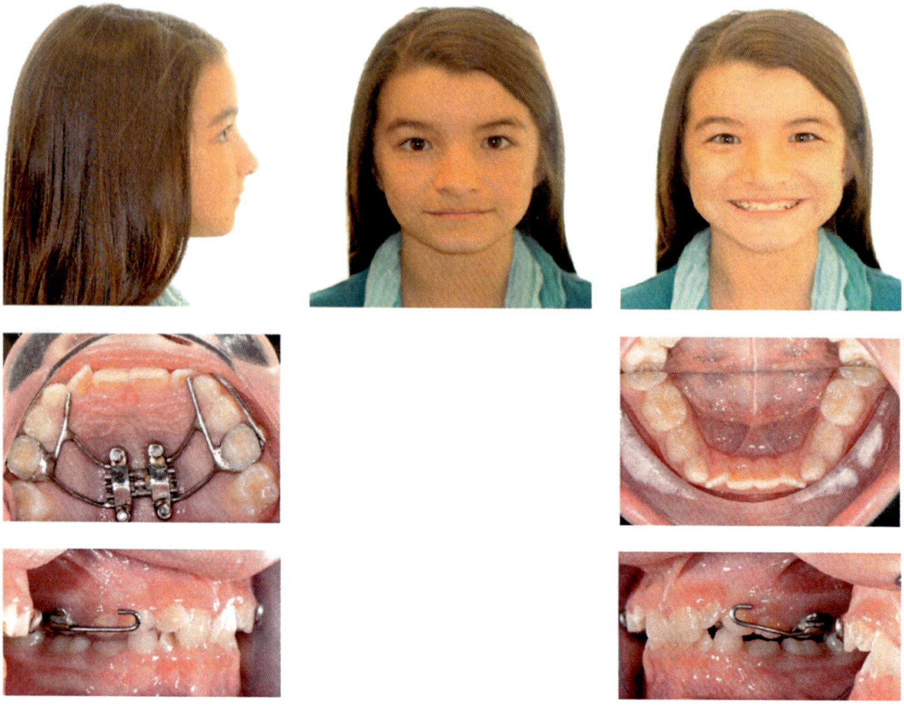

Figure 26: Composite of Patient 2, after 14 months of facemask wear.

Fig. **28** shows the lateral cephalogram after 14 months of orthopedic treatment: SNA angle increased by over 4 degrees and ANB angle also increased by 6 degrees. As the skeletal relationship improved, the U1-SN angle decreased from 94 to 86

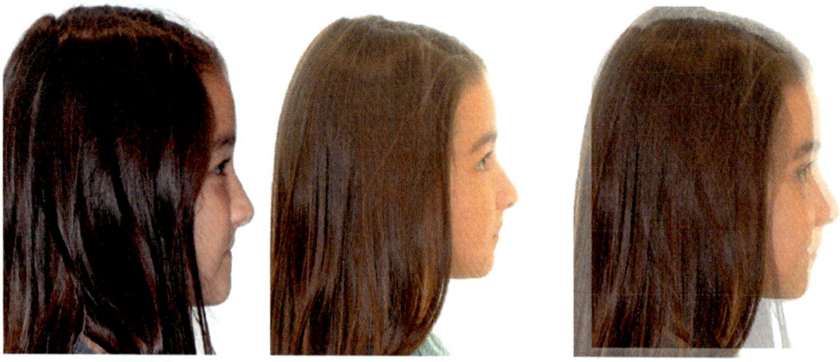

Figure 27: A comparison of the facial profiles shows a change from a straight profile (pretreatment, image on the left) to a slightly convex profile (after 14 months of facemask treatment, image on the right). Superimposition of the two profiles (the bottom image) shows a significant facial change.

degrees and the L1-MP angle increased from 79 to 89 degrees. As with the previous case, the dental compensation decompensated as skeletal harmony was achieved (Fig. **29**). Her dental relationship exhibited characteristics of a Class II Division 2 malocclusion. At this time the patient was instructed to stop the facemask wear.

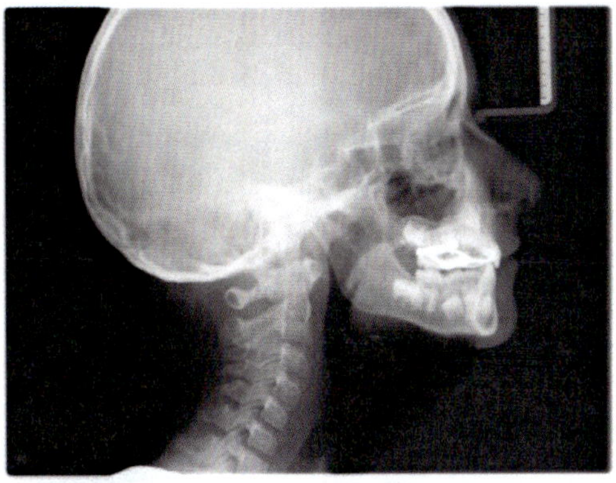

Figure 28: Lateral cephalogram of Patient 2, posttreatment.

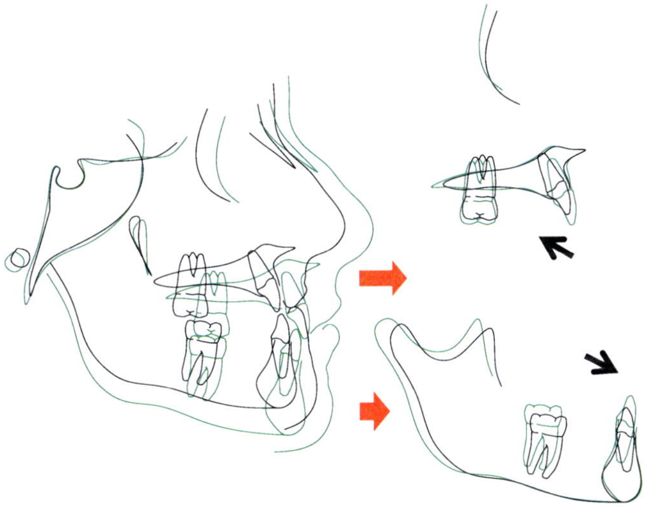

Figure 29: Superimposition showing significant downward and forward movement of maxilla after 14 months of facemask wear (green), when compared with pretreatment timepoint (black). Dental decompensations were also noted as the skeletal relationship has changed.

Growth and Development After Facemask

The patient stopped wearing the facemask for 15 months.

Results

After 15 months, the facial profile became slightly straighter (Figs. **30** and **31**). The SNA angle decreased by 1 degree and the U1-SN increased by 5 degrees, indicating that there may be a slight reversal of the skeletal relationship changes from the Phase 1 treatment. The cephalometric measurements are shown in Table **2**. When the

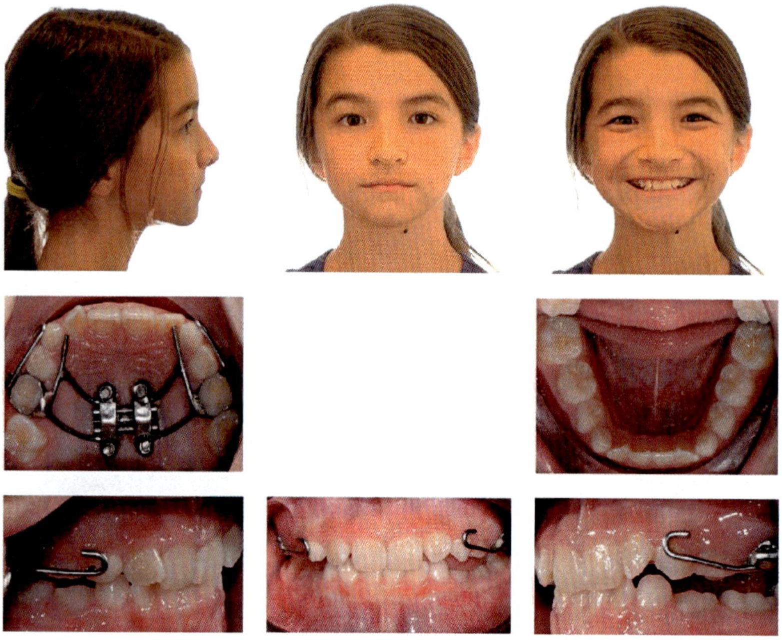

Figure 30: Composite of Patient 2, without facemask wear for 15 months.

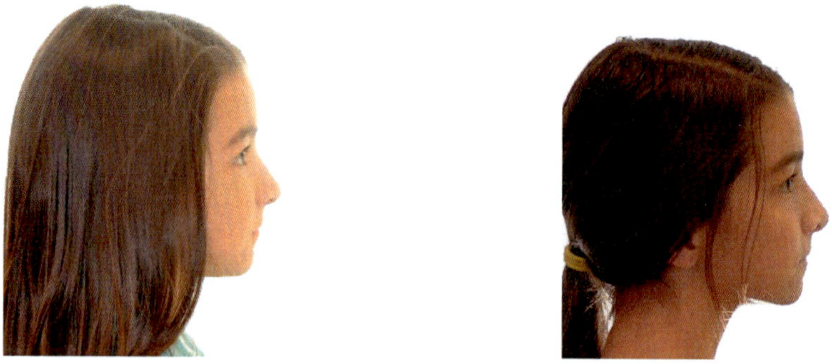

Figure 31: Comparison of facial profile shows a change from a slightly convex profile (after 14 months of facemask wear, image on the left) to a slightly straighter profile (without facemask wear for 15 months, image on the right).

superimpositions were evaluated, her maxilla actually grew in a forward direction but the mandible grew slightly more (Figs. **32** and **33**). It seems the skeletal growth achieved by the orthopedic correction did not experience a relapse, but rather the patient continued to grow in a Class III pattern, meaning the magnitude of the mandibular growth was greater than that of the maxilla. This phenomenon is well supported by many studies [28-31]. Some suggest overcorrection to accommodate for further Class III growth pattern of these patients [32]. The maxillary incisors proclined slightly as mandibular growth exceeded maxillary growth (Fig. **33**). This brings up an interesting question, "When is the optimal time for treatment?" There is no short answer for this question [33]. Generally the treatment duration increases when the treatment is started early but the patients' compliance is significantly better with younger patients. One must consider many factors: the severity of the problem, existence of traumatic occlusion, airway problems, *etc.*

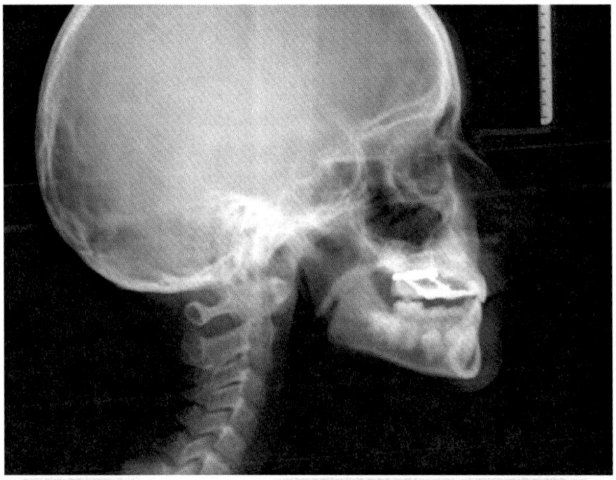

Figure 32: Lateral cephalogram of Patient 2, 15 months without facemask wear.

The patient was instructed to wear a facemask again for 3 months to manage her growth patterns. After 3 months of wearing the facemask, the patient's facial convexity returned (Figs. **34** and **35**). The mandible continued its growth but the maxilla grew slightly more, and the maxillary incisor decompensated again (Figs. **36** and **37**). Again, this illustrates the phenomena that the incisor position is largely dictated by the skeletal relationship. This means that by correcting the skeletal imbalance, the dental problem can be self-limiting. Table **3** illustrates the changes.

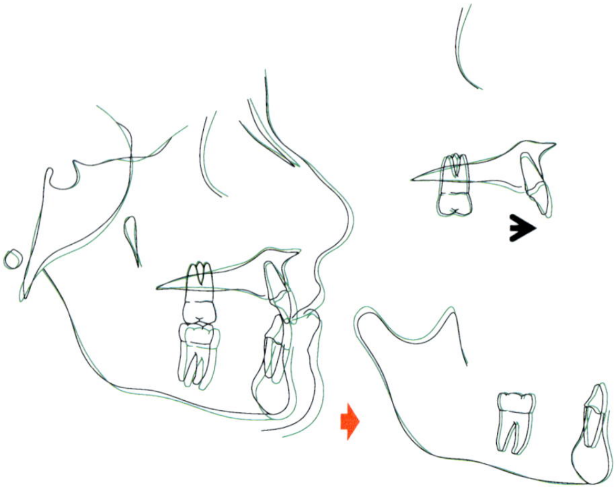

Figure 33: Superimposition shows a slight growth in the maxilla, but a comparatively increased growth in the mandible: after 14 months of facemask wear (black) and without facemask wear for 15 months (green).

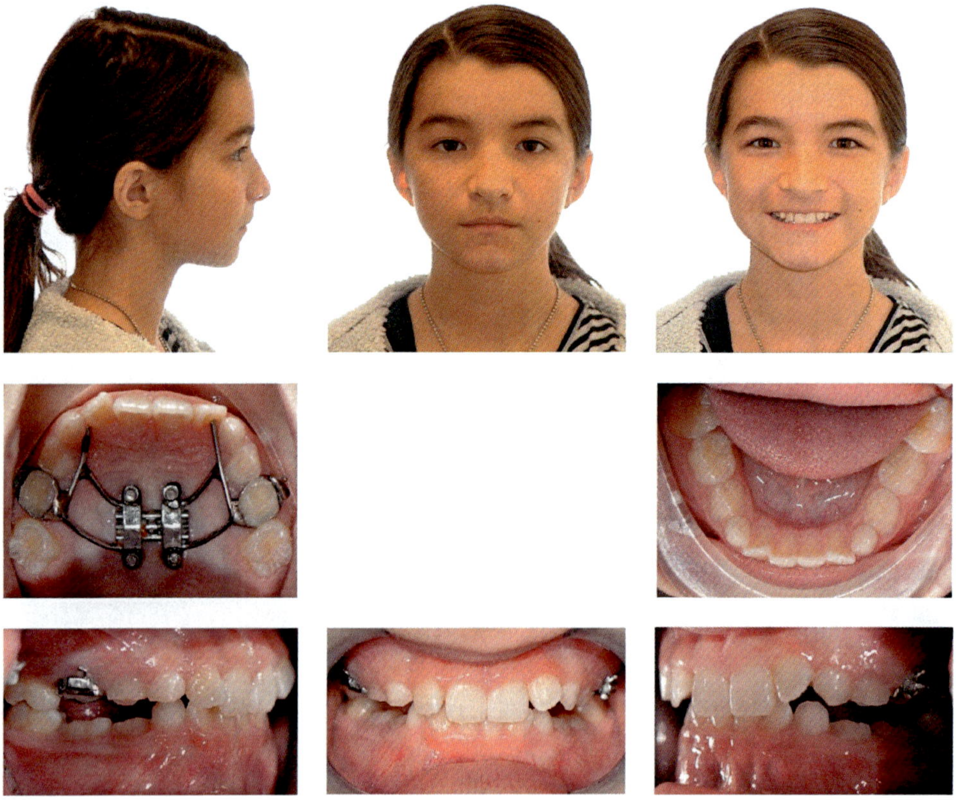

Figure 34: Composite of Patient 2, after resuming treatment with facemask for 3 months.

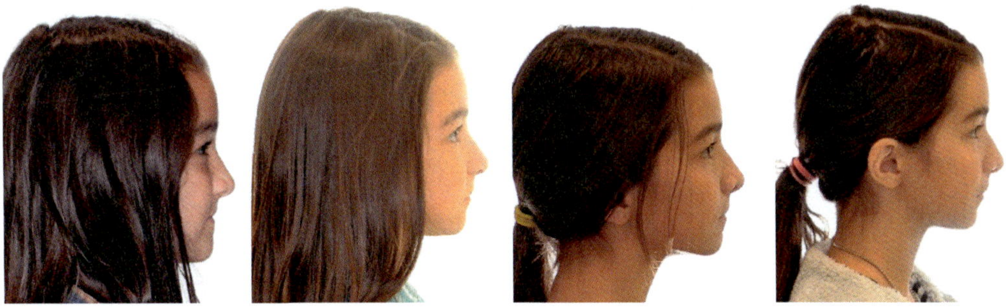

Figure 35: Comparison of facial profile after 15 months of facemask wear (two images on the left), no facemask wear for 14 months (two images in the middle), and facemask wear again for 3 months (two images on the right).

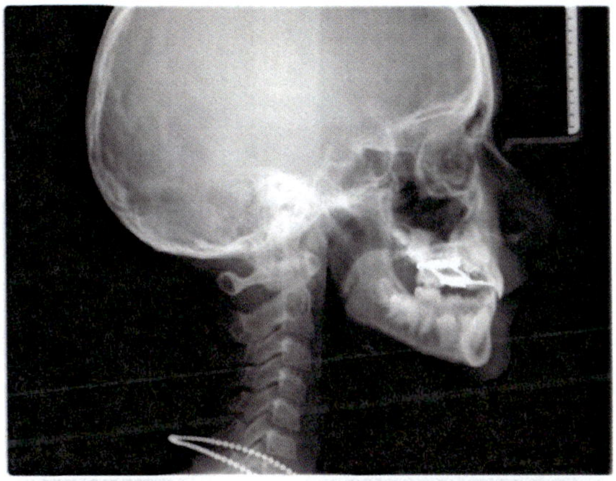

Figure 36: Lateral cephalogram of Patient 2, 3 months after reinstating facemask treatment.

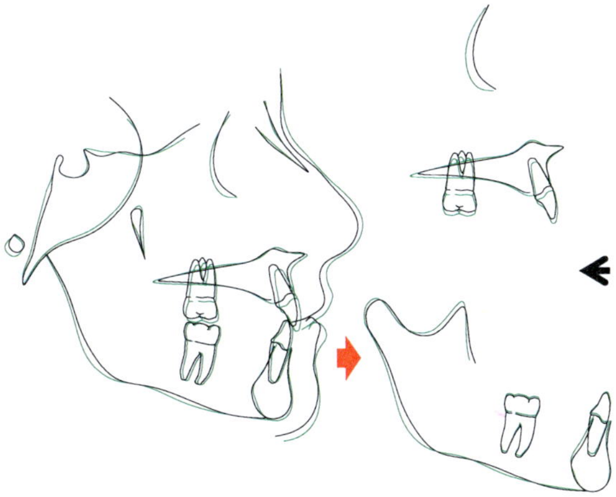

Figure 37: Superimposition shows a slight growth in the mandible, but a comparatively increased growth in the maxilla after 3 months of facemask wear (green).

Table 3: Comparison of cephalometric measurements for Patient 2.

Measurement	Initial	Phase I (14 Months with Facemask)	15 Months Without Facemask	10 Months with Facemask
SNA (°)	75.0	79.4	79.3	79.7
SNB (°)	77.1	75.5	76.4	76.3
ANB (°)	-2.1	3.8	2.9	3.5
Wits (mm)	-7.1	2.7	-1.3	0
U1-SN (°)	93.8	86.2	91.5	88.9
L1-GoGn (°)	78.8	89.2	89.6	90.8
FMA (°)	22.2	23.5	23.9	23.5
SN-GoGn (°)	27.7	29.3	30.4	30.3

Conclusion

This treatment protocol is highly effective in creating a Class II relationship in younger patients, but patients must be followed through until the growth is complete.

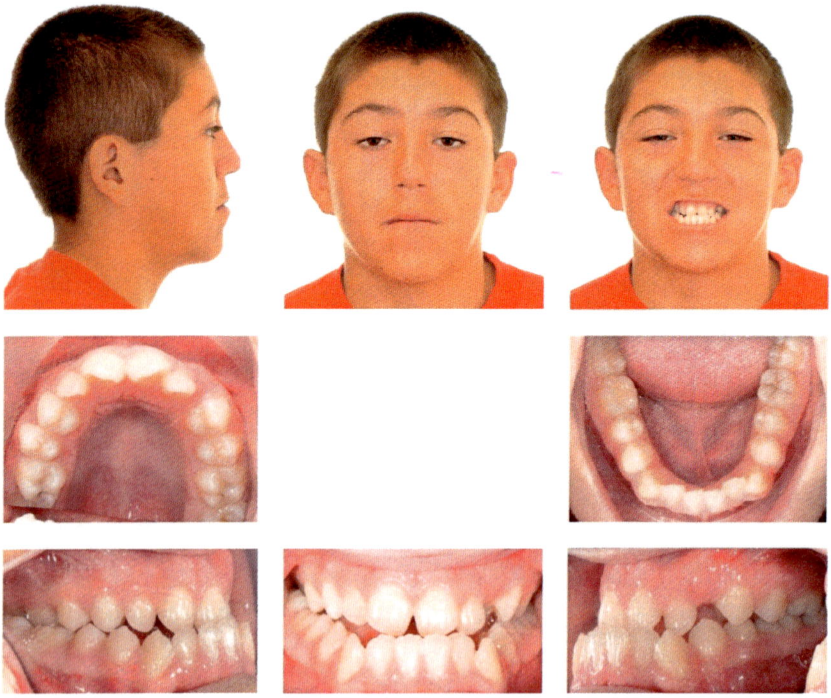

Figure 38: Composite of Patient 3, before initiation of orthopedic treatment.

CASE STUDY 3

A 12 year old male patient was presented with a dental and skeletal Class III relationship (ANB: -3.3° and Wits: -27 mm), and anterior/posterior crossbite. He had a straight facial profile with high mandibular plane angle (FMA: 32 degrees, SN-GoGn: 39 degrees) (Figs. **38** and **39**).

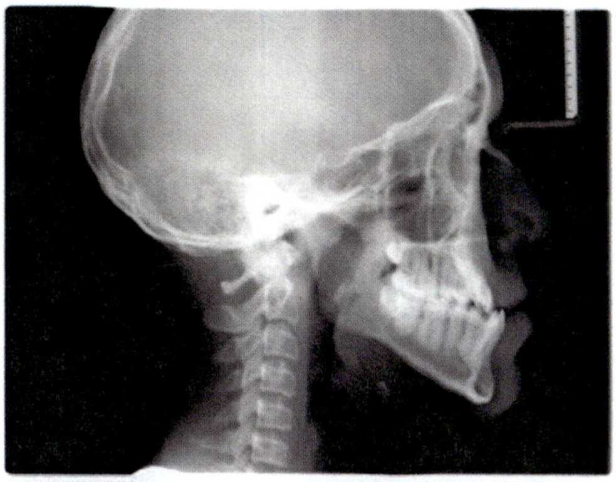

Figure 39: Lateral cephalogram of Patient 3, pretreatment.

Treatment Plan

The treatment plan consisted of Phase I orthopedic treatment utilizing with MARPE facemask and subsequent Phase II orthodontic treatment.

Phase I Treatment (Orthopedic Treatment):

The same treatment protocol was used as in the Case Study 1.

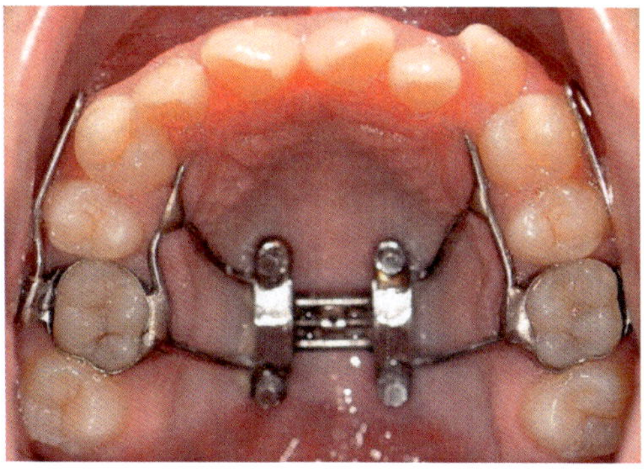

Figure 40: Micro-Implant supported Rapid Palatal Expander was used in Patient 3.

Results

After 20 months of treatment, a slight facial change was noted (Figs. **41** and **42**). The dental relationship improved to Class I, and the anterior/posterior crossbite was eliminated. Despite the extreme skeletal discrepancy (Wits: -27mm), patient's facial profile was slightly concave due to vertically displaced mandible. After improving his AP relationship to a Class I occlusion from a full Class III relationship entirely by orthopedic movements, the facial change was relatively minimal. However, when the cephalograms were examined, a significant amount of maxillary skeletal movement occurred: the ANB angle increased by 6 degrees and the Wits value improved by 17 mm (Figs. **43** and **44**; Table **4**). As the maxillary position improved, the maxillary incisors decompensated as we have seen from the previous cases. Despite this large magnitude of maxillary movement, the FMA and SN-GoGn angles did not change.

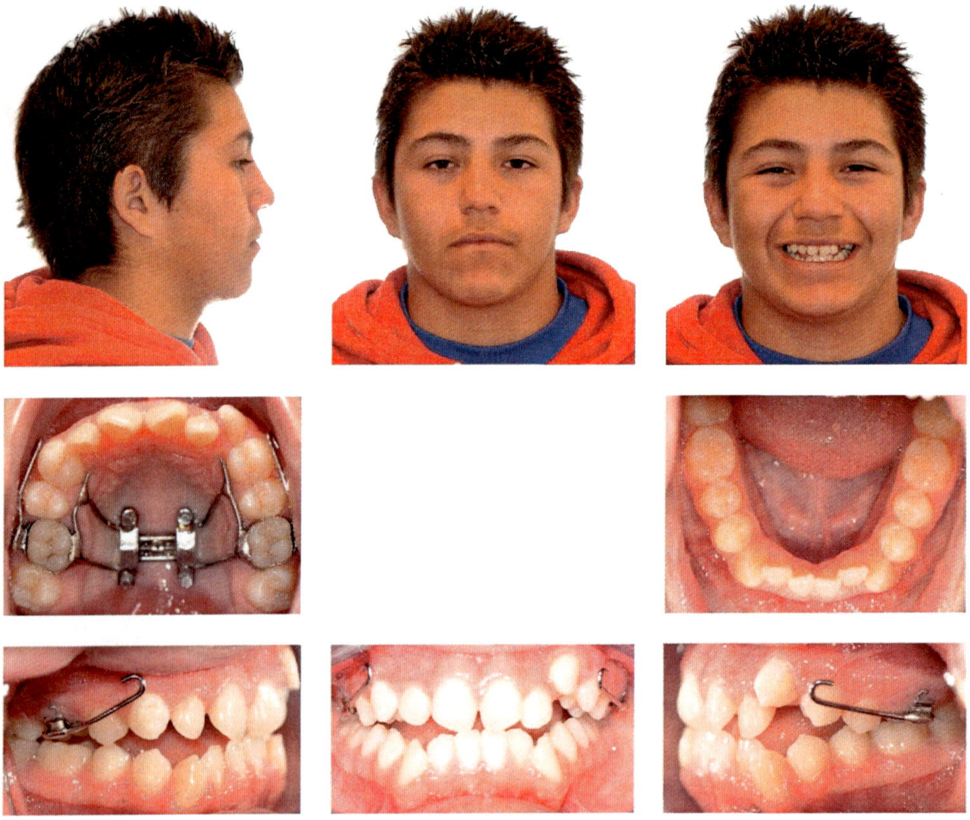

Figure 41: Composite of Patient 3, after 20 months of orthopedic treatment.

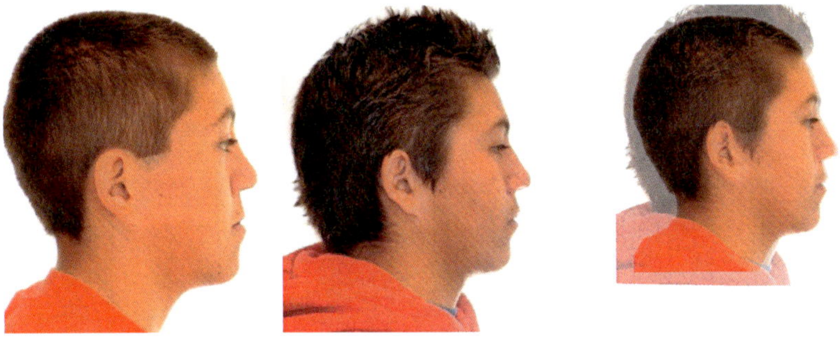

Figure 42: Composite of Patient 3 after 20 months of facemask wear. Comparison of facial profile shows change from a slightly concave profile before treatment (image on the left) to a slightly convex profile after 20 months of treatment (image in the middle).

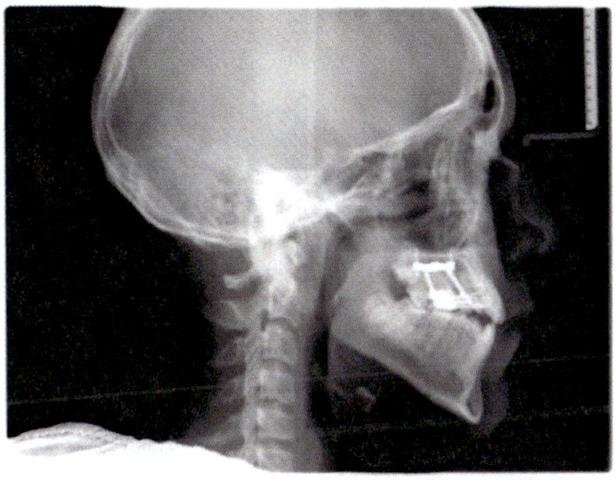

Figure 43: Lateral cephalogram for Patient 3, after 20 months of treatment.

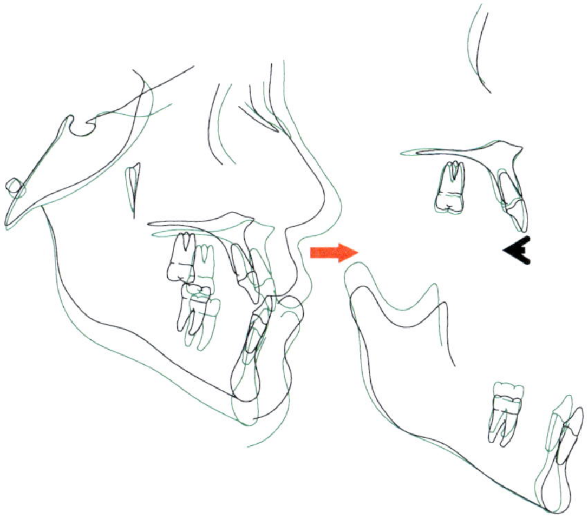

Figure 44: Superimposition showing significant skeletal change in maxilla and dental decompensation of upper dentition: pretreatment (black) and 20 months posttreatment (green).

Table 4: Comparison of cephalometric measurements for Patient 3.

Measurement	Initial	Phase I (20 months with facemask)
SNA (°)	74.1	76.9
SNB (°)	77.4	74.5
ANB (°)	-3.3	2.5
Wits (mm)	-27.3	-10.5
U1-SN (°)	97.2	94.5
L1-GoGn (°)	83.2	83.9
FMA (°)	31.8	31.8
SN-GoGn (°)	39.3	40.1

Phase II (Orthodontic Treatment):

Upper first bicuspids will be extracted to alleviate the severe arch-length deficiency. The lower arch will be intruded and distalized utilizing micro-implants as anchors. The VTO illustrates the final treatment goal (Figs. **45** and **46**). In a high angle case, the VTO is helpful in deciding how much protraction is necessary to compensate for the counterclockwise rotation of the mandible during the phase II treatment. The protocol is similar to that of surgical treatment planning.

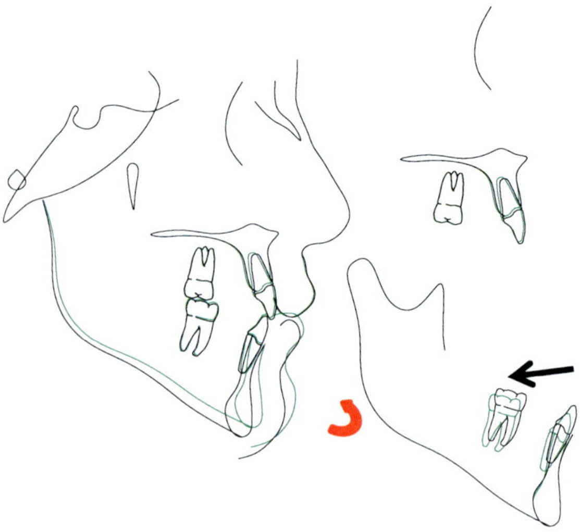

Figure 45: VTO showing the counterclockwise rotation of the mandible (green) and the amount of intrusion and distalization needed in the lower dentition (green).

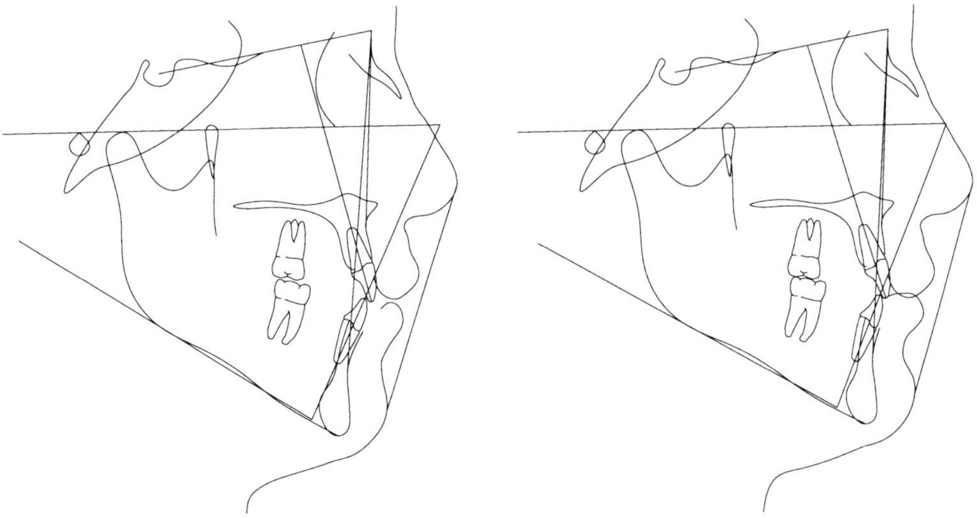

Figure 46: Comparison between preorthodontic tracing and VTO

Conclusion

The Class III high angle cases can be treated with a good control of the vertical dimension utilizing MARPE and facemask. The vertical reduction is necessary in order to achieve facial harmony after the Phase I treatment, and more protraction of maxilla is required as the mandibular plane increases in order to accommodate for the counterclockwise rotation of the mandible during the Phase II orthodontic treatment.

CONCLUDING REMARKS

Correction of Class III malocclusion with significant skeletal discrepancy, especially in high angled individuals, can be difficult without orthognathic surgery. Although growth modification techniques have been tried over the years, the results were often unreliable. The main obstacles against the traditional orthopedic correction were undesired dental movements, lack of vertical control, and patient compliance. The first two problems can be managed when micro-implants are incorporated. By utilizing such a technique, it was confirmed that a pure orthopedic correction is not only possible but also that the existing dental compensation due to skeletal disharmony can be reversed. Further study can shed some more light in the areas of proper timing of the treatment, elimination of patient compliance factors, *etc.* Hong and Moon explored the possibility of applying orthopedic force directly to the novel micro-implant design developed by Moon, and the results were promising [34, 35]. Development of an Intra-oral fixed orthopedic device can eliminate the use of facemask, and the orthopedic Class III correction can be far more predictable in the future.

SUMMARY POINTS

- The traditional early treatments of Class III malocclusion include an orthopedic correction utilizing a facemask (FM) and rapid palatal expander (RPE). Although this approach provides some improvements in skeletal relationship, a significant amount of unwanted dental movement cannot be avoided.
- The above mentioned dental movements include excessive anterior flaring of the maxillary incisors as well as buccal tipping and extrusion of the maxillary molars, causing the increase in lower face height especially in high angle cases.
- By incorporating the micro-implants into a RPE, the expansion force is concentrated near the suture according to the FEM study. This approach reduces bone bending, eliminates dental tipping, and aids in disarticulating the circummaxillary sutures connecting the maxilla to the skull.
- By applying FM force directly to microimplant-assisted RPE, the unwanted dental movements can be eliminated completely. Furthermore, the preexisting dental compensation (flared maxillary incisors and retroclined mandibular incisors) decompensates as the skeletal relationship improves.
- When this approach is used for very young patients, skeletal correction can be achieved quickly. After the orthopedic force is terminated, patient's Class III growth pattern resumes and the mandible grow at a faster rate than the maxilla. Overcorrection and long-term follow up are suggested.

- When this approach is used for patients with high mandibular plane angles, the vertical dimensions can be controlled. After the AP correction, vertical reduction through orthodontic intrusion is necessary in order to achieve a facial harmony.

- In a high angle case, the VTO is helpful in deciding how much protraction is necessary in order to compensate for the counterclockwise rotation of the mandible during the phase II orthodontic treatment.

ACKNOWLEDGEMENTS

Declared none.

CONFLICT OF INTEREST

The authors confirm that this chapter contents have no conflict of interest.

REFERENCES

[1] Nukatska S. The longitudinal study of orthopedic effects caused by chin cap treatment. Tohoku Univ Dent J 2000;1:1-17.
[2] Mitani H, Sakamoto T. Chin cap force to a growing mandible. Long-term clinical reports. Angle Orthod 1984;54:93-122.
[3] Mitani H. Recovery growth of mandible after chin cup therapy: Fact or fiction. Semin Orthod 2007;13:186-199.
[4] Sakamoto T, Iwase I, Uka A and Nakamura S. A roentgenocephalometric study of skeletal changes during and after chin cup treatment. Symposium on "Clinical and Bioengineering Aspects of Dentofacial Orthopedics", Hartford, Connecticut, 1981
[5] Ngan P, Hu AM, Fields Jr., HW. Treatment of Class III problems begins with differential diagnosis of anterior crossbites. American Academy of Pediatric Dentistry 1997;19(6): 386-395.
[6] Deguchi T, Kuroda T, Hunt NP, Graber TM. Long-term application of chincup force alters the morphology of the dolichofacial Class III mandible. Am J Orthod Dentofac Orthop 1999;116(6):610-615.
[7] Chong YH, Ive JC, Artun J. Changes following the use of protraction headgear for early correction of Class III malocclusion. Angle Orthod 1996;66:351–362.
[8] Filho OGS, Magro AC, Filho LC. Early treatment of the Class III malocclusion with rapid maxillary expansion and maxillary protraction. Am J Orthod Dentofac Orthop 1998;113(2):196-203.
[9] Turley PK. Orthopedic correction of Class III malocclusion with palatal expansion and custom protraction headgear. J Clin Orthod 1988;22:314-25.

[10] Gautam P, Valiathan A, Adhikari R. Skeletal response to maxillary protraction with and without maxillary expansion: A finite element study. Am J Orthod Dentofac Orthop 2009;135(6):723-28.

[11] Nanda R. Biomechanical and clinical considerations of a modified protraction headgear. Am J Orthod 1980;78:125-139.

[12] Wisth PJ, Tritapunt A, Rygh P, *et al.* The effect of maxillary protraction on front occlusion and facial morphology. Acta Odontol Scand 1987;45:227-237.

[13] Ngan P, Wei SHY, Hagg U, *et al.* Effect of protraction headgear on Class III malocclusion. Quintessence Int J 1992;23:197-207.

[14] Wilmes B, Nienkemper M, Drescher D. Application and effectiveness of a mini-implant- and tooth-borne rapid palatal expansion device: the hybrid hyrax. World J Orthod 2010; 11(4):323-30.

[15] B Ludwig *et al.* Mini-implants in Orthodontics, Quintessence Publishing 2008

[16] Brett J. Garrett,a Joseph M. Caruso,b Kitichai Rungcharassaeng, c James R. Farrage,c Jay S. Kim,d and Guy D. Taylore. Skeletal effects to the maxilla after rapid maxillary expansion assessed with cone-beam computed tomography. Am J Orthod Dentofac Orthop 2008;134(1):8.e1-8.e11.

[17] Macdonald KE, Kapust AJ, Turley PK. Cephalometric changes after the correction of Class III malocclusion with maxillary expansion/facemask therapy. Am J Orthod Dentofac Orthop 1999;116(1):13-24.

[18] Paul W. Major DDS, MSc, MRCD(CH).E. EIBadawy, MS, HDD, DDS. Maxillary protraction for early orthopedic correction of skeletal Class III malocclusion. Pediatr Dent 1993;15(3):203-7.

[19] Harzer W, Schneider M, Gedrange T. Rapid maxillary expansion with palatal anchorage of the hyrax expansion screw--pilot study with case presentation. J Orofac Orthop 2004;65(5):419-24.

[20] Liou EJ. Effective maxillary orthopedic protraction for growing Class III patients: a clinical application simulates distraction osteogenesis. Prog Orthod. 2005;6(2):154-71.

[21] Liou EJ and Tsai WC. A new protocol for maxillary protraction in cleft patients: Repetitive weekly protocol of alternate rapid maxillary expansions and constrictions. Cleft Palate Craniofac J 2005;42:121-127.

[22] Borzabadi-Farahani A, Lane CJ, Yen SL. Late Maxillary Protraction in Patients With Unilateral Cleft Lip and Palate: A Preliminary Study. Cleft Palate Craniofac J. 2012 Dec 13. [Epub ahead of print]

[23] Ramezanzadeh B, Pousti M, Bagheri M. Cephalometric Evaluation of Dentofacial Features of Class III Malocclusion in Adults of Mashhad, Iran. JDent Res, Dent Clin, Dent Prosp 2007;1(3).

[24] Showkatbakhsh R, Jamilian A, and Behnaz M. Treatment of Maxillary Deficiency by Miniplates: A Case Report. ISRN Surgery Volume 2011 (2011), Article ID 854924, 8 pagesdoi:10.5402/2011/854924.

[25] Şar C, Arman-Özçırpıcı A, Uçkan S, Yazıcı AC. Comparative evaluation of maxillary protraction with or without skeletal anchorage. Am J Orthod Dentofac Orthop 2011;139(5):636-49.

[26] Kircellia BH, Pektasb ZO. Midfacial protraction with skeletally anchored face mask therapy: A novel approach and preliminary results. Am J Orthod Dentofac Orthop 2008; 133(3):440-449.

[27] Mossey PA. The Heritability of Malocclusion: Part 2. The Influence of Genetics in Malocclusion. Br J of Orthod 1999;26(3):195-203.

[28] Franchi L, Baccetti T, McNamara Jr, JA. Post-pubertal assessment of treatment timing for maxillary expansion and protraction therapy followed by fixed appliances. Am J Orthod Dentofac Orthop 2004;126:555-68.

[29] Baccetti T, McGill JS, Franchi L, McNamara Jr. JA and Tollaro I. Skeletal effects of early treatment of Class III malocclusion with maxillary expansion and face-mask therapy. Am J Orthod Dentofac Orthop 1998;113:333-43.

[30] McGill J. Orthopedic alteration induced by rapid maxillary expansion and facemask therapy [thesis]. Ann Arbor: University of Michigan;1995.

[31] Shanker S, Ngan P, Wade D, Beck M, Yui C, Ila¨gg IJ, *et al.* Cephalometric A point changes during and after maxillary protraction and expansion. Am J Orthod Dentofac Orthop 1996;110:423-30.

[32] Turley PK. Managing the developing Class III malocclusion with palatal expansion and facemask therapy. Am J Orthod Dentofac Orthop 2002;122:349-52.

[33] Ngan P, Hagg U, Yiu C, and Wei SHY. Treatment Response and Long-Term Dentofacial Adaptations to Maxillary Expansion and Protraction. Semin Orthod 1997;3(4):255-64.

[34] Hong C, Lee H, Webster R, Kwak J, Wu BM, Moon W. Stability comparison between commercially available mini-implants and a novel design: Part 1. Angle Orthod 2011;81(4):692-9.

[35] Hong C, Truong P, Song HN, Wu BM, Moon W. Mechanical stability assessment of novel orthodontic mini-implant designs: Part 2. Angle Orthod 2011;81(6):1001-9.

CHAPTER 6

Stability of Class III Treatment Strategies in Growing Patients: A Systematic Review of the Literature

Toshio Deguchi[1,*] and Toru Kageyama[2]

[1]Professor Emeritus of Graduate Orthodontics, Matsumoto Dental University and Adjunct Professor, Department of Orthodontics and Oral Facial Genetics, Indiana University School of Dentistry and [2]Associate Professor, Department of Orthodontics, Hard Tissue Research Institute, Graduate School, Matsumoto Dental University, Nagano, Japan

Abstract: It has been reported that mandibular growth that was retarded and/or redirected during growth modification therapy could not be maintained during the retention period. However, research is necessary to substantiate these findings. During the last 15 years, the authors have studied the morphology, growth, function and treatment effects in Class III malocclusion. For patients with Class III malocclusion, the growth of the mandible is already 3 mm larger than its Class I counterpart by 4-5 years of age. It is also generally accepted that skeletal Class III malocclusions worsen with age, with 3 to 4 mm (or 0.5-1.0mm/year) greater increase in mandibular length compared to Class I mandibles in both genders, during the growth period. Facemask therapy is currently an accepted approach to treatment of Class III malocclusion with maxillary deficiency in young patients. On the other hand, two years of chin cup application showed a more effective orthopedic treatment and a diminished skeletal relapse at the post-retention period. Previous publications by the authors have compared the growth, TMJ response and treatment strategies with reverse headgear or chin cap compared to untreated subjects. In the current article, a systematic review was conducted to provide an evidence-base for the following orthodontic questions: Are there differences in mandibular growth between Class III and normal individuals? If so, what is its magnitude and is it clinically relevant? How is mandibular growth changed following orthopedic treatment in Class III malocclusion? Are these changes stable?

Keywords: Upper incisor lingual inclination, Moderate retrusive of the maxilla, optimal age for treatment, Concave profile, Increased length of the mandible, Cross-sectional growth studies, Longitudinal studies of mandibular growth, Anterior cross bite with functional shift of the mandible, Backward rotation of mandible, N-vertical (N-A, N-B), Chin cup appliance, Reverse-pull headgear, Non-extraction treatment, growth reduction, mandibular shape and size, Experienced orthodontist, Duration of treatment, Patient treatment choice, Magnitude and duration of loading, Stability, TMJ effect.

***Address correspondence to Toshio Deguchi:** Indiana University School of Dentistry (IUSD), Jarabak Scholar Award, Department of Orthodontics, IUSD, Matsumoto Dental University, Nagano, Japan; Tel: 317-278-3860; Fax: 317-278-1438; E-mail: deguchit@iu.edu

Peter W. Ngan, Toshi Deguchi and Eugene W. Roberts (Eds)

INTRODUCTION

A number of animal and clinical studies have been carried out over the past four decades to investigate the orthopedic effects in growing patients with Class III malocclusion. Previous research suggests that Class III orthopedic appliances may retard and redirect mandibular growth in a more downward and backward direction [1].

Approximately 60-70% of anterior cross bites in the 8-12 year-old age group are diagnosed as pseudo-Class III malocclusion [2]. Anterior cross bite and mild skeletal Class III malocclusion cases can be corrected with a variety of treatment approaches, including chin cup, orthopedic facial masks, and partial fixed appliances used for a short duration (6-12 months) [3].

Protraction of the maxilla with either a facemask or reverse-pull headgear, is currently a well-accepted approach for the treatment of Class III malocclusion, this approach tends to be more successful than classic chin cup therapy in managing young Class III patients [4-11].

The characteristic features associated with Class III malocclusion are present at the age of 4-5 years [12]. Class III mandible is 3 mm longer than the Class I mandible in both females and males subjects [13]. Baccetti *et al.* reported that individuals with skeletal Class III malocclusion showed a greater increase in mandibular length and longer mandibular growth intervals than Class I individuals [14]. That cross-sectional study was based on large sample size (n > 1000) measured at different age intervals. The results showed substantial increases in mandibular length for Class III subjects compared to those with normal occlusion, even at the more mature age of 12 to 16 years [15-17]. On the other hand, similar growth increments were observed between prognathic and normal mandibles during the prepubertal (7-10 years old) [18] and postpubertal (14-17 years old) stages [19].

A systematic review by Toffol *et al.* [20] reported that 75% of the subjects treated with facemasks had generally successful outcomes, 15% had acceptable outcomes, and 10% required surgery after 5 years of observation. Early treatment (before the age of 8 years) was highly successful in 80% of subjects.

The present Class III subjects were treated with Chin cup and Reverse pull HG. There are more than two thousand cases with full post-retention records collected from 1982-1995 (600 cases at MDU hospital) and 1970-2005 (1200 cases form Dr. Takao Kuroda, Tokushima, Japan). At post-retention, less than 5% of the cases are candidates for camouflage. There were no post-retention candidates requiring orthognathic surgery after age of 20 years. A clinical trial is indicated to determine the ratio of surgery to camouflage candidates after orthopedic treatment.

The present review paper provides an overview of the evidence regarding mandibular growth of untreated Class III individuals and the changes in Class III mandibular growth following orthopedic treatment.

SEARCH STRATEGY

A literature search was conducted using Medline/PubMed. The primary search terms used were: "Class III malocclusion," "Mandibular prognathism" and "Mandibular growth." Hand searching was also conducted to identify any studies that may have been missed during the electronic search. Fifty articles were identified, but only 30 articles, that were most relevant with respect to Class III malocclusion and mandibular growth, were included in this review.

STUDY DESIGNS

Table **1** summarizes the data from 11 studies considered in the present review. Most studies showed significant differences in mandibular growth between Class III and normal individuals. Class III patients presented more pronounced and prolonged mandibular growth, such that the severity of prognathism increased with age. However, other reports have demonstrated no difference in the extent of mandibular growth between Class III and normal subjects.

Table 1: Summary of the 11 studies related to mandibular growth in Class III individuals.

Author	**Study Design**	**Sample**	**Methods**	**Conclusion**
Jacobson *et al.* [21].	CS	149 Class III dental malocclusion patients (6-16 y)	Co-Gn	Burgeoning growth of the Class III mandible with age.
Mitani [18]	L	26 girls with true anterior crossbite (7 y to 10 y)	Ar-Pog	Similar growth increment in prognathic mandible and normal mandible during pre-pubertal period.

Table 1: contd...

Guyer *et al.* [22]	CS	144 patients with Class III molar relationships (5-15 y)	Co-Gn	No difference in mandibular growth, characteristic features associated with Class III already present at an early age
Battagel [23]	CS	285 children with Class III BSI incisor relationship (7-15 y)	Ar-Pog	Facial growth in female remained active after growth in control female had ceased (delayed growth spurt)
Mitani *et al.* [19]	L	14 males (15 y followed till 18 y) and 20 females (14 y followed till 17 y) Class III subjects	Co-Gn	Mandibular growth of Class III individuals and normal individuals similar after pubertal growth peak
Tollaro *et al.* [20]	CS	69 Class III children (36 males, 33 females, 4-6 y)	Ar-Go	Class III skeletal imbalances were already present during the deciduous dentition phase
Mijayama *et al.*	CS	1376 Class III Japanese females (2.7-47.9 y)	Co-Gn, SNB	Mandible was prognathic at an early age and increased more significantly from stage IIIC to stage IVA
Baccetti *et al.* [14]	CS	32 untreated Class III patients (7-10 y)	Co-Gn	Greater forward movement of mandible (1.3 mm) compared to untreated Class I subjects
Deguchi *et al.* [24]	CS	562 untreated Class III subjects (3, 13, 17 y)	Cd-Gn ANB, WITS	Worsened along with growth, mainly due to excessive mandibular growth in a forward direction
Reyes *et al.* [17]	CS	949 Caucasian Class III patients with Class III molar and incisor relationships (6-16 y)	Co-Gn	Mandibular growth in Class III individuals more pronounced, delayed peak and lasts longer than normal subjects
Baccetti *et al.* [13]	CS and L	1091 Class III patients (3-57 y) and 22 Class III subjects (8-15 y)	Co-Gn	1) Mandibular projection tends to worsen with age 2) Peak in mandibular growth at same maturation stage as normal individuals (CS3-CS4) 3) Longer duration of peak interval 4) More prolonged mandibular growth period

CS, cross-sectional; L, longitudinal.

MANDIBULAR GROWTH RELATED TO PUBERTAL GROWTH

Baccetti *et al.* [13, 14] found that in Class III individuals, mandibular growth peaked at the same maturation stage as normal individuals (CS3 through CS4 in cervical vertebral maturation), but the duration of the peak interval was more prolonged. However, Reyes *et al.* [17] found that the largest increase in mandibular length occurred, on average, 1 year later in both female and male Class III subjects, compared to subjects with normal occlusion. Battagel [23] also showed evidence of delayed growth in Class III individuals.

Table **2** summarizes the data derived from nine of the papers included in the present systematic review. Two studies (Deguchi 1999; Levin *et al.* 2008) were excluded because they utilized only a maxillary protraction appliance and the Frankel FR-3 appliance.

Table 2: Summary of 9 studies related to post-orthopedic treatment effects on mandibular growth in Class III individuals.

Author	**Study Design**	**Sample**	**Materials**	**Treatment Time**	**Conclusion**
Graber [25]	CCT CO-CR: no	30 patients 5-8 y	Chin cup 150-300-450 g/side, 10-12 h/day	3 y	1) Retardation of vertical ramus growth 2) Redirection of mandibular growth pattern to a more vertical direction and gonial angle closure
Mitani [26]	CCT 3 Cases	3 Japanese F	500-600 g	9 y, 3 y and 3 y	1) Inherited growth direction recovered after treatment 2) Reduction of gonial angle, deepening of antegonial notch.
Asano [27]	Animal study	Wistar rats	30g of mandibular retractive force 8 h/day	4 w	1) Mandibular retractive force resulted in shorter anteroposterior length of mandible and mandible did not show any catch-up growth after treatment
Sugawara *et al.* [15]	CCT CO-CR; no	63 Japanese F 7, 9, 11 y	250-300 g/side, 14 h/day	4-5 y	Skeletal profiles were significantly improved during the initial stages of treatment, but were not maintained thereafter in severe skeletal Class III.
Lu *et al.*[28]	CCT CO-CR; no severe case	30 Japanese children (F, M 9y)	500-600 g	5 y	1) Pre-treatment craniofacial morphology similar to post-treatment morphology 2) Backward and downward repositioning of the mandible
Deguchi, Kitsugi [29]	CCT CO-CR; yes Moderate case	24 Japanese F. G1: 8 y 10 m G2: 10 y10 m	500 g/side, 10 h/day	6-12 m. Long-term follow-up	Skeletal changes with a original Class III profile remained stable during post-treatment
Ko Y-II *et al.*[30]	CCT CO-CR; no G2: severe case	40 patients (F,M) G1: 8 yl m G2; 8 y 4 m	Chin cup, 300-500 g/side, 12-14 h/side	G1: 2 y 9 m G2: 3 y 1 m Long-term follow-up	Group 1; Stable G2; 1) More severe Class III at T0; 2) More forward rotation and forward growth of the mandible
Yoshida *et al.*[6]	CCT & RP CO-CR; no severe case	28 Japanese F 10 y 4 m	600 g at chin	14 m Long-term follow up	Retardation of mandibular growth during the treatment period, but excessive forward and downward, rebound-like growth during post-treatment period

Table 2: contd...

Deguchi *et al.* [24]	CCT CO-CR; yes G2: severe case	G1:20 Japanese F (8 y 4 m, fair-good compliance) G2: 36 (8 y 4 m, excellent)	G1: 500 g, 10 h/day for 2.5 y G2: 300 g. 14 h/day for 2 y and 1 more year at night	G1: >1 y G2: 3 y Long term follow-up	1) G1 showed some orthopedic effects of mandible and the changes maintained 2) G2 showed significantly orthopedic effects on shape and size of mandible. The changes obtained maintained at 18 year old

CC, chin cup; RPHG, reverse-pull HG; CO-CR, long centric; yes, checked; ns, not studied; F, female; M, male.

STUDY DESIGNS

Most studies evaluating the orthopedic treatment of Class III individuals were controlled clinical trials (CCTs). Randomized clinical trials (RCTs) are considered to be the gold standard for assessment of treatment outcomes and growth changes. However, no RCTs on Class III malocclusion have been reported. This lack of RCTs could be due to ethical or logistical factors. Patients in RCT are unable to choose their treatment; therefore, some subjects in the untreated control group may refuse to participate in the trial. In addition, it is impossible to blind patients or operators to the treatments in such studies. Nevertheless, a few studies have highlighted individual variations. Thus, RCTs may not reflect the true treatment outcomes.

DIFFERENCES IN SKELETAL MORPHOLOGY OF STABLE AND UNSTABLE CASES

An advantage of a chin cup appliance is that it can apply force in both the horizontal and vertical directions. Once an anterior cross bite is corrected and an acceptable posterior occlusion is obtained, the occipital direction for the chin cup stimulates bone remodeling in the maxillary and mandibular posterior segments. This allows for good intercuspation, which maintains a Class I molar relationship during the retention period. In addition, the occipital force could lead to closure of the obtuse gonial angle and the steep mandibular plane angle, which is generally maintained.

However, unstable or poor cases show increased gonial angles, a counterclockwise rotation of the mandible and unpredictable growth of the mandible at post-retention [31, 32]. These changes are characteristic of the unfavorable aspects of Class III malocclusion. Prior to the mid-1980s, the mandibular sagittal setback operation was not performed in Japan. Therefore, orthodontists and general dentists in Asian regions were reluctant to treat severe skeletal Class III cases with orthopedic appliances [33, 34].

FREQUENTLY ASKED QUESTIONS

1. *Is there a difference in mandibular growth between Class III individuals and normal individuals?*

Yes. At the age of 3-4 years, the mandible in Class III malocclusion or in anterior cross bite is 3-4 mm longer than that for patients in normal occlusion. [12, 13]. All cross-sectional data indicated more growth of the mandible in Class III malocclusion, which worsened with age [15-17, 24].

2. *If there is a difference in growth between Class III and normal subjects, what is its magnitude and is it clinically relevant?*

Yes. A longitudinal study [13] reports that the post-pubertal growth of the Class III mandible (mixed gender) is more prolonged than that of the counterpart normal occlusion. The growth for subjects with a Class III malocclusion is 3.5–7mm more, than for a normal occlusion group, between 8 and 15 years. Clinically, advancement of the maxillary dentition and the maxilla results in 4 mm of anteroposterior (A-P) correction. Backward rotation of the mandible also contributes to 2 mm of A-P correction. One year use of the face mask achieves 6 mm of Class III correction, which is retained as a significant treatment effect after five years [10].

If there is no difference in growth between Class III and normal subjects, as reported in the pre-pubertal and post-pubertal longitudinal data. However, catch-up growth** or rebound growth of the mandible could be a factor, that explains more growth of the mandible after treatment. As discussed before, more growth of the Class III mandible is a reliable factor that may explain the post-treatment changes.

3. *How does mandibular growth change following orthopedic treatment for Class III malocclusion? Are such changes stable?*

The answer is unknown. The treatment outcome varies. In a systematic review, Liu PH *et al.* [35] reported that there is insufficient data in previous studies to clarify the recommendations regarding the efficacy of chin cup therapy in the retardation of mandibular growth. Interestingly, changes in the shape of the mandible in Class III treated cases lead to smaller increments in mandibular length, and significant changes in mandibular size due to a forward reorientation of the condyle and a closing of the gonial angle [36-39].

4. *Is there a difference between the types of orthopedic treatments and the protocols used for* treatment with respect to the corrective effect on Class III mandible?

Face-mask treatment may be the best effective appliance for correction of anterior cross bite and Class III skeletal discrepancy. One year wearing this orthopedic appliance is a good choice because it would be quite difficult for young patients to wear it longer than 1 year. However, the author(s) understand that patients are often willing to use the appliance for 1 or 2 years. Once the anterior cross bite is corrected, most of the patients are willing to continue wearing it. We recommend the use of face-masks for 2 years to attain a better treatment outcome and reduce the post-treatment changes, if the patient is compliant.

** "Catch-up growth" in medicine and orthodontics. Catch-up growth of the mandible has been cited in the orthodontic literature [40]. The term "recovery growth" or "catch-up growth" was originally used by Tanner [41] to describe a phenomenon that occurs in patients during their recovery from diseases or illnesses. He stated, that it took almost 100 years for the pubertal growth spurt to be recognized for what it was. Previously, it was commonly confused with catch-up growth, the abnormally rapid growth that occurs following a period of growth retardation due to illness or starvation. It has been hypothesized that the restricted mandibular growth that occurs during initial chin cup application can return to natural levels during the retention period. "Recovery" or "catch-up growth" might cause recurrence of the original Class III features. An animal model study indicated that the mandibles in the experimental groups did not grow more than those in the control groups, nor did they reach the sizes of control mandibles after orthopedic chin cap application [27]. Sugawara *et al.* [15] previously discussed the concept of catch-up growth in chin cap-treated patients, and they were unable to ascertain whether the mandible showed any signs of catch-up growth following cessation of chin cap therapy.

CLINICAL TRIALS FOR CHIN CUP TREATMENT

Classic Strategy for Chin Cup Treatment: 1 Year Use of Chin Cup, Night-Time only with a Force of 500 gm/Side if the Patient is Fairly Cooperative

Forty female Japanese subjects with the potential for either non-extraction and extraction therapy were included in a prospective clinical trial [29]. Twenty-four patients, treated non-extraction at the Department of Orthodontics, Matsumoto Dental University Hospital (MDUH), had chin cup therapy initiated during the period 1981 to 1983. These patients were divided into pre-pubertal (n=11, Group 1) and pubertal (n=13, Group 2) groups. The criteria for selection were overclosure on maximum interdigitated occlusion, non-prominent skeletal Class III profile in rest position, possible edge-to-edge bite on posterior guided position of the mandible, incisors normally inclined, and normal orofacial function. There is no significant difference in the analysis variables in extraction and non-extraction subjects. All patients were instructed to wear a chin cup appliance for a minimum of 10 hours per day, until the anterior cross bite was corrected. Chin cup therapy was continued for another 6 months after correction of the anterior cross bite with acceptable posterior occlusion. A force of 500 grams was applied on each side, directed at the condylar head. Patients were instructed to inform the clinic if they noticed any TMJ pain or unusual movement of the mandible. The results were compared to a control group of untreated Class III female subjects (n=16).

Table 3: Age of patients for the two treatment groups (pre-pubertal and pubertal) for the various treatment periods

	Pre-Treatment	End of active Treatment	Post-Treatment	Active Treatment	Retention	N
Group 1	8y10m	13y7m	17y6m	4y9m	3y11m	11
Group 2	10y10m	14y1m	18y4m	3y3m	4y 3m	13

Group 1: pre-pubertal group, Group 2: pubertal group.

Table 4: Cephalometric values of the treatment group (n=24) for the pretreatment, end of treatment, and post-treatment periods

Values	Pre-Treatment		End of Active Treatment		Post-Treatment	
	Mean	SD	Mean	SD	Mean	SD
SNA	81.6	3.3	82.8	3.5	83.0	3.5
SNB	80.6	3.0	81.6	4.2	81.8	4.5
ANB	1.0	2.0	1.2	2.1	1.2	3.0
SN-MP	38.2	6.1	36.5	7.5	36.0	7.9
NPg-FH	86.4	3.5	88.1	4.6	88.2	4.8
IMPA	86.3	8.3	88.3	8.7	87.7	6.5
FMA	31.1	5.6	29.5	7.1	29.0	7.6
Gonial angle	127.6	8.9	124.9	8.3	123.7	8.5
Ramus angle	6.8	6.1	5.4	4.3	4.6	4.4
A-B(OP)	-6.4	1.9	-4.9	1.9	-4.7	2.0
U1 to NA	25.2	9.6	29.2	6.3	28.5	6.8
U1 to NA(mm)	3.2	2.7	6.5	2.3**	6.0	2.8
L1 to NB	25.8	7.9	26.6	8.3	26.0	6.5
L1 to NB(mm)	5.4	2.0	5.8	2.9	5.5	2.6
Interincisal angle	128.5	8.4	123.1	11.9	124.4	8.3
ANS-Me(mm)	61.4	4.5	69.0	5.7**	70.6	5.7**
S-N(mm)	64.1	1.7	67.9	2.0**	69.0	2.2
PNS-ANS(mm)	46.1	1.9	49.5	3.0**	51.0	2.5**

$^*P<0.05$; $^{**}P<0.01$.

Table 5: Comparison of cephalometric values for the treatment group (n=24) and control group (n=16) for the pre-treatment (T0), post-treatment (T1) and post-retention (T2) periods

	T0 (8y10m)	T1 (13y7m)	T2 (17y6m)
	Mean	Mean	Mean
SNA	81.6 (78.7)	82.8 (79.0)	83.0 (79.6)

Table 5: contd…

SNB	80.6 (77.8)	81.6 (80.6)	81.8 (81.8)
ANB	1.0 (0.9)	1.2 (-1.6)	1.2 (-2.2)
Wits	-6.4 (-6.6)	-4.9 (-10.0)	-4.7 (-11.1)
Ramus A	83.2 (83.6)	84.6 (82.8)	85.4 (81.5)
ArGoMe	127.6 (132.1)	124.9 (133.4)	123.7 (134.7)
FMA	31.1 (31.8)	29.5 (32.6)	29.0 (32.7)

();untreated Class III.

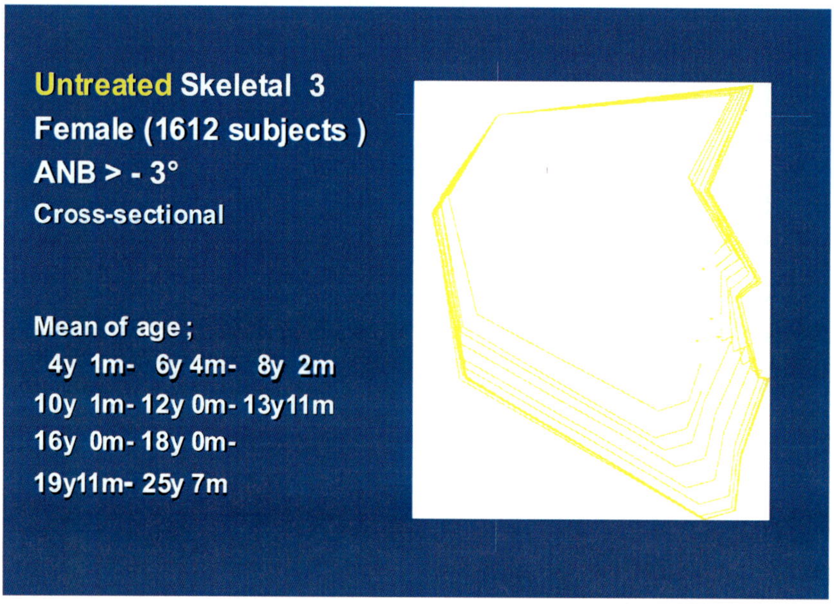

Figure 1: Profilogram of cross-sectional date in untreated female Class III.

In summary, the initial Class III skeletal components maintained the pre-treatment Class III features but showed 2.0° increase of SNA and 1.8° increase of ANB during the post-retention period. Class I normal subjects served as controls.

A typical case is presented. Note that there is skeletal improvement at T1 and T2. In the present study, chin cup-treated subjects were also compared with the untreated Class III subjects. The data shows that chin cup treatment helped to limit the growth of Class III mandible, while the maxilla continues to grow anteriorly. None of the patients showed significant skeletal changes at T0, T1 and T2. The normal Class I patients seem to be more suitable control data than that of the untreated Class III data.

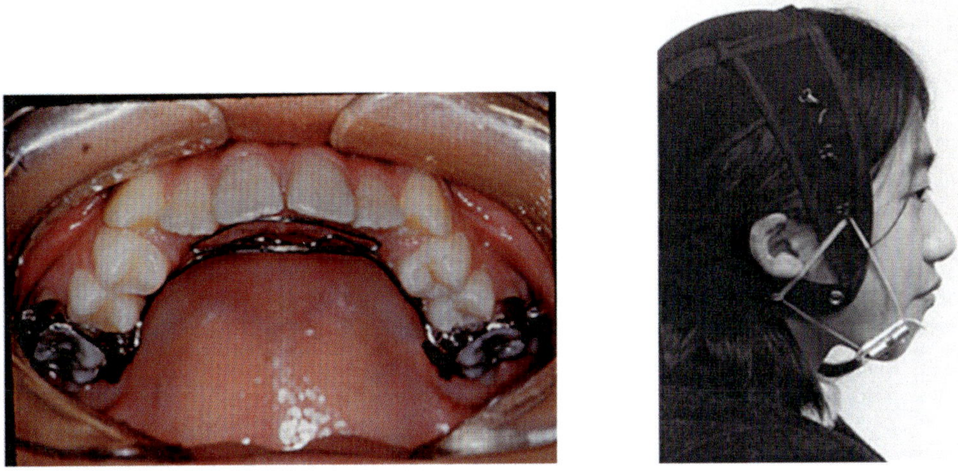

Figure 2: Maxillary lingual arch (0.9 mm) with soldered auxiliary wire (0.5 mm) and chin cup for treatment of mild and moderate skeletal Class III malocclusion. The anterior cross bite was corrected in 6 months due to labial movement of upper incisors and backward rotation of the mandible and elimination of the functional A-P shift of the mandible.

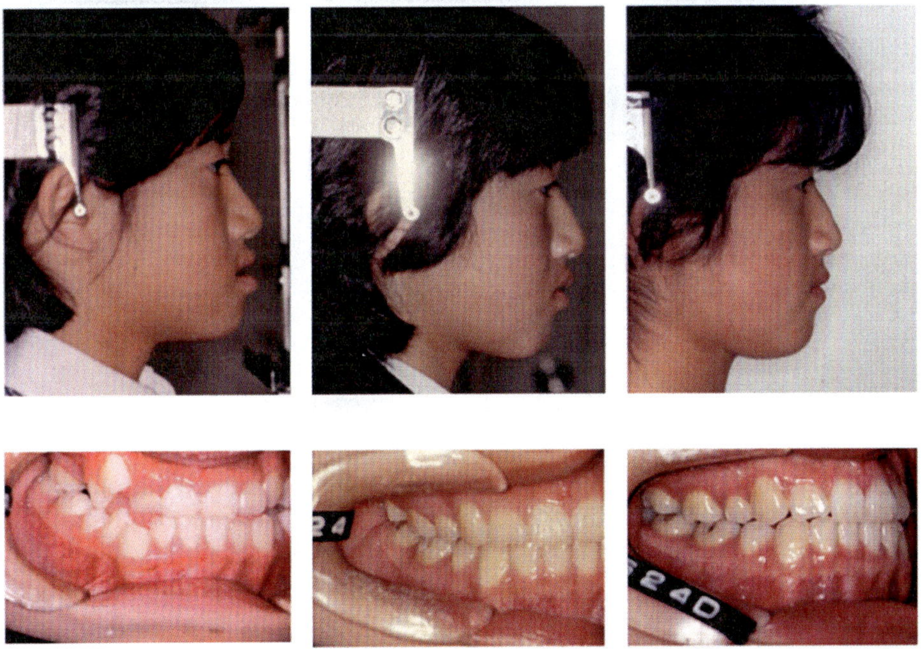

A B C

Figure 3: A female with low mandibublar plane angle was treated with extractions. A. Pre-treatment. B. Post-treatment. C. Post-retention, 4.5 years after post-treatment.

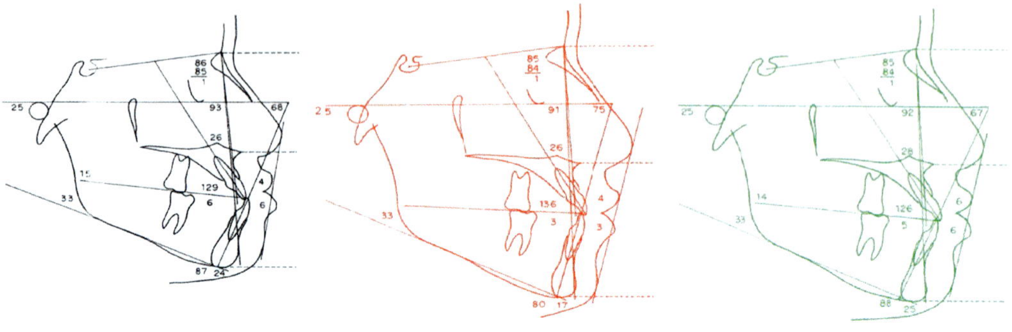

A B C

Figure 4: Cephalometric tracing of the same patient. A. Pre-treatment. B. Post-treatment. C. Post-retention, 4.5 years after post-treatment.

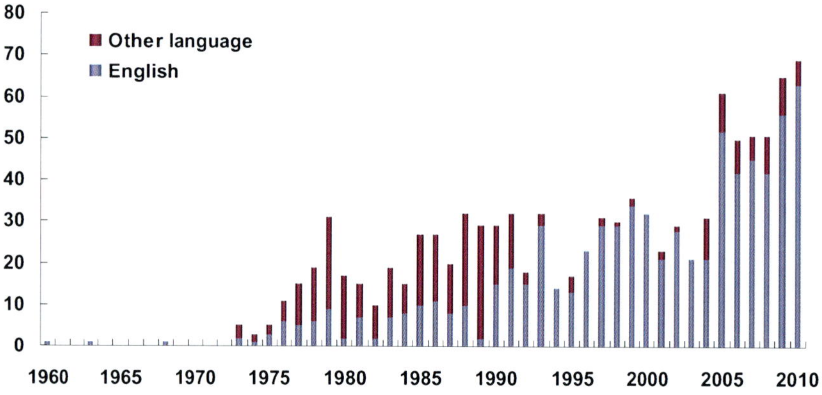

Figure 5: Year-wise comparison of published literature regarding treatment of skeletal Class III malocclusion. The term that was required for selection was "Class III malocclusion."

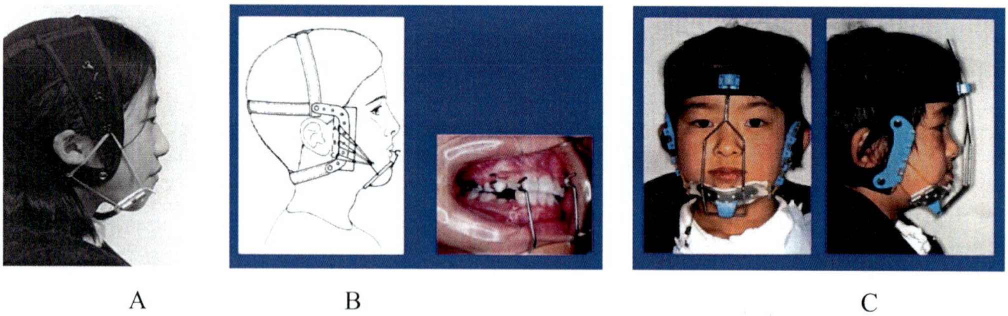

A B C

Figure 6: Appliances used for the clinical trials: A. Chin cup, B. and C. are reverse-pull headgears.

Long-Term Follow-Up of Reverse-Pull Headgear *vs.* Chin Cup Therapy

Deguchi *et al.* [24] reported that aggressive application of chin cup for 2 years resulted in effective orthopedic treatment, and skeletal relapse diminished by 0 to 40% in terms of Ramus plane to FH (Ramus angle), gonial angle, ANB, SNB and Wits during T1 compared to T2 stage at post-retention.

The Japanese female sample was selected from records of approximately 500 female patients treated for Class III malocclusion and meso-dolichofacial skeletal pattern with either reverse-pull headgear (RPHG) or chin cup (CC); there were about 250 files in each group. Selection criteria included availability of patient care records at pre-treatment (T1), immediate post Class III resolution (T2) and post retention (T3). Subjects with dental anomalies, craniofacial syndromes, and "pseudo" Class III malocclusion were excluded. The two groups were also matched for age, gender, and length of treatment. Final selection of the study sample was based upon the following steps in order of priority: 1) pre-treatment age between 6 and 8 years of age, 2) availability of diagnostically suitable records at T1, T2 and T3, and 3) age and gender matching.

Sixty-three Japanese children all treated for Class III malocclusion with either RPHG (n=33) or CC therapy (n=30) were selected. In either the RPHG or the CC group, a two-phase therapy with an edgewise appliance was included in the overall therapy when it was deemed appropriate.

Figyre 7: Soft tissue analysis

Table 6. Soft tissue analysis

	T0				T1				T2		Normal	
	mean	S.D.	T0-T1Diff		mean	S.D.	T1-T2Diff		mean	S.D.	mean	S.D.
Facial profile												
Ns-Sn-Pg angle	5.0	5.0	7.1	***	12.1	5.0	-2.3	***	9.8	5.4	9.6	4.7
N-Sn to FH angle	93.2	3.3	2.7	***	95.8	3.4	-0.7	*	95.1	3.7		
Ns-Pg to Sn	2.2	2.2	3.8	***	6.0	2.5	-1.0	**	5.0	2.8		
Lip												
Naso-Labial angle	112.8	9.8	3.0		115.8	12.0	-2.8		113.0	9.2	109.3	6.4
Z angle	80.1	5.0	-6.7	***	73.4	4.4	-0.7		72.7	4.6	69.1	4.7
Upper lip-E.plane	-1.3	1.4	-0.6		-1.9	2.1	-1.2	**	-3.1	2.0	-1.1	1.8
Lower lip-E.plane	1.7	2.3	-1.8	***	-0.1	2.4	-1.0	***	-1.2	2.0	-0.7	2.5

t-test (2sided) ; *** $p < 0.001$ ** $p < 0.01$ * $p < 0.05$

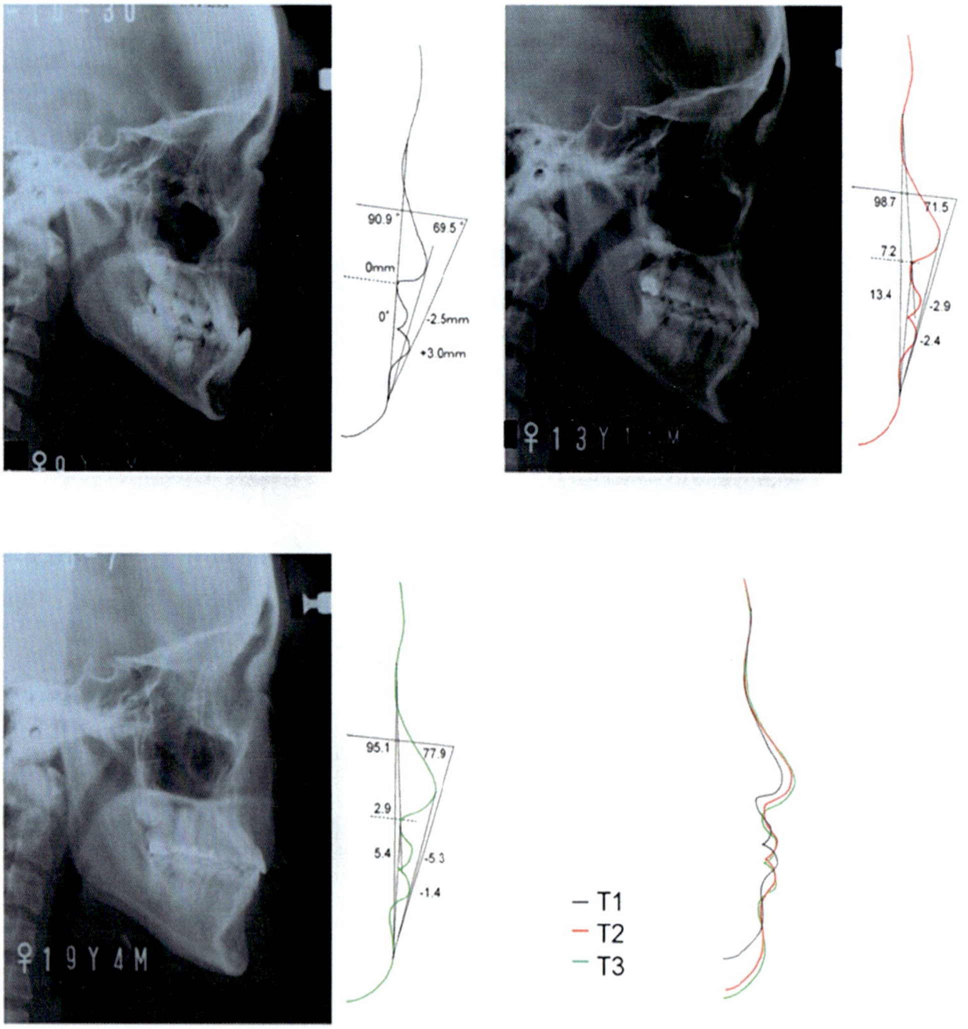

Figure 8: Soft tissue analysis with RPHG at T1, T2 and T3.

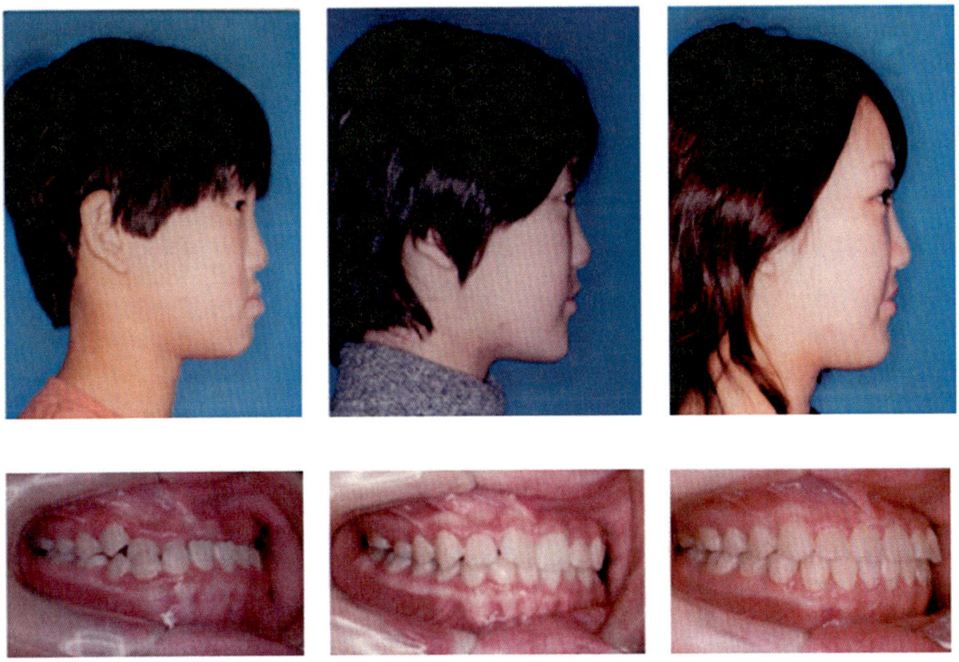

Figure 9: Chin cup therapy in a female (2 year-use, 14 h/day, 300 gm at the center of the chin).

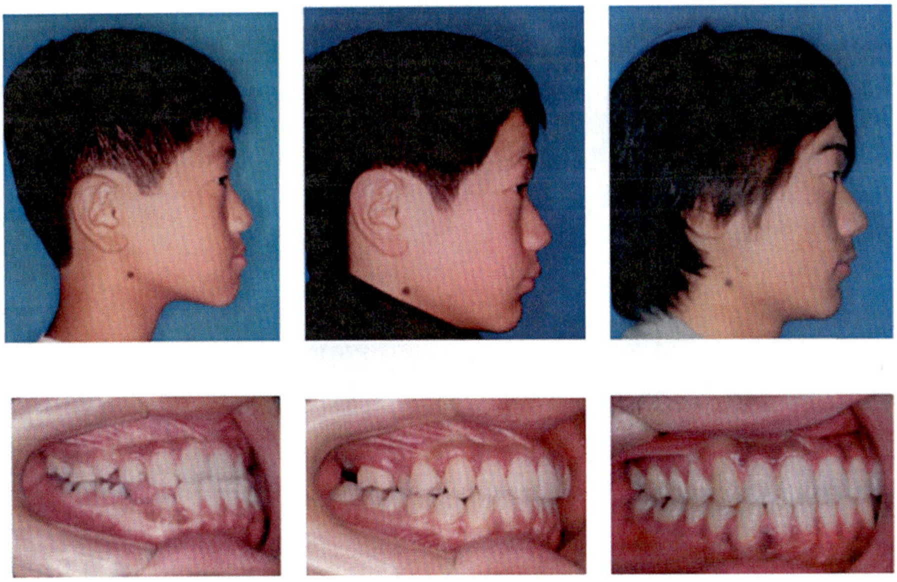

Figure 10: Chin cup therapy was performed on a male with a high mandibular plane angle.

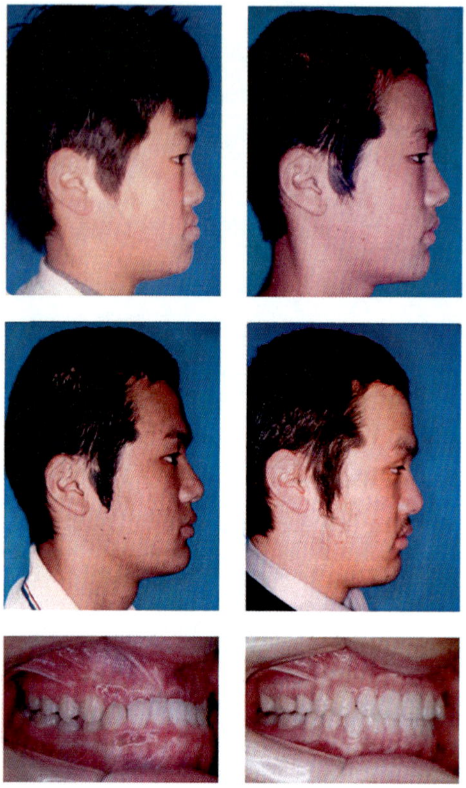

Figure 11: Chin cup therapy was performed on a male with a low mandibular plane angle.

It was hypothesized that RPHG shows more advancement of the maxillary bone and dentition post-retention. Subjects with Class III mesio-dolichofacial skeletal malocclusion pattern comprised the samples of both the RPHG (n=33) and CC (n=30) groups. All subjects of RPHG group had undergone rapid palatal expansion (RPE) for approximately 6 months. RPHG therapy included chin cup restraint of the mandible and protraction-pull of the maxilla administered during the first 6 months of RPE treatment. Chin cup therapy was continued for 2 years. Twenty-one of the 33 patients received non-extraction treatment, and all of the 33 patients underwent rapid palatal expansion. The RPHG appliance, used during rapid palatal expansion, exerted a chin cup retraction force of 300 grams, applied at the center of the chin, and maxillary protraction of 300 grams per side (Fig. **6**).

The chin cup subjects were the same patients as for the previous chin cup study [24]. Both groups showed post-treatment change (T1-T2) in the variables of ANB,

Wits and SNB, and the relapse was 22, 25 and 40%, respectively. The backward rotation (Ramus A) of the mandible was well maintained at post-retention, indicating a low frequency of relapse, and the gonial angle increased. Short use of RPHG for 6 months during RPE showed no significant difference in the CC group, although there was a slight, mean advancement of the maxilla and maxillary dentition. The hypothesis was rejected. However, the results were significantly ($p<0.5\%$) different from the untreated Class III subjects.

Conclusions: Excellent treatment and long-term retention outcomes are possible using either chin cup or reverse pull headgear for treating Class III malocclusion, if the orthopedic appliances are retained for at least 2 years.

RPHG Subjects

High Angle Case

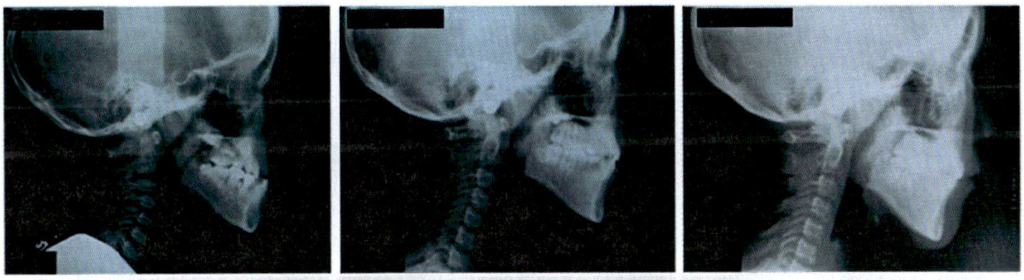

Figure 12: High angle case in a female. Non-extraction treatment. Cephalograms taken at T1, T2, and T3.

Low Angle Severe Case

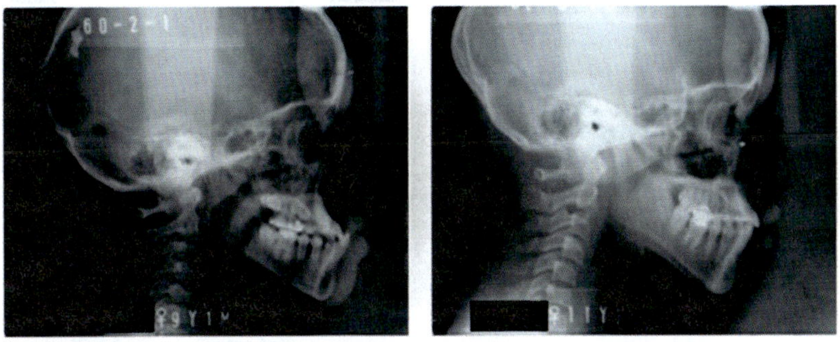

Figure 13: Cephalograms taken at pre-treatment (9 y 1 m) and immediately after active treatment (11 y 2 m). Note the bimaxillary dentoalveolar protrusion after correction of the reverse bite.

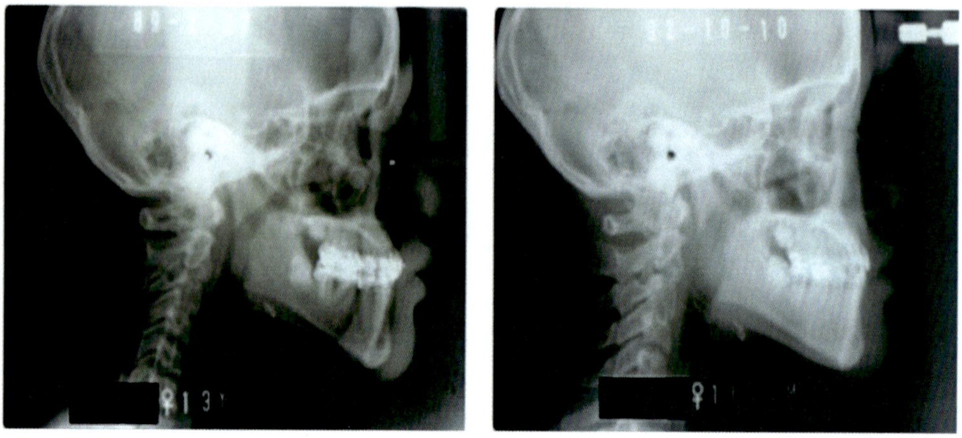

Figure 14: Phase 2 treatment included extraction of 4 first premolars to correct anterior crowding and protrusive incisors. The profile improved. The cephalogram on the right shows post-retention results.

All patients in both RPHG and CC groups showed satisfactory results with an acceptable occlusion and good profile. Cephalometric radiographs were taken at pre-treatment (T1), post-treatment (T2), and post-retention (T3). The cephalograms at T2 were selected at a time after peak mandibular growth (age of 14 y).

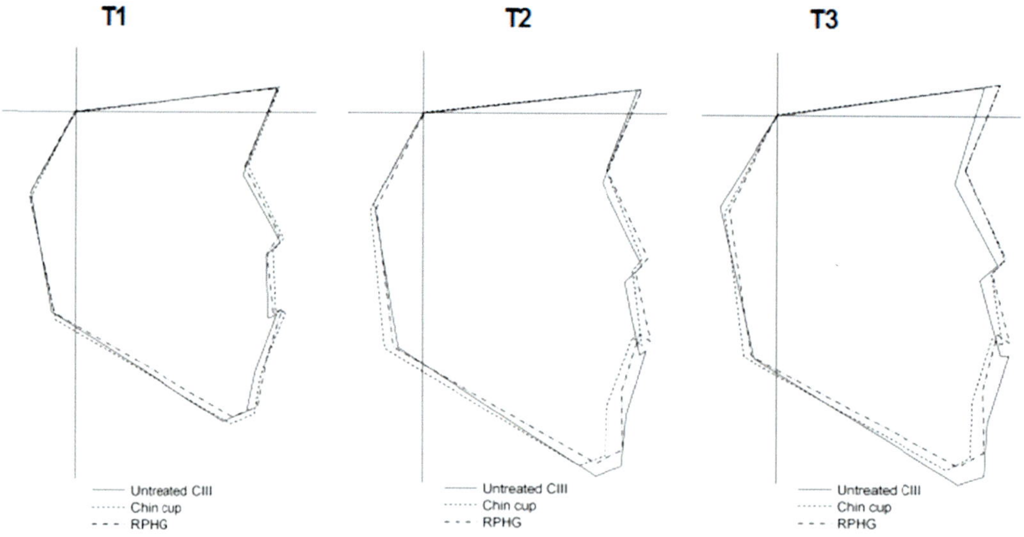

Figure 15: Profilogram of T1, T2 and T3 tracings.

Table 7: Sample size (n) and age for reverse pull headgear (RPHG) and chin cup (CC) and untreated groups at pre-treatment (T1), post-treatment (T2) and post-retention (T3).

	T1		*T2*		*T3*	
	n	*Mean (age)*	*n*	*Mean (age)*	*n*	*Mean (age)*
Untreated Class III	302	8.0	177	13.8	83	17.9
Chin Cup	36	8.2		13.6		18.4
RPHG	33	7.7		14.3		18.1

Cephalometric analysis refers to the values reported [24]. Profilogram of T1, T2 and T3 tracings (Fig. **15.**) indicated the overall treatment effects and stability of RPHG and CC groups. Note the advanced growth of the midfacial components

Table 8: Results of Student t-test comparing reverse-pull HG and chin cup study groups at pre-treatment, post-treatment and post-retention.

	RPHG						*Chin Cup*						*T-test (RPHG v.s. CC)*				
	T1		*T2*		*T3*		*T1*		*T2*		*T3*		*T1*		*T2*		*T3*
Analysis	*Mean*	*S.D.*	*Mean*	*S.D.*	*Mean*	*S.D.*	*Mean*	*S.D.*	*Mean*	*S.D.*	*Mean*	*S.D.*	*p-value*	*Signif.*	*p-value*	*Signif.*	*p-value*
N-S	64.0	2.6	68.2	3.8	69.1	3.0	64.5	2.3	68.4	2.1	68.9	2.1	0.385		0.807		0.741
N-Ba	95.6	3.7	103.1	5.5	104.9	4.4	97.7	3.4	104.6	3.1	105.9	3.4	0.020	*	0.150		0.320
N-CC	51.7	2.3	55.4	2.5	56.3	2.0	52.3	2.7	56.9	2.3	57.3	2.1	0.320		0.016	*	0.033
CC-Ba	43.9	2.8	47.7	3.5	48.6	3.3	45.3	2.9	47.8	2.6	48.5	2.9	0.038	*	0.896		0.881
NSBa	129.8	3.3	129.6	4.6	130.5	5.0	133.7	5.8	133.2	5.1	133.2	5.3	0.001	***	0.003	**	0.037
NSAr	123.2	3.0	123.6	3.9	123.5	4.0	124.4	5.5	125.0	5.3	124.9	5.7	0.264		0.217		0.250
SNA	79.8	2.9	81.0	2.8	80.8	3.0	79.8	3.2	80.2	2.9	80.4	3.2	0.995		0.272		0.622
NF to FH Pl.	2.8	3.2	3.3	2.5	3.4	3.1	5.5	2.9	5.5	2.5	5.4	2.3	0.001	***	0.001	***	0.004
SNB	80.9	3.3	79.5	3.2	79.6	3.5	79.0	3.1	77.5	2.9	78.1	3.7	0.017	**	0.007	**	0.097
ANB	-1.1	2.6	1.5	2.2	1.2	2.0	0.8	1.9	2.7	1.6	2.3	1.8	0.001	***	0.010	**	0.014
ArGoMe	132.3	5.0	128.0	5.7	127.9	5.9	133.6	5.1	128.6	5.2	128.0	5.6	0.266		0.629		0.921
Ar-Me	95.9	4.7	107.4	7.5	109.7	6.4	96.0	4.0	105.4	4.3	108.6	4.5	0.923		0.186		0.406
Ar-Go	40.2	2.8	45.8	4.5	47.7	4.0	39.6	2.9	45.3	3.2	47.4	4.2	0.395		0.549		0.735
Go-Me	64.2	3.9	73.0	5.2	73.8	4.8	64.4	3.5	71.2	3.7	73.0	4.2	0.816		0.098		0.432
Gn-Cd	104.6	4.7	117.7	7.4	120.0	6.3	103.9	3.6	114.6	3.7	118.0	4.1	0.461		0.026	*	0.116
Wits appraisal	-10.2	3.5	-3.4	2.7	-3.8	3.0	-6.2	2.7	-0.7	3.2	-2.1	3.2	0.000	***	0.000	***	0.028
FMA	29.7	3.8	29.2	4.3	28.6	5.1	31.1	4.5	30.4	5.1	29.6	5.5	0.182		0.283		0.438
Facial A.	86.7	3.0	87.0	3.3	87.3	3.8	83.1	2.5	83.3	2.5	84.2	2.7	0.000	***	0.000	***	0.000
Convexity	0.1	5.9	2.4	5.4	1.3	5.1	3.4	4.2	5.4	4.5	4.2	4.4	0.008	**	0.015	*	0.015
A-B Pl.	2.9	3.9	-2.6	3.4	-2.5	3.4	0.0	2.5	-3.8	2.1	-3.4	2.4	0.000	***	0.091		0.166
Ramus PL to FH Pl.	81.3	4.4	85.4	5.0	85.0	5.4	81.8	3.6	86.6	4.2	86.6	4.7	0.609		0.273		0.199
Y-axis	61.2	3.1	62.6	3.4	62.5	3.9	64.8	2.4	66.1	2.7	65.7	2.7	0.000	***	0.000	***	0.000
Functional occ. pl. to FH	15.8	5.1	10.8	4.8	10.8	6.5	13.9	4.0	10.2	3.2	11.2	4.3	0.089		0.581		0.758
U-1 to FH Pl.	112.5	6.2	116.2	6.6	115.5	5.5	107.5	6.6	108.0	5.7	108.2	5.3	0.002	**	0.000	***	0.000
L-1 to Mand.	87.7	5.9	86.1	6.8	86.2	7.7	91.8	5.9	87.5	6.7	88.3	6.1	0.006	**	0.393		0.217
Interincisal	130.1	8.2	128.6	8.3	129.7	8.8	127.7	9.4	132.8	9.0	132.8	8.0	0.260		0.048	*	0.136

Symbols indicate the level of significance; $P<0.05$(*), $P<0.01$(**), $P<0.001$(***)

Orthopedic treatment outcomes are based not only on growth retardation of the mandible and stimulated growth of the maxilla, but also on shape changes of the mandible. To obtain the shape change of the mandible, the force vector is an important determinant of the orthopedic effects of the chin cup, and therefore should be carefully considered in the treatment of Class III patients. The present Class III cases tended to have a hyper-divergent morphology with a high angle, which required a greater vertical force vector to correct these abnormalities [42]. The hyper-divergent Class III mandible may be biologically easier to treat orthopedically than the hypo-divergent case, because high angle cases have smaller ramus and masseter volume and less masseter muscle activity [43-47].

Three factors may contribute to unstable treatment outcomes following orthopedic treatment in severe Class III malocclusion patients: 1) upward-forward rotation of the mandible where the body or corpus of the mandible are too large to compensate the subjects with overclosure before treatment); 2) more prominent, unpredictable horizontal growth of the mandible than growth of the maxilla; and 3) obtuse gonial angle that continues to increase after treatment [31, 32].

In successfully treated patients, the gonial angle decreased, and then continued to decrease, post-treatment and during the retention phase. Yoshida *et al.* [6] found that the gonial angle increased during the post-treatment and post-retention stages at unstable subjects. Generally, the gonial angle can be maintained or tends to decrease in aging because of the increasing activity of masticatory muscles and bone apposition at the sites of gonial angle of the mandible in normal occlusion. [31, 32]. In Fig. **16**, RPHG and CC shows significant orthopedic effects of skeletal Class III treatment although there is a relapse of SNA, SNB, Wits and Ramus plane to FH (Ramus angle) at T1-T2. Advancement of the maxilla and maxillary dentition, as well as the backward positioning of the mandible are achieved and remain stable in RPHG and CC groups (Fig. **15**).

In the present study, 8 out of 63 Class III subjects required a lingual frenectomy because of the high frenum attachment with restricted tongue movement. Abnormal function and morphology of the tongue might affect long-term stability in the post-retention stage, a factor that has not been adequately addressed in the literature on Class III orthopedic treatment outcomes.

Before the mid-1980s, bilateral body split osteotomies (BBSO) have not been performed, but orthodontists and general dentists in Asian countries were reluctant to treat severe skeletal Class III cases with an orthopedic appliance, especially a chin cup [33, 34].

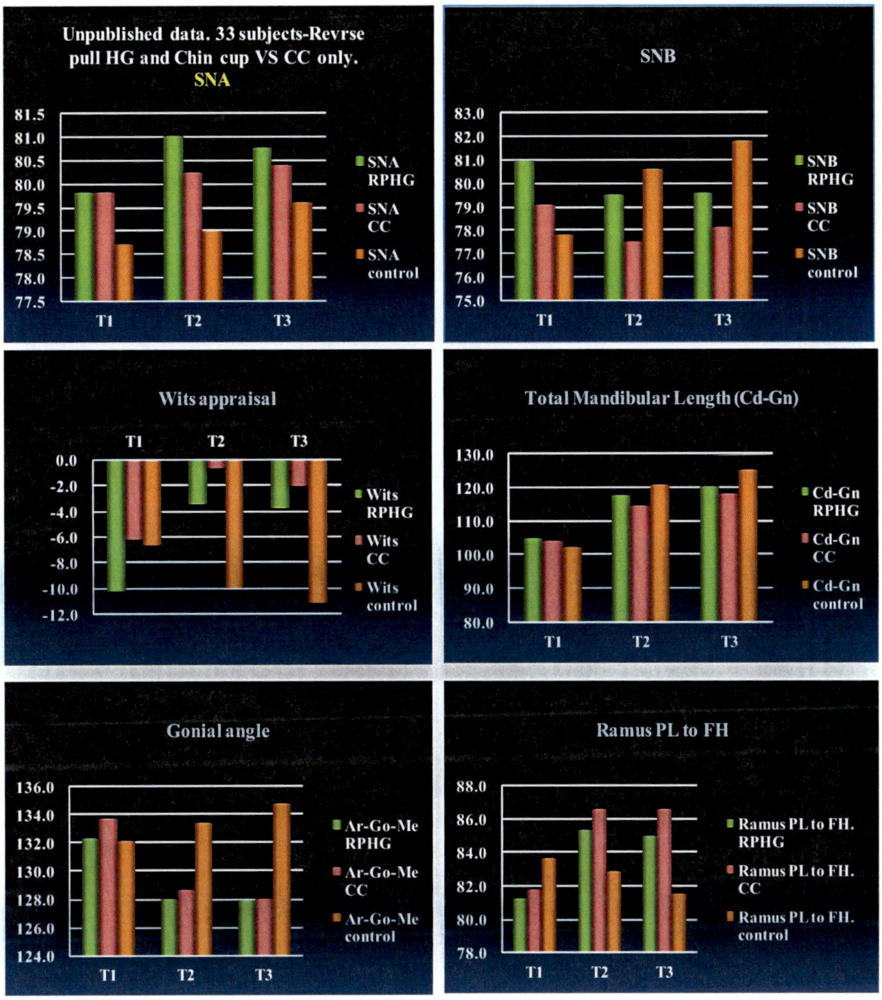

Figire 16: Bar graph showing SNA, SNB, Wits, Total mandibular length, Gonial angle and Ramus angle.

As illustrated in Fig. **17**, keys for greater success in the early correction of Class III malocclusion are:

1. Excellent cooperation can lead to overcorrection, of not only the dental but also the skeletal Class III profile, resulting in skeletal Class I (especially in meso- or hyper- divergent Class III cases).

2. The cephalometric measurements ANB, Wits, body length of the mandible, and L1-MP are useful diagnostic factors [30, 31]. Class III

malocclusion with negative open bite and either severe vertical or horizontal abnormalities should be treated with caution [6, 33, 34].

3. Orthopedic appliances used for correction of Class III malocclusion should be used for 2 years, [48] a time period that is similar to the minimum time frame for growth control with headgear. The use of CC or RPHG for 2 years or more may preclude the need for surgery in future.

Eighty-five percent of cases of severe skeletal Class III malocclusions in the United States have a maxillary hypoplasia component requiring maxillary advancement and mandibular set-back or 2 jaw surgery. A Class III malocclusion, secondary to maxillary retrognathia and mandibular prognathia in younger patients, may be treated successfully with maxillary protraction forces, thereby reducing the need for surgical maxillary advancement later in life [49]. In this scenario, a single jaw mandibular set back surgery may be all that is required, which is a great advantage for a patient.

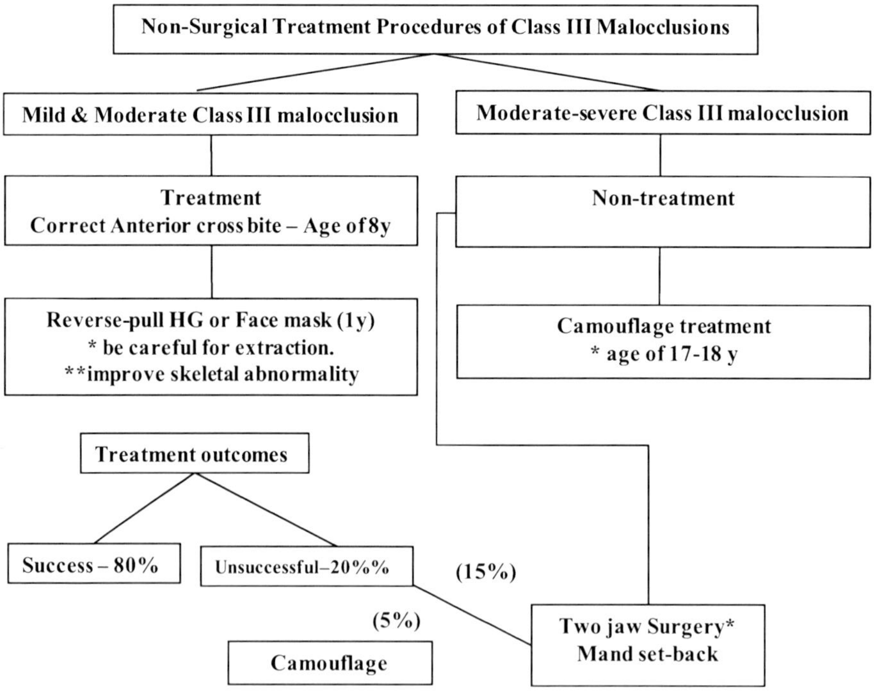

Figure 17: Diagram of diagnosis and treatment planning in class III malocclusion.

CONCLUSIONS

Early orthopedic treatment of Class III malocclusion with meso-dolichofacial skeletal pattern in 63 patients was compared using either chin cup only (n=30) or chin cup plus maxillary protraction (n=33). Active treatment with orthopedic appliances (phase 1) and Edgewise appliance (phase 2) began in mid-childhood (8 years), continued into early adolescence (13.5 years), and was followed by retention until late adolescence (18 years). Comprehensive fixed orthodontic treatment was performed if needed, and all treatment outcomes were judged successful.

Based upon the conditions of the study, both reverse pull headgear and chin cup therapies demonstrated a restraining affect on the mandible, and both affected the patients in a similar manner. Protraction forces in the RPHG and CC groups succeeded in moving the maxilla forward and proclining upper incisors compared to the untreated group. It may be concluded that the application of orthopedic force for more than 2 years will result in a successful outcome. Retention in the treatment of Class III malocclusion is a period for biological remodeling of the TMJ, muscle adaptation, remodeling of the mandible, and maintenance of the maxillary dentition in the newly adapted position.

SUMMARY POINTS

- The total mandibular length, in Class III malocclusion or anterior cross bite, is 3-4 mm longer than that for a normal occlusion at the age of 4-5 years old. All cross-sectional data indicate excessive growth of the mandible in Class III malocclusion, which worsens with age.

- The post-pubertal growth of the Class III mandible (mixed gender) is more prolonged than that of the counterpart normal occlusion. The growth in Class III malocclusion is 0.5 mm to 1.0mm/year more than that of normal occlusion between 8 to 15 years of age.

- In our "Tokushima chin cup and Reverse-pull HG treated subjects", excellent cooperation led to overcorrection of Class III dental, skeletal, and profile problems, resulting in skeletal Class I pattern. The changes were clinically well maintained at the post-retention evaluations. From post-treatment to post-retention stage, the variables of ANB, Wits, Gonial angle and Ramus angle showed from <25% relapse.

- Changes in the shape of the mandible in Class III treated cases lead to smaller-sized increments in total mandibular length (Cd-Gn), by means of a more forward orientation of the condyle and a more closed gonial angle.

- The application of orthopedic force for 2 years results in a successful outcome and stability in the treatment of Class III malocclusion. The corrected occlusion allows for biological remodeling of the TMJ, muscle adaptation, remodeling of the mandible, and maintenance of the maxillary dentition in the newly adapted position.

- Clinically, advancement of the maxillary dentition and maxilla results in 4 mm of anteroposterior (A-P) correction. Backward rotation of the mandible also contributes to 2 mm of A-P correction. One year use of the face mask allows for 6 mm of Class III correction and a 5-year follow-up observation showed the significant treatment effects were maintained.

- In our "MDU chin cup treated subjects with normal maxilla," the initial Class III skeletal components maintained the pre-treatment Class III features. The chin cup was applied for one year of nighttime wear, if patient co-operation was at least fair.

- Unsuccessful cases in severe Class III malocclusion showed: 1) forward rotation and more growth of the mandible, and 2) opening of the gonial angle at post-retention. Successful cases showed closing of the gonial angle at post-retention.

- Chin cup and lower headgear applications to the mandible were not shown to cause TMJ disorder.

ACKNOWLEDGEMENTS

Tokushima Cases are treated by Dr. Takao Kuroda, private practice, Tokushima city, Shikoku Island, Japan. These records were donated to Dr. James A.

McNamara, Center for Human Growth and Development, The University of Michigan by courtesy of Dr. Takao Kuroda and Dr. Toshio Deguchi.

CONFLICT OF INTEREST

The authors confirm that this chapter contents have no conflict of interest.

REFERENCES

[1] Graber TM. Current orthodontics concepts and techniques, Philadelphia: WB Saunders Co; 1994.
[2] Lin JJ. Prevalence of malocclusion in Chinese children age 9-15. Clin Dent (Taiwan) 1985;5:57-65.
[3] Rabie ABM, Gu Y. Diagnostic criteria for pseudo-class III malocclusion. Am J Orthod Dentofacial Orthop 2000;117:1-9.
[4] Takada K, Petdachai S, Sakuda M. Changes in dentofacial morphology in skeletal Class III children treated by a modified maxillary protraction headgear and a chincup: a longitudinal cephalometric appraisal. Eur J Orthod 1993;15:214-221.
[5] Gallagher RW, Miranda F, Buschang. Maxillary protraction: Treatment and posttreatment effects. Am J Orthod Dentofacial Orthop 1998;113:612-619.
[6] Yoshida I, Ishii H, Yamaguchi N, Mizoguchi I. Maxillary protraction and chin cap appliance treatment effects and long-term changes in skeletal Class III patients. Angle Orthod 1999;69:543-552.
[7] Ucuncu N, Ucem IT, Yukel S. A comparison of chincap and maxillary protraction appliances in the treatment of skeletal Class III malocclusions. Eur J Orthod 2000;22:43-51.
[8] Westwood PV, McNamara JA, Bacetti T, Franchi L, Sarver DM. Long-term effects of Class III treatment with rapid maxillary expansion and facemask therapy followed by fixed appliances. Am J Orthod Dentofacial Orthop 2003;123:306-320.
[9] Ghiz MA, Ngan P, Gunel P. Cephalometric variables to predict future success of early orthopedic Class III treatment. Am J Orthod Dentofacial Orthop 2005;127:301-306.
[10] Vaughn GA, Mason B, Moon HB, Turley PK. The effects of maxillary protraction therapy with or without rapid palatal expansion: A prospective, randomized clinical trial. Am J Orthod Dentofacial Orthop 2005;128:299-309.
[11] Wells AP, Saver DM, Proffit WR. Long-term efficacy of reverse pull headgear therapy. Am J Orthod Dentofacial Orthop 2006;76:915-922.
[12] Tollaro I, Baccetti T, Bassarelli V, Franchi L. Class III malocclusion in the deciduous dentition:a morphological and correlation study. Eur J Orthod 1994;16:401-408.
[13] Baccetti T, Franchi L, McNamara JA Jr. Growth in the untreated Class III subject. Semin Orthod 2007;13:130-142.
[14] Baccetti T, Reyes BC, McNamara JA Jr. Gender differences in Class III malocclusion. Angle Orthod 2005;75:510-520.
[15] Sugawara J, Asano 1, Endo N, Mitani H. Long-term effects of chin cap therapy on skeletal profile in mandibular prognathism. Am J Orthod Dentofacial Orthop 1990;98:127-133.

[16] Miyajima K, McNamara JA Jr, Sana M, Murata S. An estimation of craniofacial growth in the untreated Class III female with anterior crossbite. Am J Orthod Dentofacial Orthop 1997;112:425-434.
[17] Reyes BC, Baccetti T, McNamara JA Jr. An estimate of craniofacial growth in Class III malocclusion. Angle Orthod 2006;76:577-584.
[18] Mitani H. Prepubertal growth of mandibular prognathism. Am J Orthod 1981;80:546-553.
[19] Mitani H, Sato K, Sugawara J. Growth of mandibular prognathism after pubertal growth peak. Am J Orthod Dentofacial Orthop 1993;104:330-336.
[20] Toffol LD, Pavoni C, Baccetti T, Franchi L, Cozza P. Review article. Orthopedic treatment outcomes in Class III malocclusion. A systematic review. Angle Orthod 2008;78:561-573.
[21] Jacobson A, Evans WG, Preston CB, Sadowsky PL. Mandibular prognathism. Am J Orthod 1974;66:140-171.
[22] Guyer EC, Ellis E, McNamara JA Jr. Behrents RG. Components of Class III malocclusion in juveniles and adolescents. Angle Orthod 1986;56:7-30.
[23] Battagel JM. The etiological factors in Class III malocclusion. Eur J Orthod 1993;15:347-370.
[24] Deguchi T, Kuroda T, Minoshima Y, Graber TM. Craniofacial features of patients with Class III abnormalities: Growth-related changes and effects of short-term and long-term chin cap therapy. Am J Orthod Dentofacial Orthop 2002;121:84-92.
[25] Graber, LW. Chin cup therapy for mandibular prognathism. Am J Orthod, 1977;72:23-41.
[26] Mitani H, Sakamoto T. Chin cap force to a growing mandible. Long-term clinical reports. Angle Orthod 1984;54:93-112.
[27] Asano T. The effects of mandibular retractive force on the growing rat mandible. Am J Orthod Dentofacial Orthop 1986;90:464-474.
[28] Lu Y C-L, Tanne K, Hirano Y, Sakuda M. Craniofacial morphology of adolescent mandibular prognathism. Angle Orthod 1993;63:277-282.
[29] Deguchi T, Kitsugi A. Stability of changes associated with chin cup treatment. Angle Orthod1996;66:139-145
[30] Ko Y-II, Baek SH, Mah J, Yang WS. Determinants of successful chincup therapy in skeletal Class III malocclusion. Am J Orthod Dentofacial Orthop 2004;126:33-41.
[31] Tahmina K, Tanaka E, Tanne K. Craniofacial morphology in orthodontically treated patients of Class III malocclusion with stable and unstable treatment outcomes. Am J Orthod Dentofacial Orthop 2000;117:681-690.
[32] Baik HS. Limitations in orthopedic and camouflage treatment for Class III malocclusion. Semin Orthod 2007;13:158-174.
[33] Irie M, Nakamura S. Orthopedic approach to severe skeletal Class III malocclusion. Am J Orthod 1975;67:377-392.
[34] Watanabe M, Suda N, Ohyama K. Mandibular prognathism in Japanese families ascertained through orthognathically treated patients. Am Dentofacial Orthop 2005;128:112-116.
[35] Liu ZP, Li CJ, Hu HK, Chen JW, Li F, Zou SJ. Efficacy of short-term chincup therapy for mandibular growth retardation in Class III malocclusion. A systematic review. Angle Orthod 2011;81:162-168.
[36] Mimura H, Deguchi T. Morphological adaptation of temporomandibular joint after chin cup therapy. Am J Orthod Dentofacial Orthop 1996;110:541-546.
[37] Deguchi T. Force distribution of the temporomandibular joint and temporal bone surface subjected to the head-chincup force. Am J Orthod Dentofacial Orthop 1998;114:277-282.

[38] Franchi L, Baccetti T, McNamara JA Jr. Shape - coordinate analysis of skeletal changes induced by rapid palatal expansion and facial mask therapy. Am J Orthod Dentofacial Orthop 1998;114:418-426.

[39] Liu PH, Chang CH, Chang HP, Chang HF. Treatment effects of chin cup application on mandible in Class III malocclusion: strain tensor analysis. A pilot study. Quintessence Int 2004;35:621-629.

[40] Mitani H. Recovery growth of the mandible after chin cup therapy: Fact or Fiction. Semin Orthod 2007;13:186-199.

[41] Tanner JM. A history of the study of human growth, 1981, Cambridge: University Press.

[42] Deguchi 1, Kuroda 1, Hunt NP, Graber TM. Long-term application of chincup force alters the morphology of the dolichofacial Class III mandible. Am J Orthod Dentofacial Orthop1999;116:610-615.

[43] Tsunori M, Mashita M, Kasai K. Relationship between facial types and tooth and bone characteristics of the mandible obtained by CT scanning. Angle Orthod 1988;68:557-562.

[44] Kitai N, Fujii S, Murakami S, Furukawa S, Kreiborg S, Takada K. Human masticatory muscle volume and zygomatico-mandibular form in adults with mandibular prognathism. J Dent Res 2002;81:752-756.

[45] Ribeiro DPB, Gandelmann IHA, Medeiros PJ. Comparison of mandibular rami width in patients with prognathism and retrognathia. J Oral Maxillofac Surg 2006;64:1506-1509.

[46] Chen F, Wu LP, Terada K, Saito I. Longitudinal intermaxillary relationships in Class III malocclusions with low and high mandibular plane angles. Angle Orthodontist 2007;77:397-403.

[47] Cha BK, Kim C-H, Baek S-H. Skeletal sagittal and vertical facial types and electromyographic activity of the masticatory muscle. Angle Orthod 2007;77:463-470.

[48] Katashiba S, Deguchi T Sr, Kageyama T, Minoshima Y, Kuroda T, W. Eugene Roberts. The aggressive Chin cup protocol (14h/day for 2 years with excellent compliance) depends on commitment to overcorrection of the skeletal Class III malocclusion. Orthod Waves 2006;65:57-63.

[49] Kluemper GT, Spalding PM. Realities of craniofacial growth modification. Atlas Oral Maxillofac Surg Clin North Am 2001;9:23-51.

PART III: DIAGNOSIS AND TREATMENT IN THE NON-GROWING PATIENTS

CHAPTER 7

Anterior Crossbite Treatment with a Self-Ligating Bracket System

Mohammad Razavi*

University of Alberta, Clinical Instructor, School of Dentistry, Dept. Of Orthodontics, Edmonton Clinic Health Academy, 11405-87 Avenue NW, Edmonton, Alberta T6G1C9, Case Western Reserve University, School of Dental Medicine, Dept. Of Orthodontics, 10900 Euclid Ave., Cleveland, OH 44106, USA

Abstract: Anterior crossbite in the permanent dentition may be due to abnormal inclination of the maxillary and mandibular incisors, occlusal interferences, or skeletal discrepancies of the maxilla and/or mandible. Traditionally Class III patients are treated with lower premolar extraction. When extractions are performed only in the mandibular arch, special attention should be paid to the torque of the lower incisors to prevent excessive lingual tipping. Gingival recession may occur with excessive retraction of the lower incisors to close extraction space(s). The use of a self-ligating bracket system may have advantages for treating crossbite associated with both Class III and Class I malocclusions. The play between the main arch wire and the bracket slot provides mechanical freedom to facilitate tooth movement. Clinical cases are presented to demonstrate this technique for correcting Class III and Class I malocclusions with anterior crossbite.

Keywords: Class III malocclusions, Passive self-ligating bracket system, skeletal Class, Anterior Crossbite.

TREATMENT PRINCIPLES FOR NON-GROWING SKELETAL CLASS III PATIENTS

The treatment of Class III discrepancies continues to challenge orthodontists due to the diversity of skeletal and dental problems associated with a given malocclusion. Skeletally patients may present with an undersized maxilla, overdeveloped mandible or a combination of both [1]. When compared to skeletally balanced individuals, Class III subjects tend to have shorter anterior cranial base, longer posterior cranial base, an acute cranial base, excessive lower anterior facial height a shorter, posteriorly positioned maxilla, excessively proclined maxillary incisors, and retroclined mandibular incisors due to dentoalveloar compensations [2]. Depending on the types of Class III malocclusion, different options and treatment goals can be applied. Treatment options depend on the degree of anteroposterior and vertical skeletal discrepancy, as well as on the incisal inclination, and overall facial esthetics

***Address correspondence to Mohammad Razavi:** 205-308 Palladium Dr. Kanata, ON, Canada. K2V 1A1; Tel: 613-592-7679; Fax: 613-592-7680; E-mail: mrazavi@palladiumorthodontics.com

[2]. Communication with patients and prioritization of treatment goals is crucial for successful orthodontic treatment of these patients. The treatment goal is to obtain a functional and esthetic treatment result that is acceptable to the orthodontist, patient, and their family.

Proffit and Ackermann [3] reported on the limitation of camouflage Class III malocclusion. For successful non-surgical orthodontic treatment, the maxillary incisors should not procline more than 2 mm, and the mandibular incisor should not be retracted more than 3mm, relative to the apical base of bone. Burns *et al.* reported successful treatment of Class III malocclusions using camouflage treatment in patients who had a Wits appraisal -5.0 mm or more [4]. Rabie and Gu reported other diagnostic characteristics that are desirable for camouflage treatment of Class III malocclusions: 1. upright maxillary incisors, 2. normal to minimally retroclined mandibular incisors, 3. a forward positioned mandible of normal skeletal length, and 4. a decreased lower anterior facial height, especially in the midface region [5]. A few investigators recommended camouflage treatment of low angle Class III malocclusions by increasing the lower face height and reducing the deep overbite [2, 4]. Intermaxillary elastics or mechanics that can increase the vertical dimension can be used to achieve these goals. In high angle cases, mechanics that increase the lower face height should be avoided. In the anteroposterior dimension, the maxillary incisors should not be tipped forward because the incisors may already be compensated by excessive angulation. Therefore, maxillary incisors should be moved with adequate labial root torque to control the axial inclination of the upper incisors. For patients with skeletal Class III malocclusions, the mandibular incisors are usually already tipped lingually in skeletal Class III patients. So, if it is necessary to tip these teeth further lingually for anterior cross bite correction, it is advised to proceed with caution and carefully check the periodontal support at each appointment.

CONVENTIONAL EDGEWISE TREATMENT WITH OR WITHOUT EXTRACTION

The need for extraction of mandibular premolars or incisors depends on the severity of the malocclusion and the amount of crowding in the dental arches. Extraction of the mandibular premolars is indicated if lingual retraction of the mandibular incisors is desired. Extraction of the maxillary second and mandibular first premolars is indicated when treatment goals include correction of the molar classification. Extraction of a mandibular incisor is indicated in cases with mild crowding of the mandibular arch, associated with a favorable Bolton tooth size discrepancy, or for patients with mild mandibular crowding along with an anterior cross bite. Finally, non-extraction therapy can be used in low angle cases with the presence of an anterior cross bite by uprighting the mandibular posterior teeth and a counter clockwise rotation of the occlusal plane.

ADVANTAGES OF THE SELF-LIGATING BRACKET SYSTEM

The first self-ligating bracket was introduced in the 1930s with the presentation of the Russell Lock appliance [6]. The increased cost of these brackets was likely the reason for the vast skepticism amongst orthodontists until recent years; however, continuing claims of decreased treatment time and reduced frictional resistance compared to conventional edgewise brackets has renewed interest in these brackets. Reduced friction is of significant importance to camouflage treatment of Class III malocclusions, because they minimize anchorage requirements and undesirable tooth movement to accomplish the anterior torque requirements [7]. A systematic review of self-ligating brackets revealed a reduction of 1.5° in the proclination of mandibular incisors when compared to conventional ligation [8]. Control over mandibular incisor position is of significant importance in non-surgical correction of Class III malocclusions.

Harradine [7] reported the ideal ligation system as one with robust and secure ligation, with full engagement of the wire by the bracket, resulting in low friction between the arch wire and the bracket. Furthermore, the system should be easy to use, allow for attachment of elastic chain modules, and provide for increasing friction when desired. Above all it should provide good oral hygiene, and produce a comfortable patient experience. After an extensive search for the optimal appliance system, that could provide all of the above characteristics, the SmartClip appliance system (Trademark of 3M Unitek, 2724 S. Peck Rd, Monrovia, CA 91016; www.3Munitek.com) was used in the treatment of the following patients.

CASE REPORT 1

A 11-year-old male presented with the chief complaint of “bite problems”. Clinical examination revealed a Class I malocclusion, with complete anterior crossbite and moderate maxillary and mild mandibular tooth size/arch length discrepancy (Figs. **1A, B** & **C**). No anterior functional shift or habitual bite pattern was detected in the clinical exam. The maxillary midline was deviated to the right by 3 mm due to the labially blocked out maxillary right canine. Cephalometric analysis (Table **1**) revealed a balanced skeletal relationship, with a normal-sized mandible, retroclined maxillary incisors and protruded mandibular incisors. Soft tissue analysis revealed an obtuse nasolabial angle with mid-face deficiency. A non-extraction therapy was undertaken in an effort to improve the upper lip position.

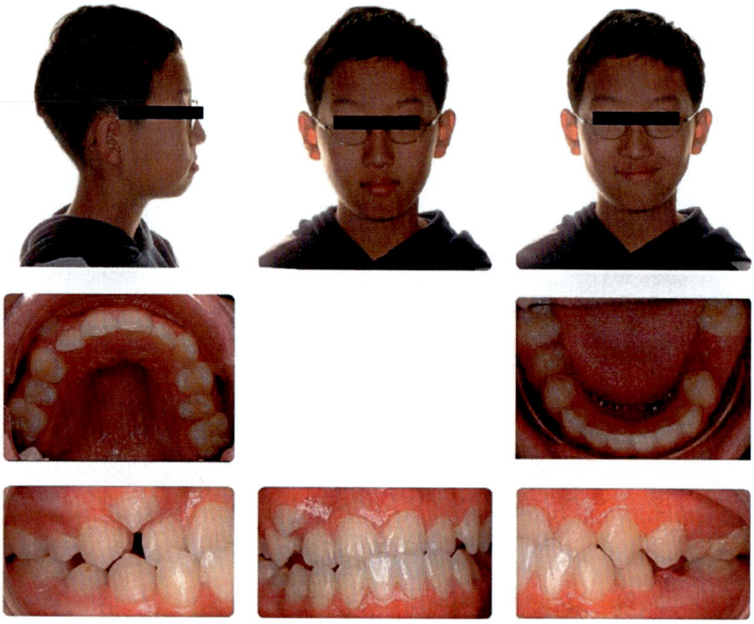

Figure 1A: Pretreatment clinical photos.

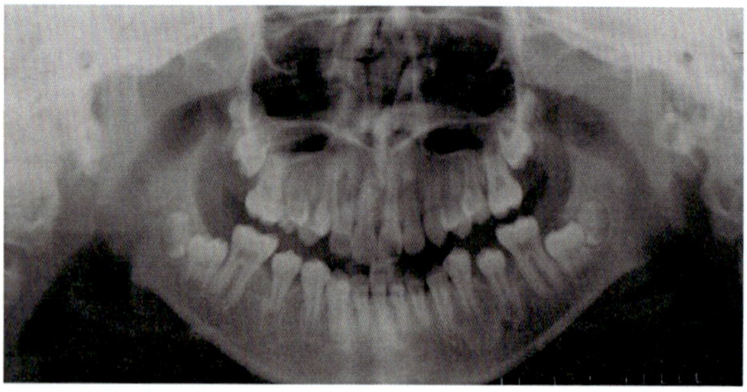

Figure 1B: Pretreatment panoramic radiograph.

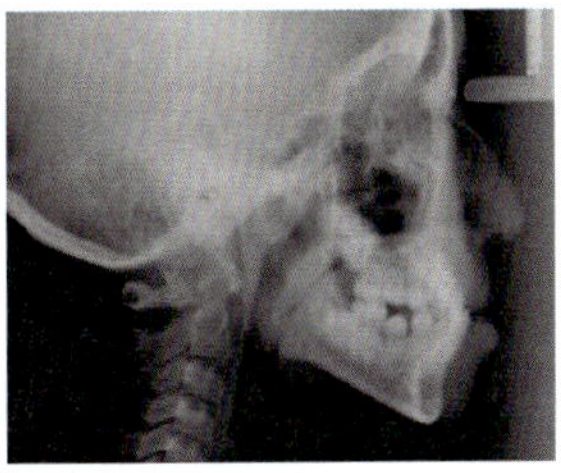

Figure 1C: Pretreatment cephalometric radiograph.

Table 1: Pretreatment cephalometric measurements

	Value	Norm	Std Dev
Maxilla to Cranial Base			
SNA (°)	79.2	82.0	3.5
Mandible to Cranial Base			
SNB (°)	77.3	80.9	3.4
SN - GoGn (°)	32.2	32.9	5.2
FMA (MP-FH) (°)	29.0	25.1	4.5
Maxillo-Mandibular			
ANB (°)	1.8	1.6	1.5
Maxillary Dentition			
U1 - NA (mm)	2.9	4.3	2.7
U1 - SN (°)	98.3	102.4	5.5
Mandibular Dentition			
L1 - NB (mm)	8.7	4.0	1.8
L1 - GoGn (°)	98.2	93.0	6.0
Soft Tissue			
Lower Lip to E-Plane (mn	4.8	-2.0	2.0
Upper Lip to E-Plane (mn	-2.8	-3.7	2.0

Fixed appliances (022x028 SmartClip™ Self-Ligating brackets, Variable Prescription Orthodontics™ (VPO) were bonded to the upper and lower arches. The use of VPO dynamic prescription allowed for the specific selection of maxillary brackets with additional labial crown torque, and mandibular brackets with lower labial crown torque. This bracket selection is ideal for correction of the anterior cross bite. The wire sequence was .014" Super Elastic Nitinol wires for 11 weeks, followed by tandem upper and lower .014"/.016" Super Elastics Nitinol wires for 15 weeks, during which time light Class III elastics were used to achieve a positive overjet. The transition to upper and lower .019"x.025" Heat Activated Nitinol and eventual .019x.025 Beta Titanium wires was used for the detailing and finishing stage of the treatment.

The entire treatment lasted for 22 months, during which the patient had a total of 12 appointments. Post-treatment records revealed a Class I molar relationship with ideal overjet and overjet (Figs. **2 A, B** & **C**). Cephalometric superimposition (Table **2**, Fig. **3**) indicated the ideal overjet was achieved by proclination of the maxillary incisors and retroclination of the mandibular incisors. Regional superimposition revealed that extrusion of maxillary molars as a result of Class III intermaxillary elastics, leading to counter clockwise rotation of the occlusal plane and correction of the malocclusion.

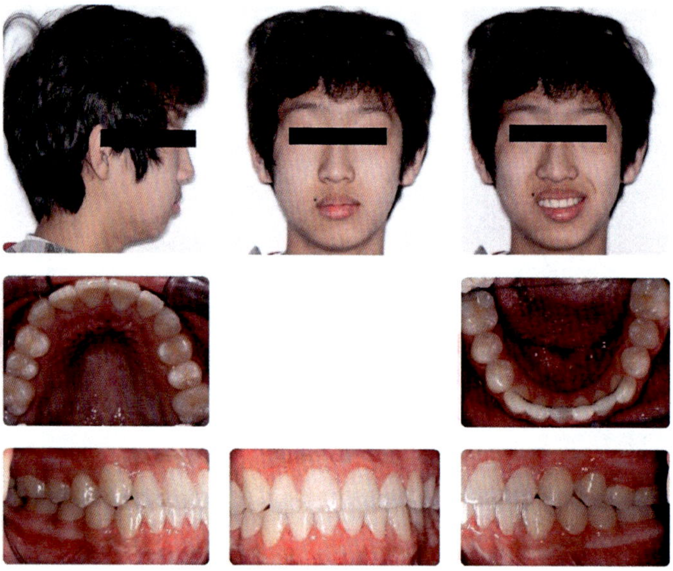

Figure 2A: Post-treatment clinical photos.

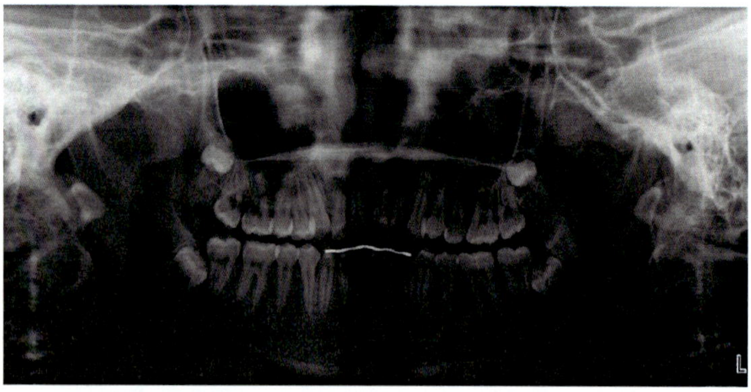

Figure 2B: Post-treatment panoramic radiograph.

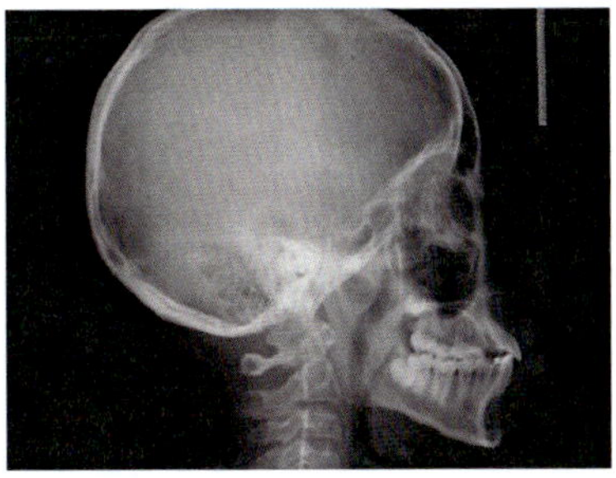

Figure 2C: Post-treatment cephalometric radiograph.

Table 2: Post-treatment cephalometric measurements

	Value	Norm	Std Dev
Maxilla to Cranial Base			
SNA (°)	73.0	82.0	3.5
Mandible to Cranial Base			
SNB (°)	70.5	80.9	3.4
SN - GoGn (°)	41.2	32.9	5.2
FMA (MP-FH) (°)	26.7	24.3	4.5
Maxillo-Mandibular			
ANB (°)	2.5	1.6	1.5
Maxillary Dentition			
U1 - NA (mm)	6.8	4.3	2.7
U1 - SN (°)	106.6	102.7	5.5
Mandibular Dentition			
L1 - NB (mm)	7.0	4.0	1.8
L1 - GoGn (°)	93.0	93.0	6.0
Soft Tissue			
Lower Lip to E-Plane (mm	5.1	-2.0	2.0
Upper Lip to E-Plane (mm	-1.6	-5.1	2.0

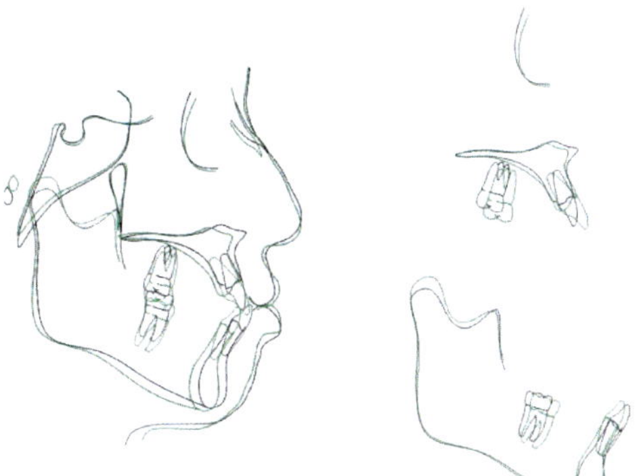

Figure 3: Pretreatment (black) and Post-treatment (green) cephalometric superimposition.

CASE REPORT 2

An 11-year-old male presented with the chief complaint of "my lower jaw is larger than my upper jaw". Clinical examination revealed a Class III molar relationship, with a complete anterior crossbite and a mild maxillary tooth size/arch length discrepancy (Figs. **4 A, B** & **C**). No functional shift was detected during the clinical exam. Cephalometric analysis (Table **3**) revealed a retrusive maxilla, with a protrusive mandible which resulted in an ANB of -4.9. The maxillary incisors were proclined, while the mandibular incisors were mildly retroclined. Soft tissue analysis revealed a posteriorly positioned upper lip, and a protrusive lower lip. Non-extraction therapy was indicated to improve the upper lip position.

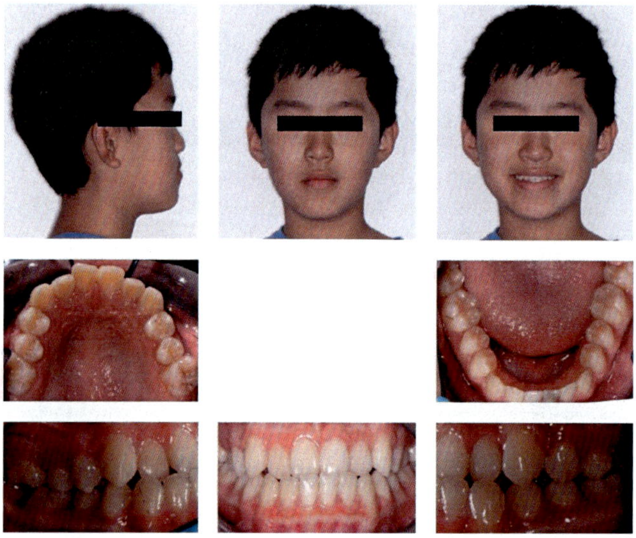

Figure 4A: Pretreatment clinical photos.

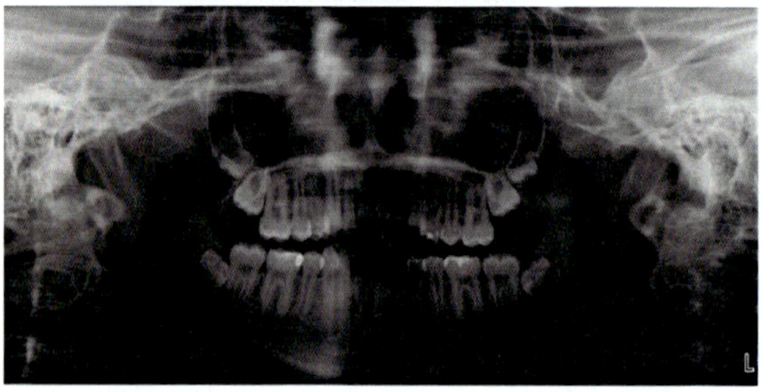

Figure 4B: Pretreatment panoramic radiograph.

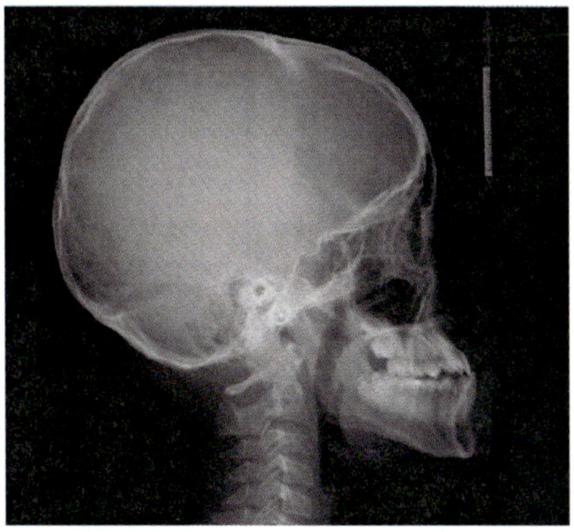

Figure 4C: Pretreatment cephalometric radiograph.

Table 3: Pretreatment cephalometric measurements

	Value	Norm	Std Dev
Maxilla to Cranial Base			
SNA (°)	79.0	82.0	3.5
Mandible to Cranial Base			
SNB (°)	83.9	80.9	3.4
SN - GoGn (°)	30.6	32.9	5.2
FMA (MP-FH) (°)	20.1	25.1	4.5
Maxillo-Mandibular			
ANB (°)	-4.9	1.6	1.5
Maxillary Dentition			
U1 - NA (mm)	9.4	4.3	2.7
U1 - SN (°)	111.6	102.4	5.5
Mandibular Dentition			
L1 - NB (mm)	5.1	4.0	1.8
L1 - GoGn (°)	86.5	93.0	6.0
Soft Tissue			
Lower Lip to E-Plane (mn	2.8	-2.0	2.0
Upper Lip to E-Plane (mn	-2.4	-3.7	2.0

Fixed appliances (022x028 SmartClip™ Self-Ligating brackets, Variable Prescription Orthodontics™) were bonded on the upper and lower arches. The VPO dynamic prescription was used including high torque maxillary incisors and low torque mandibular incisors, in order to camouflage the underlying skeletal discrepancy. Atypical bracket position was utilized to prevent excessive molar extrusion and creation of an iatrogenic open bite. Upon bracket placement, upper and lower .014" Super Elastic Nitinol wires were used for 12 weeks to resolve the maxillary crowding and final leveling was achieved by placement of upper and lower tandem .014"/.016" Super Elastics Nitinol wires for 10 weeks. Light Class III elastics were started upon placement of the tandem arch wires and continued throughout the sequence of wire changes until the .019"x.025" Heat Activated Nitinol. Detailing and finishing was accomplished with .019"x.025" Beta Titanium arch wires.

The treatment required a total of 11 appointments over a period of 18 months. Post-treatment records documented the achievement of a Class I molar relationship with an ideal overjet and overjet (Figs. **5 A, B** & **C**). Cephalometric superimposition (Table **4**, Fig. **6**) indicated the ideal overbite was achieved by extrusion of the maxillary incisors, a treatment result that was due to the atypical bracket position. There was minimal proclination of the maxillary incisors, as these teeth were already excessively proclined at the beginning of treatment. Overjet correction was mainly achieved through uprighting of the entire mandibular dentition, both in the anterior and posterior segments.

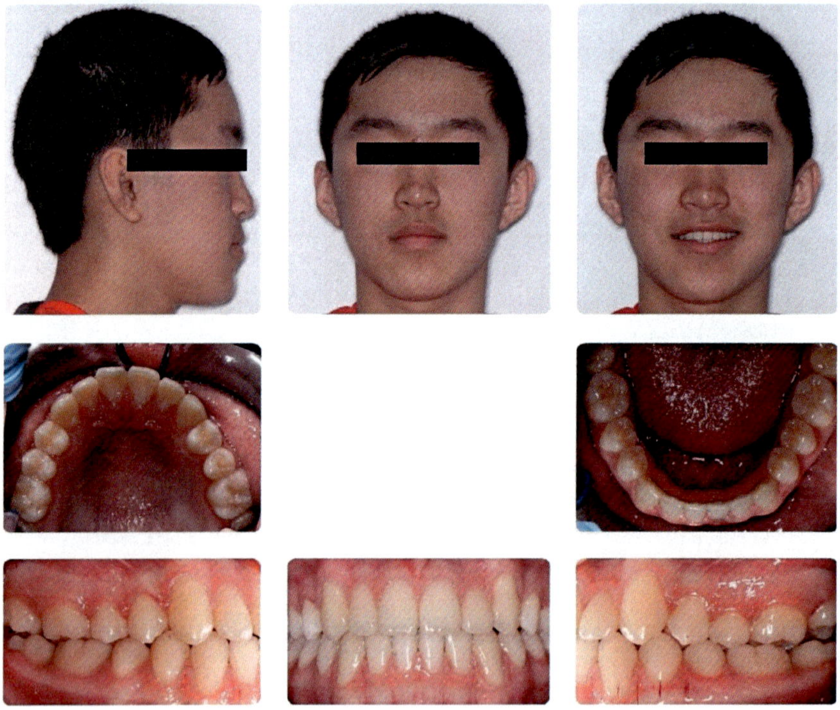

Figure 5A: Post-treatment clinical photos.

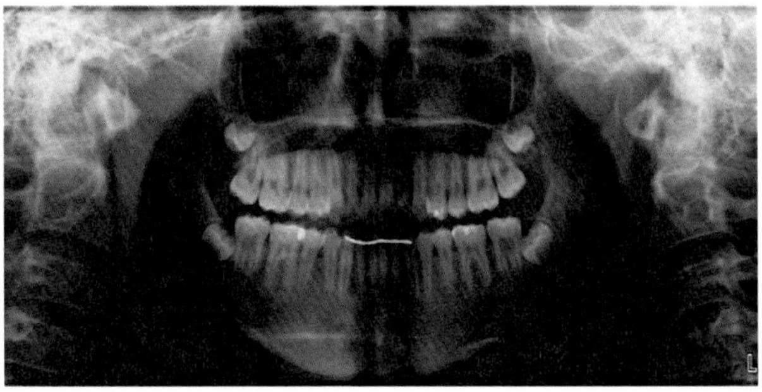

Figure 5B: Post-treatment panoramic radiograph.

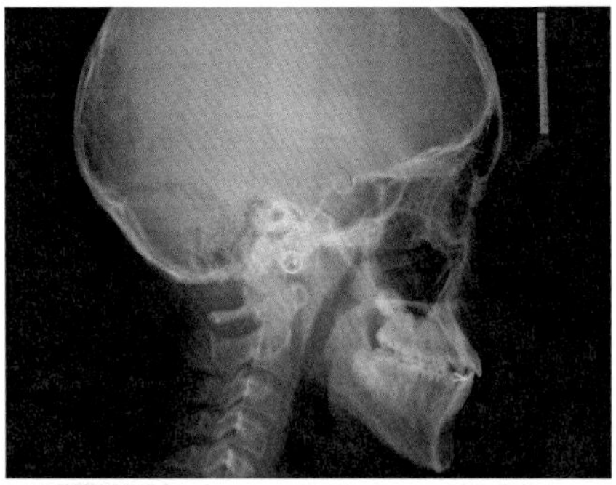

Figure 5C: Post-treatment cephalometric radiograph.

Table 4: Post-treatment cephalometric measurements

	Value	Norm	Std Dev
Maxilla to Cranial Base			
SNA (°)	80.1	82.0	3.5
Mandible to Cranial Base			
SNB (°)	80.9	80.9	3.4
SN - GoGn (°)	32.0	32.9	5.2
FMA (MP-FH) (°)	36.5	24.5	4.5
Maxillo-Mandibular			
ANB (°)	-0.9	1.6	1.5
Maxillary Dentition			
U1 - NA (mm)	10.3	4.3	2.7
U1 - SN (°)	117.2	102.6	5.5
Mandibular Dentition			
L1 - NB (mm)	5.3	4.0	1.8
L1 - GoGn (°)	84.8	93.0	6.0
Soft Tissue			
Lower Lip to E-Plane (mn	2.6	-2.0	2.0
Upper Lip to E-Plane (mr	-1.1	-4.7	2.0

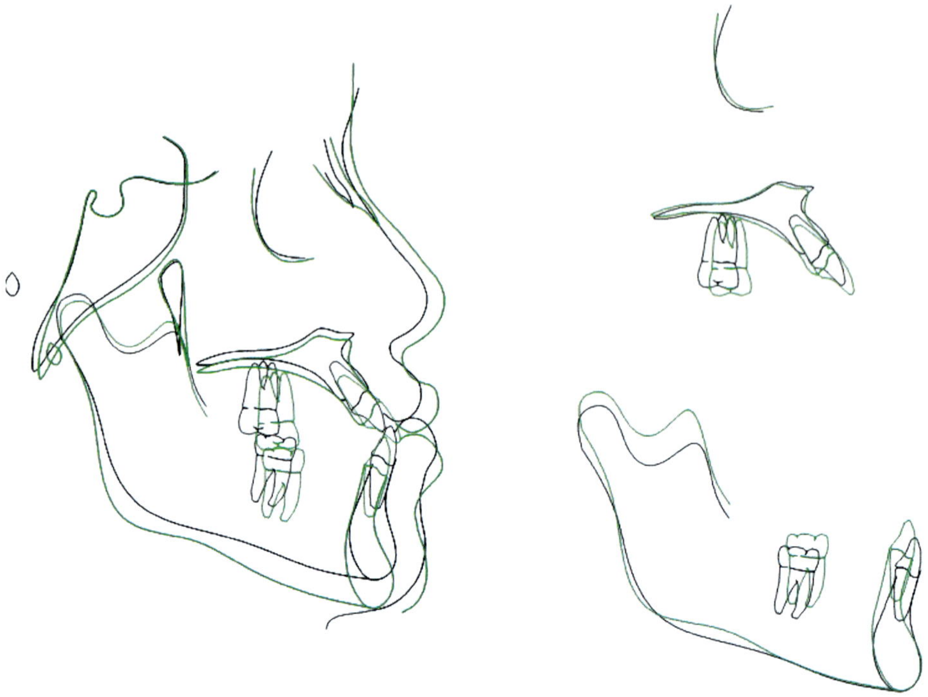

Figure 6: Pretreatment (black) and Post-treatment (green) cephalometric superimposition.

CASE REPORT 3

A 17-year-old female presented with the chief complaint of "underbite". Clinical examination revealed a Class I malocclusion, with complete anterior crossbite and minimal maxillary and mandibular tooth size/arch length discrepancy (Figs. **7 A, B** & **C**). There was an absence of a functional shift. The mandibular midline was deviated to the left by 2mm, and excess space was noted distal to the lower right lateral incisor. Cephalometric analysis (Table **5**) revealed a mildly prognathic mandible, with excessive proclination of maxillary and mandibular incisors. The excessively proclined maxillary incisors limited the correction of the anterior crossbite through further proclination of these teeth. Therefore, one of the treatment options was extraction of the maxillary premolars and a Lefort I maxillary advancement. However, the patient declined the surgical option. Since she presented with an acceptable facial profile, the treatment goal was to correct the anterior crossbite mainly through retraction of the proclined mandibular incisors.

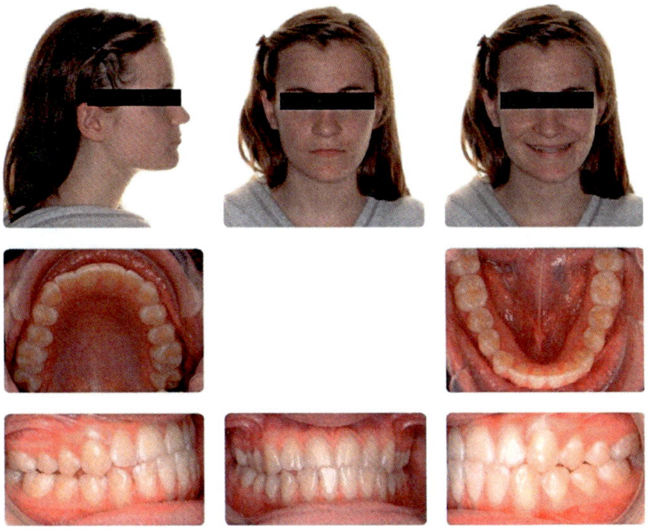

Figure 7A: Pretreatment clinical photos.

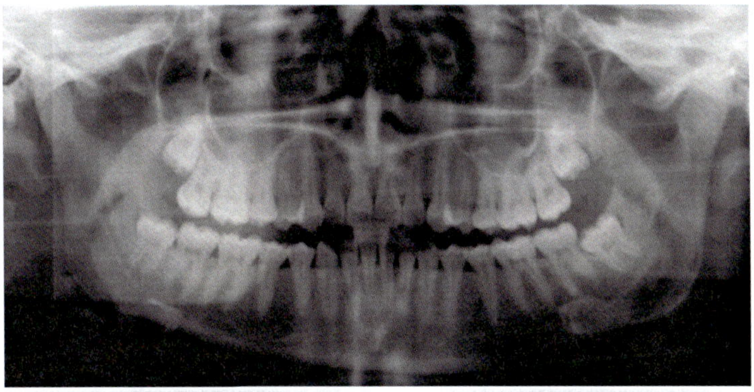

Figure 7B: Pretreatment panoramic radiograph.

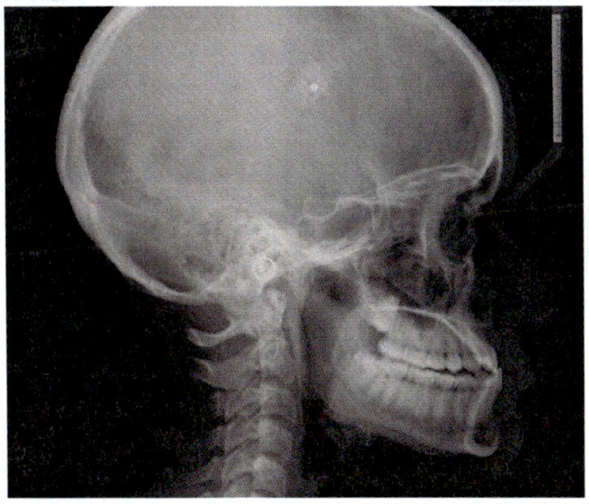

Figure 7C: Pretreatment cephalometric radiograph.

Table 5: Pretreatment cephalometric measurements

	Value	Norm	Std Dev
Maxilla to Cranial Base			
SNA (°)	84.6	82.0	3.5
Mandible to Cranial Base			
SNB (°)	87.5	80.9	3.4
SN - GoGn (°)	16.8	32.9	5.2
FMA (MP-FH) (°)	14.1	23.9	4.5
Maxillo-Mandibular			
ANB (°)	-2.9	1.6	1.5
Maxillary Dentition			
U1 - NA (mm)	4.9	4.3	2.7
U1 - SN (°)	118.5	102.8	5.5
Mandibular Dentition			
L1 - NB (mm)	3.8	4.0	1.8
L1 - GoGn (°)	100.2	93.0	6.0
Soft Tissue			
Lower Lip to E-Plane (mn	-1.2	-2.0	2.0
Upper Lip to E-Plane (mn	-6.3	-6.0	2.0

Referral was made for the extraction of the third molars prior to the initiation of orthodontic treatment. Fixed appliances (022x028 SmartClip™ Self-Ligating brackets, Variable Prescription Orthodontics™) were bonded to both the upper and lower arches. Medium torque maxillary incisor brackets were selected to avoid further proclination of the maxillary incisors, while low torque brackets were used in the mandibular arch to aid in the uprighting and reduction in proclination of these teeth. A typical bracket position was employed to prevent excessive extrusion of the molars. This approach was necessary because no mandibular growth was expected. Molar extrusion may have resulted in an anterior open bite, particularly with the use of Class III elastics. The arch wire sequence was: .014" Super Elastic Nitinol wires for 10 weeks in both arches, upper and lower tandem .014"/.016" Super Elastics Nitinol wires for 7 weeks, followed by .019"x.025" Heat Activated Nitinol in both arches. Class III elastics were used to obtain a positive overjet after placement of rectangular archwires. In this case, elastic use was delayed until full size wires were in place, in order to avoid uncontrolled tipping of the maxillary incisors. Detailing and finishing was completed with .019"x.025" Beta Titanium.

The entire treatment lasted for 16 months, during which the patient has a total of 9 appointments. Post-treatment records revealed a Class I molar relationship with an ideal overjet and overjet (Figs. **8 A, B** & **C**). Cephalometric superimposition (Table **6**, Fig. **9**) indicated the ideal overjet was mainly achieved by retroclination of the mandibular incisors. However, even though measures were taken to avoid further proclination of the maxillary incisors, the use of Class III elastics resulted in these teeth becoming more proclined at the end of treatment. The vertical dimension was well controlled through the use of atypical bracket position which minimized molar extrusion and a subsequent anterior open bite.

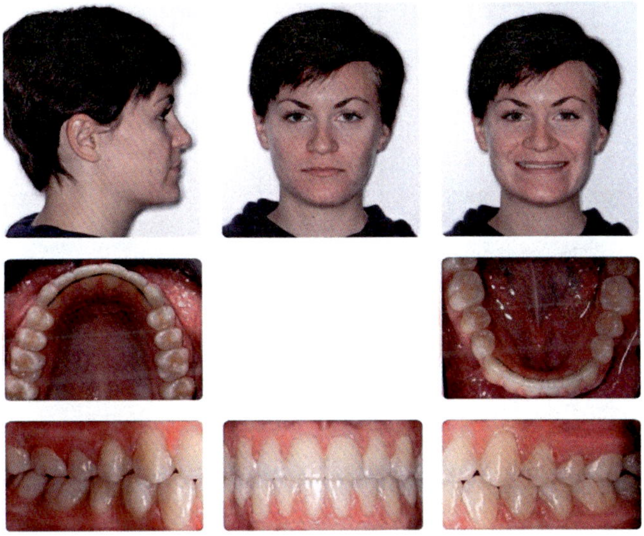

Figure 8A: Post-treatment clinical photos.

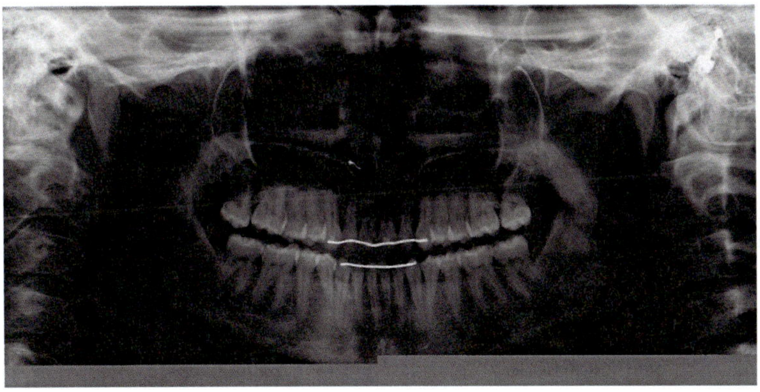

Figure 8B: Post-treatment panoramic radiograph.

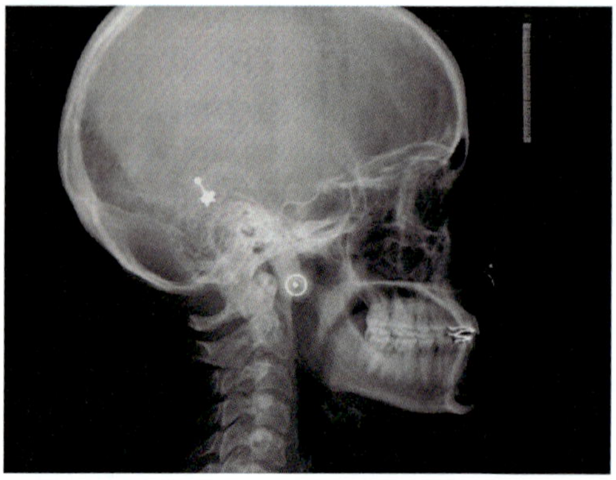

Figure 8C: Post-treatment cephalometric radiograph.

Table 6: Post-treatment cephalometric measurements

	Value	Norm	Std Dev
Maxilla to Cranial Base			
SNA (°)	79.5	82.0	3.5
Mandible to Cranial Base			
SNB (°)	82.5	80.9	3.4
SN - GoGn (°)	21.4	32.9	5.2
FMA (MP-FH) (°)	18.8	23.9	4.5
Maxillo-Mandibular			
ANB (°)	-2.9	1.6	1.5
Maxillary Dentition			
U1 - NA (mm)	9.6	4.3	2.7
U1 - SN (°)	124.2	102.8	5.5
Mandibular Dentition			
L1 - NB (mm)	2.1	4.0	1.8
L1 - GoGn (°)	92.5	93.0	6.0
Soft Tissue			
Lower Lip to E-Plane (mn	-3.4	-2.0	2.0
Upper Lip to E-Plane (mn	-6.4	-6.0	2.0

CASE REPORT 4

A 12-year-old female presented with a chief complaint of "underbite". Clinical examination revealed a Class III subdivision right malocclusion, with maxillary transverse deficiency, and a posterior right crossbite of the maxillary right first molars. The maxillary anterior teeth were in complete anterior crossbite, with moderate maxillary and mild mandibular tooth size/arch length discrepancy

(Fig. **10 A, B, C**). Clinical exam did not reveal a functional shift. The maxillary midline was deviated to the right by 2 mm, resulting in reduced space for the eruption of the maxillary right canine. Cephalometric analysis (Table **7**) revealed a reduced vertical facial height, along with a mildly prognathic mandible and retroclined mandibular incisors. Soft tissue analysis confirmed esthetically acceptable facial features.

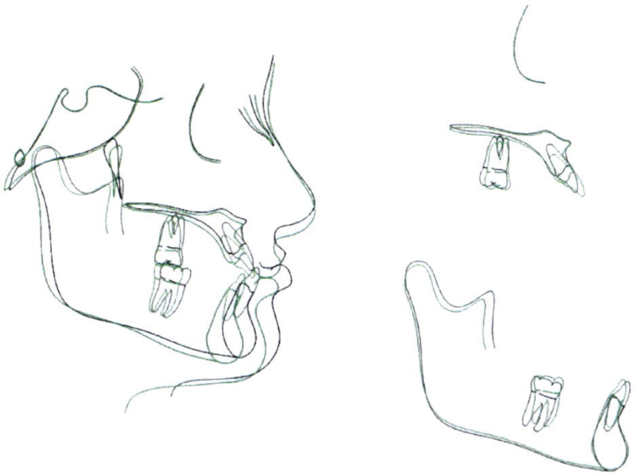

Figure 9: Pretreatment (black) and Post-treatment (green) cephalometric superimposition.

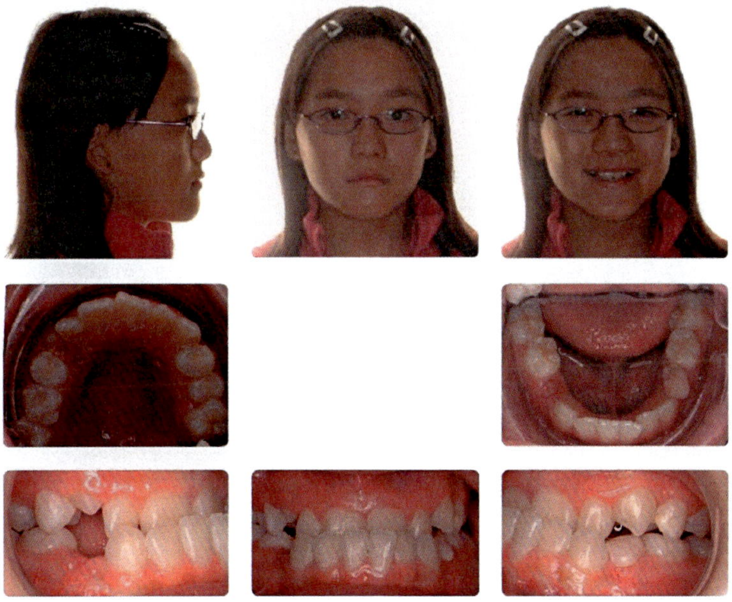

Figure 10A: Pretreatment clinical photos.

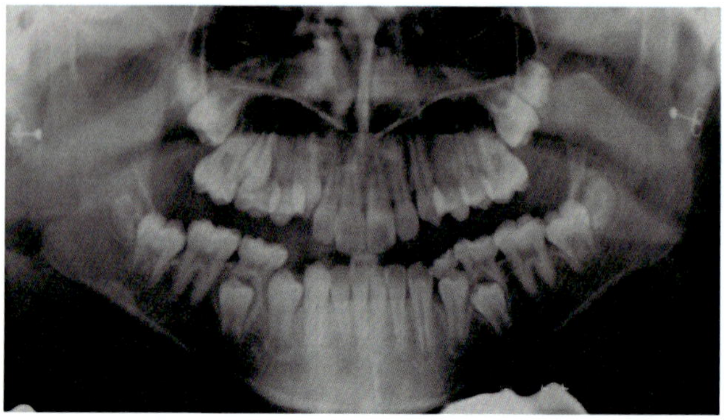

Figure 10B: Pretreatment panoramic radiograph.

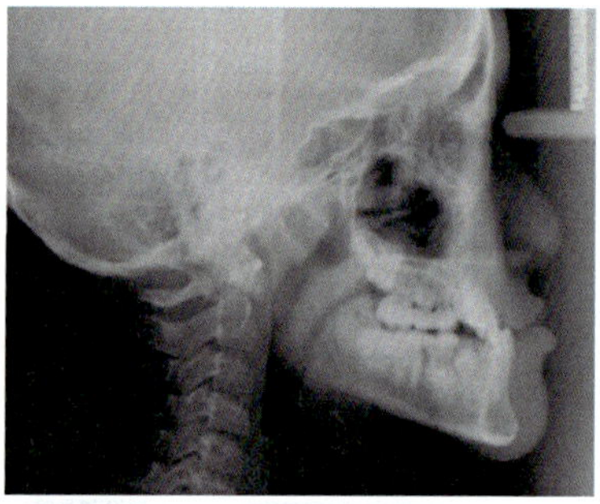

Figure 10C: Pretreatment cephalometric radiograph.

Table 7: Pretreatment cephalometric measurements

	Value	Norm	Std Dev
Maxilla to Cranial Base			
SNA (°)	82.4	82.0	3.5
Mandible to Cranial Base			
SNB (°)	89.1	80.9	3.4
SN - GoGn (°)	22.0	32.9	5.2
FMA (MP-FH) (°)	26.6	25.0	4.5
Maxillo-Mandibular			
ANB (°)	-6.7	1.6	1.5
Maxillary Dentition			
U1 - NA (mm)	5.5	4.3	2.7
U1 - SN (°)	108.7	102.5	5.5
Mandibular Dentition			
L1 - NB (mm)	1.3	4.0	1.8
L1 - GoGn (°)	80.0	93.0	6.0
Soft Tissue			
Lower Lip to E-Plane (mr	1.0	-2.0	2.0
Upper Lip to E-Plane (mr	-2.8	-3.8	2.0

Orthodontic treatment was initiated with a rapid maxillary expansion appliance to correct the posterior crossbite and create space in the maxillary arch. The maxillary expansion was stabilized for a period of six months before fixed appliances (022x028 SmartClip™ Self-Ligating brackets, Variable Prescription Orthodontics™) were bonded to both upper and lower arches. The treatment goals included proclination of the maxillary incisors, while maintaining the upright mandibular incisors in order to camouflage the underlying skeletal discrepancy. Therefore, high torque maxillary incisor and low torque mandibular incisor brackets were utilized. The arch wire sequence was initiated with upper and lower .014" Super Elastic Nitinol wires, followed by tandem upper and lower .014"/.016" Super Elastics Nitinol wires. Upper and lower .019"x.025" Heat Activated Nitinol completed the alignment of each arch. Detailing and finishing in each arch was accomplished with .019"x.025" Beta. Class III elastics were used to obtain a positive overjet.

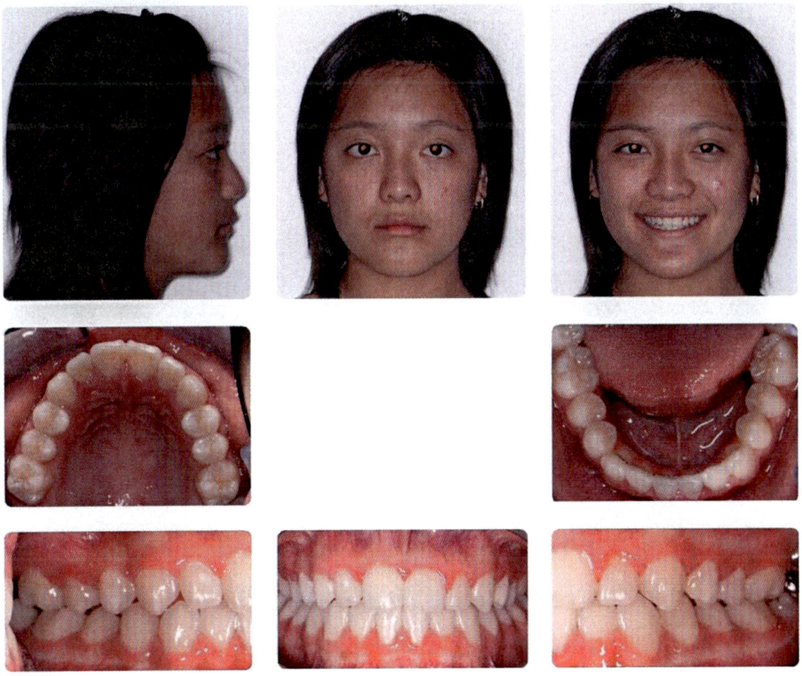

Figure 11A: Post-treatment clinical photos.

The treatment required a total of 13 appointments, with the first three appointments devoted to the fabrication and placement of the maxillary expansion appliance. The entire treatment lasted for 21 months. Post-treatment records revealed a Class I molar relationship with an ideal overjet and overjet (Fig. **11 A, B, C**). Cephalometric superimposition (Table **8**, Fig. **12**) indicated the ideal overjet was achieved by proclination of the maxillary incisors and retroclination of the mandibular incisors. Regional superimposition revealed that the entire mandibular dentition was uprighted, which assisted in the correction of the Class III malocclusion. In addition, the use of extrusive mechanics increased the vertical dimension and improved the overall facial esthetics.

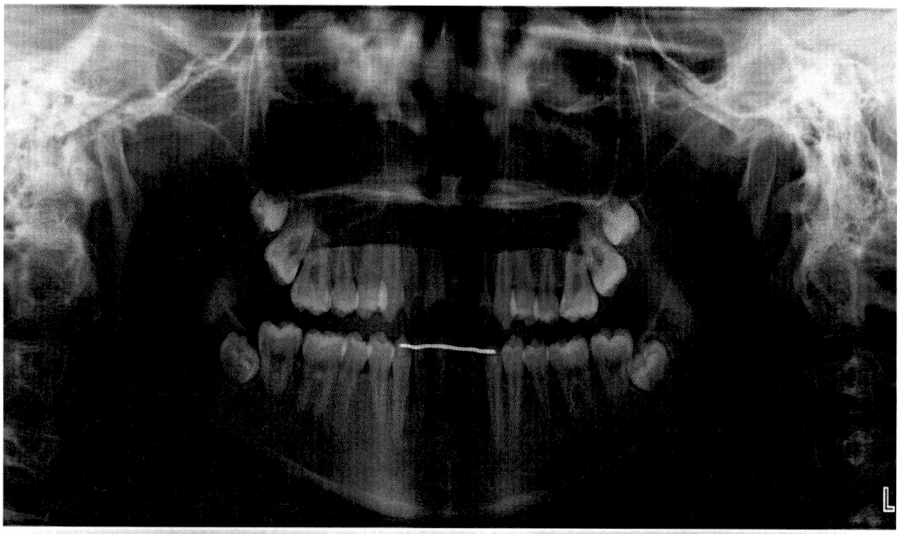

Figure 11B: Post-treatment panoramic radiograph.

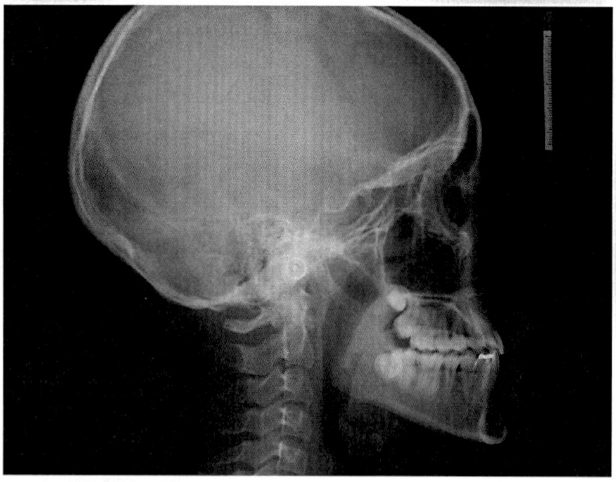

Figure 11C: Post-treatment cephalometric radiograph.

SUMMARY

The use of self-ligating brackets, in particular those of Variable Prescription Orthodontics™ provides a viable treatment option in non-surgical correction of malocclusions with an anterior crossbite. Reduced friction in this appliance system allows for predictable uprighting of the mandibular dentition, and mild retraction of the lower incisors. By choosing higher torque maxillary incisor brackets, or lower torqued mandibular incisors, or combining the two bracket types, one can help to build the dental compensations into the final treatment position of the teeth. This method is applicable for correction of anterior crossbite in both Class I and Class III malocclusions. For successful treatment, attention must be paid to the vertical dimension in order to avoid excessive extrusive mechanics which can result in anterior open bites. Patients with increased vertical dimension at the onset of treatment may best be served by including orthognathic surgery in combination with orthodontic treatment. For patients with milder anteroposterior jaw discrepancies, where the vertical dimension is normal or decreased, the above treatment protocol can provide patients with a less invasive treatment option.

Table 8: Post-treatment cephalometric measurements

	Value	Norm	Std Dev
Maxilla to Cranial Base			
SNA (°)	83.3	82.0	3.5
Mandible to Cranial Base			
SNB (°)	83.7	80.9	3.4
SN - GoGn (°)	26.6	32.9	5.2
FMA (MP-FH) (°)	27.6	24.0	4.5
Maxillo-Mandibular			
ANB (°)	-0.5	1.6	1.5
Maxillary Dentition			
U1 - NA (mm)	6.0	4.3	2.7
U1 - SN (°)	112.2	102.7	5.5
Mandibular Dentition			
L1 - NB (mm)	2.6	4.0	1.8
L1 - GoGn (°)	83.4	93.0	6.0
Soft Tissue			
Lower Lip to E-Plane (mn	-2.2	-2.0	2.0
Upper Lip to E-Plane (mn	-4.2	-5.7	2.0

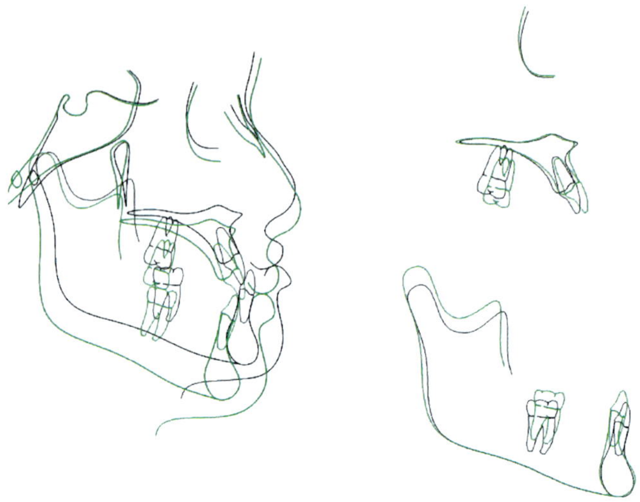

Figure 12: Pretreatment (black) and Post-treatment (green) cephalometric superimposition.

ACKNOWLEDGEMENTS

Declared none.

CONFLICT OF INTEREST

The authors confirm that this chapter contents have no conflict of interest.

REFERENCES

[1] Ngan P, Hu AM, Fields HW. Treatment of Class III problems begins with differential diagnosis of anterior crossbites. Pediatr Dent 1997;19:386-95.

[2] Stelzig-Eisenhauer A, Lux CJ, Schuster G. Treatment decision in adult patients with Class III malocclusion: Orthodontic therapy or orthognathic surgery. Am J Orthod Dentofacial Orthop 2002;122:27-38.

[3] Proffit WR, Ackermann JL. A systematic approach to orthodontic diagnosis and treatment planning. In: Graber TM, Swain BF, editors. Current orthodontic concepts and techniques. 3rd ed. Saint Louis: C. V. Mosby; 1985.

[4] Burns NR, Musich DR, Martin C, Razmus , Gunel E, Ngan P. Class III camouflage treatment: What are the limits? Am J Orthod Dentofacial Orthop 2010;137:9:e1-9.e13.

[5] Rabie ABM, Gu Y. Diagnostic criteria for pseudo-Class III malocclusion. Am J Orthod Dentofacial Orthop 2000;117:1-9.

[6] Stolzenberg J. The Russell attachment and its improved advantages. Int J Orthod Dent Child 1935; 21:837-40.

[7] Harradine NW. Self-ligating brackets: Where are we now? J Orthod 2003; 30:262-273.

[8] Chen SSH, Greenlee GM, Kim JE, Smith CL, Huang GJ. Systematic review of self-ligating brackets. Am J Orthod Dentofacial Orthop 2010;137:726.e18.

Send Orders for Reprints to reprints@benthamscience.net
Orthodontic Treatment of Class III Malocclusion, **2013, 201-227** **201**

CHAPTER 8

Treatment of Class III Cases with Temporary Anchorage Devices

Teruko Takano-Yamamoto*

Division of Orthodontics and Dentofacial Orthopedics, Tohoku University Graduate School of Dentistry, Sendai, Japan

Abstract: There are many ways of using temporary anchorage devices (TADs) to treat patients with severe Class III malocclusions. The mini-plate is one example but a surgical flap is required to place and remove the device. Miniscrews placed in the retromolar pad enjoy the advantage of being placed in dense cortical place, but it is difficult to use them to apply direct force to retract the whole lower arch. The inter-radicular mini-screw is easy to place, but the amount of whole lower arch distalization is very limited. In this article, the author will discuss the use of miniscrews placed in the buccal shelf to correct severe Class III malocclusions. As long as the patient has an orthognathic, or at least acceptable profile, most severe Class III malocclusions can be treated by this method. Buccal shelf mini-screws are placed outside the alveolar process, so extensive lower arch distalization is possible. The thick cortical plate of high density bone in the buccal shelf area offers very good skeletal anchorage for retracting the mandibular arch and/or intruding lower molar to correct an anterior openbite. When treatment is complete, the miniscrews can be removed easily, even without local anesthetic. In this chapter, the anatomic considerations, materials and size of the screws, and the clinical application will be discussed and illustrated with case reports.

Keywords: Class III malocclusion, MEAW technique, buccal shelf, mini-screw, extra-alveolar TADs, biomechanics of Class III treatment, distalization, entire mandibular dentition, unilateral posterior crossbite, nonextraction approach, a 6 degrees-of -freedom jaw movement recording system, TMD, jaw function, MRI, coronal view, facial asymmetry.

INTRODUCTION

The purpose of orthodontic treatment in adults is to improve dental and jaw functions and dentofacial aesthetics for better quality of life of patients with malocclusion. The correction of malocclusion by performing orthodontic treatment achieves harmonious occlusion with satisfactory morphology, function, and aesthetics [1-2]. A skeletal Class III malocclusion is a common corrective in a prevalence of 8%-22%

***Address correspondence to Teruko Takano-Yamamoto:** Division of Orthodontics and Dentofacial Orthopedics, Tohoku University Graduate School of Dentistry, 4-1, Seiryo-machi, Aoba-ku, Sendai, 980-8575, Japan; Tel: +81-22-717-8372; Fax: +81-22-717-8372; E-mail: t-yamamo@m.tohoku.ac.jp among all orthodontic patients [3]. Due to difficulties in predicting craniofacial growth for individuals with this problem [4-7], Class III malocclusion with mandibular prognathism is a great interest to orthodontists. It should be noted that, even now, in an adult patient with skeletal Class III malocclusion, to determine the choice of orthodontic camouflage treatment or orthognathic surgery is a clinical challenge.

For an adult patient ended growth, the orthodontic treatment approach depends on the original growth pattern, severity of the skeletal discrepancy, facial profile, and requirements of patients [8]. For borderline cases, the profile of soft tissue is an important factor for making a treatment plan [9]. It is a good choice that orthodontists do not perform the surgical correction to patients with Class III malocclusion if they present with an acceptable facial profile. However, it is difficult to treat Skeletal Class III malocclusions, by using the conventional mechanics due to basal bone discrepancies. In addition, the distal movement of the whole mandibular arch is also difficult to achieve by using traditional orthodontic mechanics. An improper transverse relation of the buccal teeth or improper lower incisor inclination may remain after completion of orthodontic treatment.

Recently, temporary anchorage devices (TADs) such as mini-screws and mini-plates have been used as clinical tools in treatment of severe Class III malocclusions. Absolute skeletal anchorage using implant permits three-dimensional tooth movement, and their use has resulted in good orofacial function and morphology. In many cases, the excellent skeletal anchorage precludes the need for orthognathic surgery [10,11]. This chapter will discuss the utility of extra-alveolar TADs for treating Class III malocclusion in adults.

CONVENTIONAL TREATMENT OF CLASS III AND RELATED PROBLEMS

During treatment with multi-bracket appliances, anchorage is clearly the most important factor leading to successful treatment. With respect to anchorage, various techniques have been devised and are used in contemporary orthodontics. Adult Class III patients without orthognathic surgery have been treated using several types of treatment methods such as. multi-brackets with Class III elastics, extraction, and multi-loop edgewise archwire therapy [12-16]. Class III elastics or extraoral anchorage applied to the mandibular anterior teeth can be used to retract the mandibular anterior teeth and control the bite depth during the treatment procedure. to achieve standard range of interincisal relations and functionally stable occlusion[17-20]. The quality of the treatment results, however, depends on the degree of using such anchorages by patients.

Class III elastics might negatively affect the inclination of the occlusal plane, vertical interincisal relation, and temporomandibular joint. Furthermore, these intermaxillary mechanics, sometimes result in undesirable side effects such as backward and downward rotation of the mandible, labial inclination of the maxillary incisors, lingual retroclination of the mandibular incisors, and molar extrusion [21]. These changes may cause the problems of dentofacial aesthetics and unstability of the retention phase, especially in patients with long-face. In such cases, the lingual crown torque and the labial crown torque should be increased for the both upper and lower incisors, respectively, to react against forces of vertical component produced by Class III elastics.

The multi-loop edgewise archwire (MEAW) has many loops with second-order bend to control the posterior teeth. It permits individual movement of each tooth and transmits the force produced by the Class III elastics throughout the upper and lower arch [22, 23]. After extraction of third molars, the entire lower dentition is then moved distally while being upright by using a MEAW technique combined with intermaxillary elastics. This combination induces counterclockwise rotation of the occlusal plane, without significant posterior rotation of the mandible. The procedure is appropriate for a long faced patient, although it often results in flaring and extrusion of the upper incisors to achieve proper inter-incisal relations.

The incorporation of a J-hook headgear to the lower arch has been used to produce sequential forces on the terminal molars, premolars, and canines for distal tooth movement [17]. The J-hook headgear promotes the distal tipping of the terminal molars, prepares mandibular anchorage with distal tipping of the first molars and second premolars, and eliminates intrusive forces on the incisors. The use of this apparatus is discontinued when a Class I molar relation is achieved along with proper overbite and overjet. The placement of a J-hook headgear to the lower arch is possibly an alternative to the use of Class III elastics for treating Class III malocclusion [24].

Options of compensatory orthodontic treatment without surgery for adult patients with skeletal Class III malocclusion include several kind of extraction patterns, such as extraction of the mandibular first premolars or incisors. Extraction of mandibular incisor is occationally indicated for moderate Class III malocclusion having an anterior crossbite or an edge-to-edge incisor relation [25]. The decision is determined by factors such as the severity of the anterior crowding of the mandible, the Bolton analysis, and the degrees of overbite and overjet.

Several reports have suggested a relation between occlusion and temporomandibular disorders (TMDs). Unilateral posterior crossbite [26,27] and anterior open bite [28] are suggested as possible factors leading to TMD. patients with mandibular deviation show functional and morphological asymmetries. related to vertical asymmetries (*e.g.*, of the frontal occlusal plane angles). Mandibular deviation is strongly associated with the path of condyle which is steeper on the non-deviated side during protrusive excursion and maximum opening and closing excurtion [26, 29]. Patients having a unilateral posterior crossbite show a reverse sequence pattern of the incisal path, whereas those with mandibular prognathism show a chopping pattern [30-32]. Asymmetrical loading on the bilateral temporomandibular joint (TMJ) seems to be an important causative factor of TMD [33-37]. Therefore, both functional improvement and morphological improvement are important after orthodontic treatment. At the initial stage of treatment, we have used splint therapy to reduce symptoms associated with TMD [11]. Use of a stabilization splint has resulted in a significant reduction in these symptoms. Thus, changing the occlusion, such as by correcting the crossbite, might alleviate any discomfort due to the TMD. However, the relationship between the use of intermaxillary elastics and TMD is still lacking any clear evidence in the literature. The presence of TMD signs and symptoms are not consistent in orthodontic patients any treatment mechanics, such as headgear, intermaxillary elastics, extraction, and nonextraction [38]. On the contrary, it is reported that loading of backward direction on the condyle induces anterior disk displacement [39]. Therefore, environmental factors that might cause upward and backward pressure on the condyle should be suppressed its expression to be a minimize [40]. Further studies are needed to demonstrate if orthodontic treatments using fixed appliance raise the prevalence of TMD [41]. Nevertheless, some past reports suggested a correlation between orthodontic treatment and TMD [42, 43], so it is possible that orthodontic treatment may be effective in treating TMD.

Because oral conditions have been shown to decline with age [44]. Various considerations are required for adult patients during comprehensive orthodontic treatment. They may require prosthetic restorations for missing teeth, have periodontal problems, or experience TMD [45]. Orthodontic treatment is certainly more challenging for older adults than for children and adolescents [46]. Aged adults suffer from the most common periodontal diseases such as gingivitis and chronic periodontitis [46]. The pathological periodontal condition sometimes causes undesirable tooth migration and cuspal interferences.

Thus, the mandibular position in some patients is forced to change for accommodation of these situation. These patients may be benefited from orthodontic treatment with TADs to establish the physiological position of the mandible, an appropriate and stable occlusion, and facial esthetics.

USEFULNESS OF TADs FOR CLASS III TREATMENT

Control of anchorage is one of the most important factors for obtaining an ideal orthodontic outcome. For example, the use of an osseointegrated implant as anchorage [47-51] has opened up a variety of treatment options for patients with Class III malocclusion. In contrast to extra-oral or intermaxillary anchorage, TADs do not require patient cooperation. Also, the TADs preclude any undesirable reciprocal force with tooth movement [17, 46, 52-54]. Therefore, TADs are another highly useful addition to the orthodontic armamentarium. The use of TADs and their simple mechanics allows us to avoid complicated wire bending, and there is minimal loss of anchorage. Also, Class III elastics are not required. Tooth movement using TADs can be regulated precisely according to the treatment plan [55].

Dental implants [47], miniscrews [48-51], and mini-plates [51] have been used for orthodontic anchorage. These medical equipment can provide the absolute and stable anchorage for various direction of tooth movements without the need for patient's cooperation of using headgear or Class III elastics. Dental implants used for orthodontic anchorage, however, do have a few disadvantages: they are too expensive for temporary use; and their use is limited to a narrow region, such as the area of a missing tooth, the retromolar region, or the maxillary tuberosity.

In an effort to circumvent these problems, titanium screws and mini-plates have been used for providing stationary anchorage during orthodontic treatment. The mini-plate allows us to apply stronger orthodontic force. The disadvantage is that it is surgically more invasive than placement of a titanium screw alone.

Titanium mini-screws are currently popular because they allow various orthodontic tooth movements with minimal anatomical limitations for placement. They are less costly and simpler to place, because there is no incision or mucogingival flap reflection [53]. Hence, the patient experiences less discomfort after implantation [53]. In spite of their small diameter and short length, mini-screws can produce stable anchorage for various tooth movements including intrusion, retraction, and protraction [11, 40, 56-61]. Furthermore, it is possible to reduce the failure rate by taking into consideration the implantation method, site of implantation, timing for applying orthodontic force [51], the design of the screw [62], and among others. The success rates for mini-plates and mini-screws are not significantly different [51]. Although there is still the possibility of loosening, mini-screw implants have a success rate of approximately 90 % [53, 63, 64].

Mini-screws are generally implanted either between the first and second molars or between the second premolar and the first molar in the mandibular arch [10, 51, 53]. Then intra-arch elastics or coil spring is attached on mini-screws, and, the whole mandibular arch can be moved distally with no movement of the maxillary dentition. Extraction of mandibular teeth may even be avoided by the use of mini-screws. Therefore, treatment with TADs for distalization of mandibular dentition might become a new treatment strategy for patients with Class III malocclusion. The range of orthodontic treatment options should be enlarged by using TADs in patients with skeletal deformity and the aging.

PLACEMENT SITES FOR TADS TO RETRACT THE ENTIRE MANDIBULAR DENTITION

TADs can be placed in many osseous sites in the alveolar process and palate. They can be placed in different sites relative to the occlusal plane. In the mandibular arch, mini-screws can be placed in the retromolar area as well as in inter-radicular spaces between the second and first molars, or between the first molars and second premolars [21, 51, 53, 65, 66].

For most clinicians, the concerns about placement of miniscrews are success rates, the risk factors for failure and damaging roots. In human and animal research, it was indicated that the success rates of miniscrews in the mandible were significantly lower than in the maxilla, dental implants in the mandible have a success rate higher than that in the maxilla [52, 53, 61, 67]. The correlation between success rate and the proximity of the miniscrew to a neighboring tooth root were evaluated [67]. As a result, a major risk factor for failure of screw anchorage is the proximity of mini-screws to the neighboring tooth root, especially in the mandible. The screw placement not to be closer to root is the significant factor for the stability of the miniscrews for orthodontic anchorage [67].

It is also important to choose the acceptable size, length and diameter of and the optimal location and angulation for miniscrews to avoid injury to the tooth roots. The preliminary study demonstrated an approximately 5-7% possibility of injury to the roots or nerve tissue during the placement of miniscrews in dogs. We quantitatively evaluated cortical bone thickness in various location in the maxilla and the mandible using cone-beam CT to determine the optimal locations and angulations for placement and acceptable length and diameter of the miniscrews to be used as anchorage in orthodontic treatment [66]. As a result the most stable location for a miniscrew is mesial or distal to the first molar, and the best angulation is 30° from the long axis of the tooth. Based on the data of the distance from the cortical bone surface to the root surface, cortical bone thickness and the root proximity, Thus, the safest size for a mini-screw is less than approximetry 1.5 mm in diameter and 6 to 8 mm in length [66]. For palatal side, the optimal location for placement is mesial to the first molar at 30°, and the safest size is 8 to 10 mm in length of mini-screw [68]. Furthermore, the quality of alveolar bone surrounding the mini-screw might be also an important factor influencing on stability and success rate of mini-screw. However, our findings using cone beam computed tomography scans (CBCT) showed bone density did not exert major effect on mini-screw failure in adult patients [69].

The retromolar area is the best site for mini-screws to retract the lower dentition without interference of tooth roots. However, it is difficult to place mini-screws in retromolar area primarily due to abundant movable soft tissue and limited space. However, various types of tooth movement can be accomplished by adjusting the position of the mini-screws and the height of the hook for attaching the Nickel Titanium coil spring or power chain.

TREATMENT PROCEDURE

As efficient tooth movement is possible with the use of mini-screws, effective control in the anterior-posterior, vertical, and transverse direction can be achieved that is well beyond what is possible with conventional methods [10, 11, 70, 71]. Miniscrews are effective anchorage for moving the mandibular arch distally in a Class III cases [18, 21], intrusion of molars in patients with an open bite [11, 56], and moving the maxillary arch distally in a Class II case [46, 71]. To correct mild Class III malocclusions, mini-screws with intra-arch elastics have been used to retract the entire lower arch. For the non-surgical correction of a Class III malocclusion the entire mandibular dentition can be retracted with no movement of the maxillary dentition. In addition, the extraction of mandibular teeth may be avoided with the use of mini-screws. Sometimes the extraction of a single incisor is required to eliminate an anterior crossbite, reverse overjet or edge to edge anterior occlusion. Two different techniques for lower arch retraction will be discussed: 1. entire dentition retraction, and 2. sequential retraction.

Entire Dentition Retraction: Two mini-screws are placed posterior to the most distal teeth, that is in the retromolor area of the mandibular arch. After leveling the arches, a stainless steel rectangular archwire is placed, with hooks mesial to the canines. A retraction force is applied from the mini-screws to the hooks, using NiTi coil springs or power chains.

Sequential Retraction: In general, interradicular mini-screws are placed between the first and second molars. After posterior teeth are moved to a Class I molar relationship by flattening the occlusal plane, the first mini-screws are removed if there is proximity of the mini-screw to root surface. The second mini-screws are placed distal to the second premolars and the anterior teeth are further retracted by additional flattening of the occlusal plane.

BIOMECHANICAL CONSIDERATIONS

The type of tooth movement produced by a TAD is determined by biomechanical principles as well as considerations such as force direction (line of action), moment, center of resistance (CR) and center of rotation [72].

If the line of force passes through the CR of a lower dentition, that is engaged with a rigid archwire, the entire arch is subjected to bodily movement. Uprighting of mandibular anterior teeth and mild distal *en masse* retraction of the entire mandibular dentition are achieved by direct anchorage from the mini-screws. The mandibular occlusal plane usually can be maintained during retraction of entire lower dentition. Therefore, this type of mechanics is useful for a case with normal overbite (Fig. **1**).

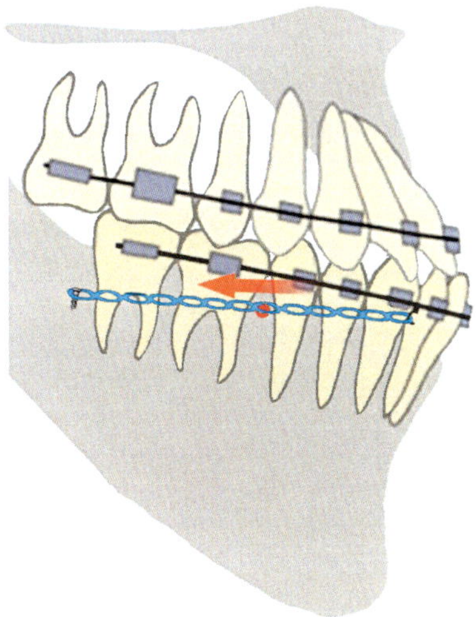

Figure 1: Distalization of the entire mandibular dentition is achieved by placing mini-screws in retromolar pad area. Note the line of force passes through the CR of the lower dentition.

If the line of force passes occlusal to the CR, the mandibular occlusal plane will rotate counter clockwise during *en masse* retraction. The lower anterior teeth will be extruded. This type of mechanics is useful for a case with anterior open bite or an open bite tendency (Fig. **2**).

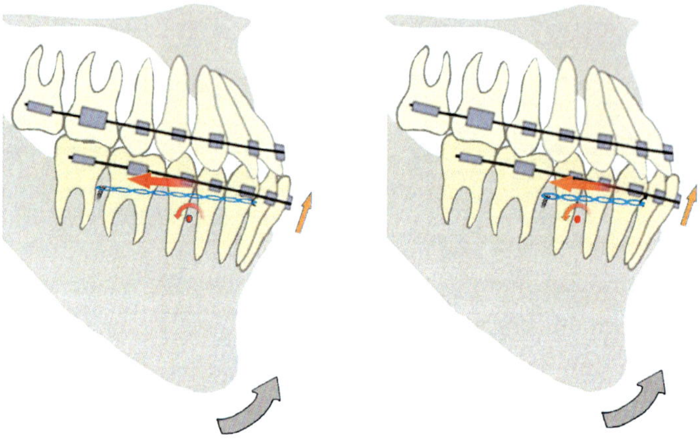

Figure 2: (A) Distalization of the lower arch is achieved by placing mini-screws between the first and second molars. (B) Retraction of teeth in the lower arch can also be anchored by placing mini-screws between the premolars. Note the line of action passes above the CR of the lower dentition.

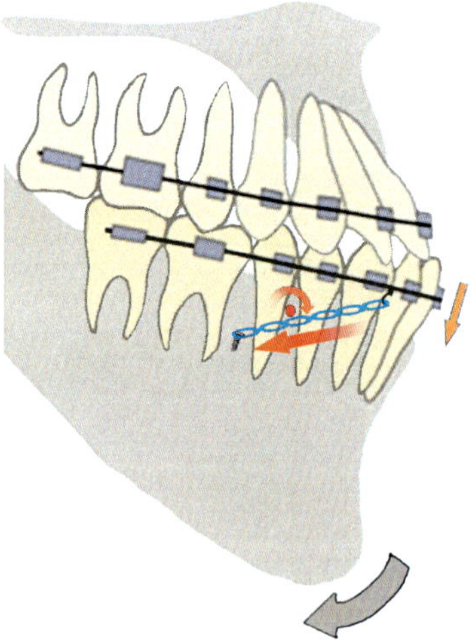

Figure 3: Distalization of the lower arch between the premolar and molar. Note the line of action passes below the CR of the lower dentition.

If the line of force passes apically to the CR, the mandibular occlusal plane will rotate in a clockwise direction during *en masse* retraction (Fig. **3**). This type of mechanics is useful for a case of a deep bite or deep bite tendency. Molar teeth will be extruded.

CASE REPORTS

CASE 1: SKELETAL CLASS III WITH ANTERIOR AND UNILATERAL POSTERIOR CROSSBITE

A patient with Angle Class III molar relationship and skeletal Class III skeletal base desired a nonsurgical, nonextraction approach to treatment. Therefore, mini-screws were used for anchorage to correct the anterior and unilateral posterior crossbite by moving the total mandibular dentition distally with an edgewise appliance.

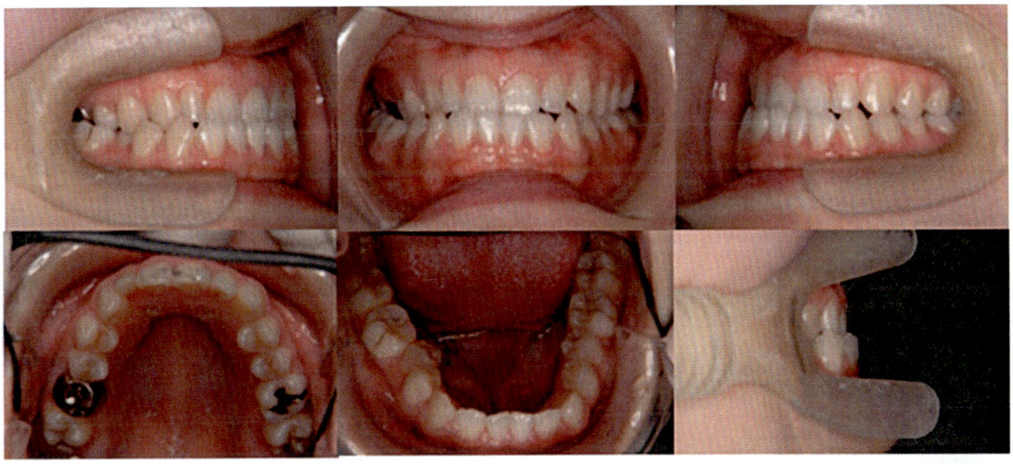

Figure 4: Intraoral photographs show anterior and posterior crossbites.

Diagnosis and Etiology

A 19 years 7 months female had a chief complaint of mandibular protrusion with a straight profile due to mandibular excess. She also had anterior and right molar crossbites with an unbalanced anterior tooth size ratio due to peg lateral incisors. Intraorally, she had a decreased axial inclination of mandibular incisors and an Angle Class III molar relationship. Cephalometrically, the patient had a skeletal Class III jaw-base relation [ANB angle -2.5°] compared with the Japanese norm

[73], slight mandibular deviation to the right, circumoral musculature strain during lip closure, overjet of -2.4 mm, and overbite of 2.6 mm (Figs. **4-6**, Table **1**). No TMJ symptoms were noted. By evaluating the jaw movement with a 6 degrees-of-freedom jaw movement recording system, it was found that during anterior jaw movement the left condylar movement was partially limited, and the movement of the central incisors shifted to the left.

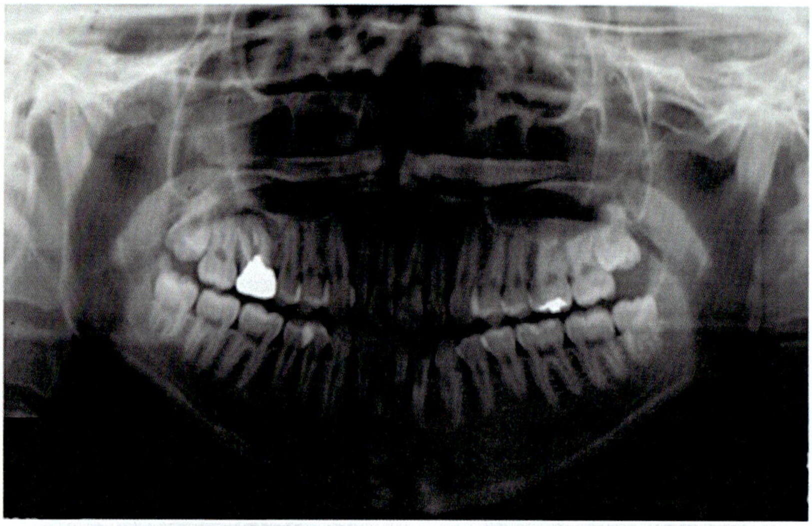

Figure 5: Panoramic radiograph of the patient.

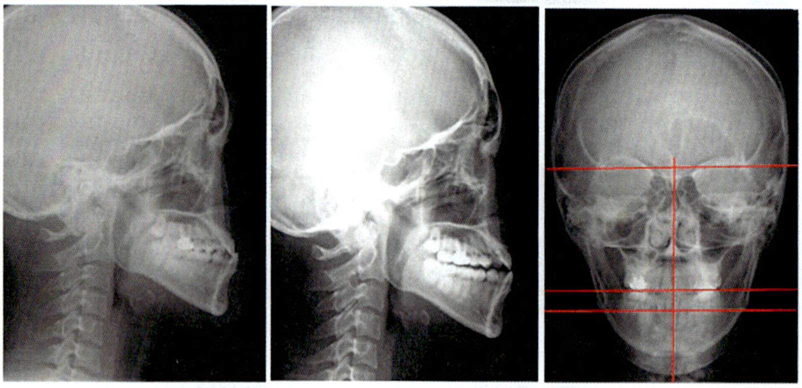

Figure 6: (A) Lateral cephalogram in centric occlusion (B) Lateral cephalogram in centric relation (C) PA cephalogram of the patient.

Table1. Cephalometric Summary

Variables	Mean	SD	Pretreatment	Posttreatment
Angle (°)				
ANB	2.8	2.44	-2.6	0.2
SNA	80.8	3.61	79.8	82.4
SNB	77.9	4.54	82.3	82.2
Mp-FH	30.5	3.60	35.4	29.0
Gonial, A	122.1	5.29	128.0	126.4
U1-FH	112.3	8.26	109.8	121.3
U1-NF	115.0	6.99	116.0	130.0
L1-Mp	93.4	6.77	85.1	81.9
IIA	123.6	10.64	134.1	121.0
Occlusal, P	16.9	4.40	12.4	9.7
Linear (mm)				
S-N	67.9	3.65	70.2	70.2
N-Me	125.8	5.04	125.6	126.3
Me/NF	68.6	3.71	71.8	72.7
Go-Me	71.4	4.14	78.3	78.7
Ar-Me	106.6	5.74	115.5	113.7
Ar-Go	47.3	3.33	47.4	45.3
OJ	3.1	1.07	-2.1	1.9
OB	3.3	1.89	2.6	0.5
U1/NF	31.0	2.34	30.6	28.6
U6/NF	24.6	2.00	27.5	27.6
L1/Mp	44.2	2.68	44.7	46.0
L6/MP	32.9	2.50	31.7	31.9

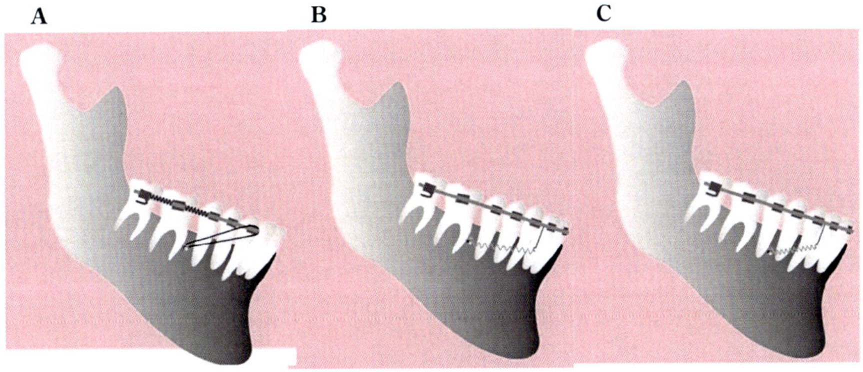

Figure 7: Schematic distalization of mandibular arch.

Treatment Procedure

The mandibular third molars were extracted before orthodontic treatment. An 0.018-inch slot preadjusted edgewise appliance was used for all the teeth in the maxilla and for the canines, premolars, and molars in the mandible. After 5 months of leveling, 0.016 × 0.022-inch stainless steel archwires were placed, and mini-screws (6 mm length, 1.4 mm diameter) were inserted between the second premolar and first molar on both sides of the mandible. The mandibular molars were then moved distally with elastics between the screws and hooks from the canines for 3 months (Fig. **7A**). After brackets were placed on the mandibular central and lateral incisors, the mandibular anterior teeth and premolars were moved distally for 4 months with a nickel-titanium closed-coil spring (200 g) (Fig. **7B**). During this process, mini-screws were replaced at the attached gingivae between the first and second premolars because of their proximity to the tooth root, and retraction of the anterior teeth continued until a positive anterior tooth overlap was obtained (Fig. **7C, 8**). The total active treatment period was 19 months. After removing the edgewise appliances, wrap-around-type retainers were placed in both arches.

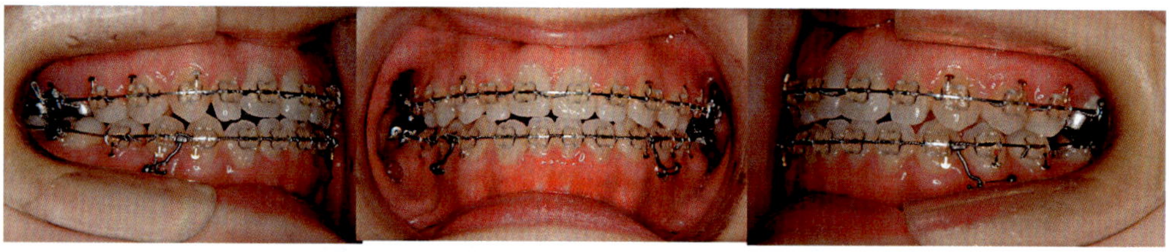

Figure 8: Miniscrews were placed to retract the mandibular arch.

Treatment Results and Discussion

Lateral cephalogram in the rest position of the mandible showed a large freeway space as well as a short vertical height of the maxilla and the alveolar bone (Fig. **6**). Therefore, both sides of the upper molars were somewhat extruded which affected the physiological position of the mandible (Figs. **8** and **9**). Post-treatment records showed significant improvements of the facial profile having a retracted lower lip from the E-line (Fig. **9**). The slight mandibular deviation improved, and the strain of the circumoral musculature during lip closure was corrected.

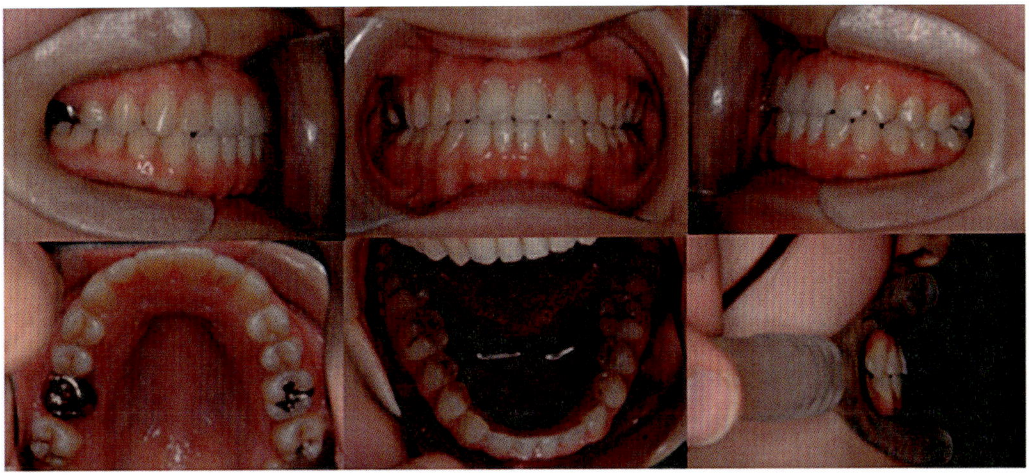

Figure 9: Post-treatment photographs show the correction of anterior and posterior crossbites and a good interdigitation of the dentition.

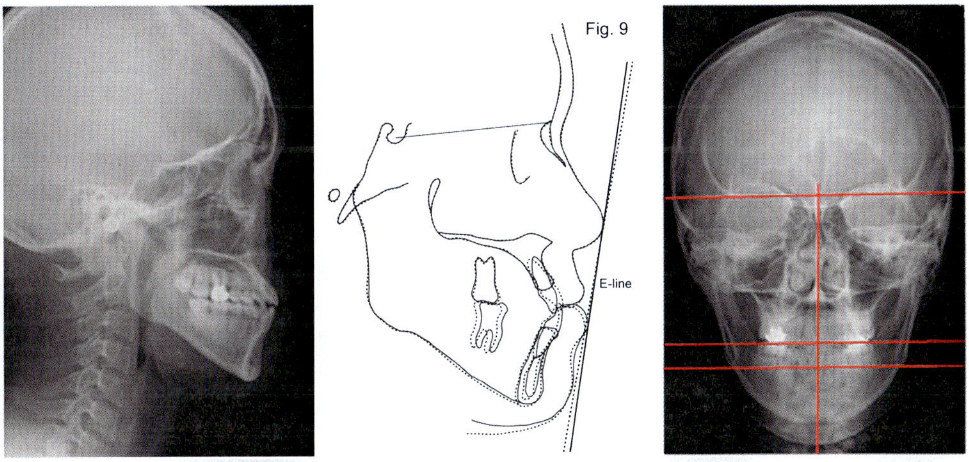

Figure 10: (A) Post-treatment lateral cephalogram, (B) Superimposition of the pre- and post-treatment lateral cephalograms, and (C) Post-treatment PA cephalogram.

The occlusion showed acceptable interdigitation and canine guidance (Fig. **9**). Labial inclination of the maxillary anterior teeth, slight lingual inclination of the mandibular anterior teeth, and a positive relation of the anterior tooth overlap (overjet 1.6 mm, overbite 1.5 mm) were obtained. There was a slight clockwise rotation of the mandible, which increased the ANB angle thereby improving the skeletal Class III jaw-base relation (Fig. **10**, Table **1**). Horizontally, the intermaxillary dental midline was in accordance with the cranial midline. Post-treatment PA cephalogram documents the symmetrical correction. (Fig. **10C**). The former discrepancy in the anterior tooth size ratio was diminished by restoration of the peg lateral incisors (Fig. **9**).

The post-treatment panoramic radiograph showed good parallel positions of the tooth roots, without marked root resorption (Fig. **11**). No TMJ symptoms were noted during the dynamic treatment or the retention period. A three-dimensional 6 degrees-of-freedom jaw movement recording system showed an increased range of condylar movement during lateral excursive and anterior jaw movement. Also, the incisal path during right and left lateral excursive movement had stabilized.

In conclusion, using mini-screws for anchorage to correct Class III malocclusion with anterior and molar crossbite resulted in stable occlusion, improvement in jaw function and facial aesthetics. The results were maintained at the 2 years of retention evaluation.

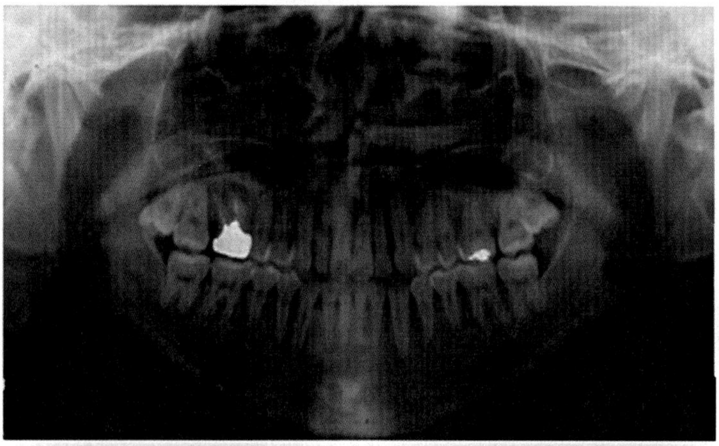

Figure 11: Post-treatment panoramic radiograph of the patient.

CASE 2: MANDIBULAR PROTRUSION ASSOCIATED WITH FUNCTIONAL PROBLEMS

A young man presented with a skeletal Class III jaw-base relation and Angle Class III molar relation, associated with crossbite of the incisors and right molars. Functional problems were noted: reciprocal clicking at the left TMJ and a mandibular shift during opening and closing. However, the skeletal discrepancy was insignificant. The chief complaint of the patient was the functional problem. He wanted it corrected without changing his profile. Class III elastic might have a negative influence on the TMJ [74]. Therefore, mini-screws were used for orthodontic anchorage to move the mandibular arch distally. Ideal occlusion was achieved, and the crossbite and functional problems were alleviated without orthognathic surgery.

Diagnosis and Etiology

This male patient, age 18 years 5 months, complained of unstable occlusion and jaw discomfort. He had an Angle Class III molar relation with overjet -1 mm, overbite 0 mm, and skeletal Class III jaw-base relation (ANB angle -0.4°) which is beyond the Japanese norm [73] (Figs. 1**2-14**, Table **2**). There was also a slight deviation of the mandible to the left, a concave profile due to mandibular excess, and strain of the circumoral musculature on lip closure. The maxillary teeth had 3mm of crowding. Anterior and right posterior crossbites were observed (Fig. 1**2**). There was a tendency for an increased mandibular plane. There was no skeletal asymmetry or occlusal plane cant (Fig. **14**). With regard to jaw function, the TMJ clicked when the mouth was opened and closed (reciprocal click). Also, mandibular deviation to the right during closure was observed using a three-dimensional, 6 degrees-of-freedom jaw movement recording system. MRI of the TMJ showed normal disk position on the sagittal views, whereas medial displacement with reduction on the left side was observed on the coronal views (Fig. **15**).

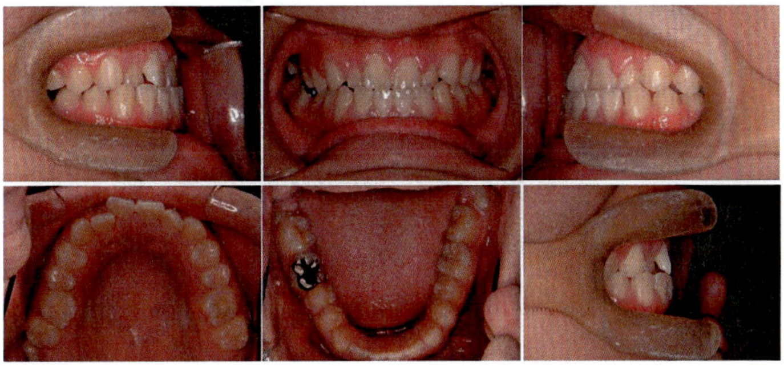

Figure 12: Pre-treatment intraoral photographs show an anterior crossbite.

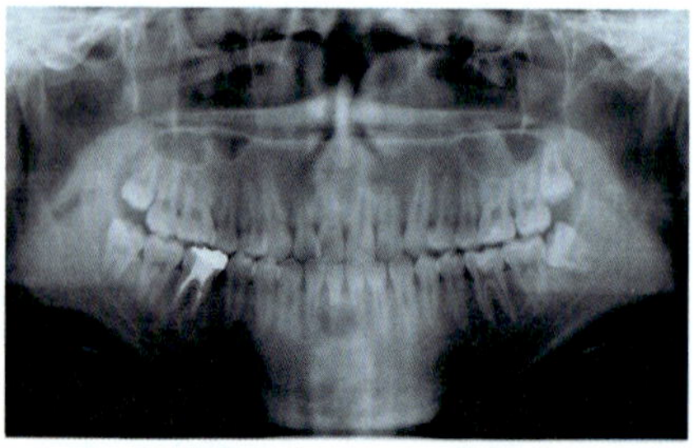

Figure 13: Pre-treatment panoramic radiograph.

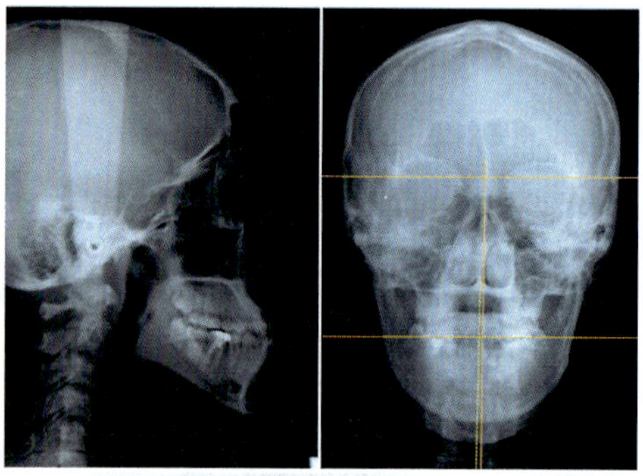

Figure 14: Pre-treatment cephalograms were exposed in the lateral (A) and Posteriro-Anterior projections (B).

Table 2: Cephalometric Summary

Variables	Mean	SD	Pretreatment	Posttreatment
Angle (°)				
ANB	2.8	2.44	-0.4	-0.3
SNA	80.8	3.61	75.8	76.2
SNB	77.9	4.54	76.3	76.5
Mp-FH	30.5	3.60	33.7	32.9
Gonial, A	122.1	5.29	125.1	123.5
U1-FH	112.3	8.26	116.4	115.3
U1-NF	115.0	6.99	32.8	32.3
L1-Mp	93.4	6.77	90.0	84.8
IIA	123.6	10.64	120.0	127.0
Occlusal, P	16.9	4.40	18.9	17.8
Linear (mm)				
S-N	67.9	3.65	71.8	71.9
A´-Ptm´	47.9	2.80	49.3	49.8
N-Me	125.8	5.04	141.0	147.5
Me/NF	68.6	3.71	80.3	81.7
Go-Me	71.4	4.14	79.5	81.9
Ar-Me	106.6	5.74	123.5	125.6
Ar-Go	47.3	3.33	56.9	58.0
OJ	3.1	1.07	-0.5	2.0
OB	3.3	1.89	0.0	1.5
U1/NF	31.0	2.34	32.8	32.3
U6/NF	24.6	2.00	28.0	29.0
L1/Mp	44.2	2.68	49.0	51.0
L6/MP	32.9	2.50	37.7	38.6

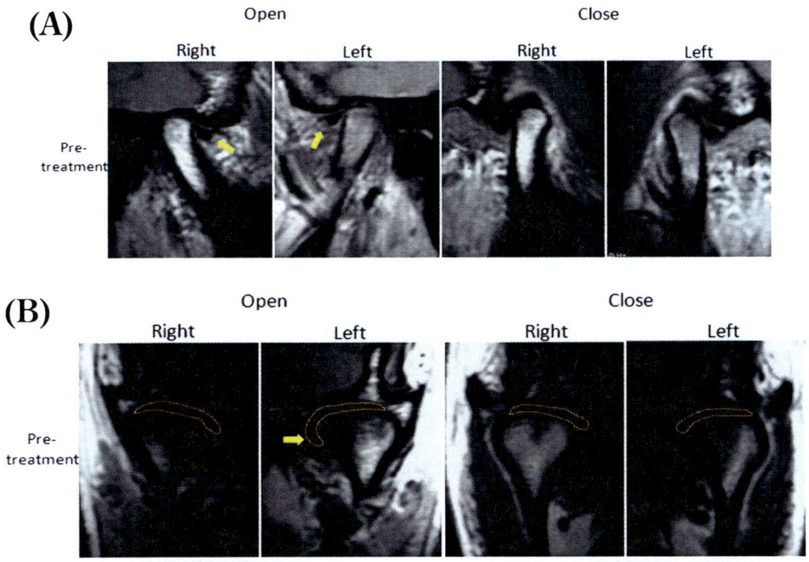

Figure 15: (A) A pre-treatment MRI of the TMJs showed normal disk positions in the sagittal views. (B) Pre-treatment MRI of the TMJs in the coronal view show medial displacement with reduction on the left side.

The patient was diagnosed with a Angle Class III malocclusion and skeletal Class III jaw-base relation associated with anterior and posterior crossbite on the right side and TMD. Treatment objectives were to relieve TMD symptoms, correct the anterior and unilateral posterior crossbite, achieve Angle Class I molar relation, and correct the profile.

Treatment Progress

Prior to active treatment, a stabilization splint (orthotic) was placed in the mandibular arch to stabilize the mandibular position. Three months later, the TMD symptoms were alleviated, and active treatment was initiated. A preadjusted edgewise appliance with 0.022-inch slots was placed on the maxillary teeth. The initial archwire was 0.016-inch nickel-titanium. After 2 months of leveling of the maxillary arch, a preadjusted edgewise appliance with 0.022-inch slots was placed on the mandibular teeth, and a 0.014-inch nickel-titanium archwire was placed. A few weeks later the mandibular third molars were extracted. About 3 months into treatment, titanium mini-screws (8 x 1.5 mm) were implanted in the buccal alveolar bone, between the mandibular second premolar and the first molar (Fig. **16**).

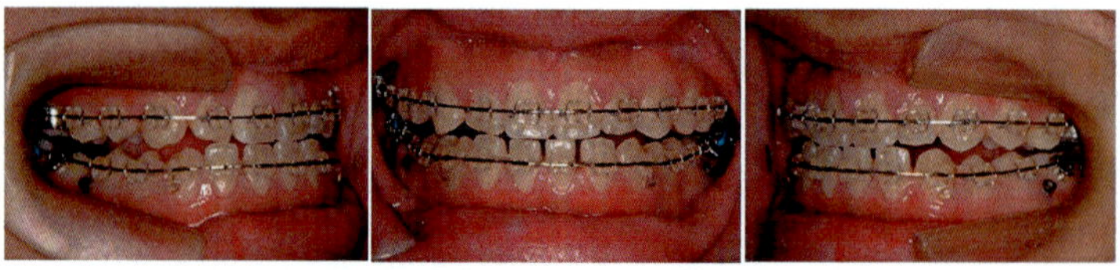

Figure 16: Progress intraoral photographs shows the position of the miniscrews in buccal shelf area.

Because there was no occlusal interference, the mandibular arch was moved distally *en masse* with elastic chains delivering 200 g of force between the screw head and canine bracket hook, bilaterally. After 6 months of traction, an overjet and overbite of 2 mm each was achieved (Fig. **16**). The edgewise appliances and mini-screws were removed after 12 months (Figs. **17** and **18**). The total active treatment duration was 24 months. Circumferential removable retainers were placed in both arches. A stable occlusion with coincident maxillary and mandibular dental midlines was maintained after 2 years of retention.

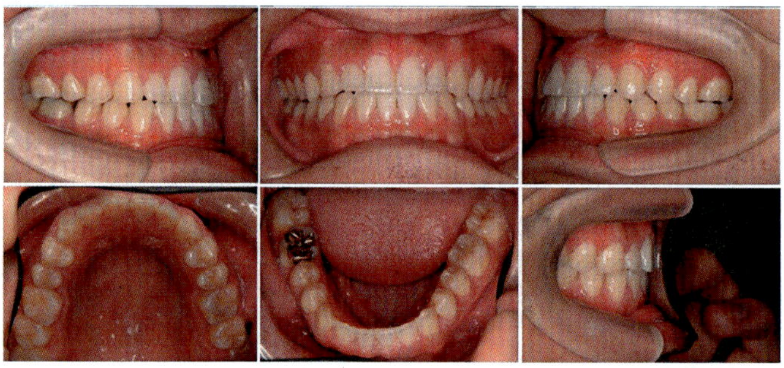

Figure 17: Post-treatment intraoral photographs show a Class I buccal occlusion.

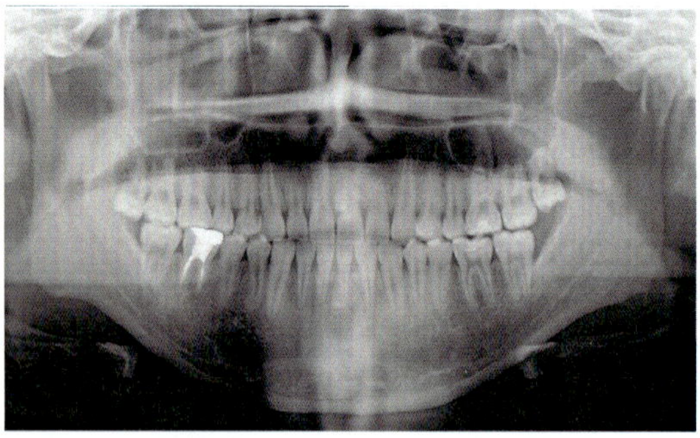

Figure 18: Post-treatment panoramic radiograph.

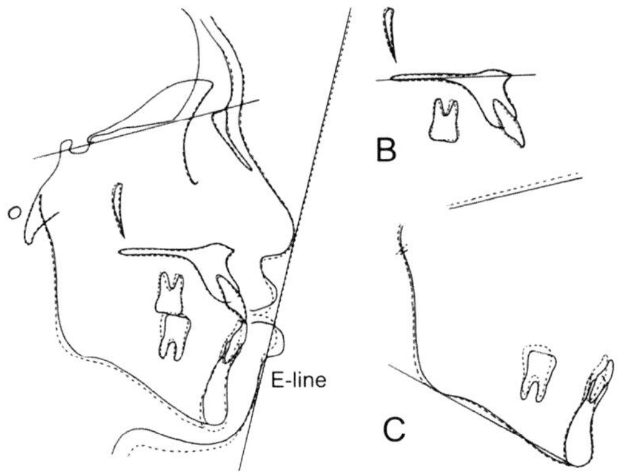

Figure 19: Treatment is documented with pre- and post-treatment lateral cephalogram tracings superimposed on: (A) anterior cranial base , (B) maxilla, and (C) mandible.

Treatment Results and Discussion

Nonsurgical orthodontic treatment was selected because the patient did not wish to change his profile. Because he had a history of TMD, the use of Class III elastics was contraindicated [73] because they may distally position the mandibular condyle in the TMJ fossa. Controlled distal movement of the mandibular arch was required. Mini-screws were used to reinforce the anchorage for maximizing the distal movement of the molars, and they also helped control the vertical dimension to prevent extrusion of the tipped molars. The mandibular incisors were lingually inclined after 3 mm of retraction, and the mandibular first molar was moved 2.5 mm distally (Fig. **19**, Table **2**). Despite slight maxillary first molar extrusion, clockwise rotation of the mandibular plane was not observed, because of the vertical growth of the mandibular ramus.

The axial inclination of the anterior teeth, which was within the normal range on the initial cephalometric radiograph, was maintained by torque control during distal movement of the mandibular arch (Table **2**). In addition, the torque was carefully controlled to avoid contact of the incisor roots with cortical bone due to the thin symphysis (Fig. **20**). Thus, reliable control of the incisors in the anterior-posterior and vertical directions by using mini-screws resulted in an ideal incisor relation without unwanted flaring of the maxillary incisors, which is often seen with camouflage Class III treatment.

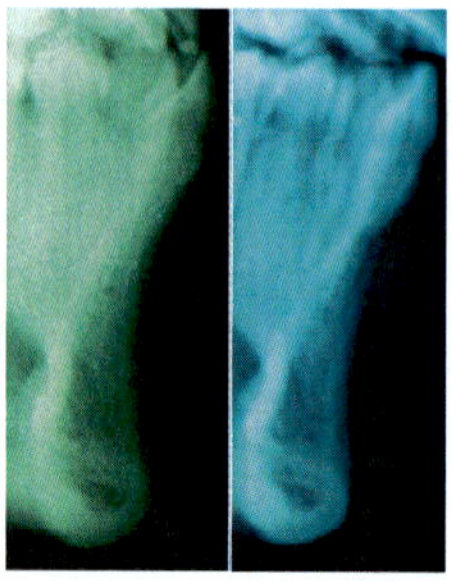

Figure 20: Pre- and Post-treatment cephalometric radiographs show the axial inclination of the lower incisors.

Anterior disk displacement was not observed on the initial sagittal MRI scan, although the coronal view indicated medial disk displacement. Thus, it is recommended that not only sagittal but also coronal views be obtained for evaluating the lateral-medial position of the disk, which may help diagnose any internal derangement of the TMJ.

There was also crossbite in the right molar region, which may have contributed to the occurrence of TMD [26]. After orthodontic treatment, frontal cephalometric radiography showed that the maxillary and mandibular dental midline coincided with the cranial midline (Fig. **21**). Also, TMJ clicking during jaw opening had disappeared. Thus, correcting the occlusion (*i.e.*, the anterior and unilateral posterior crossbite) appeared to have alleviated the TMD.

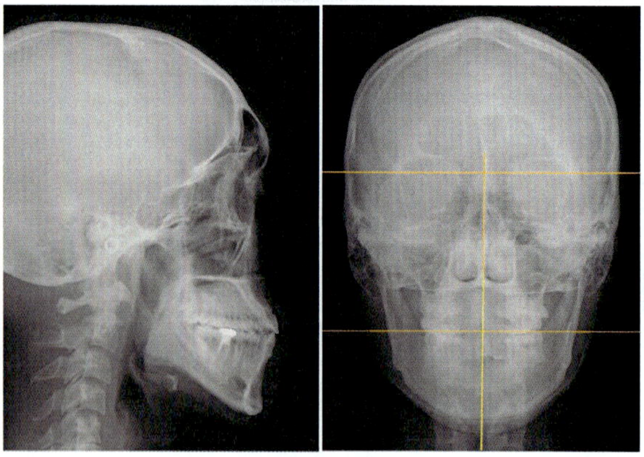

Figure 21: PA cephalogram documents the skeletal symmetry of the patient.

Based on the present case, it is suggested that the use of mini-screws as anchorage leads to efficient, optimized tooth movement that corrects anterior and posterior crossbite. This approach is consistent with physiological positioning of the jaw, and relief of TMD. Furthermore, a stable occlusion is expected to help stabilize the functional movement of the jaw, diminishing clinical symptoms of TMD.

SUMMARY POINTS

- Class III patients with anterior and posterior crossbites can be treated successfully with placement of TADs in the mandibular buccal shelf area.
- The use of mini-screws as anchorage for tooth movement is useful for achieving physiological positioning of the jaw, and relief of TMD.
- Mini-screws have proven useful for *en masse* distal movement of mandibular teeth in adult patients with TMD.
- Patients with Class III problems and facial asymmetry can be treated with TADs to resolve dental problems supplemented by orthognathic surgery to resolve the skeletal problem.

ACKNOWLEDGEMENTS

Declared none.

CONFLICT OF INTEREST

The author confirms that this chapter contents have no conflict of interest.

REFERENCES

[1] Throckmorton GS, Johnston CP, Gonyea WJ, *et al.* A preliminary study of biomechanical changes produced by orthognathic surgery. J Prosthet Dent 1984; 51:252-261.

[2] Ehmer U and Broll P. Mandibular border movements and masticatory patterns before and after orthognathic surgery. Int J Adult Orthodon Orthognath Surg1992;7:153-159.

[3] Proffit WR, Fields HW and Sarver DM. Contemporary orthodontics. 4th ed. St Louis: Mosby-Year Book; 2007. p. 689-693.

[4] Baccetti T, Franchi L and McNamara JA Jr. Cephalometric variables predicting the long-term success or failure of combined rapid maxillary expansion and facial mask therapy. Am J Orthod Dentofacial Orthop. 2004;126:16-22.
[5] Ishikawa H, Nakamura S, Kim C, *et al*. Individual growth in Class III malocclusions and its relationship to the chin cup effects. Am J Orthod Dentofacial Orthop.1998;114:337-346.
[6] Auconi P, Scazzocchio M, Defraia E, *et al*. Forecasting craniofacial growth in individuals with class III malocclusion by computational modelling. Eur J Orthod. 2013 Jun 18.[Epub]
[7] Khatoon T, Tanaka E and Tanne K. Craniofacial morphology in orthodontically treated patients of Class III with stable and unstable treatment outcomes. Am J Orthod Dentofacial Orthop. 2000;117:681-690.
[8] Kerr WJ and Ten Have TR. Changes in soft tissue profile during the treatment of Class III malocclusion. Br J Orthod 1987;14:243-249.
[9] Proffit WR. Interarch elastics: their place in modern orthodontics. In: Hosl E, Baldauf A, editors. Mechanical and biological basics in orthodontic therapy. 1991. p. 173-178.
[10] Takano-Yamamoto T and Kuroda S. Titanium screw anchorage for correction of canted occlusal plane in patients with facial asymmetry. Am J Orthod Dentofacial Orthop 2007;132:337-342
[11] Kuroda S, Sugawara Y, Tamamura N, *et al*. Anterior open bite with temporomandibular disorder treated with titanium screw anchorage: Evaluation of morphological and functional improvement. Am J Orthod Dentofacial Orthop 2007;131:550-560
[12] Kuroda S, Sakai Y, Tamamura N, Deguchi T, Takano-Yamamoto T. Treatment of severe anterior open bite with skeletal anchorage in adults: comparison with orthognathic surgery outcomes. Am J Orthod Dentofacial Orthop. 2007;132:599-605.
[13] Kim YH, Han UK, Lim DD, *et al*. Stability of anterior openbite correction with multiloop edgewise archwire therapy: a cephalometric follow-up study. Am J Orthod Dentofacial Orthop 2000;118:43-54.
[14] Lin J and Gu Y. Preliminary investigation of nonsurgical treatment of severe skeletal Class III malocclusion in the permanent dentition. Angle Orthod 2003;73:401-410.
[15] Janson G, de Souza JE, Alves Fde A, *et al*. Extreme dentoalveolar compensation in the treatment of Class III malocclusion. Am J Orthod Dentofacial Orthop 2005;128:787-794.
[16] Glenn G. An American Board of Orthodontics case report: the nonsurgical orthodontic correction of a Class III malocclusion. Am J Orthod Dentofacial Orthop 1997;111:149-155.
[17] Cozzani G. Extraoral traction and class III treatment. Am J Orthod. 1981;80:638-650.
[18] Merrifield LL. Edgewise sequential directional force technology. J Charles H. Tweed Int Found. 1986;14:22-37.
[19] Lin J and Gu Y. Lower second molar extraction in correction of severe skeletal class III malocclusion. Angle Orthod. 2006; 76:217-225.
[20] Faerovig E and Zachrisson BU. Effects of mandibular incisor extraction on anterior occlusion in adults with Class III malocclusion and reduced overbite. Am J Orthod Dentofacial Orthop. 1999;115:113-124.
[21] Sugawara Y, Kuroda S, Tamamura N, *et al*. Adult patient with mandibular protrusion and unstable occlusion treated with titanium screw anchorage. Am J Orthod Dentofacial Orthop 2008;133:102-111
[22] Hu H, Chen J, Guo J, *et al*. Distalization of the mandibular dentition of an adult with a skeletal Class III malocclusion. Am J Orthod Dentofacial Orthop. 2012;142:854-62.
[23] Park EW. Treatment of severe skeletal Class III malocclusions with MEAW therapy. Int J MEAW. 1997;4:75-93.

[24] Kuroda Y , Kuroda S, Alexander RG, *et al.* Adult Class lll Treatment Using a J-Hook Headgear to the Mandibular Arch. Angle Orthod 2010;80:336-343

[25] Canut JA. Mandibular incisor extraction: indication and long-term evaluation. Eur J Orthod 1996;18:485-489.

[26] Pirttiniemi P, Kantomaa T and Lahtela P. Relationship between craniofacial and condyle path asymmetry in unilateral cross-bite patients. Eur J Orthod 1990;12:408-413.

[27] Miyawaki S, Tanimoto Y, Araki Y, *et al.* Movement of the lateral and medial poles of the working condyle during mastication in patients with unilateral posterior crossbite.Am J Orthod Dentofacial Orthop. 2004;126:549-554.

[28] Pullinger AG, Seligman DA and Gornbein. A Multiple logistic regression analysis of the risk and relative odds of temporomandibular disorders as a function of common occlusal features. J Dent Res 1993;72:968-979

[29] Oguri Y, Yamada K, Fukui T, *et al.* Mandibular movement and frontal craniofacial morphology in orthognathic surgery patients with mandibular deviation and protrusion. J Oral Rehabil 2003;30:392-400.

[30] Hashimoto T, Kuroda S, E L, Tanimoto Y *et al.* Correlation between craniofacial and condylar path asymmetry. J Oral Maxillofac Surg. 2008; 66:2020-2027

[31] Kambylafkas P, Kyrkanides S and Tallents RH. Mandibular asymmetry in adult patients with unilateral degenerative joint disease. Angle Orthod. 2005; 75:305-310.

[32] Ahlgren J. Pattern of chewing and malocclusion of teeth. A clinical study. Acta Odontol Scand. 1967; 25:3-13.

[33] Takeshita N, Ishida H, Watanabe H *et al.* Improvement of asymmetric stomatognathic functions, unilateral crossbite, and facial esthetics in a paient with askeletal Class III malocclusion and mandibular asymmetry, treated with orthognathic surgery. Am J Orthod Dentofacial Orthop. 2013, ; 144:441-454

[34] Trpkova B, Major P, Nebbe B, *et al.* Craniofacial asymmetry and temporomandibular joint internal derangement in female adolescents: a posteroanterior cephalometric study. Angle Orthod 2000;70:81-88.

[35] Ahn SJ, Lee SP and Nahm DS. Relationship between temporomandibular joint internal derangement and facial asymmetry in women. Am J Orthod Dentofacial Orthop 2005;128:583-591.

[36] Hatala MP, Macher DJ, Tallents RH, *et al.* Effect of a surgically created disk displacement on mandibular symmetry in the growing rabbit. Oral Surg Oral Med Oral Pathol Oral Radiol Endod 1996;82:625-633.

[37] Inui M, Fushima K and Sato S. Facial asymmetry in temporomandibular joint disorders. J Oral Rehabil 1999; 26:402-406.

[38] Owen A. Unexpected temporomandibular joint findings during fixed appliance therapy. Am J Orthod Dentofacial Orthop 1998;113:625-631.

[39] Farrar WB and McCarty WL. A clinical outline of temporomandibular joint diagnosis and treatment. Montgomery, Ala: Walker Printing; 1983. p. 84-85.

[40] Wyatt WE. Preventing adverse effects on the temporomandibular joint through orthodontic treatment. Am J Orthod Dentofacial Orthop 1987;91:493-499.

[41] Kim MR and Graber TM. Orthodontics and temporomandibular disorder: a meta-analysis. Am J Orthod Dentofacial Orthop 2002;121:438-446.

[42] Egermark I, Magnusson T and Carlsson GE. A 20-year follow-up of signs and symptoms of temporomandibular disorders and malocclusions in subjects with and without orthodontic treatment in childhood. Angle Orthod 2003;73:109-115.

[43] Henrikson T and Nilner M. Temporomandibular disorders, occlusion and orthodontic treatment. J Orthod 2003;30:129-137.

[44] DeBiase CB and Austin SL. Oral health and older adults. J Dent Hyg 2003;77:125-145.

[45] Proffit WR and Fields HW Jr. Contemporary orthodontics. 3rd ed. St Louis: Mosby; 1999.

[46] Fukunaga T, Kuroda S, Kurosaka H, *et al.* Skeletal anchorage for orthodontic correction of maxillary protrusion with adult periodontitis. Angle Orthod 2006;76: 148-155.

[47] Roberts WE, Helm FR, Marshall KJ, *et al.* Rigid endosseous implants for orthodontic and orthopedic anchorage. Angle Orthod. 1989; 59:247-256.

[48] Creekmore TD and Eklund MK. The possibility of skeletal anchorage. J Clin Orthod. 1983; 17:266-269.

[49] Costa A, Raffaini M and Melsen B. Miniscrews as orthodontic anchorage: apreliminary report. Int J Adult Orthod Orthognath Surg. 1998; 3:201-209.

[50] Park HS, Bae SM, Kyung HM, *et al.* Micro-implant anchorage for treatment of skeletal Class I bialveolar protrusion. J Clin Orthod. 2001; 35: 417-422.

[51] Miyawaki S, Koyama I, Inoue M, *et al.* Factors associated with the stability of titanium screws placed in the posterior region for orthodontic anchorage. Am J Orthod Dentofacial Orthop. 2003 ; 124:373-378.

[52] Deguchi T, Takano-Yamamoto T, Kanomi R, *et al.* The use of small titanium screws for orthodontic anchorage. J Dent Res 2003;82: 377-381.

[53] Kuroda S, Sugawara Y, Deguchi T, *et al.* Clinical use of miniscrew implants as orthodontic anchorage: success rates and postoperative discomfort. Am J Orthod Dentofacial Orthop 2007; 131:9-15.

[54] Kanomi R. Mini-implant for orthodontic anchorage. J Clin Orthod. 1997;31:763-767

[55] Roberts WE, Engen DW, Schneider PM, *et al.* Implant- anchored orthodontics for partially edentulous malocclusions in children and adults. Am J Orthod Dentofacial Orthop 2004;126: 302-304.

[56] Kuroda S, Katayama A and Takano-Yamamoto T. Severe anterior open-bite case treated using titanium screw anchorage. Angle Orthod 2004;74:558-567.

[57] Kuroda S, Sugawara Y, Yamashita K, *et al.* Skeletal Class III oligodontia patient treated with titanium screw anchorage and orthognathic surgery. Am J Orthod Dentofacial Orthop 2005;127:730-738.

[58] Park HS, Kwon TG and Kwon OW. Treatment of open bite with microscrew implant anchorage. Am J Orthod Dentofacial Orthop 2004;126:627-636.

[59] Park HS, Kwon TG and Sung JH. Nonextraction treatment with microscrew implants. Angle Orthod 2004;74:539-549.

[60] Kyung HM, Park HS, Bae SM, *et al.* Development of orthodontic micro-implants for intraoral anchorage. J Clin Orthod 2003;37:321-328.

[61] Cheng SJ, Tseng IY, Lee JJ, *et al.* A prospective study of the risk factors associated with failure of mini-implants used for orthodontic anchorage. Int J Oral Maxillofac Implants 2004;19:100-106.

[62] Cha JY, Takano-Yamamoto T and Hwang CJ. The effect of miniscrew taper morphology on insertion and removal torque in dogs. Int J Oral Maxillofac Implants. 2010; 25:777-83.

[63] Crismani AG, Bernhart T, Schwarz K, *et al.* Ninety percent success in palatal implants loaded 1 week after placement: a clinical evaluation by resonance frequency analysis. Clin Oral Implants Res 2006;17:445-450.

[64] Park HS, Lee SK and Kwon OW. Group distal movement of teeth using microscrew implant anchorage. Angle Orthod 2005;75:602-609.

[65] Suzuki,M, Deguchi T, Watanabe H *et al.* Evaluation of optimal length and insertion torque for miniscrew Am J Orthod Dentofacial Orthop 2013; 144:251-259.

[66] Deguchi T, Nasu M, Murakami K *et al.* Quantitative evaluation of cortical bone thickness with computed tomographic scanning for orthodontic implants. Am J Orthod Dentofacial Orthop 2006;129:721.e7-721.e12

[67] Kuroda S, Yamada K, Deguchi T *et al.* T Root proximity is a major factor for screw failure in orthodontic anchorage. Am J Orthod Dentofacial Orthop. 2007;131:S68-73.

[68] Deguchi T, Kurosaka H, Oikawa H, *et al.* Comparison of orthodontic treatment outcomes in adults with skeletal open bite between conventional edgewise treatment and implant-anchored orthodontics. Am J Orthod Dentofacial Orthop. 2011:139:S60-68.

[69] Watanabe H, Deguchi T, Hasegawa M,et al. Orthodontic miniscrew failure rate and root proximity, insertion angle, bone contact length, and bone density.Orthod Craniofac Res. 2013;16:44-55.

[70] Kuroda S, Yamada K, Deguchi T *et al.* Class II malocclusion treated with miniscrew anchorage: comparison with traditional orthodontic mechanics outcomes. Am J Orthod Dentofacial Orthop. 2009;135:302-309.

[71] Yamada K, Kuroda S, Deguchi T, *et al.* Distal movement of maxillary molars using miniscrew anchorage in the buccal interradicular region. Angle Orthod. 2009; 79: 78-84.

[72] Brandon N. Meyer Jie Chen and Thomas R. Katona. Does the center of resistance depend on the direction of tooth movement? Am J Orthod Dentofacial Orthop 2010; 137:354-61.

[73] Wada K, Matsushita K, Shimazaki S, *et al.* An evaluation of a new case analysis of a lateral cephalometric roentgenogram. J Kanazawa Med Univ 1981;6:60-70

[74] Grummons D. Orthodontics for the TMJ-TMD patient. 1st ed. :Wright;1994

Send Orders for Reprints to reprints@benthamscience.net

CHAPTER 9

Class III Facial Asymmetry, Mandibular Deviation and Its Related Surgical Orthodontic Treatment

Isao Saito* and Naoko Watanabe

Division of Orthodontics, Niigata University Graduate School of Medical and Dental Sciences, Niigata, Japan

Abstract: The Class III facial asymmetry, mandibular deviation and its related surgical orthodontic treatment will be discussed in this chapter. The number of orthodontic patients with a diverted bite and/or facial asymmetry has been increasing recently. Diagnosis and treatment for Class III patients with facial asymmetry and/or mandibular deviation tend to be more complex than those without asymmetric mandible are. Orthodontists have to discriminate between asymmetric problems of dental nature as opposed to skeletal origin. For instance, the amount of dentoalveolar compensation in the molar region should be part of the diagnosis. Management of the developing Class III malocclusion with mandibular deviation is important since malocclusion tends to deteriorate with growth. On the other hand, skeletal Class III patients are frequently accompanied by facial asymmetry or midline deviations and some eventually need surgical orthodontic treatment. In this chapter, the authors will review the literatures on prevalence of orthodontic asymmetries, possible changes in Class III mandibular deviation with age, morphological features of Class III mandibular deviation, including three-dimensional evaluation and perception of facial asymmetry. In addition, Class III facial asymmetry cases treated with orthognathic surgery will be introduced. Since two-jaw surgery has been recently indicated, more often than before for better outcomes, surgical orthodontic cases corrected with one-jaw or two-jaw surgery will be discussed. Postoperative changes of the frontal facial appearances in skeletal Class III patients with deviation will be compared between one-jaw and two-jaw surgeries as well as postoperative stability of Class III cases with facial asymmetry that surgically treated.

Keywords: Facial asymmetry, Mandibular deviation, Prevalence of facial asymmetry and morphological deviation, Etiology of facial asymmetry and morphological deviation, Analysis and evaluation of facial asymmetry, Frontal cephalogram, Superimposition of frontal cephalograms, Perception of facial asymmetry, Questionnaire investigation of facial asymmetry, CT mages, Three-dimensional (3D) analysis of morphological asymmetry, 3D deviation ratio, 3D morphological symmetry ratio, Deterioration of mandibular deviation with growth beyond prediction, Surgical Orthodontic treatment of Class III facial asymmetry, 3D analysis of dental casts using laser scanner, SSRO, IVRO, two-jaw surgery, 3D analysis of postoperative soft tissue changes.

***Address correspondence to Isao Saito:** 2-5274 Gakkocho-dori, Chuo-ku, Niigata 951-8514, Japan; Tel: +81-25-222-1620; Fax: +81-25-222-1620; E-mail: isao@dent.niigata-u.ac.jp

Peter W. Ngan, Toshi Deguchi and Eugene W. Roberts (Eds)

INTRODUCTION

In orthodontic treatment, sufficient consideration has been given to soft tissue around the mouth and other parts of face since the paradigm shift from "Angle paradigm" to "Soft tissue paradigm" occurred in the early 20th century [1]. Improvement of facial appearance is a major concern among patients seeking treatment. Orthodontists are thus required to treatment plan based on understanding the characteristics and adaptation limits of each patient's soft tissue and to correct teeth and jaw positions to achieve acceptable facial harmony and oral function [2].

Fig. **1** shows the change in age distribution in patients newly registered at the orthodontic clinic of Niigata University Medical and Dental Hospital (NUMDH) over the past 15 years. Adult patients aged 20 years or more at the first examination account for 30.6% on average (23.5-37.4%). Since 1998, subjects with age 30 years or more have accounted for 10-15% of all new patients. In addition to those presenting with malalignment, many adult patients also present with disharmony around the mouth and other problems related to facial appearance [3]. Attempts have been made to investigate the changing distribution of reasons for receiving treatment among patients with jaw deformity at the orthodontic clinic of NUMDH during a 10-year period from 1990 [4] and another 10-year period from 2000 [5]. The proportion of patients who decided to receive treatment because of dissatisfaction with facial appearance increased by 10.3% between 2000 [4] and 2010 [5] reaching 79.4% in the latter decade. This indicates that a very large proportion of patients with jaw deformity receive treatment partially because they want to have their facial appearance improved.

Since ancient times, psychologists and philosophers have wondered why humans prefer symmetry. A possible explanation can be that we are genetically programmed to prefer symmetry. Facial symmetry is a major concern among humans. While facial or dental occlusion asymmetry is considered a common finding [6, 7], the frequency of patients with facial asymmetry or mandibular/occlusal deviation is gradually increasing, particularly among orthodontic patients. This chapter provides an overview of facial asymmetry and mandibular/occlusal deviation by presenting some of our research findings in this area, supplemented with a review of literature. Furthermore, Class III facial asymmetry cases treated with orthognathic surgery are introduced. Postoperative stability for Class III cases with facial asymmetry surgically treated is discussed as well.

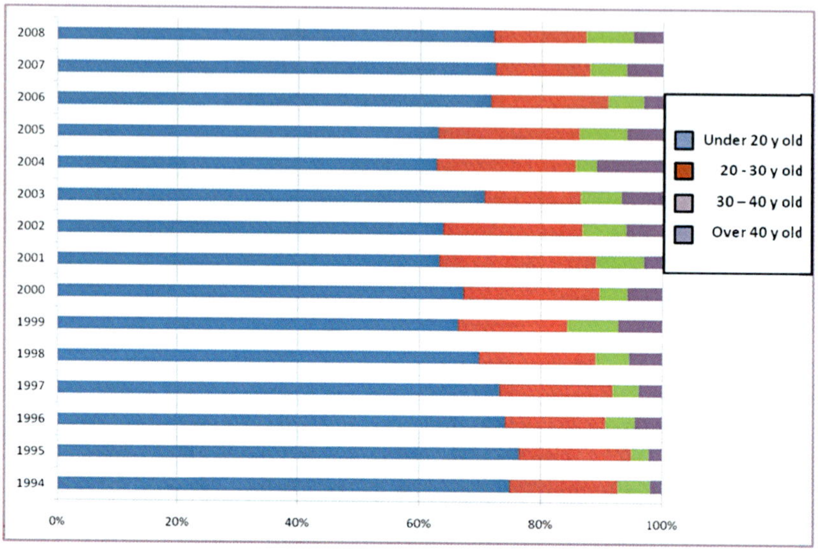

Figure 1: Yearly change in age distribution of new orthodontic outpatients at Niigata University Medical and Dental Hospital (1994-2008) (Citation from Saito *et al.,* [42]).

Prevalence of Facial Asymmetry and Its Etiology

1. Prevalence of Facial Asymmetry or Morphological Deviation

Letzer *et al.* [7] examined frontal cephalograms of 50 patients with ideal occlusion or malocclusion for symmetry of maxillofacial structures. In patients with ideal occlusion, the anterior cranial base and the mandible were significantly symmetric overall, although partial asymmetry was observed in some patients. A clinical investigation involving school children without orthodontic history by Sheats *et al.* [8] identified facial asymmetry in 12% of children with permanent dentition. These findings suggest that facial asymmetry can also be found in healthy individuals without malocclusion at relatively high frequency. Sheats and colleagues also identified, through review of data at initial presentation of orthodontic patients, facial asymmetry in 6%, molar anteroposterior asymmetry in 22%, deviations of the maxillary and mandibular dental midlines from the facial midline in 39% and 62%, respectively, and unmatched maxillary and mandibular dental midlines in 46% [8]. In patients with permanent dentition without orthodontic history, the prevalence of unmatched maxillary and mandibular dental midlines was 21% and that of molar asymmetry was 23% [8]. Thus, unmatched maxillary and mandibular dental midlines was more prevalent among orthodontic patients. The prevalence of lateral deviations, such as cross bite and scissors bite, although varies depending on the chronological age and dental age of the patients studied and the population in each study area, ranging from 5 to 21% [9-11], with a higher prevalence of cross bite than that of scissors bite [12].

Previous statistical surveys involving Japanese patients with jaw deformity have revealed an 11-25% prevalence of facial asymmetry [13, 14]. Our clinical statistical surveys involving jaw deformity patients showed that deviation and/or open bite were found in nearly 50% of skeletal Class II/III cases [4] and that deviation of maxillary and mandibular dental midlines were found in 47.6% of jaw deformity patients studied [5]. In a previous study involving patients with skeletal mandibular protrusion surgically treated [15], maxillofacial skeletal asymmetry was found in approximately 80% of patients through analysis of frontal cephalograms, while the prevalence of soft tissue asymmetry as determined by analysis of facial photographs was only 56%. A recent survey on the current status of jaw deformity treatment conducted by the Japanese Society for Jaw Deformities [16] also reported the proportion of patients with both anteroposterior deviation and asymmetry relative to the total number of patients who had undergone orthognathic surgery was approximately 28% for those with mandibular protrusion and 18% for those with mandibular retrusion or maxillary protrusion. The inconsistent prevalence of asymmetry among institutions is probably attributed to differences in the type of data on which each survey was based, measurement methods, and evaluation criteria. In a survey conducted in patients with jaw deformity outside Japan [17], clinically apparent facial asymmetry was found in 34% of all patients studied; the prevalence of asymmetry being 28% among Class II cases and 40% among Class III cases or Class I long face cases. These findings indicate that a relatively large proportion of patients with jaw deformity also have facial asymmetry both in and outside Japan, and that skeletal Class III cases are frequently associated with facial asymmetry.

2. Etiology of Facial Asymmetry or Mandibular Deviation

This includes congenital and acquired factors [6]. Congenital factors include genetic factors and congenital disorders. Even if such abnormalities are not identified, craniofacial asymmetry may be present in some fetuses and infants before the onset of chewing investigating the morphometry of skull, and they might be exacerbated with growth [18]. However, since phenomena related to lateral deviation and asymmetry during the course of growth and development are complicated, obvious evidences have not been fully provided despite attempts to identify relevant genetic factors [12].

There are two major acquired factors contributing to facial asymmetry or deviation. The first factor is asymmetric endochondral ossification occurring in the mandibular condyle, the growth center of the mandible. Unilateral decrease or failure in the ossification of cartilage in the mandibular condyle leads to asymmetric growth of the mandible and consequent facial asymmetry [19, 20]. Given the experimental finding that cutting of the unilateral mandibular condyle results in a significant decrease in the size of the mandible on the affected side [21], it is likely that unilateral damage to the mandibular condyle due to trauma or other causes leads to mandibular deviation and/or facial asymmetry.

The second acquired factor is functional mandibular deviation due to occlusal interference or unilateral cross bite observed in the posterior dentition [22]. Prolonged functional occlusal deviation leads to quantitative and qualitative changes in the overall load on the mandibular condyle and the entire mandible during functioning, and thus is likely to develop into structural asymmetry. This trend is particularly evident in growing children. This is supported by the experimental finding reported by Fuentes *et al.* that artificially induced functional occlusal deviation by forward displacement of the unilateral mandibular condyle caused increased thickness of condylar cartilage and cellular proliferation potential [23]. Langberg *et al.* have also discussed that leaving unilateral cross bite untreated during school age possibly yields compensatory asymmetry of the positional relationship between the mandibular condyle and mandibular fossa, and subsequent positional deviation of the mandible and persistent unilateral cross bite even into adulthood [24]. Furthermore, Mongini *et al.* [25] and Schmid *et al.* [26] reported that jaw orthopedic treatment of mandibular asymmetry in growing children, which was considered due to adaptational change to functional deviation, induced compensatory change in the growth of the mandible and temporomandibular joint, followed by remission of the deviation. Therefore, dentists should be aware that in patients with asymmetric congenital factors, the degree of asymmetry may worsen as they grow, so they are likely to eventually require surgical orthodontic intervention. For patients with facial asymmetry primarily associated with acquired factors, such as functional occlusal deviation, active intervention should be carried out before structural deviation becomes evident.

Analysis and Evaluation of Facial Asymmetry

1) Analysis Using Frontal Facial Photographs and Frontal Cephalograms

For analysis of facial asymmetry and mandibular/occlusal deviation, it is important to obtain as much information as possible on the structural characteristics of asymmetry *via* clinical examinations [27, 28]. Clinical examinations include evaluation of the facial midline, inclination and positions of the nasal dorsum and apex, philtrum and mentum, symmetry when viewed from the lower part of the mentum, inclination of the occlusal plane due to asymmetry of the vertical height of the molars, presence or absence of occlusal interference and twisted maxillary and mandibular dental arches.

There have been many reports regarding the definitions of midlines on frontal cephalograms [29-32]. Asami conducted a biometric study using front facial photographs of 204 adults taken with closed lips to evaluate the usefulness of the midline defined as a line passing through the following 3 points: the center of nasal apex, the deepest point of the V-shape notch of the upper vermilion border, and the center of the line connecting the right and left medial canthuses [29]. These 3 points were on a single straight line in 60% of patients while deviations were observed in the remaining 40%, although the deviations were mild, ranging from 1.2 mm to 1.3 mm. Watanabe [30] defined the line passing through the supranasal point, which is relatively resistant to disease-related change [31], and perpendicular to the line passing through the superior borders of the ear rods on both sides and orbital points on either side (the Frankfurt Horizontal plane) as the midline; then he evaluated its usefulness in 30 volunteers with normal occlusion, and compared to 5 different midlines defined by moiré topography in previous studies. The highest rate of matching with Watanabe's midline (90%) was demonstrated by the line passing through the center of the right and left medial canthuses and perpendicular to the FH plane.

As mentioned above, "Normal asymmetry" resulting from slight differences in the size of facial structures on both sides can be found in laypersons without malocclusion [28]. It is thus difficult to define a definitive midline over facial soft tissue from a frontal view. In clinical practice, however, since symmetry is usually evaluated in the middle and lower parts of the face; the midline is commonly defined as the line passing through the center of the line connecting the right and left medial canthuses and perpendicular to the line connecting the right and left lateral canthuses, or the line drawn from the center of the line connecting the right and left medial canthuses to pass through the nasal dorsum and apex, philtrum, and mentum [32]. Sufficient care should still be taken when setting the midline in patients with facial asymmetry, since these patients may have asymmetry in the vertical positions of right and left optic fissures and/or significantly inclined optic fissure.

A frontal cephalogram is essential for identifying asymmetry in maxillofacial hard tissue [32-36]. Facial parts should be selected as measurement points or reference lines that are easily measured used for analysis. Fig. **2** shows the measurement points and reference lines routinely employed for analyses and evaluations using frontal cephalograms [27]. A median reference line is defined as the line passing through the crista galli (CG) and that perpendicular to the line connecting the right and left latero-orbitales (Lo-Lo') [27, 33]. Another investigator has used the line passing through the ANS as the median reference line [36], but this line is not very appropriate since a certain proportion of patients with facial asymmetry also have midface deformity. The Lo (Lo') is more easily recognizable than the Z or FM point adjacent to the Lo (Lo'), but it tends to be displaced when the head is rotated. However, since head rotation on cephalogram is almost limited to up-down motion (pitching), the Lo-Lo' line is considered appropriate in the setting of the midline for analysis.

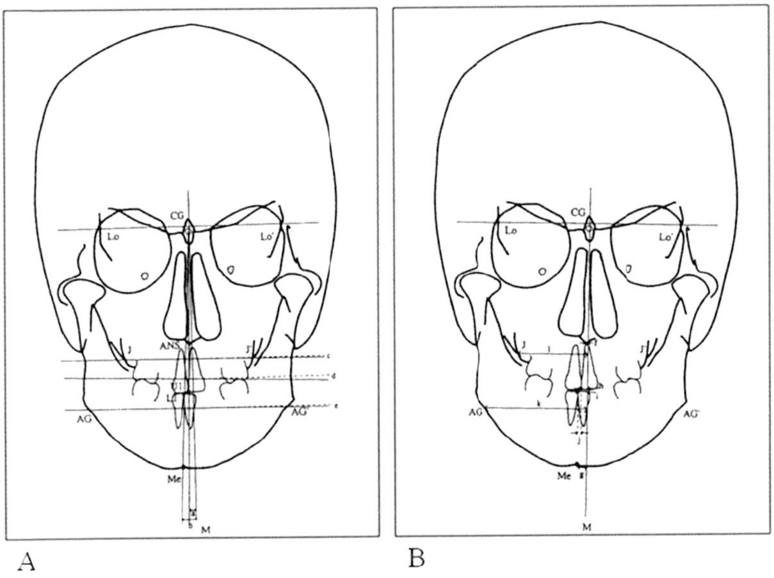

Figure 2: Landmarks and reference lines for morphometry using posteroanterior cephalogram (citation from Kobayashi *et al.* [27]).

Horizontal reference line: A line connecting the latero-orbitale on the right side (Lo) and on the left side (Lo').

Median reference (M) line: A line perpendicular to the horizontal reference line through crista galli (CG).

A : Angular measurements

a) Maxillary deviation angle: formed by M line and the connecting line of CG and ANS.
b) Mandibular deviation angle: formed M line and the connecting line of CG and Me.
c) Maxillary plane angle: formed by horizontal reference line and the connecting line of J and J'.
d) Horizontal occlusal plane angle: formed by horizontal reference line and the connecting line of the occlusal surface of the right and left first molars.
e) Mandibular plane angle: formed by M line and the connecting line of AG and AG'.

B : Linear measurements

f) Maxillary deviation distance: perpendicular distance from M line to ANS.
g) Mandibular deviation distance: perpendicular distance from M line to Me.

h) Upper midline deviation: perpendicular distance from M line to the contact point of the upper central incisors.
i) Lower midline deviation: perpendicular distance from M line to the contact point of the lower central incisors.
j) Difference between the upper and lower midlines: perpendicular distance from the upper midline to the lower one.
k) Mandibular width: perpendicular distance from M line to AG or AG'.
l) Maxillary width: perpendicular distance from M line to J or J'.

Measurement points and reference lines used to identify asymmetric portions and evaluate the degree of asymmetry are shown in Fig. **2** (A: angular, B: linear). The measured length of the line vertically projected from points J (J') and AG (AG'), which are set bilaterally, to median reference line M, maxillary asymmetry index (|JM-JM'|/JM+JMx100), and mandibular asymmetry index (|AG-AG'| / AG+AGx100) [27, 37] are also useful for evaluating the degree of asymmetry.

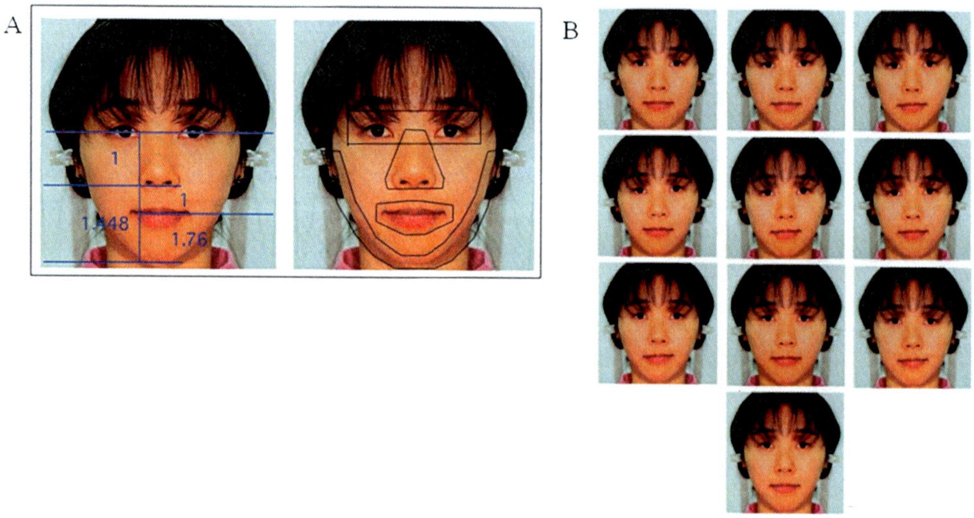

Figure 3: Investigation on perception of facial asymmetry by a WWW questionnaire (modified citation from Saito *et al.* [42]) A : A mirror symmetry image with golden proportion was created as the reference image. To create asymmetric images, four facial parts were rotated by 3 degrees counterclockwise. B : 9 asymmetric images created and a mirror symmetry image were randomly arranged.

Superimposed frontal cephalograms are useful for evaluating change in the degree of facial asymmetry over time or before and after treatment in growing children. However, as mentioned above, head pitching around ear rods may occur during imaging. We therefore conducted a study using dry skulls to examine how the difference in head position is reflected in superposed cephalograms, especially the mandibular contour. The results demonstrated that a head rotation angle of 0° or head slightly tilted downward permits accurate superposition in the entire mandible, with little deviation around the gonial regions [38]. Therefore, when a frontal cephalogram is taken, the head position should be such that it makes the FH plane as parallel with the floor as possible. Even with the head tilted slightly downward, the accuracy of superposition should not be significantly affected.

Fig.4

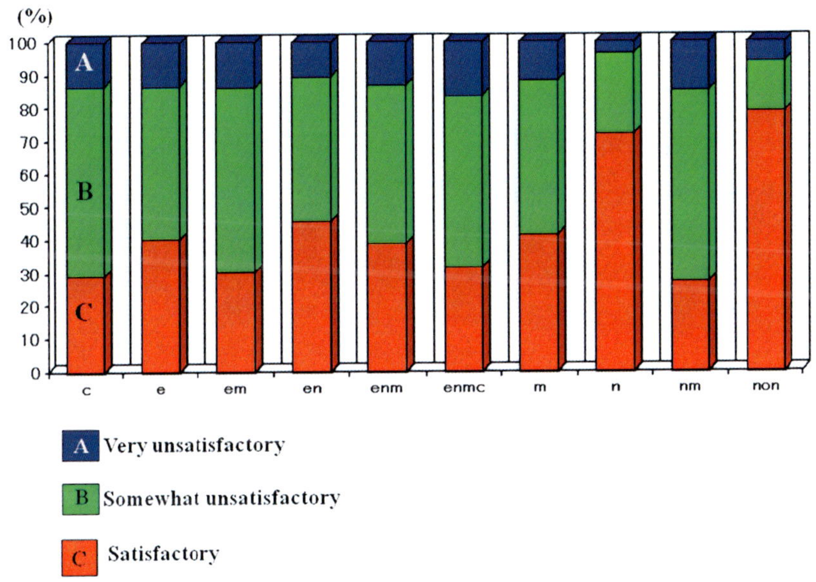

Figure 4: Results of investigation on perception of facial asymmetry (modified citation from Saito *et al.* [42]). Rotated parts are as follows. c : only chin, e : only pupil line, em : pupil line and oral fissure, en : pupil line and nose, enm : pupil line, nose and oral fissure, enmc : pupil line and nose, enm : pupil line, nose, oral fissure and chin, m : oral fissure, n : nose, nm : nose and oral fissure, non : a mirror symmetry.

2) Identification and Evaluation of Facial Asymmetry

Several studies have been conducted to determine the facial parts that influence the identification and evaluation of asymmetry [39-41]. We tried to conduct an internet survey to examine how people feel about asymmetric facial appearance

[42]. A completely mirror-symmetric frontal facial photographs was created and used as the reference image (Fig. **3A**, left). Nine asymmetric images were created by rotating one or more of the following 4 facial parts by 3 degrees counterclockwise: the pupil line, nose, oral slit and chin (Fig. **3A**, right). The 10 images, including 9 asymmetric and 1 completely mirror symmetry images, were randomly arranged (Fig. **3B**) and subjects were asked to select an answer from 3 options. The results are as shown in Fig. **4**. When a single part was rotated, more subjects selected the answer "I have somewhat or very unsatisfactory" to asymmetric oral fissure (m) and chin (c) than to asymmetric pupil line (e) or nose (n). When multiple parts were rotated simultaneously, more subjects answered that they had strange feeling with asymmetric facial images with than without rotated oral fissure.

Lee *et al.* [39] used asymmetric frontal facial photographs to identify factors affecting the subjective rating of asymmetry (mild, moderate, or severe), and identified inclination of the oral slit, displacement of the chin, inclination of the lower mandibular edge and asymmetry of the jaw angles as significant factors. Meyer-Marcotty *et al.* [40] reported that in face-to-face facial evaluation, subjects had a more negative impression of facial images with asymmetric parts located closer to the facial midline. An eye fixation analysis using subjective evaluation and the eye tracking method was performed to determine what parts of the face oral surgeons and orthodontists look at when evaluating facial asymmetry [41]. The findings demonstrated the gazing duration was relatively longer at the chin, nose, and lips, suggesting the degree of mental deviation and inclination of oral fissure influence the evaluation of asymmetry. When diagnosing or treating patients with facial asymmetry, sufficient consideration should be given to how much improvement can be made to inclined oral fissure and asymmetry in the lower part of face, especially chin, for better patient satisfaction.

Orthodontists may find it difficult to define the maxillary and mandibular dental midlines and in some cases, the presence of facial asymmetry makes it difficult to match the dental midline and the facial midline. Defining the degree of midline deviation regarded as "deviation" and the acceptable range of deviation is helpful when providing treatment. Beyer *et al.* [43] presented 8 smile photographs with the maxillary dental midline shifted by increments of 0.7 mm to orthodontists, general dentists, and adolescent orthodontic patients and their parents and asked them to evaluate the photographs. The maximum acceptable deviation of the maxillary dental midline was 2.2 ±1.5 mm. Johnston *et al.* [44] also presented facial photographs with the maxillary dental midline shifted from the philtrum to the right and left by increments of 1 mm to orthodontists and regular individuals and reported that 56 % of them answered that they had strange feeling to photographs with 2 mm deviation. In both studies, orthodontists were more sensitive to deviation than laypersons. Pinho *et al.* [45] presented 5 facial photographs with 0-4.0 mm deviations of maxillary and mandibular dental midlines to orthodontists, prosthodontists and laypersons and examined whether they can identify deviation. Orthodontists and prosthodontists identified 1.0 mm and 3.0 mm deviations as esthetically abnormal, respectively, while laypersons did not recognize deviation even in photographs with 4.0 mm deviation. These findings may be useful in designing treatment plans for facial asymmetry with midline deviation. In clinical practice, sufficient consideration should also be given to individual differences in the recognition of and sensitivity to midline deviation.

Morphological and Functional Characteristics of Facial Asymmetry

It has recently become possible to three-dimensionally construct the maxillofacial structure from CT images. This has also made it possible to three-dimensionally identify complicated deformities of craniofacial bones, such as asymmetry, twist, and distortion of facial structures, which could not be analyzed by two-dimensional imaging modalities [46, 47]. We evaluated three-dimensional asymmetric morphology of the maxilla and the mandible (ratio of three-dimensional asymmetry) and three-dimensional positions of the maxilla and the mandible relative to the skull (ratio of three-dimensional deviation) by the volume rendering (VR) method in 15 skeletal Class III patients with jaw deformity accompanied by facial asymmetry, in an attempt to classify patterns of deviation [48]. Figs. **5A-D** illustrates the procedures to measure ratio of three-dimensional asymmetry and ratio of three-dimensional deviation for the maxilla and the mandible. Fig. **6** shows measurement results for individual patients in the study.

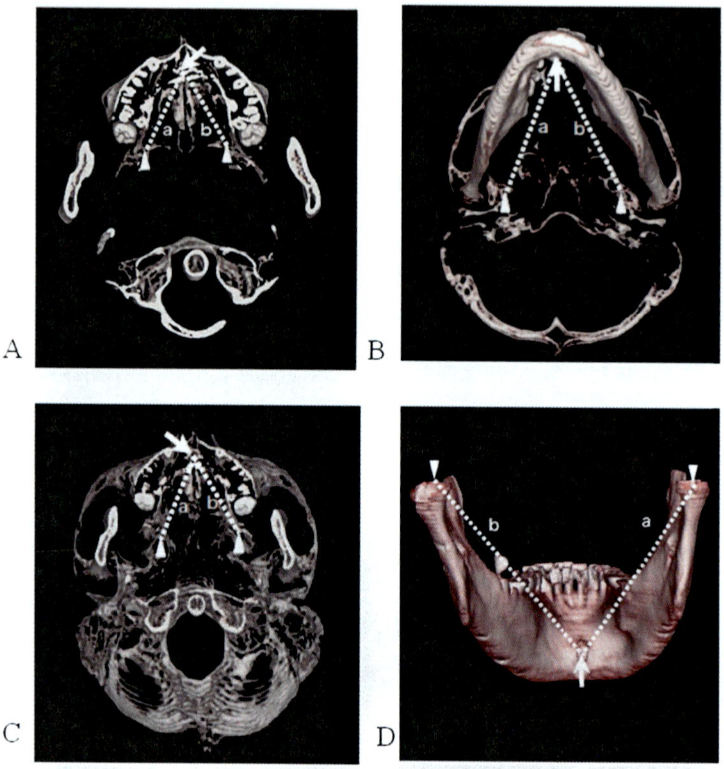

Figure 5: Measurement methods for 3D deviation ratio and 3D morphological asymmetry ratio of the maxilla and the mandible in jaw deformity patients with facial asymmetry (modified citation from Wakamatsu *et al.* [48]) A. Ratio of 3D deviation of the maxilla in the craniofacial complex. arrow heads: Foramen palatinum majus arrow: Foramen incisivum Ratio of 3D deviation of the maxilla=$[(a-b/a+b)\times 100]$. B: Ratio of 3D deviation of the mandible in the craniofacial complex. arrow heads: Foramen spinosum arrow: Spinae mentale. Ratio of 3D deviation of the mandible=$[(a-b/a+b)\times 100]$. C: Ratio of 3D morphological asymmetry of the maxilla. arrow heads: Foramen spinosum arrow: Foramen incisivum. Ratio of 3D morphological asymmetry of the maxilla=$[(a-b/a+b)\times 100]$. D: Ratio of 3D morphological asymmetry of the mandible. arrow heads: Mandibular condylion arrow: Spinae mentalis. Ratio of 3D morphological asymmetry of the mandible=$[(a-b/a+b)\times 100]$.

Only a few patients showed significant asymmetry of the maxilla, with small variations. In the mandible, asymmetry was more evidently observed than positional deviation relative to the skull, with rather large variations among patients. This supports the previous report that in many cases of facial asymmetry, asymmetric growth of the mandible leads to the gradual manifestation of asymmetry in the lower facial region [12]. In contrast, in a study conducted by

Langberg *et al.* of adult patients with unilateral cross bite [24], mandibular positional deviation or horizontal asymmetry of teeth/alveolar bone, but not structural asymmetry of the mandible, was significantly greater in those with unilateral cross bite than the control group. These results suggest that the deviation pattern varies among subjects selected or individual patients.

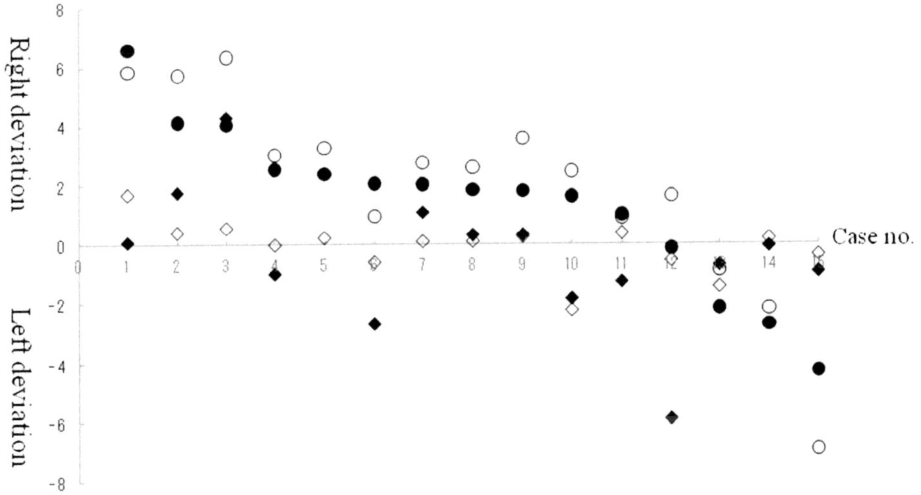

Figure 6: Three-dimensional ratio of morphological asymmetry and deviation in individual cases (modified citation from Wakamatsu *et al.* [48]); ◇Ratio of 3D morphological asymmetry of the maxilla; ◆Ratio of 3D deviation of the maxilla in the craniofacial complex; ○Ratio of 3D morphological asymmetry of the mandible; ●Ratio of 3D deviation of the mandible in the craniofacial complex.

Studies have suggested a close relationship between mandibular deviation and the structure and/or function of the temporomandibular joint. We have also addressed this issue [49-51]. Sato and colleagues found that patients with mandibular deviation had a smaller angle between the long axes of the mandibular condyle in the deviated side than that in the non-deviated side and a backward displacement of the mandibular condyle in the mandibular fossa [49]. Another study to determine the three-dimensional position of the mandibular condyle in the mandibular fossa and the relationship between the shape of the articular eminence and mandibular deviation using helical CT [50] also revealed an outward deviation of the mandibular condyle in the mandibular fossa and a significantly greater inclination of the posterior slope of the articular eminence in the deviated side compared to the non-deviated side.

The structural characteristics of temporomandibular joint affect jaw movement in patients with mandibular deviation. This is supported by the fact that both the distance of mandibular condyle movement and curvature of mandibular movement trace are larger in the deviated side compared to the non-deviated side; *i.e.*, greater mandibular deviation is associated with greater asymmetry [51], and there is a significant correlation of the degree of mandibular deviation to asymmetry of condyle path angles and condyle path curvature during mandibular protrusive movement [49]. These observations suggest that patients with mandibular deviation may have developed so-called adaptation change resulting from a close interaction between structural asymmetry of the right and left temporomandibular joints and asymmetry of mandibular movement.

Three-dimensional analyses have been performed to examine the relationship between hard tissue morphology and masticatory muscles in patients with facial asymmetry or mandibular deviation [52-56]. Kondo [52] measured the cross-sectional areas of masseter and medial pterygoid muscles on CT scans and analyzed masseter muscle activity during maximum biting, and then identified positive correlations between asymmetry in the cross-sectional area of the masseter muscle and that for medial pterygoid muscle and between the degree of mandibular deviation and asymmetry of masseter muscle activity. Kwon *et al.* [53] divided patients with skeletal mandibular protrusion into two groups according to the presence or absence of asymmetry, measured masseter muscle volume on CT scans and examined its relationship with mandibular asymmetry. They found that asymmetry in the volumes of masseter and medial pterygoid muscles was associated with structural asymmetry of the mandible, and discussed that the asymmetry of muscle volume was not a cause of asymmetric development, but a consequence of adaptation. We have also examined the relationship between masseter volume in the resting state and deviation pattern by the VR method in patients with skeletal mandibular protrusion (Figs. **7-9**) and found little correlation between three-dimensional deviation rate of the mandible and asymmetry in masseter volume [54] (Fig. **9**).

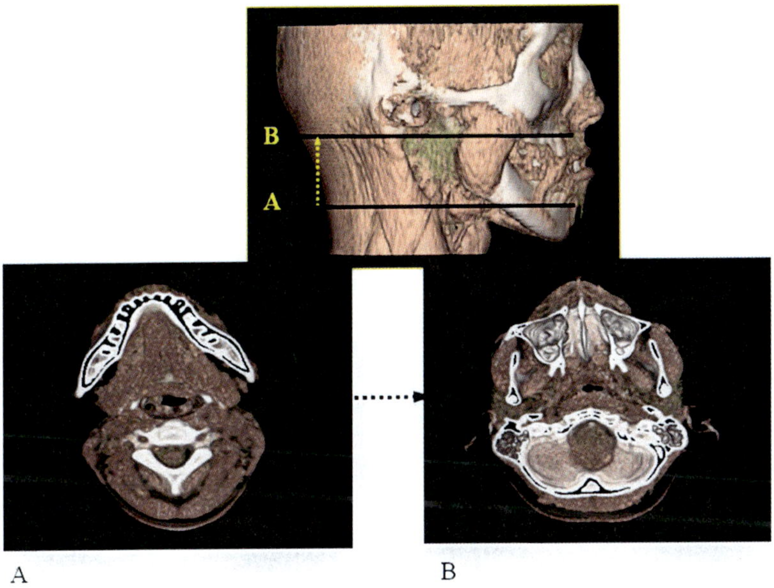

Figure 7: Range for volume measurement of masseter muscle on 3D-CT (citation from Wakamatsu *et al.* [54]) A: An initiation point of measurement. B: An end point of measurement.

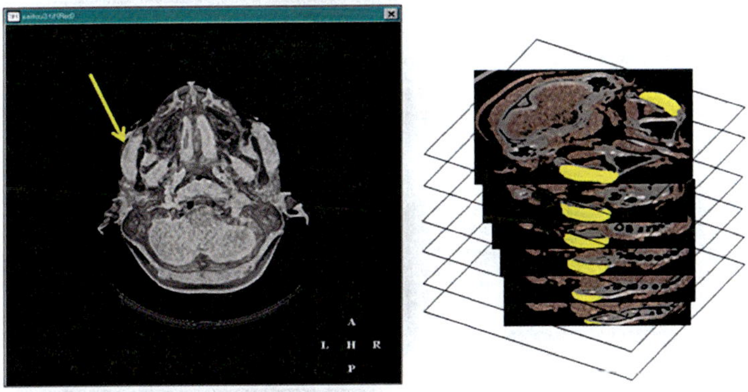

Figure 8: Volume measurement of masseter muscle (citation from Wakamatsu *et al.* [54]) The cross section of the left masseter muscle (arrow) and data sliced at intervals of 2mm were shown. Masseter volume was calculated from the total area of the cross sections obtained.

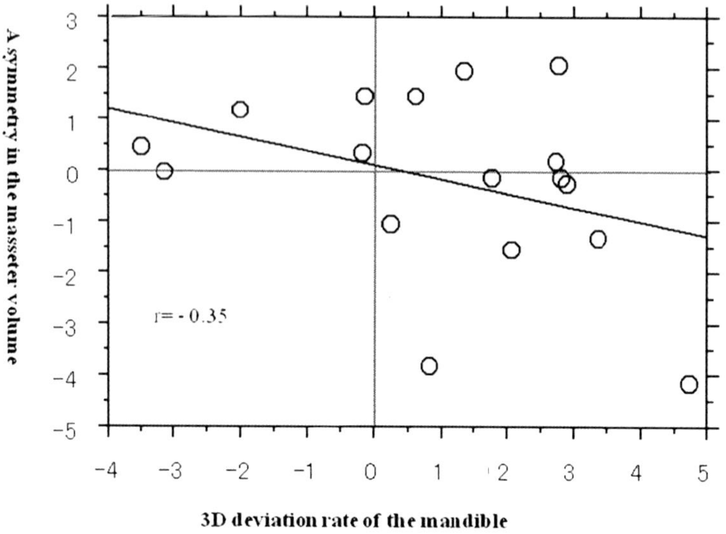

Figure 9: Correlation between three-dimensional deviation rate of the mandible and asymmetry in masseter volume (Wakamatsu *et al.* [54]) The mandibular deviation was defined as negative and positive for deviation to the right and the left respectively.

Asymmetry in masseter volume was calculated by subtraction from a volume of the right masseter to that of the left masseter. An insignificant correlation coefficient of -0.35 was attained.

It has also been reported that patients who experienced exacerbation of mandibular asymmetry as they grew and developed show impaired symmetric mandibular movement and reduced cervical muscle activities [55]. In growing children with functional molar cross bite, a significant increase in temporal muscle volume was found following improvement of cross bite [56]. However, the relationship between the structure and function of these muscles in patients with facial asymmetry has not been fully elucidated yet.

Orthodontic Treatment for Mandibular Deviation and Skeletal Class III with Facial Asymmetry

In some growing children, asymmetry may not become evident owing to compensatory changes in teeth and alveolar bone but often develops into skeletal deviation during growth and development [57]. For those patients in whom repositioning of the mandible and course correction to symmetric growth/development can be achieved by early treatment, phase II treatment is relatively easily performed in the permanent dentition. For those patients who have undergone extraordinarily imbalanced mandibular development (Fig. **10**),

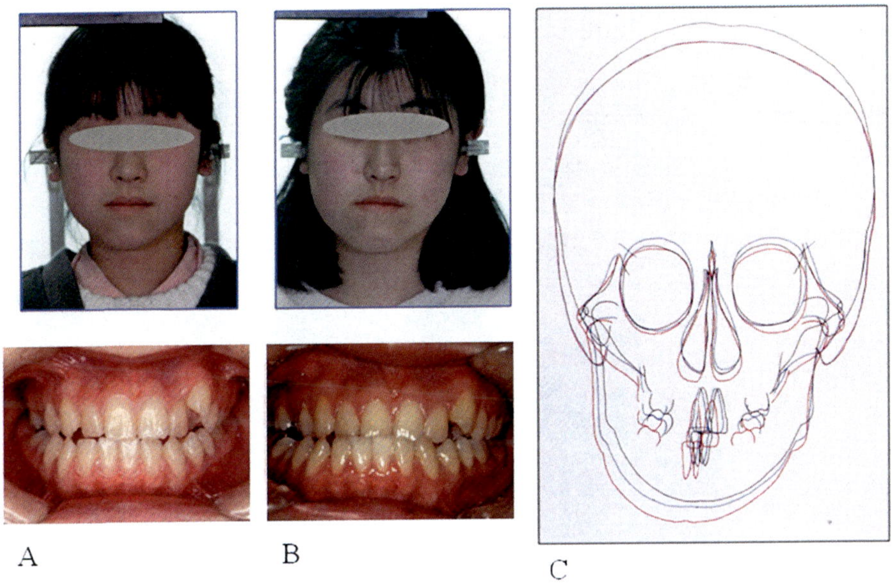

Figure 10: A mandibular deviation case deteriorated with growth and development beyond prediction (modified citation from Kobayashi *et al.* [27]) A: At the first visit (11-year and 4-month old) B: At the reevaluation after periodical follow-up (15-year and 6-month old) C: The superimposition of posteroanterior cephalograms during periodical observation.

considerations should be given to various treatment options for asymmetry, such as asymmetric tooth extraction, use of asymmetric intermaxillary elastics and application of asymmetric torque, even if improvement can be expected by orthodontic treatment alone [58, 59]. In orthodontic diagnosis for patients with facial asymmetry or mandibular/occlusal deviation, it is essential to determine whether the main cause is dental problems as reflected in abnormalities in teeth/alveoli or dentition, or skeletal ones as reflected in abnormalities in jaw morphology or malposition [59, 60]. For differential diagnosis, it is important to accurately identify compensatory changes such as tooth axis inclination and alveolar deformity. These changes specifically include buccolingual inclination of the molars and/or premolars in the presence of cross bite and mesiodistal inclination of the maxillary and mandibular anterior teeth in the presence of midline deviation. The author tries to develop a continuous whole dentition analysis system based on dental model measurement using a three-dimensional laser scanner, in order to enable clinically relevant three-dimensional morphological evaluation of teeth and alveolar bone [61]. This system will enable superimposition of the cross-sectional images of the right and left dental arches using dental casts prepared in daily clinical practice, allowing for detailed, visual, and objective evaluation of compensatory changes in the dentition (Fig. **11**).

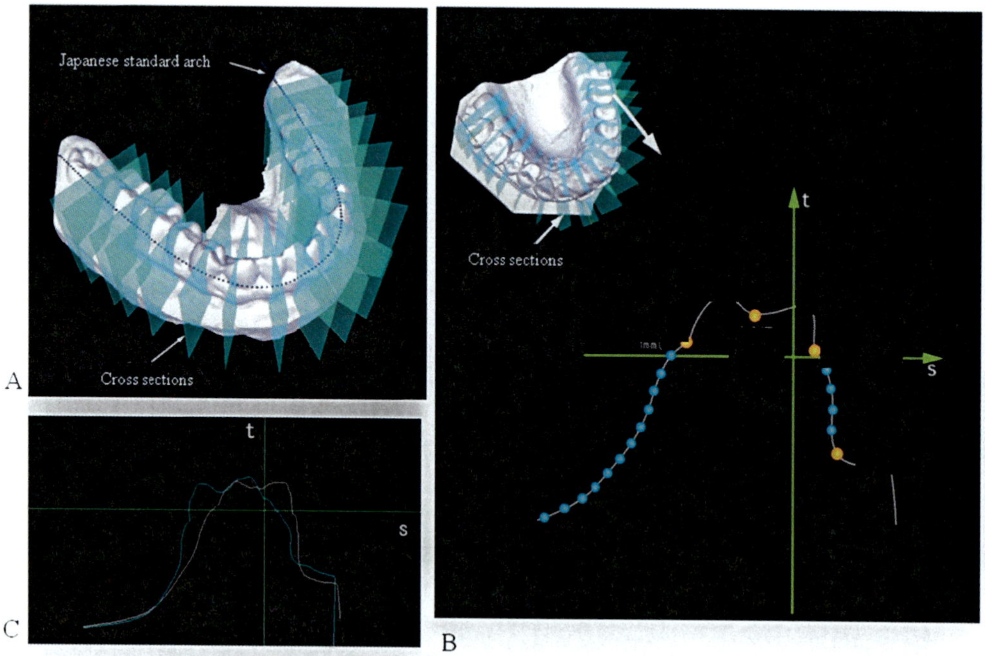

Figure 11: A three-dimensional analyzing system for dental casts using laser scanner (modified citation from Ochi *et al.* [61]); A: Calculation of arbitrary cross sections; B: Extraction of characteristic points on each two-dimensional cross section C: The superimposition on the contralateral outline at the first molar for symmetric analysis.

Surgical orthodontic treatment is indicated in severe and combined cases of deviation of the maxillary and mandibular dental midlines and asymmetric molar dentition [32] with significant structural jaw asymmetry. Fig. **12** shows a male adult patient with chief complaints of facial asymmetry, lack of incisal contact and midline deviations. The mandible skeletally shifted to the right with slight protrusion of the lower lip (Fig. **12A** and **B**). Pretreatment panoramic radiograph indicated late existence of three primary second molars along with concomitant 3 congenitally missing second premolars except the upper left one (Fig. **12A**). According to frontal cephalogram and reconstructed 3D-CT image before treatment, morphological asymmetry was limited in the mandible (Fig. **12B**). This patient was diagnosed as severe mandibular deviation with anterior open bite, proclination of the lower incisors, slight lower crowding and three congenitally missing second bicuspids. 3 primary second molars and the upper left second premolar were extracted for presurgical orthodontic treatment. Because the amount of mandibular setback was very different on the left and the right in this case, sagittal split ramus osteotomy on the left and intraoral vertical ramus osteotomy on the right were undergone to improve facial asymmetry as suitably as possible. Further, simultaneous genioplasty was indicated to obtain more symmetric face. Symmetric face and balanced facial profile were accomplished with proper occlusal interdigitation. Dental midline deviation was successfully corrected with adequate overjet and overbite after treatment (Fig. **12C**).

A

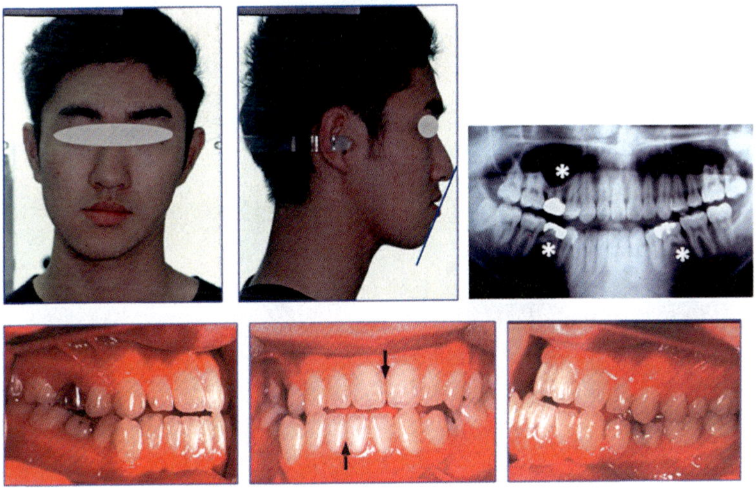

Figure 12A: A case of mandibular prognathism accompanied by facial asymmetry treated with mandibular surgery alone. A: Facial and intraoral pictures before treatment Late development of 3 second primary molars, with concomitant congenitally missing 2nd premolars, was observed in all quadrants except for the upper left.

B

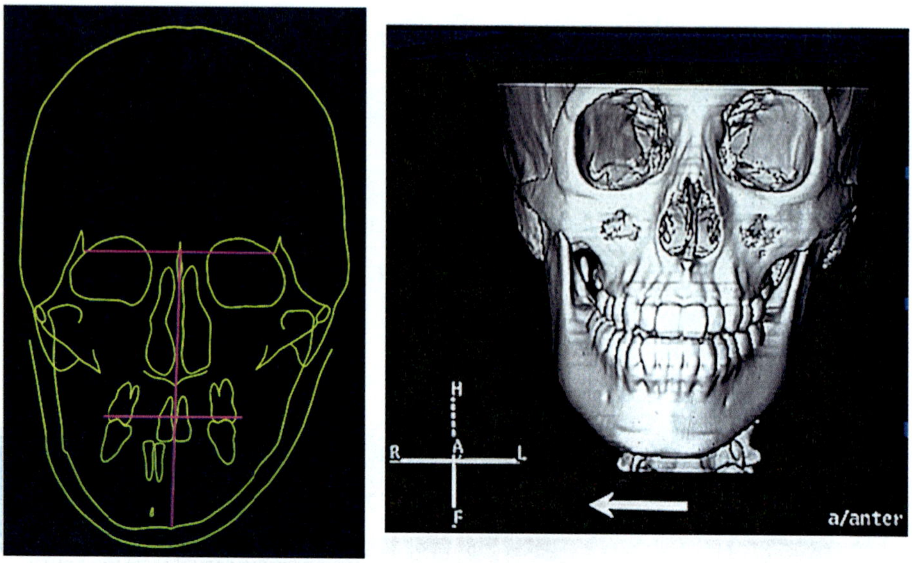

Figure 12B: Pretreatment posteroanterior cephalogram and reconstructed 3D-CT image.

C

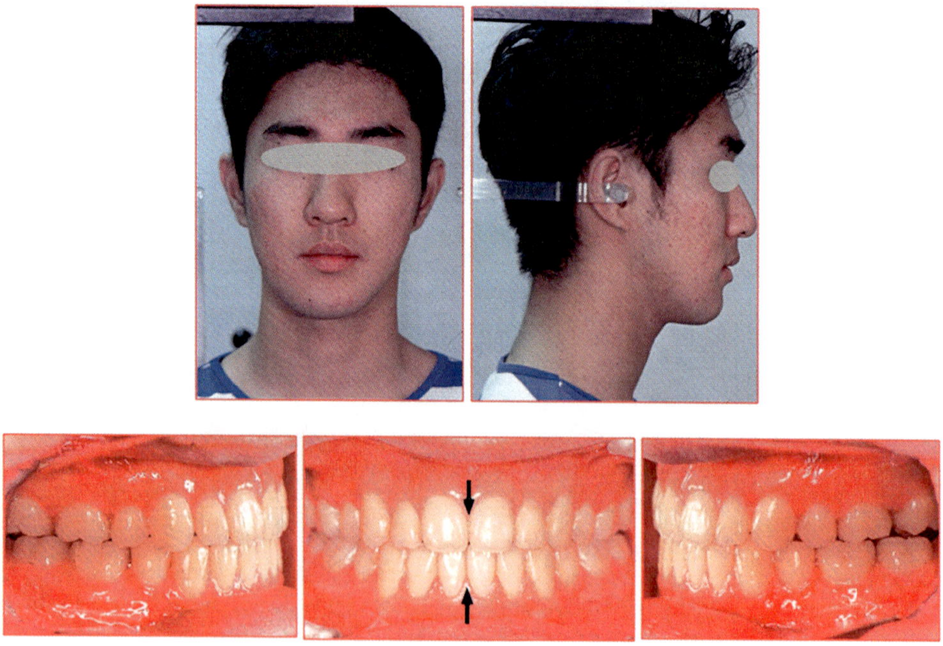

Figure 12C: Facial and intraoral pictures after treatment.

Fig. **13** shows a patient with skeletal mandibular protrusion accompanied by facial asymmetry treated with surgical orthodontic treatment. The patient was diagnosed as skeletal mandibular protrusion accompanied by horizontal inclination of the maxilla and occlusal plane and mandibular deviation to the right (Fig. **13A**). Presurgical orthodontic treatment involving extraction of the bilateral upper and lower first premolars was followed by two-jaw surgery. Reduction in facial asymmetry, improved facial profile and suitable occlusion were attained along with a coincidence of dental midlines after treatment (Fig. **13B**).

A

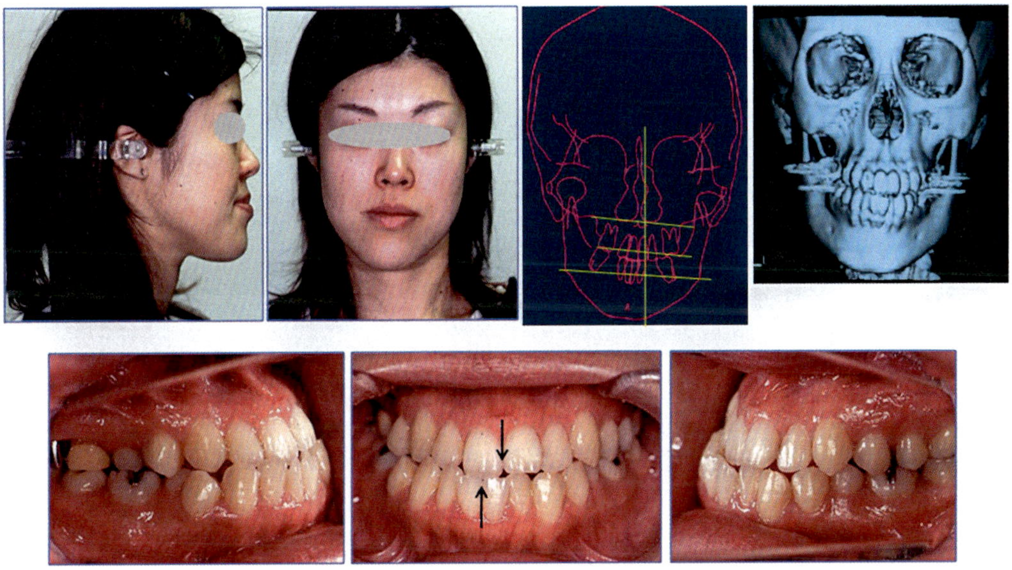

Figure 13A: A case of mandibular prognathism accompanied by facial asymmetry treated with two-jaw surgery. A: Facial and intraoral pictures, posteroanterior cephalometric tracing and reconstructed 3D-CTimage before treatment. B: Facial and intraoral pictures, and superimposition of pre- and posttreatment frontal cephalometric tracing after treatment (Citation from Saito *et al.*, [42]).

Two-jaw surgery is required in patients with deformities extending across the mandible to the maxilla, as represented by this case. We have demonstrated that patients treated with two-jaw surgery have shown significant improvement in Me deviation and reduction in nasal width asymmetry compared to those treated with sagittal split ramus osteotomy alone [62]. A review of the data obtained in Niigata University Medical and Dental Hospital in the past 10 years revealed that the patients who underwent two-jaw surgery accounted for about 50-65% of all patients treated with orthognathic surgery [5] and showed favorable outcomes [63].

B

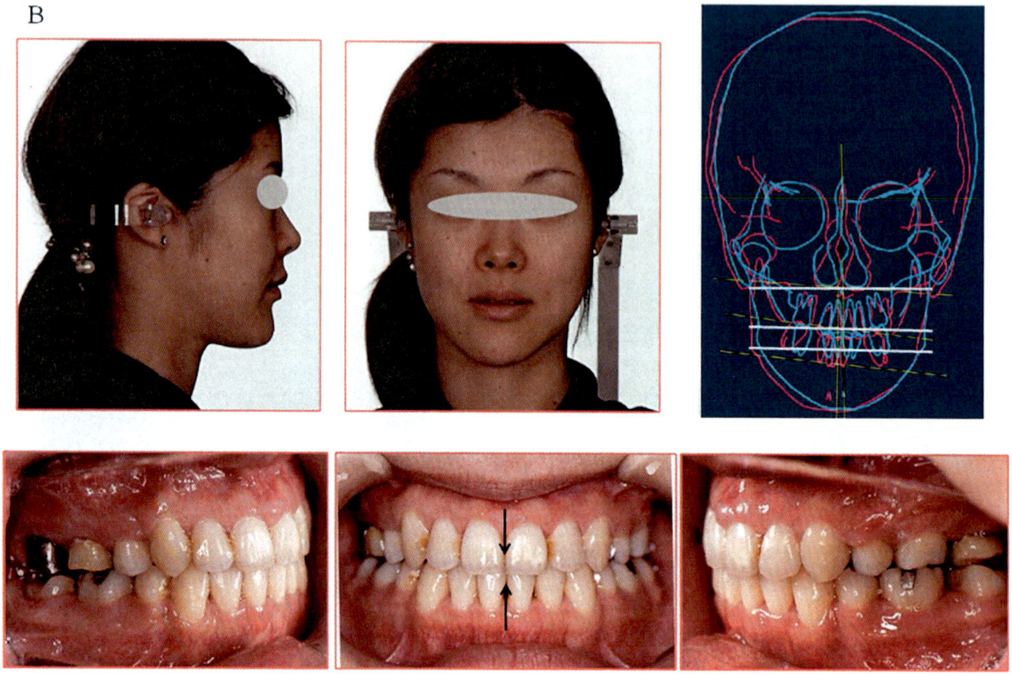

Figure 13B: Facial and intraoral pictures, and superimposition of pre- and post-treatment frontal cephalometric tracing after treatment (Citation from Saito *et al.,* [42]).

Postoperative prediction is prerequisite when performing surgical orthodontic correction. In addition to two-dimensional cephalometric prediction, the usefulness of three-dimensional analysis has also been demonstrated in recent studies [64, 65]. Troulis *et al.* [64] have developed software that improves the accuracy of three-dimensional analysis to treatment planning, such as "Cutting Tool" to slice maxillofacial structures and move them to planned surgical sites on a CT scan, and "Collision Tool" to detect interference by bone fragments during surgical movement. Xia *et al.* [65] have developed a new preoperative three-dimensional prediction technique where an orthognathic surgery plan is designed using reconstructed 3-D CT images and a facial model is created by coloring of changes in soft tissue caused by surgery with a 3-D color texture mapping method. We have also analyzed relative changes in soft tissue against hard tissue following orthognathic surgery using three-dimensional images reconstructed from CT scans in patients with skeletal mandibular protrusion accompanied by facial asymmetry [66]. Fig. **14A** and **B** exhibit the setting of the vertical and horizontal measurement axes and the measurement procedure. The preoperative thickness of soft tissue and soft tissue compliance rate are measured and calculated for four regions; *i.e.*, the cheek and chin on both the deviated and non-deviated sides (Fig. **14C**). As shown in Table **1A** and **B**, the three-dimensional analysis performed in this study demonstrated excellent means to detect asymmetry and a potential for extensive and objective evaluation of soft tissue compliance rate in patients with facial asymmetry.

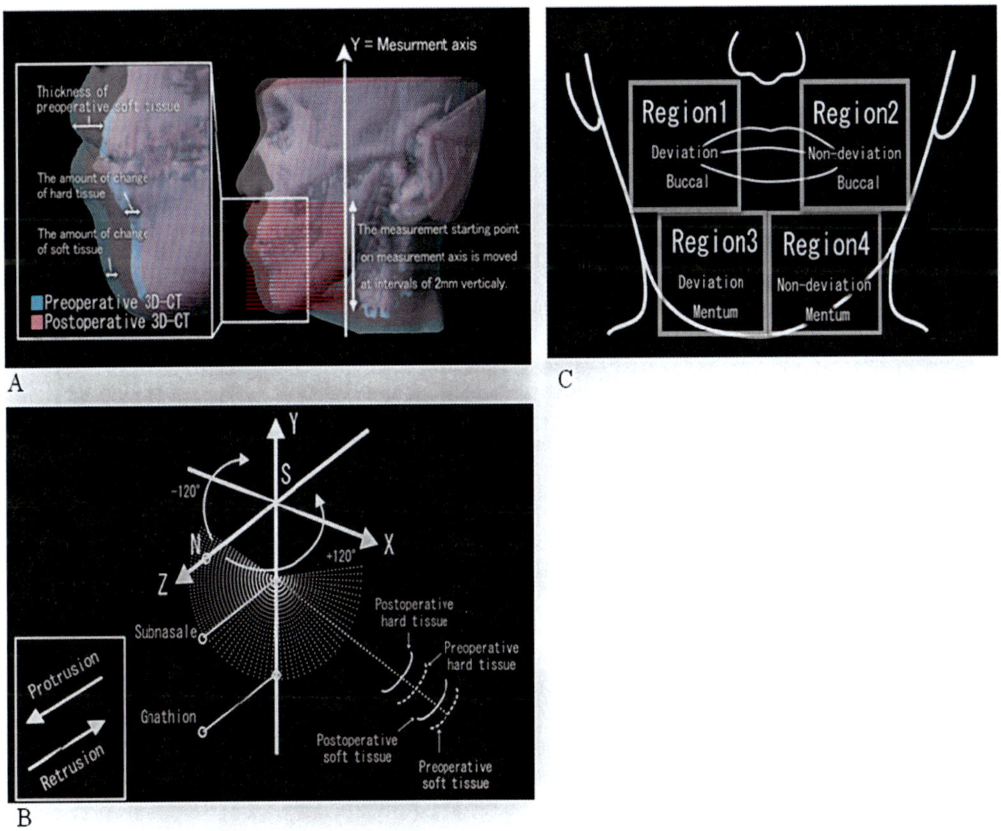

Figure 14: The method for three-dimensional analysis of postoperative soft tissue changes in skeletal Class III patients with facial asymmetry (citation from Yamazaki *et al.* [66]) A: Setup of measurement axis and measurements procedure (vertical). B: Setup of measurement axis and measurements procedure (horizontal). C: Setup of four measurement regions.

Table 1A: Regression parameters and R^2 in retrusion points of each region. (citation from Yamasaki *et al.* [66])

Region (retraction change)	Regression parameter	Coefficient of determination (R^2)
Region 1 deviation side in buccal region	0.678*	0.879
Region 2 non-deviation side in buccal region	0.426*	0.749
Region 3 deviation side in mentum	0.873*	0.957
Region 4 non-deviation side in mentum	0.738*	0.895

By simple linear regression analysis (target variable : soft tissue change, explaining variable : hard tissue change)
* significant value with $P < .01$

Table 1B: Regression parameters and R^2 in protrusion points of each region. (Citation from Yamasaki *et al.* [66])

Region (protrusion change)	Regression parameter	Coefficient of determination (R^2)
Region 1 deviation side in buccal region	0.370 *	0.560
Region 2 non-deviation side in buccal region	0.372 *	0.639
Region 3 deviation side in mentum	–	–
Region 4 non-deviation side in mentum	0.856 *	0.687

By simple linear regression analysis (target variable : soft tissue change, explaining variable : hard tissue change)
* significant value with $P < .01$

Attempts have also been made to predict postoperative changes in soft tissue following orthognathic surgery using three-dimensional data for facial soft tissue in two forms (on lip closure or anterior teeth exposure) and dental casts in daily practice [67], or three-dimensional digital dental model data, using a noncontact 3-D measurement system without X-ray exposure [68]. Both strategies provide clinically sufficient integration accuracy. Further application and evaluation of these strategies in various types of patients will enable their application to three-dimensional prediction of soft tissue morphology and comparison of pre- and postoperative soft tissue morphology.

CONCLUSIONS

This chapter discussed various aspects of facial asymmetry and mandibular/occlusal deviation, such as development, evaluation and identification of asymmetry, structural/functional characteristics of mandibular deviation, and treatment of asymmetry. The relevant literature was reviewed and discussed. Recent advances in testing equipment and analysis software have led to rapid progress in techniques for the analysis/evaluation of hard and soft tissues from two-dimensional to three-dimensional techniques. We clinicians should be committed to improving patient satisfaction by providing quality care and better treatment outcomes, while actively incorporating new findings, based on a full understanding of traditional techniques for basic clinical examination, tests, and analysis.

SUMMARY POINTS

- A clinical investigation identified that facial asymmetry in school children without orthodontic treatment could be as high as 12%, suggesting facial asymmetry can be found in healthy individuals without malocclusion at a relatively high frequency.

- Several surveys indicated that a relatively large proportion of patients with jaw deformity have facial asymmetry both in and outside Japan and patients with skeletal Class III malocclusions were frequently associated with facial asymmetry.

- There are two major acquired factors contributing to facial asymmetry or deviation. One is asymmetric endochondral ossification occurring in the mandibular condyle and the site of growth of the mandible, and the other is functional mandibular deviation due to occlusal interference or unilateral cross bite observed in the lateral dentition and molar region.

- In many cases of facial asymmetry, asymmetric growth of the mandible leads to the gradual manifestation of asymmetry in the lower region, and a close relation between mandibular deviation and temporomandibular joint exists.

- In clinical practice, the midline is most commonly defined as the line passing through the center of the line connecting the right and left medial canthuses and perpendicular to the line connecting the right and left lateral canthuses, or the line drawn from the center of the line connecting the right and left medial canthuses to pass through the nasal dorsum and apex, philtrum, and mentum.

- According to several studies on the facial parts that influenced the identification and evaluation of asymmetry, more subjects answered that they have strange feeling with asymmetric facial images with rotated oral fissure.

- The relationship between hard tissue morphology and masticatory muscles in patients with facial asymmetry or mandibular deviation has been examined with 3D technology, but to date the results are still not clear.

- Surgical orthodontic treatment is indicated in patients with severe jaw asymmetry with deviation of the maxillary and mandibular dental midlines and asymmetric molar dentition. Two-jaw surgery is required in patients with deformities extending across the mandible to the maxilla.

- Clinicians should be committed to improving patient satisfaction by providing quality care and better treatment outcomes while actively incorporating new findings, based on full understanding of traditional techniques for basic clinical examination, tests, and analysis.

ACKNOWLEDGEMENTS

Declared none.

CONFLICT OF INTEREST

The authors confirm that this chapter contents have no conflict of interest.

REFERENCES

[1] Proffit WR: Malocclusion and dentofacial deformity in contemporary society. In: Proffit WR, Fields HW Jr., Sarver DM, Eds. Contemporary Orthodontics. 4th ed., St. Louis, Mosby, 2007; pp. 3-23.

[2] Ackerman JL, Proffit WR and Sarver DM. The merging soft tissue paradigm in orthodontic diagnosis and treatment planning. Clin Orthod Res 1999; 2: 49-52.

[3] Saito I. What is the proportional face?-From the point of view of Orthodontists-. J Kouhokushinetsu Orthod Soc 2007; 15: 13-9.

[4] Machida N, Saito I, Terada K, *et al.* Clinico-statistical investigation on jaw deformity patients in the past ten years at Orthodontic Clinic of Niigata University Dental Hsp. J Kouhokushinetsu Orthod Soc 2000; 8 : 31-34.

[5] Oguri Y, Naganuma K, Harada F, *et al.* Clinical survey of surgical-orthodontics cases treated in the past decade at the Orthodontic Department, Niigata University Medical and Dental Hospital. Jpn J Jaw Deform 2010; 20: 297-04.

[6] Bishara SE, Burkey PS, Kharouf JG. Dental and facial asymmetries: a review. Angle Orthod 1994; 64: 89-98.

[7] Letzer GM, Kronman JH. A postero-anterior cephalometric evaluation of craniofacial asymmetry. Angle Orthod 1967; 37: 205-11.

[8] Sheats RD, McGorray SP, Musmar Q, Wheeler TT, King G. Prevalence of orthodontics asymmetries. Semin Orthod 1998; 4: 138-45.

[9] Melsen B, Stensgard K, Pedersen J. Sucking habits and their influence on swallowing pattern and prevalence of malocclusion. Eur J Orthod 1979; 1: 271-80.

[10] Larsson E. The effect of dummy-sucking on the occlusion: a review. Eur J Orthod 1986; 8: 127-30.

[11] Kürol J, Berglund L. Longitudinal study and cost-benefit analysis of the effect of early treatment of posterior cross-bites in the primary dentition. Eur J Orthod 1992; 14: 173-9.

[12] Pirttiniemi P. Association of mandibular and facial asymmetries—a review. Am J Orthod Dentofac Orthop 1994; 106: 191-200.

[13] Minami K, Sugawara T, Mori Y, *et al.* Clinico-statistical study of orthognathic surgery. J Jpn Stomatol Soc 1997; 46: 165-70.

[14] Yunoki H, Nakajima M, Hayashi H, *et al.* Clinico-statistical study on orthognathic surgery for 11 years at second department of oral and maxillofacial surgery, Osaka Dental University. Jpn J Jaw Deform 1999; 9: 51-6.

[15] Haraguchi S, Takada K, Yasuda Y. Facial asymmetry in subjects with skeletal Class III deformity. Angle Orthod 2002; 72: 28-35.

[16] Kobayashi T, Saito C, Inoue N, *et al.* Treatment of jaw deformity: A nationwide survey of the situation in Japan. Jpn J Jaw Deform 2008; 18: 237-50.

[17] Severt TR, Proffit WR. The prevalence of facial asymmetry in the dentofacial deformities population at the University of North Carolina. Int J Adult Orthodon Orthognath Surg 1997; 12: 171-6.

[18] Rossi M, Ribeiro E, Smith R. Craniofacial asymmetry in development: An anatomical study. Angle Orthod 2003; 73: 381-5.

[19] Sarnat BG. Developmental facial abnormalities and the temporomandibular joint. J Am Dent Assoc 1969; 79: 108-17.

[20] Erickson GE, Waite DE. Mandibular asymmetry. J Am Dent Assoc 1974; 89: 1369-73.

[21] Spyropoulos MN, Tsolakis AI. Altered mandibular function and prevention of skeletal asymmetries after unilateral condylectomy in rats. Eur J Orthod 1997; 19: 211-8.

[22] Mongini F, Schmid W. Craniomandibular asymmetries. In: Mongini F, Schmid W, Eds. Craniomandibular and TMJ orthopedics. Stomatognathic dysfunction. Chicago, Quintessence Pub Co, 1989; pp.47-66.

[23] Fuentes MA, Opperman LA, Buschang P, *et al.* Lateral functional shift of the mandible: Part I. Effects on condylar cartilage thickness and proliferation. Am J Orthod Dentofacial Orthop 2003; 123: 153-9.

[24] Langberg BJ, Arai K, Miner M. Transverse skeletal and dental asymmetry in adults with unilateral lingual posterior cross bite. Am J Orthod Dentofacial Orthop, 127 2005; 6-16.

[25] Mongini F, Schmid W. Treatment of mandibular asymmetries during growth: A longitudinal study. Eur J Orthod 1987; 9: 51-67.

[26] Schmid W, Mongini F, Felisio A. A computer-based assessment of structural and displacement asymmetries of the mandible. Am J Orthod Dentofacial Orthop 1991; 100: 19-34.

[27] Kobayashi M, Saito I, Ishii K, *et al.* Lomg-term observation of mandibular protrusion cases worsen in pubertal growth spurt. J Jpn Orthod Soc 1996; 55: 234-45.

[28] Proffit WR, Sarver DM, Ackerman JL. Orthodontic diagnosis: The development of a problem list. In: Proffit WR, Fields HW Jr., Sarver DM, Eds. Contemporary Orthodontics. 4th ed., St. Louis, Mosby, 2007; pp.167-233.

[29] Asami K. Anatomical study on the frontal view of the face of Japanese by gauged photography of the face: 1. Face with closed mouth. J Tokyo Dent College Soc 1978; 78: 835-78.

[30] Watanabe K. A study on facial asymmetry –Consideration on the establishment of the so called "madi line"-. Nihon Univ Dent J 1979; 53: 1037-47.

[31] Beorkowitz S, Cussi J. Biostereometric analysis of surgically corrected abnormal faces. Am J Orthod 1977; 72: 526-38.

[32] Arnett GW, Bergman RT. Facial keys to orthodontic diagnosis and treatment planning —part II. Am J Orthod Dentofacial Orthop 1993; 103: 395-411.

[33] Sassouni V, Ed. Orthodontics in dental practice. 1st ed., St. Louis, Mosby, 1971; pp. 325-55.

[34] Ricketts RM. Cephalometric analysis and synthesis. Angle Orthod 1961; 31: 141-56.

[35] Kondo E. Posteroanterior cephalometric study of cranio-facial and arch width. J Jpn Orthod Soc 1972; 31: 117-36.

[36] Aoshima O. Investigation of the facial symmetry of cases with cross bites needing surgical orthodontic treatment using postero-anterior Roentgenographic cephalometrics. J Jpn Orthod Soc 1990; 49: 256-62.

[37] Haraguchi Y, Nkata S, Watanabe M, Komiya C. Functional analysis of the masticatory muscle in a patient with progressing facial asymmetry. J Jpn Orthod Soc 1994; 53: 183-91.

[38] Fuki T, Morita S, Hanada K. Study on new method for superimposition of mandibular outline on frontal cephalograms. J Jpn Orthod Soc 1996; 55: 364-71.

[39] Lee MS, Chung DH, Lee JW, Cha KS. Assessing soft-tissue characteristics of facial asymmetry with photographs. Am J Orthod Dentofacial Orthop 2010; 138: 23-31.

[40] Meyer-Marcotty P, Alpers GW, Gerdes ABM, Stellzig-Eisenhauer A. Impact of facial asymmetry in visual perception: A 3-dimensional data analysis. Am J Orthod Dentofacial Orthop 2010. 137: 168.e1-168.e8.

[41] Kato Y, Kobayashi T, Hasebe D, Kano H, Saito C. A study in subjective evaluation and gaze point analysis of facial asymmetry: Analysis using eye-tracking-. Jpn J Jaw Defor 2009; 19: 184-92.

[42] Saito I, Watanabe N, Yamaki M. Facial asymmetry and deviated jaw and/or occlusion. Niigata Dent J 2010; 40: 111-23.

[43] Beyer JW, Lindauer SJ. Evaluation of dental midline position. Semin Orthod 1998; 4: 146-52.

[44] Johnston CD, Burden DJ, Stevenson MR. The influence of dental to facial midline discrepancies on dental attractiveness ratings. Eur J Orthod 1999; 21: 517-22.

[45] Pinho S, Ciriaco C, Faber J, Lenza MA. Impact of dental asymmetries on the perception of smile esthetics. Am J Orthod Dentofac Orthop 2007; 132: 748-53.

[46] Terada K, Saito I, Hanada K. Study on the simulation in planning for orthognathic surgery by using a personal computer. J Jpn Orthod Soc 1990; 49: 331-40.

[47] Cavalcanti MG, Haller JW, Vannier MW. Three-dimensional computed tomography landmark measurement in craniofacial surgical planning: experimental validation *in vitro*. J Oral Maxillofac Surg 1999; 57: 690-4.

[48] Wakamatsu T, Yamaki M, Hanada K, Hayashi T, Saito I. Three-dimensional evaluation of morphological asymmetry of maxillofacial complex in patients showing mandibular prognathism with facial asymmetry. Jpn J Jaw Deform 2007; 17 : 29-36.

[49] Sato Y, Fukui T, Hara S, *et al.* Relationship among mandibular deviation, condylar morphology and condylar movement. J Jpn Soc TMJ 1993; 5: 58-68, 1993.

[50] Yahata M, Yamada K, Hayashi T, Saito I: Unilateral condylar bone deformity and slope of articular eminence related to mandibular asymmetry. J Craniomandib Pract 2009; 27: 261-7.

[51] Fukui T, Sato Y, Yamada K, Morita S, Hanada K. Relationships between mandibular lateral deviation and bilateral condylar paths on mandibular protrusive movement. J Jpn Orthod Soc 1992; 51: 203-9.

[52] Kondo H. A study of the masticatory muscles morphology and function on asymmetric prognathism –used by computer tomography-. SHIGAKU 1991; 78: 1261-70.

[53] Kwon TG, Lee KH, Park HS, *et al.* Relationship between the masticatory muscles and mandibular skeleton in mandibular prognathism with and without asymmetry. J Oral Maxillofac Surg 2007; 65: 1538-43.

[54] Wakamatsu T, Hanada K, Hayashi T, Saito I. Volume measurement of masseter muscle using volume rendering technique in jaw deformity patients with mandibular deviation. Niigata Dent J 2006; 36: 233-38.

[55] Dong Y, Wang XM, Wang MQ, Widmalm SE: Asymmetric muscle function in patients with developmental mandibular asymmetry. J Oral Rehabil 2008; 35: 27-36.

[56] Castelo PM, Gavião MB, Pereira LJ, Bonjardim LR. Evaluation of changes in muscle thickness, bite force and facial asymmetry during early treatment of functional posterior crossbite. J Clin Pediatr Dent 2010; 34: 369-74.

[57] Hanson PR, Melugin B. Surgical orthodontic treatment of mandibular asymmetries. Semin Orthod 2009; 15: 268-78.

[58] Nanda R, Margolis MJ. Treatment strategies for midline discrepancies. Semin Orthod 1996; 2: 84-9.

[59] Burstone CJ. Diagnosis and treatment planning of patients with asymmetries. Semin Orthod 1998; 4: 153-64.

[60] Legan HL. Surgical correction of patients with asymmetries. Semin Orthod 1998; 4: 189-98.

[61] Ochi K, Yamzoe K, Morita S, Saito I. Development of a three-dimensional analyzing system for dental casts. Niigata Dent J. 2008; 38: 23-4.

[62] Takemura F, Morita S, Yamaki M, *et al.* Postoperative changes of he frontal facial soft tissues in patients with mandibular prognathism and mandibular deviation. Jpn J Jaw Deform 2007; 17 : 238-46.

[63] Al-Gunaid T, Yamada K, Takagi R, Saito C, Saito I. Postoperative stability of bimaxillary surgery in Class III patients with mandibular protrusion and mandibular deviation; a frontal cephalometric study. J Oral Maxillofac Surg 2008; 37: 992-8.

[64] Troulis MJ, Everett P, Seldin EB, Kikinis R, Kaban LB. Development of a three-dimensional treatment planning system based on computed tomographic data. Int J Oral Maxillofacial Surg 2002; 31: 349-57.

[65] Xia J, Samman N, Yeung RW, *et al.* Computer-assisted three-dimensional surgical planning and simulation. 3D soft tissue planning and prediction. Int J Oral Maxillofac Surg 2000; 29:250-8.

[66] Yamazaki K, Terada K, Nakamura J, *et al.* Three-dimensional analysis comparing changes in soft tissue with those in hard tissue following orthognathic surgery in patients showing mandibular prognathism with facial asymmetry. Jpn J Jaw Deform 2005; 15 : 87-94.

[67] Kohara A, Terada K, Matsubara T, *et al.* Examination of precision of integrating three-dimensional facial and dental data. Jpn J Jaw Deform 2009; 19 : 193-8.

[68] Rangel FA, Maal TJJ, Berge SJ, *et al.* Integration of digital dental casts in 3-dimensional facial photographs. Am J Orthod Dentofac Orthop 2008; 134 : 820-6.

CHAPTER 10

Combined Surgical Approaches in Class III Malocclusion

Hyoung-Seon Baik*

Department of Orthodontics, College of Dentistry, Yonsei University, Seoul, South Korea

Abstract: Young Class III patients with deficient maxilla can be treated with maxillary orthopedic appliances such as the facemask. Patients with an over-developed mandible require orthodontics, in combination with orthognathic surgery to correct the underlying skeletal and dental discrepancy, after growth is completed. For Class III patients, craniofacial morphology varies among different racial groups and it is important to understand the cephalometric characteristics of these different ethnic groups. For example, in Northeast Asian countries such as Korea and Japan, there are more Class III patients with mandibular excess rather than maxillary deficiency, compared to the Caucasian populations. In treatment planning for orthognathic surgery, 3-dimensional analysis using CBCT provides more detailed information than a conventional 2-dimensional cephalogram. Also, for orthognathic surgery patients, laser scanning may show 3-dimenisonal information on soft tissue as well as hard tissue changes. Therefore, soft tissue changes in facial profile as well as mid-facial area can be quantitatively calculated. The best orthognathic surgery cases result from a close interaction with the oral surgeon and a well planned pre-surgical orthodontic phase. This can simplify the orthognathic surgical plan and result in good long-term stability. In this chapter, 3-dimensional analysis of the hard and soft tissue will be introduced for both pre- and post-surgical consideration of Class III patients treated by combined orthodontics/orthognathic surgery.

Keywords: Orthognathic surgery, 3D CT, Laser Scanning, 3D analysis, Pre-surgical orthodontics.

INTRODUCTION

The prevalence of Class III malocclusion is higher in Northeast Asian countries compared to the western countries [1-3]. In patients with severe maxillomandibular skeletal discrepancies, orthodontic treatment in combination with orthognathic surgery is usually recommended; pre-surgical orthodontic treatment is usually started when the growth is completed [4]. The distribution of

***Address correspondence to Hyoung-Seon Baik:** Department of Orthodontics, College of Dentistry, Yonsei University, 50 YONSEI-RO SEODAE MUN KU, Seoul, South Korea; Tel: +82-10 5311-8794; E-mail: baik@yuns.ac

Peter W. Ngan, Toshi Deguchi and Eugene W. Roberts (Eds)

the skeletal pattern was examined in 1439 patients who had undergone orthodontic treatment combined with orthognathic surgery at the Department of Orthodontics, Yonsei University Dental Hospital, over a 10 year-period from 2001 to 2010. The number of patients was found to increase each year, and the ratio between female and male patients was consistently 1:1 over the ten year-period. The proportions of Class III, Class II and Class I patients were 84.7%, 11.3% and 4.0%, respectively. The average age of patients who received surgery increased slightly from the age of 22.2 in 2001 to 23.0 in 2010. The proportion of patients over 30 years of age increased, as a result of an increase in the aged population of the country, and growing demand for esthetic improvement in aged group [1].

Cephalometric Characteristics of Surgical Class III Patients

Understanding the cephalometric characteristics of Class III surgical patients is crucial for planning the proper surgical approach. Baik *et al.* [3] compared the cephalometric measurements of 222 (106 male, 116 female) patients with skeletal Class III malocclusion with 100 normal adults (50 male, 50 female, Table **1**). Surgical Class III patients were found to have a shorter anterior and posterior cranial base, with a smaller saddle angle; a shorter maxillary length (Co-A), but a normal SNA angle, related to the shorter anterior cranial base; a longer mandibular length (Co-Gn) and an increased SNB angle; an increased lower facial height and a larger gonial angle; protrusive maxillary incisors and upright mandibular incisors; and a retrusive upper lip to the Ricketts' E line.

Table 1: Comparisons (mean and SD) between the normal and surgical groups

Measurement	**Male**		**Female**	
	Normal Group (n = 50)	**Surgical Group (n = 106)**	**Normal Group (n = 50)**	**Surgical Group (n = 116)**
Cranial base				
Anterior cranial base (mm)	73.4 (2.8)	72.3 (3.5)*	70.0 (3.1)	68.6 (3.5)†
Posterior cranial base (mm)	41.0 (3.7)	38.5 (3.7)†	36.6 (2.6)	34.5 (3.2)‡
Cranial base angle	126.1 (4.7)	122.0 (5.5)‡	127.3 (4.6)	123.1 (9.3)‡
Maxillary position				
Co-A (mm)	94.97 (4.79)	89.66 (4.56)‡	89.01 (3.30)	86.13 (4.53)‡

Table 1: contd...

SNA angle	81.84 (3.16)	80.99 (3.76)	80.85 (3.06)	80.26 (3.13)
Mandibular position				
Co-Gn (mm)	130.99 (5.20)	140.42 (6.94)‡	120.95 (4.6)	129.83 (6.68)‡
SNB angle (deg)	80.18 (3.04)	85.86 (3.78)‡	78.92 (3.35)	83.23 (3.40)‡
Maxilla/mandible relationship				
ANB angle	1.92 (1.28)	-4.89 (3.01)‡	2.29 (1.24)	-3.20 (2.20)‡
Wits appraisal (mm)	-1.83 (2.10)	-14.65 (6.14)‡	-2.71 (1.90)	-11.02 (4.49)‡
Maxillomandibular differential (mm)	36.02 (4.16)	50.81 (7.04)‡	31.94 (4.01)	43.70 (6.33)‡
Vertical relationships				
Mandibular plane angle	31.79 (3.47)	32.61 (6.09)	33.39 (3.45)	35.63 (5.97)*
Lower anterior facial height	75.31 (4.32)	78.92 (6.52)‡	69.14 (3.98)	73.29 (5.55)‡
Gonial angle	118.65 (6.12)	124.85 (9.20)‡	118.61 (5.42)	123.95 (8.87)‡
Dentition				
Max. 1 to SN (deg)	107.08 (5.32)	113.80 (6.53)‡	104.14 (4.80)	111.92 (7.41)‡
IMPA	95.91 (5.22)	82.23 (9.08)‡	94.84 (4.64)	83.62 (7.90)‡
Soft tissue				
Esthetic line to upper lip	0.35 (2.31)	-4.01 (2.94)‡	-0.23 (1.95)	-3.24 (2.33)‡
Esthetic line to lower lip	1.81 (2.45)	1.77 (2.77)‡	1.45 (2.36)	1.60 (2.61)

Maxillomandibular differential = (Co-Gn)-(Co-A).

$^{*}P<0.05$; $^{\dagger}P<0.01$; $^{\ddagger}P<0.001$.

1) Anteroposterior Relationship

Table **2** shows the comparison of the anteroposterior skeletal pattern of Class III surgical group with normal adults. The mean values of maxillary length (Co-A) and mandibular length (Co-Gn) in the adults with normal occlusion were used as the norm. The maxillary or mandibular component was given ‘0 (normal)’, when the measurement was within 1 standard deviation from the mean value, ‘+ (greater than normal)’, when they exceeded the normal range, and ‘- (smaller than normal) ’, when it was smaller than the normal range. The results were 38.7% of the male and 42.2 % of the female Class III patients had normal maxilla and prognathic mandible,

36.8% of the male and 25% of the female patients had retrognathic maxilla and a prognathic mandible, and 17.9% of the male and 25% of the female patients displayed retrognathic maxilla and normal mandible.

Table 2: Comparison of sagittal components

Co-A / Co-Gn	Male (n = 106)		Female (n = 116)	
	n	%	n	%
Max 0, Mand +	41	38.7	49	42.2
Max -, Mand +	39	36.8	29	25.0
Max -, Mand 0	19	17.9	29	25.0
Max 0, Mand 0	7	6.6	0	0.0
Max +, Mand +	0	0.0	9	7.8

Max=maxilla, Mand=mandible.
Mean values of the normal patients were used as the norm, and their standard deviation was used to indicate the normal range of measurements. The surgical patients were classified as normal (0) when the measurement was within 1 standard deviation, greater range (+) when it exceeded the normal range, and smaller range (-) when it was smaller than the normal range.

Fig. **1** shows the anteroposterior relations of the maxilla and mandible according to the SNA and SNB angle. These results were in contrast with that of Ellis and McNamara in 1984 [2]. Caucasian Class III patients had primarily a maxillary deficiency, while Korean patients had primarily a mandibular prognathism.

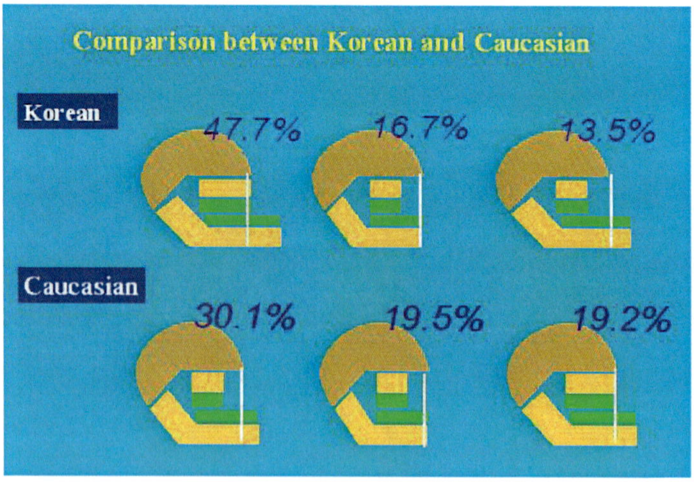

Figure 1: Comparison between Korean and Caucasian in AP relationship by SNA and SNB angles.

2) Vertical Relationship

Table **3** compares the average gonial angle between surgical Class III patients and normal adults. Patients were classified as either normal (0), greater than normal (+) or smaller than normal (-). It was found that 50.3% of males and 53.4 % of females had greater gonial angle than the normal, 43.4 % of males and 38.8 % of females were in normal range, and only 5.7% of males and 7.8% of females had smaller gonial angle. Therefore, Korean surgical Class III patients may have a more hyperdivergent facial pattern.

Table 3: Comparison of vertical position

Gonial angle	Male		Female	
	N	%	N	%
Greater than normal	54	50.9	62	53.4
Normal	46	43.4	45	38.8
Smaller than normal	6	5.7	9	7.8

3) Morphological Characteristics of the Symphysis in Skeletal Class III Patients

The morphology of the mandibular symphysis in skeletal Class III patients is important because it serves as the primary reference for the esthetics of the facial profile and is a determinant in planning the lower incisor position during orthodontic and orthognathic surgery treatment. Chung & Baik [5] evaluated the basal and symphyseal widths, along with the alveolar and symphyseal heights, using lateral cephalograms of 28 skeletal Class III patients with crossbites, 41 skeletal Class III patients with openbite, and 32 patients with normal occlusion (Fig. **2** and Table **4**). The width of the symphyseal region including the basal width, point B width, Id width, symphyseal thickness and pogonion width were similar in adult Class III crossbite and normal occlusion groups, but significantly less in the adult Class III openbite group. The symphyseal height was similar in all three groups. These results implied that the openbite rather than the negative overjet may be the major factor influencing symphyseal morphology in the adult Class III malocclusion.

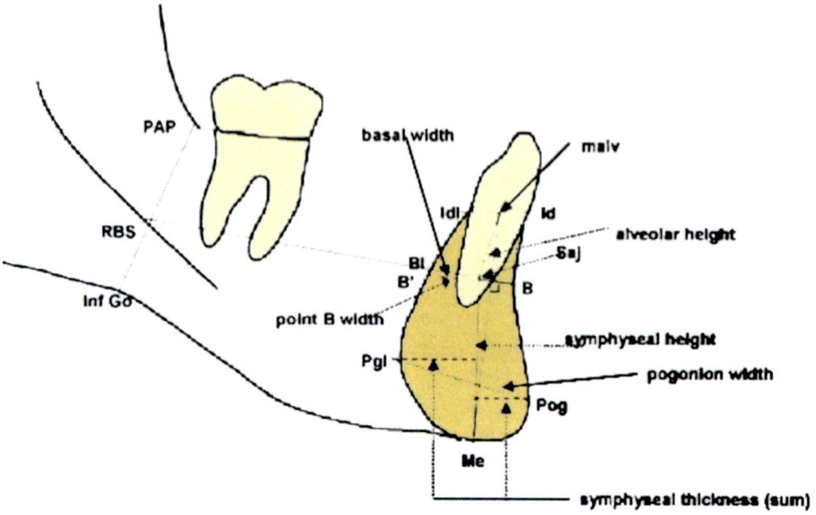

Figure 2: Landmarks and measurements of the symphyseal region. Conventional mandibular landmarks: *Me*, menton; *Pg*, pogonion; *B*, supramentale; *Id*, infradentale; *Idl*, lingual point infradentale. Landmarks based on Suri *et al.*: *PAP*, posterior alveolar point, most posteroinferior midplaned point on the anterior border of the ascending ramus; *Inf Go*, inferior gonion, midplaned point on the lower border of the mandible where the convexity at Go merges with the concavity of the antegonial notch; *RBS*, ramus body syncline, the point of intersection of a line drawn from Inf Go to PAP with the cortical outline of the midplaned mandibular nerve; *Bl*, lingual point B, the point of intersection of a line drawn from RBS to B, with the lingual contour of symphysis; *saj*, symphysis-alveolar junction, the midpoint of a line drawn from Bl to B; *Pgl*, lingual point pogonion, the highest point on the lingual contour of the symphysis, located by the greatest perpendicular distance from a line drawn from the saj to Me; *malv*, (midpoint of anterior alveolus), midpoint of a line drawn from Idl to Id. Landmark base on Nojima *et al.*: *B*, point on the lingual outline of the symphysis drawn from B perpendicular to a line connecting malv to Me. Mandibular measurements: *alveolar height*, length of a line drawn from malv to saj; *symphyseal height*, length of a line drawn from saj to Me; *symphyseal thickness*, the sum of the lengths of the perpendiculars dropped from Pg and Pgl to a line drawn from saj to Me; *basal width*, length of a line drawn from Bl to B.

Table 4: Symphyseal dimension of the control, Class III with crossbite, and Class III with openbite groups (Mean and SD)

Measurements	**Control (n = 32)**	**Crossbite (n = 28)**	**Openbite (n = 41)**
	Mean (SD)	**Mean (SD)**	**Mean (SD)**
Basal width (B-Bl)	9.58 (1.85)	8.88 (1.84)	6.74 (1.64)‡
Point B width (B-B')	9.76 (1.77)	9.08 (1.94)	6.98 (1.93)‡
Id width (Id-Idl)	6.98 (0.76)	6.71 (0.94)	5.83 (1.20)‡
Symphyseal thickness (sum)	16.35 (1.32)	15.82 (1.48)	14.22 (1.45)‡

Table 4: contd...

Pogonion width (Pog-Pgl)	16.29 (1.47)	15.79 (1.58)	14.38 (1.49)‡
Alveolar height (malv-Saj)	12.45 (2.08)	10.88 (2.87)	10.12 (4.01)*
Symphyseal height (Saj-Me)	25.48 (1.83)	25.39 (1.93)	25.06 (2.49)
Total height (malv-Me)	36.93 (2.78)	35.52 (2.52)	34.78 (3.49)*

*$P<0.05$; †$P<0.01$; ‡$P<0.001$.

3-D ANALYSIS IN CLASS III MALOCCLUSION

1) 3-Dimensional Computed Tomography

To understand the morphology of the skeletal Class III patients, and develop a better diagnostic tool for surgery, 3-dimensional CT can be used to overcome the limits of a 2-dimensional lateral cephalogram. Three dimensional computed tomography (3-D CT) is widely used in dentistry for many reasons: a spatial image of the craniofacial structures can be produced, the image can be viewed three-dimensionally by changing the rotational axis, and the inner structures can be observed independently by adjusting the image density of the organs. The use of spiral (medical) CT has been limited because of the high radiation dose. In contrast, the cone beam CT exposes patients to less radiation, so it is more practical for routine usage.

In 2006, Park & Baik *et al.* [6] took CT images of 30 subjects with normal occlusion using medical CT, and the axial images were reconstructed into a 3D model by computer software. The V works^{R} 4.0 and V surgery^{R} (Cybermed, Seoul, Korea) software programs were used to measure the 3D models. The authors proposed 19 reproducible landmarks along with the horizontal reference plane parallel to the FH plane, the midsagittal plane, the coronal reference plane as well as several linear and angular measurements. This constituted a new 3D analysis method for the diagnosis of patients with craniofacial deformity (Fig. **4**).

Fig. **3** shows a 19 year-old woman who came to the department with the chief complaints of mandibular proganthism and facial asymmetry. In addition to the conventional 2-dimensional lateral cephalogram, 3D CT images were taken to gain more comprehensive and useful information, to facilitate treatment planning for orthognathic surgery. The patient had a protrusive chin, and menton was deviated to the left. From the intraoral view, she had bilateral Class III canine and molar relationships and the lower dental midline was shifted to the left. She had a concave profile as a result of the mandibular prognathism. From the lateral cephalogram, she was diagnosed as skeletal Class III, with mandibular prognathism (SNA: 76°, SNB: 81.2° ANB: -5.1°, Wits: -12.4mm, Mand. body length: 84.6 mm), and hyperdivergent facial profile (Gonial angle: 129.7°, SN-GoMe: 34.7°). The upper and lower anterior teeth were compensated according with the skeletal pattern (U1 to SN 107.5° and IMPA 79.3°). From the PA cephalogram, the vertical measurements did not show any significant differences between the right and left sides; however, horizontal measurements revealed that the right side was longer than the left. Unlike the clinical findings, the deviation of menton was not evident on the PA cephalogram, which may be attributed to the errors in establishment of reference planes and possible compensatory camouflage. Two-dimensional cephalogram and facial photographs do not normally enable precise assessment of asymmetry. A 3D CT was taken and the image (Fig. **4**) was reconstructed in 3D model to be analyzed by Park & Baik's method [6].

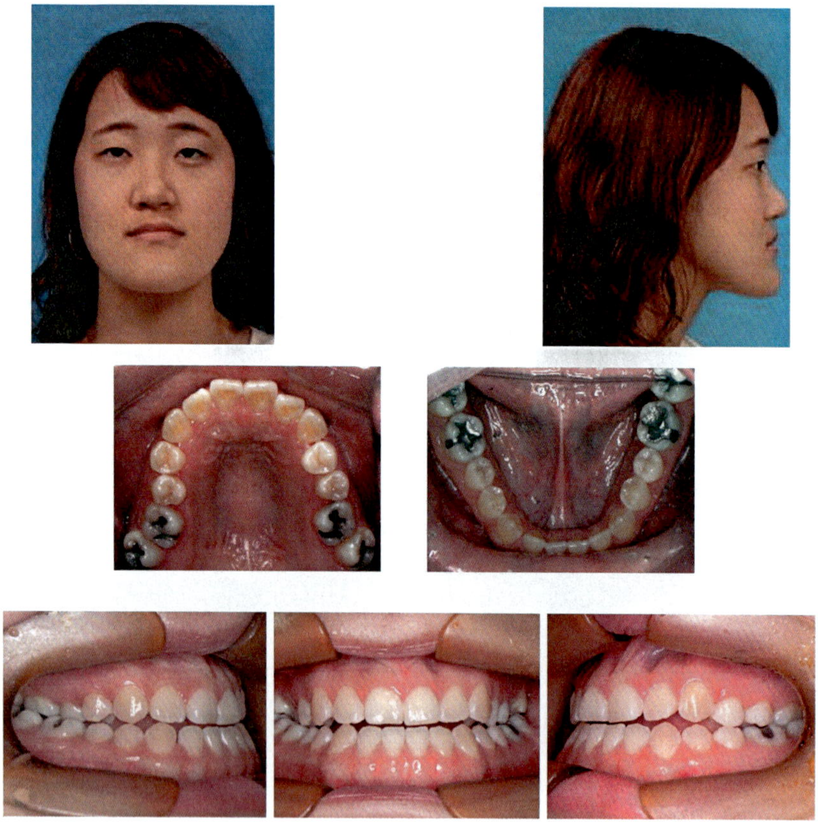

Fig. 3: contd….

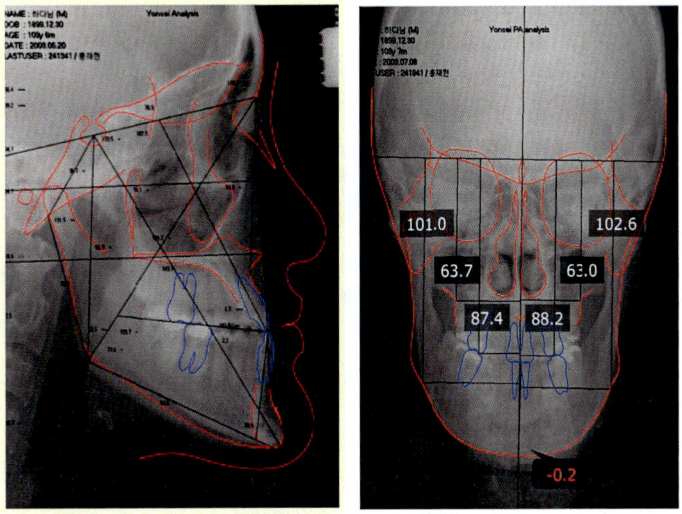

Figure 3: Initial photos and x-ray/.

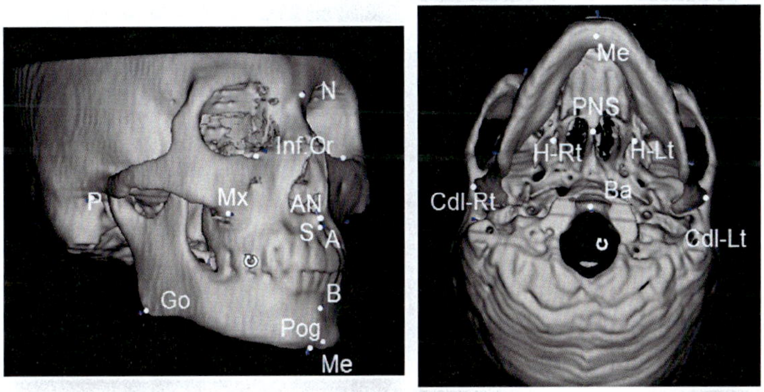

Figure 4-1: Landmarks on the 3-D structure. For reference planes: Nasion, Basion, Infraorbitale, Porion; for A-P & vertical relation: ANS, A, B, Pog, Me, PNS; for maxillomandibular symmetry: Maxillare, Hamular process, Condylion laterale, Gonion.

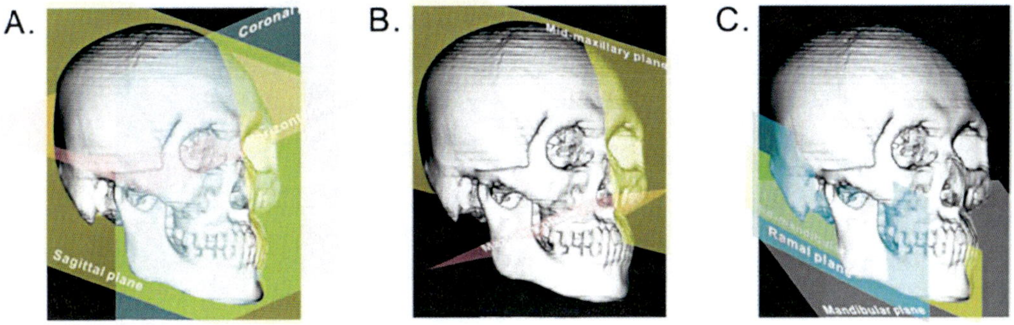

Figure 4-2: Reference planes used in this study.

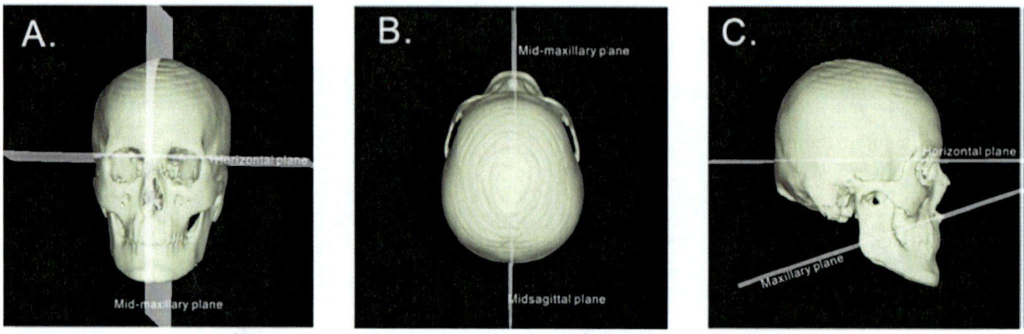

Figure 4-3: Maxillary measurements: A, canting; B, rotation; C, divergence.

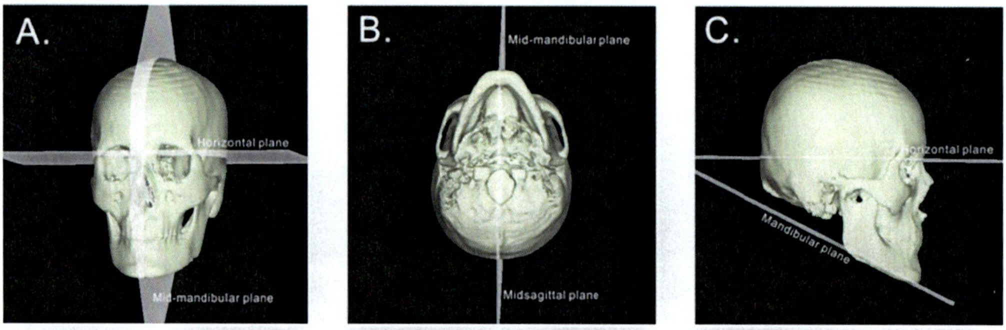

Figure 4-4: Mandibular measurements: A, canting; B, rotation; C, divergence.

Figure 4: Landmarks and reference planes of 3-D analysis.

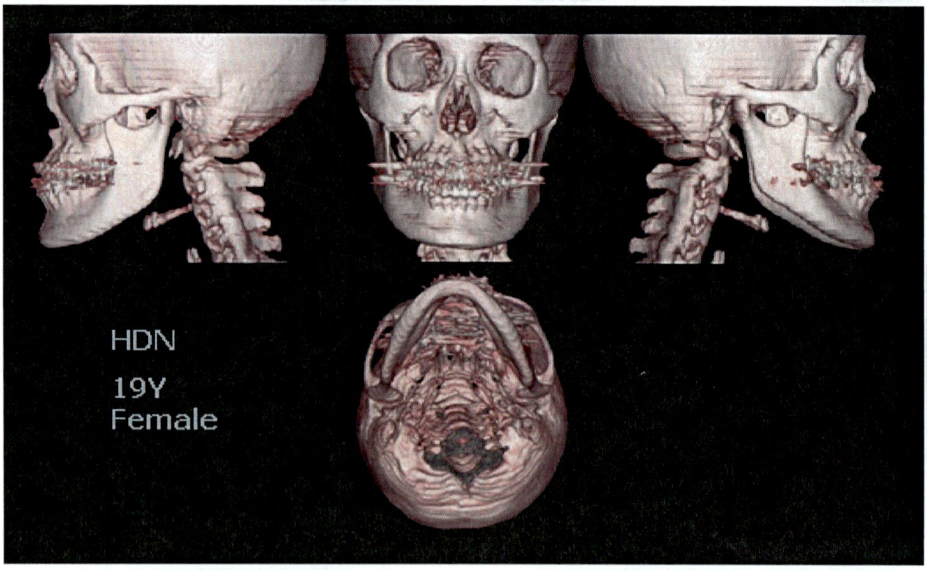

Fig. 5: contd….

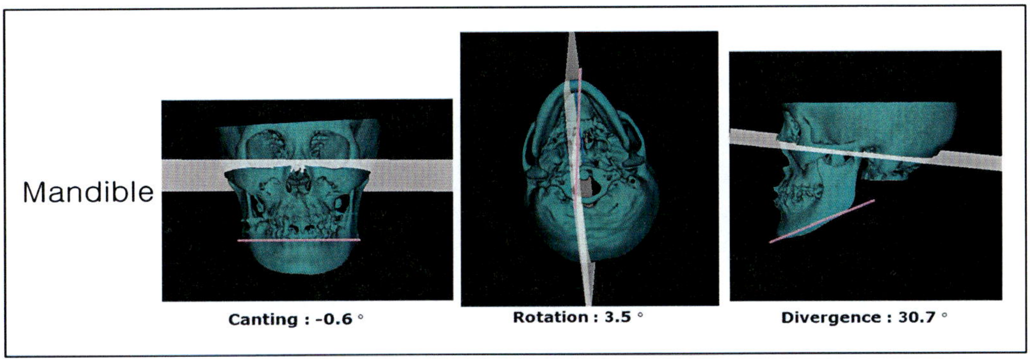

			Female norm	Pre-Op	
			Mean ± S.D.	Measurement	Dev.
Zygoma					
	Facial index		88.8 ± 5.9	93.5	-
	Midface angle				
		Rt	129.0 ± 8.5	**120.7**	↓
		Lt	130.6 ± 6.8	**123.2**	↓
		diff.	0.1 ± 2.7	2.5	-
Maxilla					
	Canting(°)	Rt	0.4 ± 1.2	2.3	↑
	Rotation(°)	Lt	-0.6 ± 0.9	3.4	↑
	Divergence(°)	diff.	-21.3 ± 3.6	-13.8	↑
Mandible					
	Canting(°)	Rt	0.3 ± 1.5	-0.6	-
	Rotation(°)	Lt	-0.8 ± 1.4	3.5	↑
	Divergence(°)	diff.	30.9 ± 5.8	30.7	-

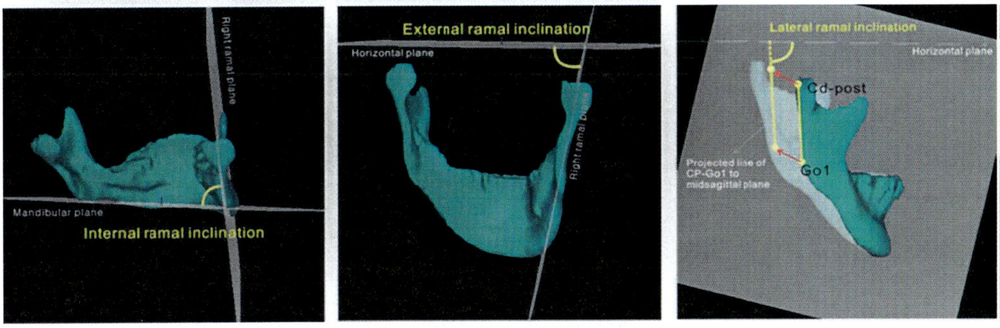

Fig. 5: contd….

Mandibular shape analysis			
Body length	Rt	96.6	↑
	Lt	95.4	↑
Gonial angle	Rt	131.9	↑
	Lt	124.8	
Ramal height	Rt	52.3	
	Lt	57.4	↑
Internal ramal Inclination	Rt	95.2	
	Lt	83.5	↓
External ramal inclination	Rt	77.1	↓
	Lt	82.9	
Lateral ramal Inclination	Rt	81.7	
	Lt	84.7	

Figure 5: 3-D analysis of the patient.

From the frontal CT image (Fig. **5**), the maxilla was canted 2.3 degrees in the counterclockwise direction to the horizontal reference plane. Viewing from the bottom of the image, the maxilla was rotated 3.5 degrees to the left, relative to the midsagittal plane. Divergence between the nasal plane and the mandibular plane - 13.8 degrees with ANS located 9 degrees above the norm. Viewing from the bottom, menton was rotated 3.5 degrees to the left and the mandibular body lengths were greater than the norms, with the right mandibular body 1.2 mm longer than the left. The Gonial angle was greater on the right side but the ramal height was longer on the left; this was the reason why the deviation of menton was not notable from the PA cephalogram. Internal ramal inclination was smaller on the right side than the left, but the external ramal inclination was smaller on the right side than the left.

As mentioned before, 3D CT can give more helpful information than a 2-dimensional cephalogram in treatment planning. You and Baik [7] investigated 50 adult patients with mandibular prognathism, and the patients were divided into symmetry group (n=20) and asymmetry group (n=30) according to the degree of menton deviation (Fig. **6**). The 3D CT scans were obtained using a spiral CT scanner. Landmarks were designated on the reconstructed 3D surface model. Lines to represent the condylar, coronoid, angular, body, and chin units were used. Ramal and body volumes were measured in the hemi-mandibles. The results showed that both condylar and body units appear to contribute to the mandibular asymmetry.

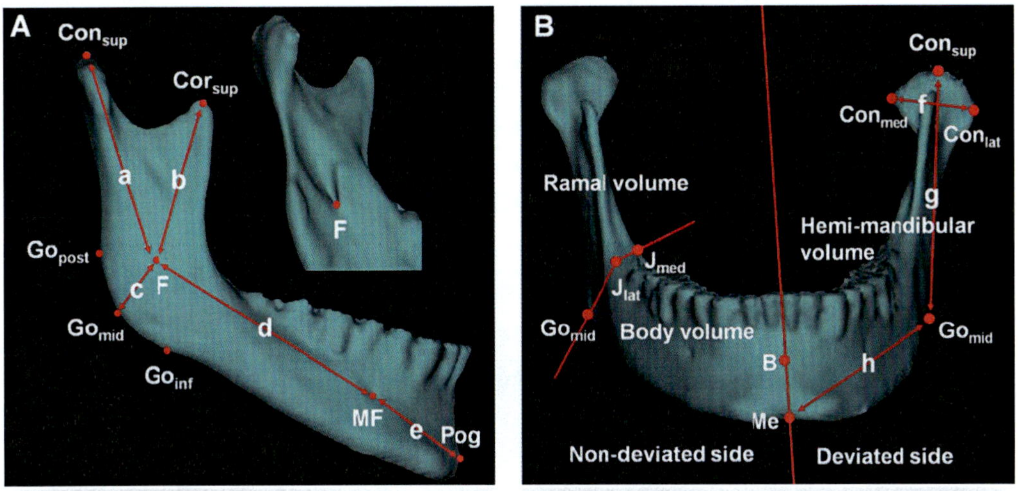

Figure 6: Landmarks and measurements used in this study: A, a, condylar unit length; b, coronoid unit length; c, angular unit length; d, body unit length; e, chin unit length. B, f, condylar width; g, ramal height; h, body length.

2) 3-D Soft Tissue Analysis

In orthognathic surgery patients, the importance of soft tissue analysis increases as much as hard tissue analysis. In the past, soft tissue changes could only be evaluated with a 2-dimensional cephalogram, but recent advances in imaging technology have enabled the use of moire stripe, stereophotogrammetry, 3D CT, and a CCD camera for 3 dimensional analysis. We used the laser scanning system to evaluate the soft tissue.

Baik *et al.* [8] scanned a mannequin head with Vivid 900 (Minolta, Tokyo, Japan) laser scanner to propose reproducible soft tissue landmarks of facial structures (Fig. 7). Korean adults with normal occlusion (male 30, female 30) were scanned by a 3D laser scanner, then 3D facial images of the subjects were constructed by the Rapidform 2004 program (Inus Technology Inc., Seoul, Korea). Reference planes in the facial soft tissue 3D images as well as a 3D coordinate system (X axis-left/right, Y axis-superior/inferior, Z axis-anterior/posterior) were established on the 3D image (Fig. **8**). A total of 43 linear measurements, 8 angular measurements, 29 linear distance ratios were defined. 3D facial models of Korean adults with normal occlusion were obtained [9]. These data could be used as a reference for 3-D diagnosis and treatment planning for patients with Class III malocclusion and dentofacial deformity, as well as for 3D analysis of facial soft tissue changes after orthodontic treatment and orthognathic surgery.

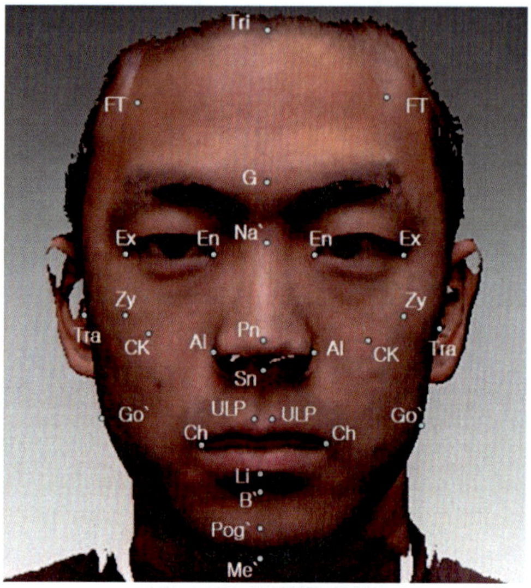

Figure 7: Soft tissue landmarks.

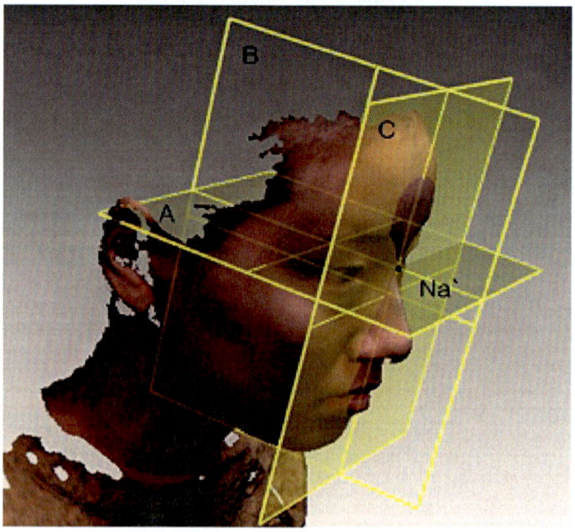

Figure 8: Reference planes: A, axial plane passing through N'; B, midsagittal plane; C, coronal pane.

Fig. **9** shows a 19 year old man who was seen in the department with the chief complaints of mandibular protrusion. The patient underwent a 2-jaw surgery, after pre-surgical orthodontic treatment. 3D laser scanning was taken before and after surgery and a superimposition was performed to evaluate soft tissue changes before and after surgery.

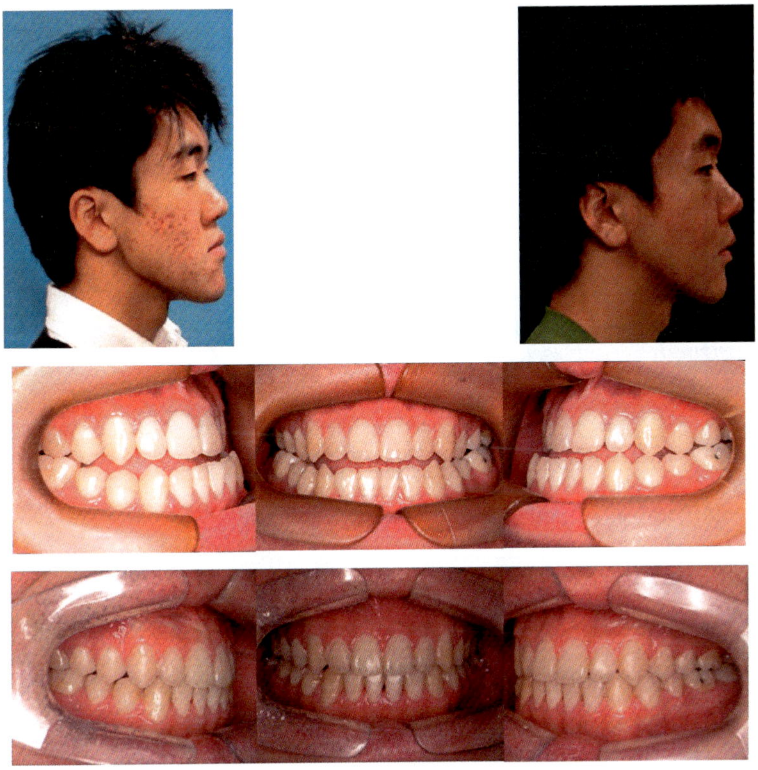

Figure 9: Before and after treatment.

Using the laser scanner, Baik and Kim [10] evaluated the soft tissue changes of 20 Class III patients who underwent 2-jaw surgery (Max.: advancement and PNS impaction, Mand.: set back with an intraoral vertical ramus osteotomy) to correct skeletal Class III malocclusions. Ten patients had 2-jaw surgery with genioplasty, and the other 10 had 2-jaw surgery without genioplasty. The ratios of soft tissue changes to hard tissue movement were calculated and compared between two groups. The result showed no significant difference in the horizontal ratios of the soft tissue to hard tissue changes between the two groups. In both groups, the ratios of the horizontal changes in the paranasal area were higher than in the subnasale area

(Fig. **10** and Table **5**). There were more changes in the subalar area than in the supracommissural area, and more changes in the chin and labiomental areas than in the subcommissural area. Ala moved anterolaterally, and cheilion moved posteroinferiorly. The distance between upper-lip point and cheilion increased significantly ($p<0.05$). Fig. **11** shows in the 3D angles the transverse nasal prominence and transverse upper lip prominence increased significantly ($p<0.05$).

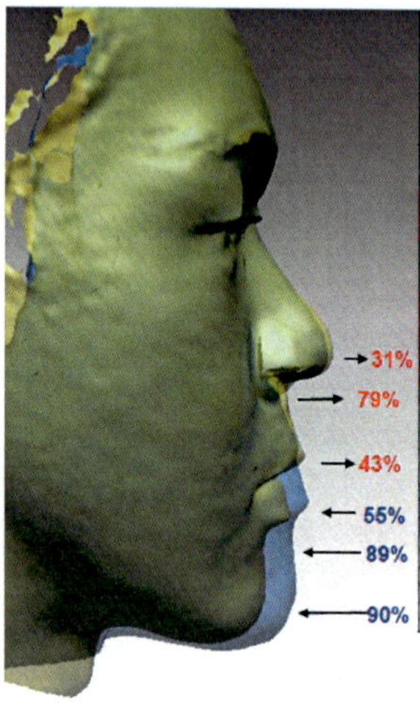

	Present study			Soncul et at*
	Mean(mm)	SD	% Movement	% Movement
nasal tip	0.80	1.50	31	29
paranasal	1.94	0.86	75	79
subnasal	2.03	0.88	79	81
subalar	1.78	0.84	69	79
supracommissural	1.19	2.17	46	45
upper vermilion	1.10	2.72	43	66
lower vermilion	-5.63	3.29	55	64
subcommissural	-7.42	3.13	73	46
Labiomental groove	-9.05	4.97	89	90
chin	-9.19	5.68	90	97

Figure 10 and Table 5: Ratios of the soft tissue changes to the hard tissue changes.

A 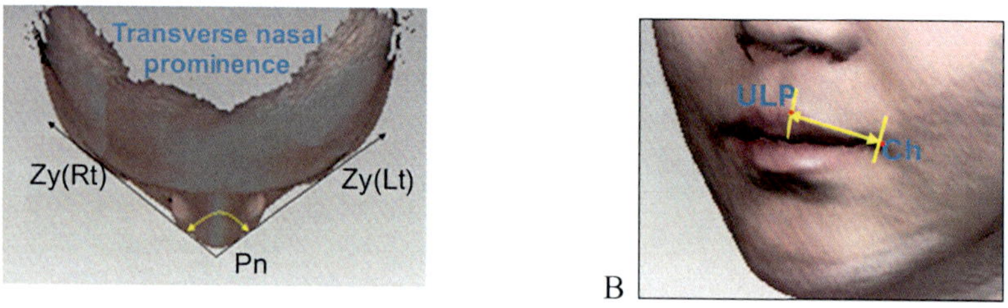

Figure 11: A, Transverse nasal prominence angle. B, The distance between upper-lip point and cheilion increased.

Pre- and Post Orthodontic Treatment Considerations

1) Pre-Orthodontic Treatment Considerations

The objectives of pre-surgical orthodontic treatment are to coordinate upper and lower dental arches, align teeth in their own supporting bone, decompensate upper and lower incisors, in addition to maintaining inter-molar and canine widths for a stable occlusion after surgery. Pre-surgical orthodontic treatment should be accomplished according to the surgical plan, and confirmed by the collaborating surgeon, before starting treatment. Leveling should be accomplished together with alignment. Vertical displacement is better corrected and more stable when treated by surgery rather than by orthodontic tooth movement. In Class III patients, anterior teeth flaring and/or crowding is often a finding due to maxillary deficiency. Extraction of premolars bilaterally and Class II elastics may be indicated to improve the axial inclination of upper anterior teeth and decompensate retroclined lower anterior teeth. If posterior impaction of the maxilla is planned, the axial inclination of upper anterior teeth should be controlled in pre-surgical phase because the axial inclination will be decreased due to posterior impaction during surgery (Fig. **12**).

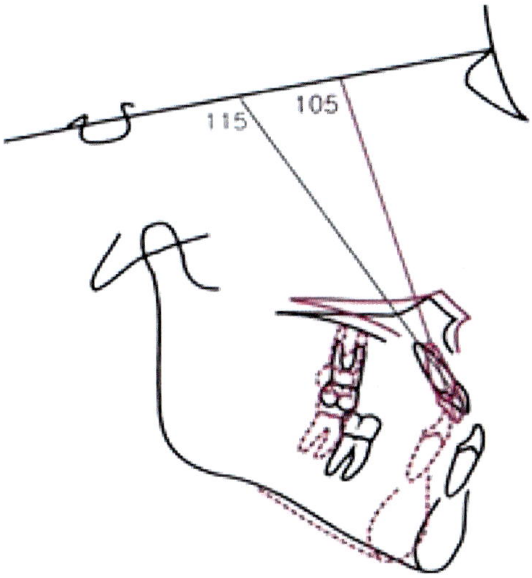

Figure 12: The axis of upper anterior tooth is changed by posterior impaction of maxilla.

For posterior anchorage preparation, stabilizing lingual arches or extraoral appliances such as headgear were used in the past, but recently mini-screws are gradually replacing these appliances. Burstone's precision lingual arch can be used for molar width control. At the end of pre-surgical orthodontic treatment, it is helpful to take impressions and examine the occlusal compatibility. A full dimension stainless steel rectangular wire should be placed at least 1 month before the surgery (Fig. **13**).

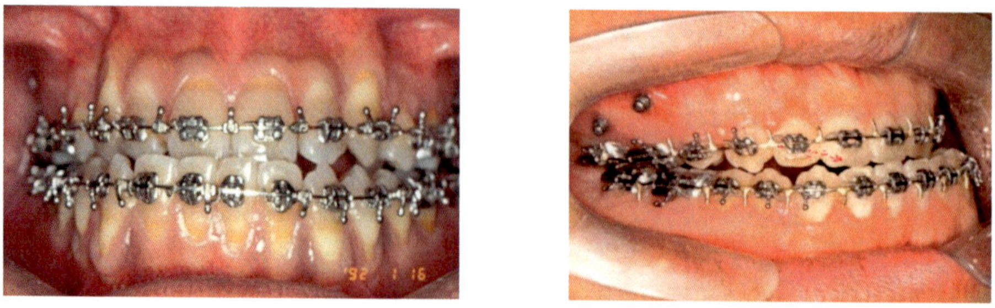

Figure 13: Surgical wire with crimpable hook and soldered brass wire.

A patients' appearance may worsen during presurgical treatment. Even if upper premolars were extracted, the pre-surgical orthodontic treatment phase does not necessarily last more than a year.

2) Surgery

When orthodontic preparation for surgery has been completed, manual cephalometric or computerized prediction with a video-imaging program should be done with a cephalometric radiograph taken just before surgery. The surgical treatment plan should be reviewed and simulated with model surgery. From the repositioned dental casts, simulating the actual surgery, wafer splints are fabricated. In 2-jaw surgery cases, dental casts can be mounted on a semi-adjustable articulator, after a face bow transfer.

In Korea, the percentage of 2-jaw surgeries in Class III patient surgery cases is higher than for 1-jaw surgery *via* mandibular set-back, because mandibular prognathism is more prevalent than maxillary deficiency (Table **6**). Compared to the cases performed in the United States, few cases in Korea undergo maxillary advancement alone [3]. Most of the maxillary surgeries for Class III patients were performed by a LeFort I osteotomy to move the maxilla forward, or up and forward. For maxillary expansion, surgical assisted rapid palatal expansion (RPE) or a surgical widening procedure can be done. Recently, mini-screws were applied to assist in the widening of the maxilla [11]. Maxillary surgery *via* LeFort I surgery has some negative effects including widening of the alar base. Therefore, a cinch suture is recommended after LeFort I surgery especially for the many Asian patients with wide alar bases. In borderline cases between 2-jaw and 1-jaw surgery, more esthetic results can be obtained when performing mandibular set back alone, because there is no change in the nose. However, individual characteristics should definitely be considered (Fig. **14**).

Table 6: Comparison of Class III surgery prevalence

Procedure	Korean patients (n = 299)		American patients (n = 99)	
	n	%	n	%
Mandibular setback only	59	19.7	5	5.1
Maxillary advancement only	2	0.7	32	32.2
Bimaxillary	238	79.6	62	62.6

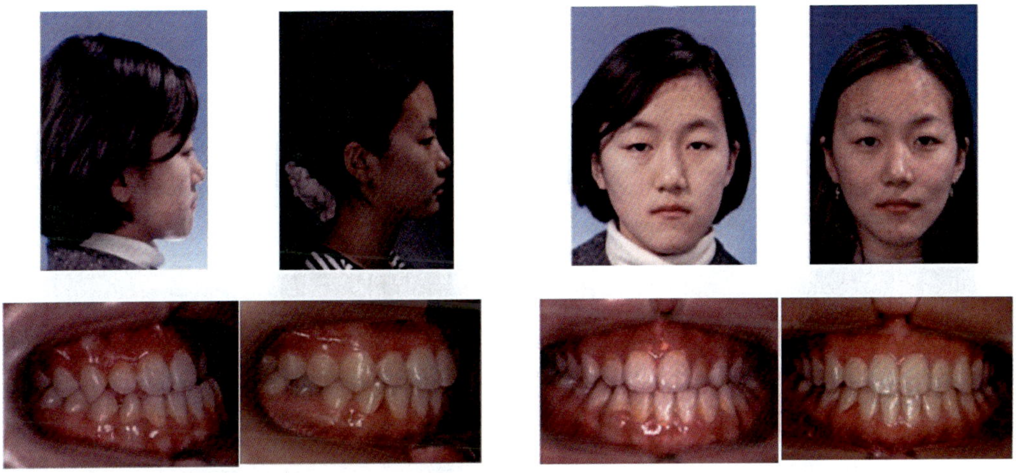

Figure 14: Mandible only surgery case: no changes in nose.

For mandibular surgery, the mandibular body ostectomy or anterior subapical osteotomy may be chosen, but bilateral sagittal split ramal osteotomy (SSRO) or intraoral vertical ramus osteotomy (IVRO) are the most common procedures. Advancement genioplasty is effective for avoiding a double chin after mandibular set-back. Recently, the demands for a surgery-first approach to achieve a rapid esthetic improvement are increasing. However, appropriate case selection, precise prediction and accurate wafer fabrication are crucial to avoid possible extension of treatment time and poor results.

3) Post –Surgical Orthodontic Treatment

Post-surgical orthodontic treatment is generally started 3-4 weeks after jaw surgery, once the surgeon confirms initial bone healing and appropriate jaw movement. Any failed brackets should be rebonded before resuming the post-surgical treatment. Rigid surgical wires and the wafer splint are then removed, and replaced by round wires. Light box elastics can be used for occlusal seating (Fig. **15**).

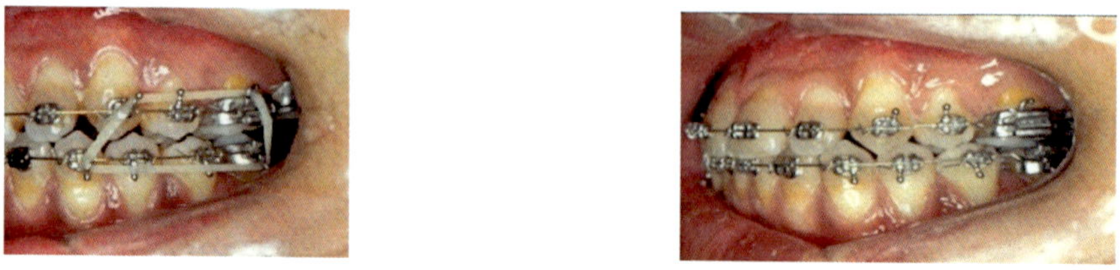

Figure 15: Box elastics for occlusal seating.

4) Debonding and Retention

Usually 3-6 months after surgery, post-orthodontic treatment can be completed once the teeth settle into full occlusion. Since the full dimensional surgical wire was inserted, at the end of the pre-surgical treatment, brackets may be removed after occlusal seating with the round working wire. In open bite patients, wire components in the retainer should not pass through the occlusal area or the extraction site. Considering that the orthognathic surgery patients are generally adults, retainers should be worn for longer periods of time (Fig. **16**).

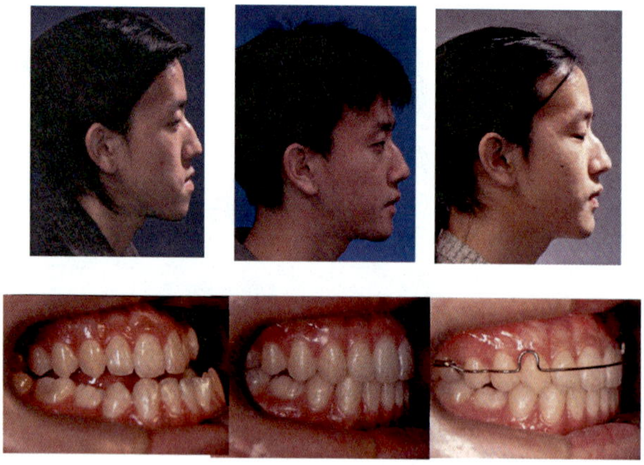

Figure 16: Before, after, and post 2 years retention.

5) Considerations in Class III Surgery

The amount of the maxillary advancement is dependent on the resistance of the upper lip. In general, advancement of more than 10 mm is not advisable.

Excessive maxillary advancement may impede the velopharyngeal system and affect speech. According to Dr. Proffit, the combination of maxillary advancement and mandibular setback is more stable than isolated mandibular setback surgery [12]. Although 2-jaw surgery is more common than one jaw surgery, 2-jaw surgery is not recommended when the maxillary position is considered normal. After mandibular set back, the volume of the oral cavity may be decreased. Accordingly, there may bc concerns about the obstruction of the respiratory tract due to tongue volume. In most actual cases, however, the tongue moves downward rather than backward, so there is no need for surgery to reduce tongue volume. When the maxilla is advanced or superiorly repositioned, the alar base gains more support and therefore dilates. This opens the laminal valve and enhances nasal breathing [12]. A concern may arise for sleep apnea patients, because a set-back osteotomy of mandible can reduce the dimension of airway space. For these patients, combining anterior segmental subapical osteotomy may be recommended to avoid excessive mandibular set back.

CASES

Case 1: Kang S Y - Long Face, Non-Extraction Therapy

Diagnosis and Treatment plan

Fig. **17** shows a 24 year-old woman who came to the Department of Orthodontics, Dental Hospital, Yonsei University, with the chief complaint of mandibular protrusion. The extraoral examination indicated a concave facial profile and a long anterior facial height. From the intraoral and dental cast examination, molar and canine relationships were Class III on both sides. Anterior and posterior cross-bite was noted as well as mild anterior crowding in the lower arch.

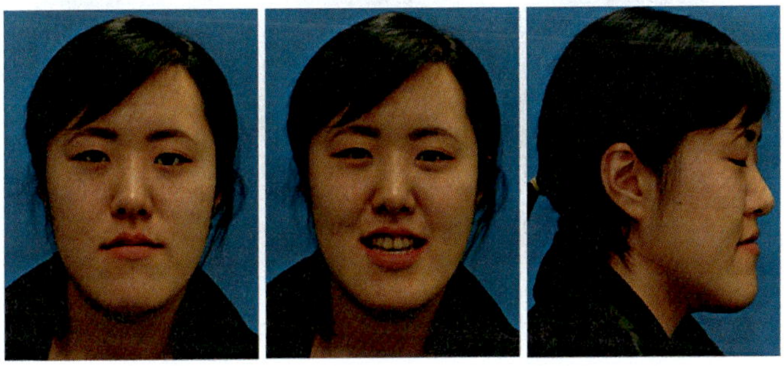

Fig. 17: contd....

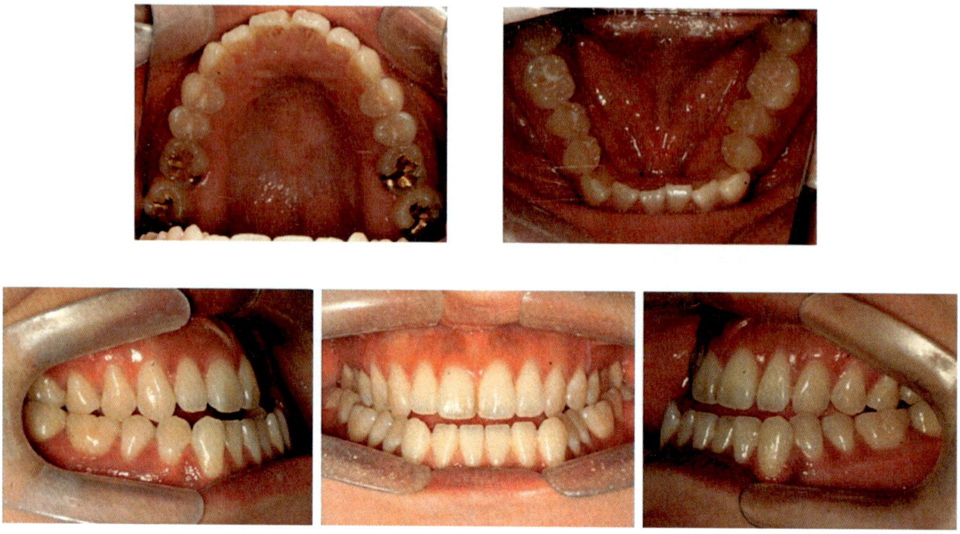

Figure 17: Initial photos.

Fig. **18** shows the lateral cephalometric analysis which revealed a skeletal Class III with maxillary deficiency, mandibular prognathism (SNA angle; 75.9°, SNB angle;79.3°, ANB angle; -3.4°, Wits; -19.8, mandibular body length; 92.1mm), and a hyperdivergent facial profile (SN-MP angle; 43.0°). The axial inclination of the upper anterior teeth was within normal range, but the lower anterior teeth were retroclined (IMPA; 74.0°). The patient had excessive upper incisal exposure (U1 to Stomion superius: 4mm). On the panoramic radiograph, the sizes of the left and right condylar head were different (Fig. **18**).

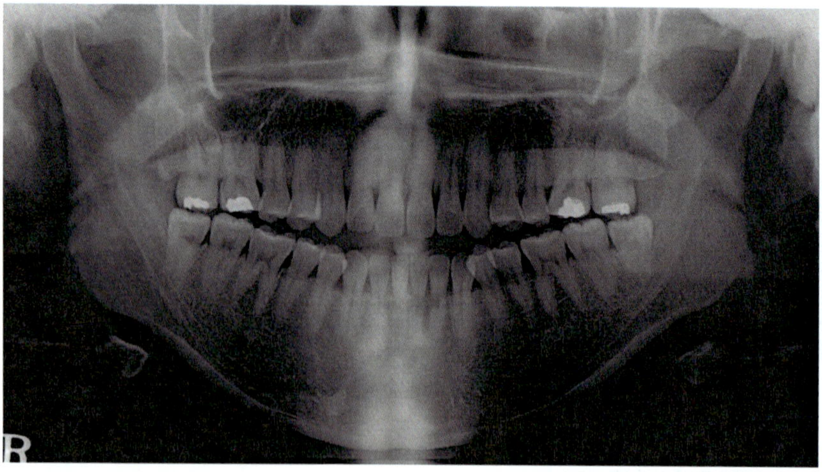

Fig. 18: contd....

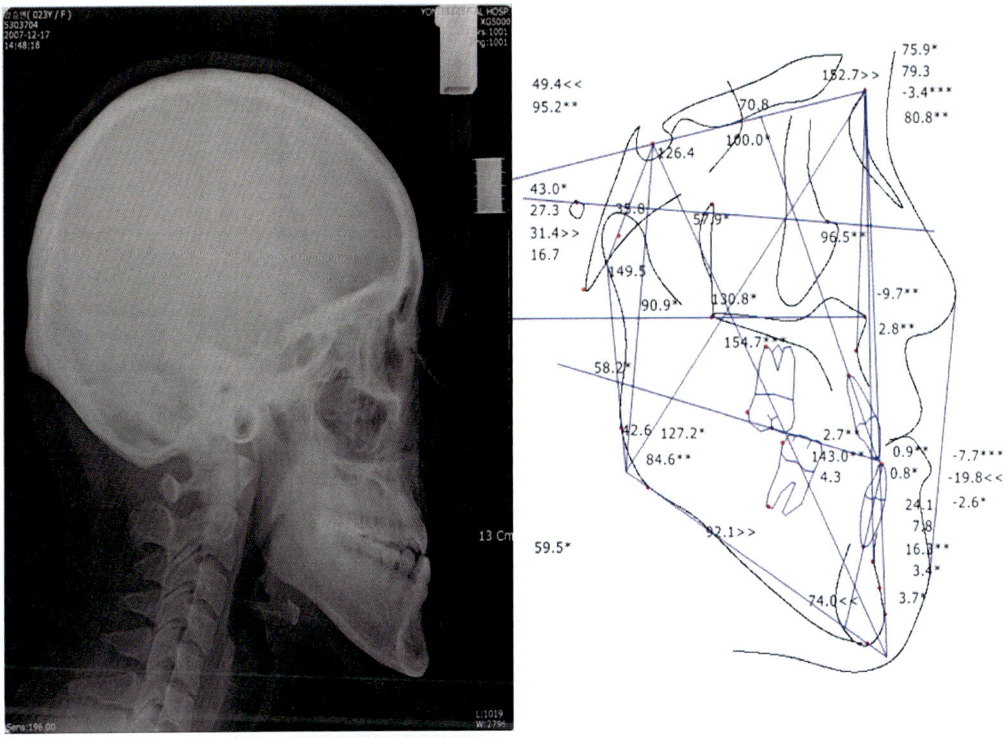

Figure 18: Initial X-ray.

The pre-surgical orthodontic treatment objectives were to decompensate the retroclined lower anterior teeth and to coordinate upper and lower arches. A 2-jaw surgery, impaction and advancement of maxilla as well as a set back of mandible, was planned to reduce the long anterior facial height and correct the concave profile.

Treatment

At pre-surgical treatment phase, tooth #18, 38 and 48 were extracted, the lingually tipped mandibular premolars were expanded and the retroclined lower anterior teeth were corrected with Class II elastics (Fig. **19**). A LeFort 1 osteotomy was performed on the maxilla for an advancement of 4.0mm, plus an impaction of 5.0mm at ANS and 7.0mm at PNS. Bilateral intraoral vertical ramus osteotomy was performed to set back the protruded mandible. For additional reduction of the anterior facial height and a more esthetic chin profile, a 3mm reduction genioplasty was done.

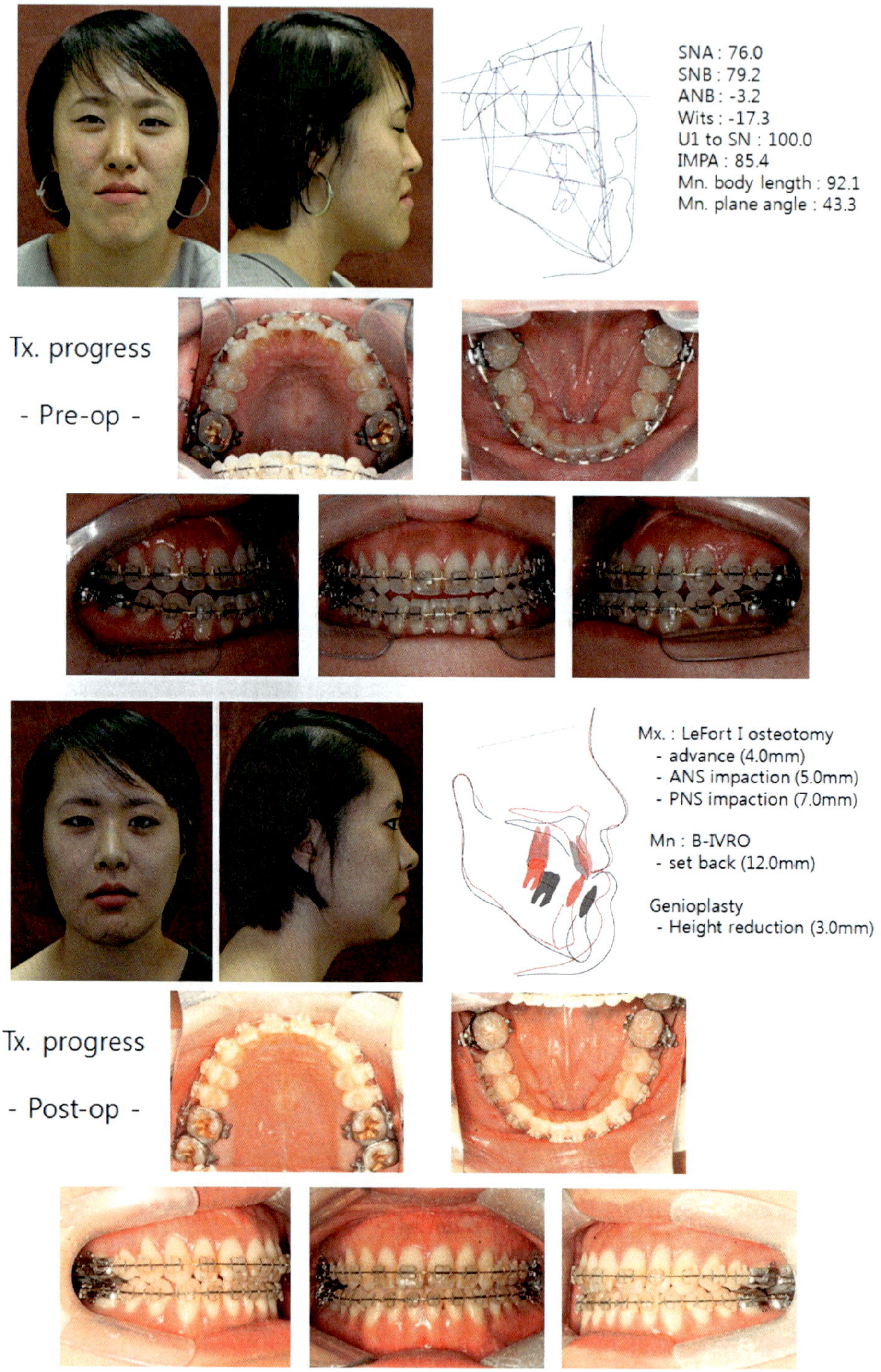

Figure 19: Treatment progress.

Treatment Results and Comments

Anterior and posterior cross-bites were corrected and a satisfactory occlusion was achieved. Improvement of the concave profile and a reduction of the long anterior facial height were noted (Figs. **20** and **21**).

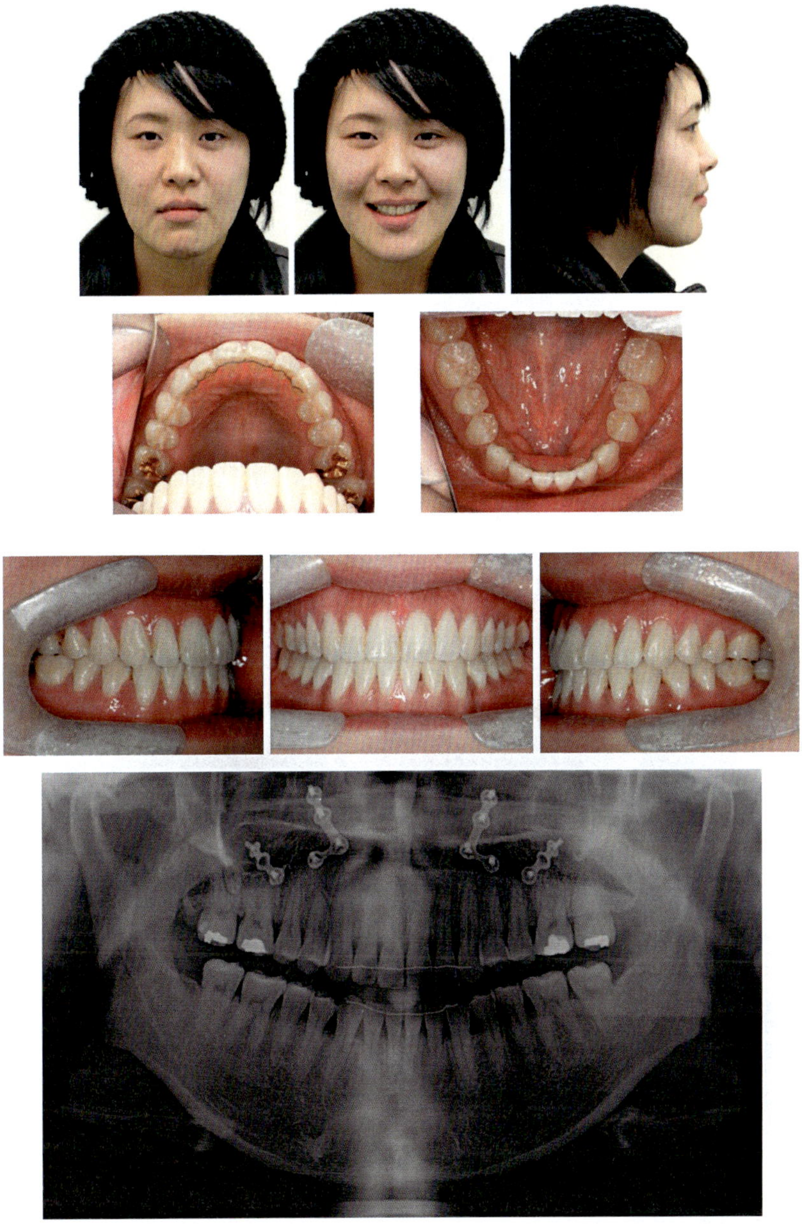

Fig. 20: contd….

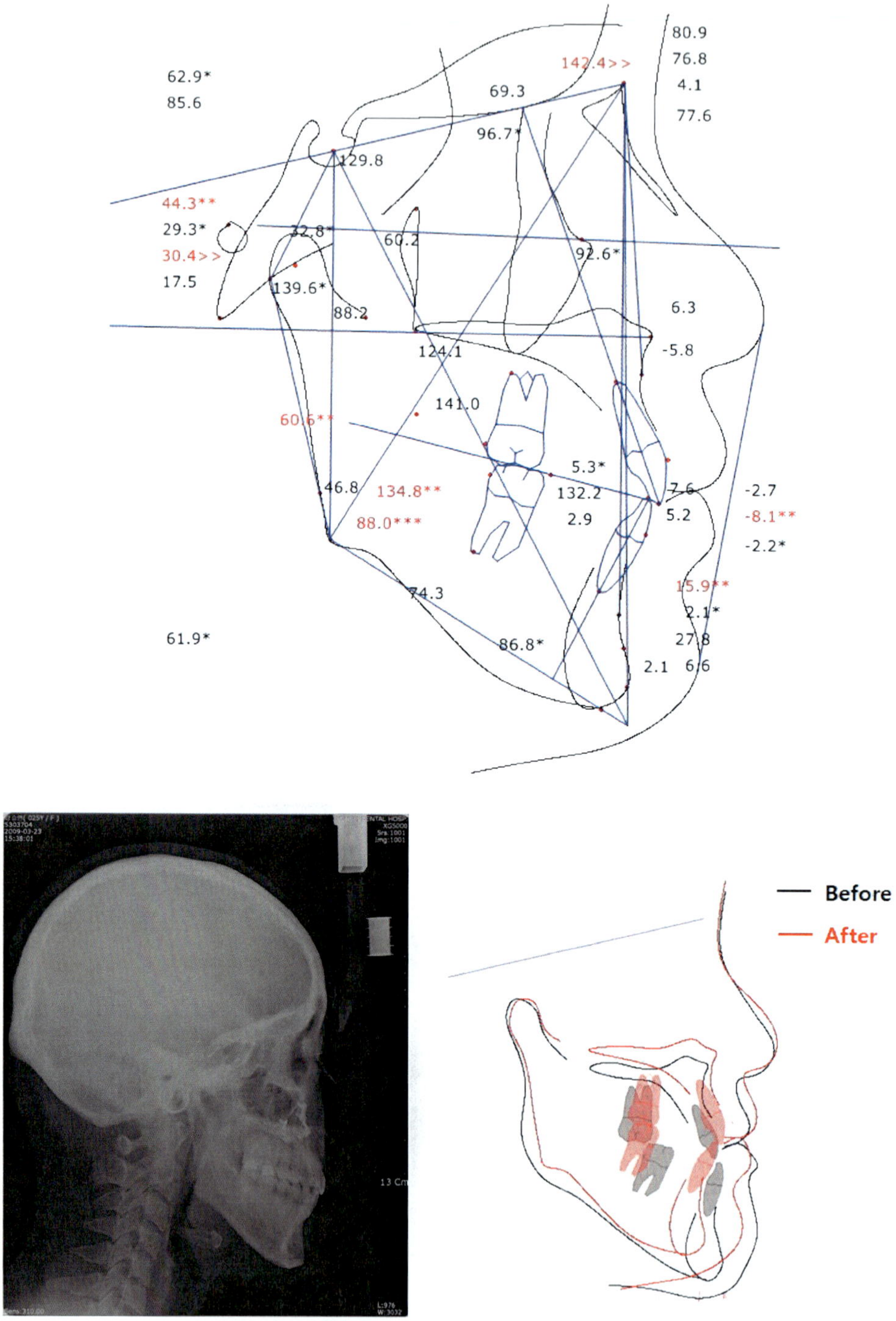

Figure 20: After debonding photos and X-ray.

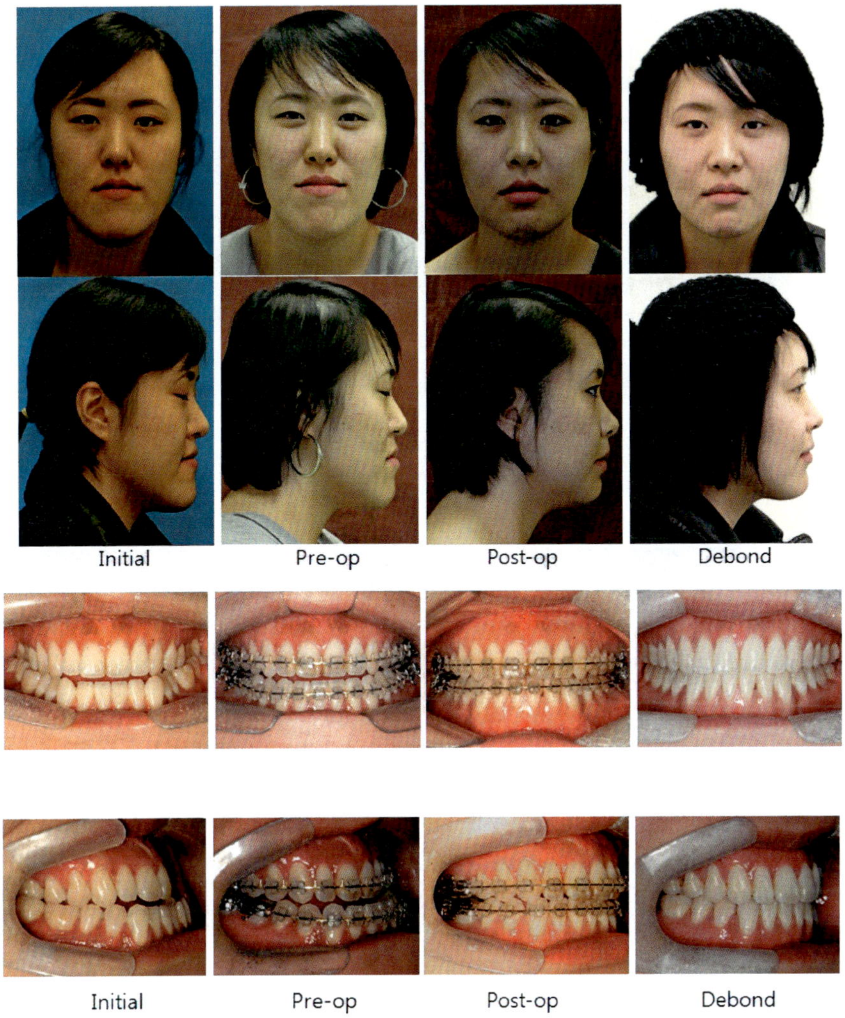

Figure 21: Before and after treatment.

Case 2: Kim B Y - Class III, Extraction of #14 and 24

Diagnosis and Treatment Plan

Fig. **22** shows a 25-year-old male patient who presented to the Department of Orthodontics with the chief complaint of anterior crossbite. The patient had a protruded mandible and a long facial height. The frontal view showed a mild asymmetry, with the chin deviated to the patient's left. From the intraoral view, the patient had bilateral Class III canine and molar relationships with an anterior crossbite. The lower dental midline was shifted 3.5mm t o the left.

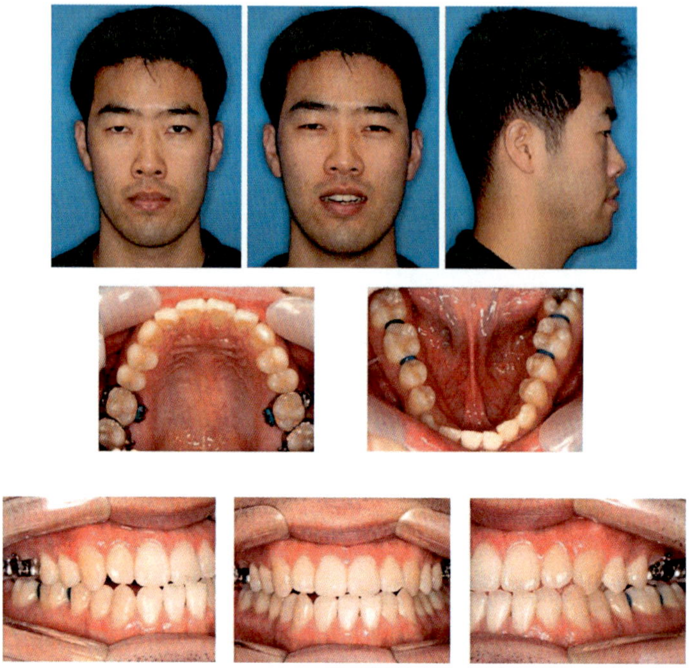

Figure 22: Initial photos.

The lateral cephalogram (Fig. **23**) showed that the patient has a skeletal Class III pattern with bimaxillary protrusion (A-point to Nasion perpendicular: 4.9mm, SNA angle: 86.7°, SNB angle: 87.8°, ANB angle: -1.1°, Wits: -13.1, mandibular body length: 91.2mm). The upper and lower anterior teeth were compensated to the skeletal discrepancy with U1 to SN 111.6°, and IMPA 84.9°. On the panoramic radiograph, the size of the left and right condylar heads was different.

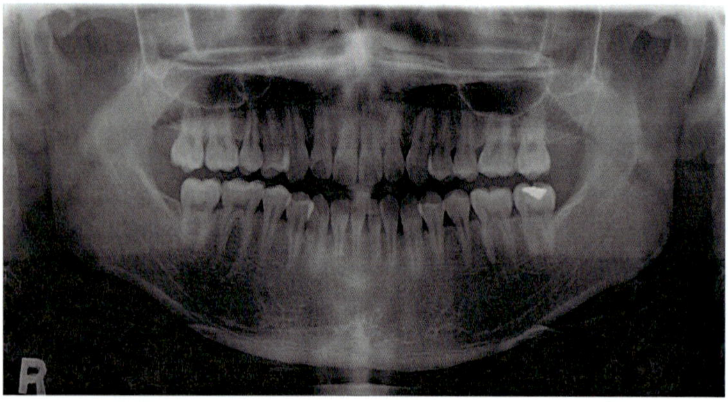

Fig. 23: contd….

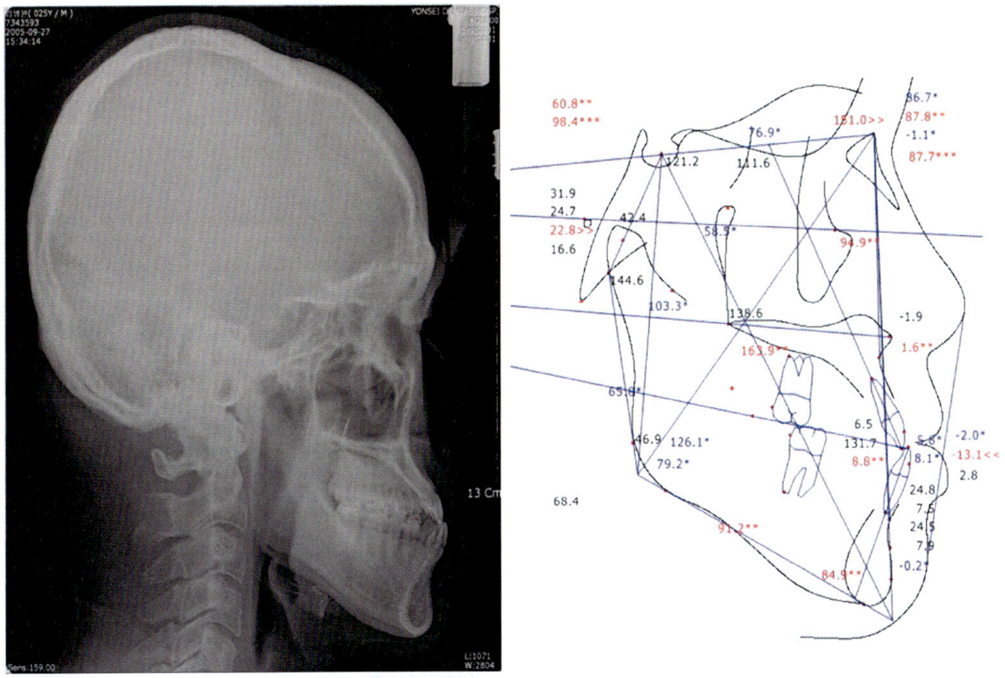

Figure 23: Initial X-ray.

Pre-surgical orthodontic treatment objectives were to decompensate the proclined upper anterior teeth and the retroclined lower anterior teeth as well as to coordinate the upper and lower arches. A 2-jaw surgery with impaction of the maxilla was planned to reduce the excessive facial height, and a mandibular set back was indicated to correct the protrusion of the mandible.

Treatment

Before placement of orthodontic brackets, both maxillary first premolars (#14 and 24) were extracted for retraction of the upper anterior segment. During the pre-surgical orthodontic phase, compensatory tipping of the upper and lower anterior teeth was corrected by wearing Class II elastics (Fig. **24**). The maxilla was set back by 3.0 mm, as well as impacted by 3.0 mm at ANS and 4.0 mm at PNS, with a LeFort I osteotomy. The mandible was set back by 13 mm with an intraoral vertical ramus osteotomy.

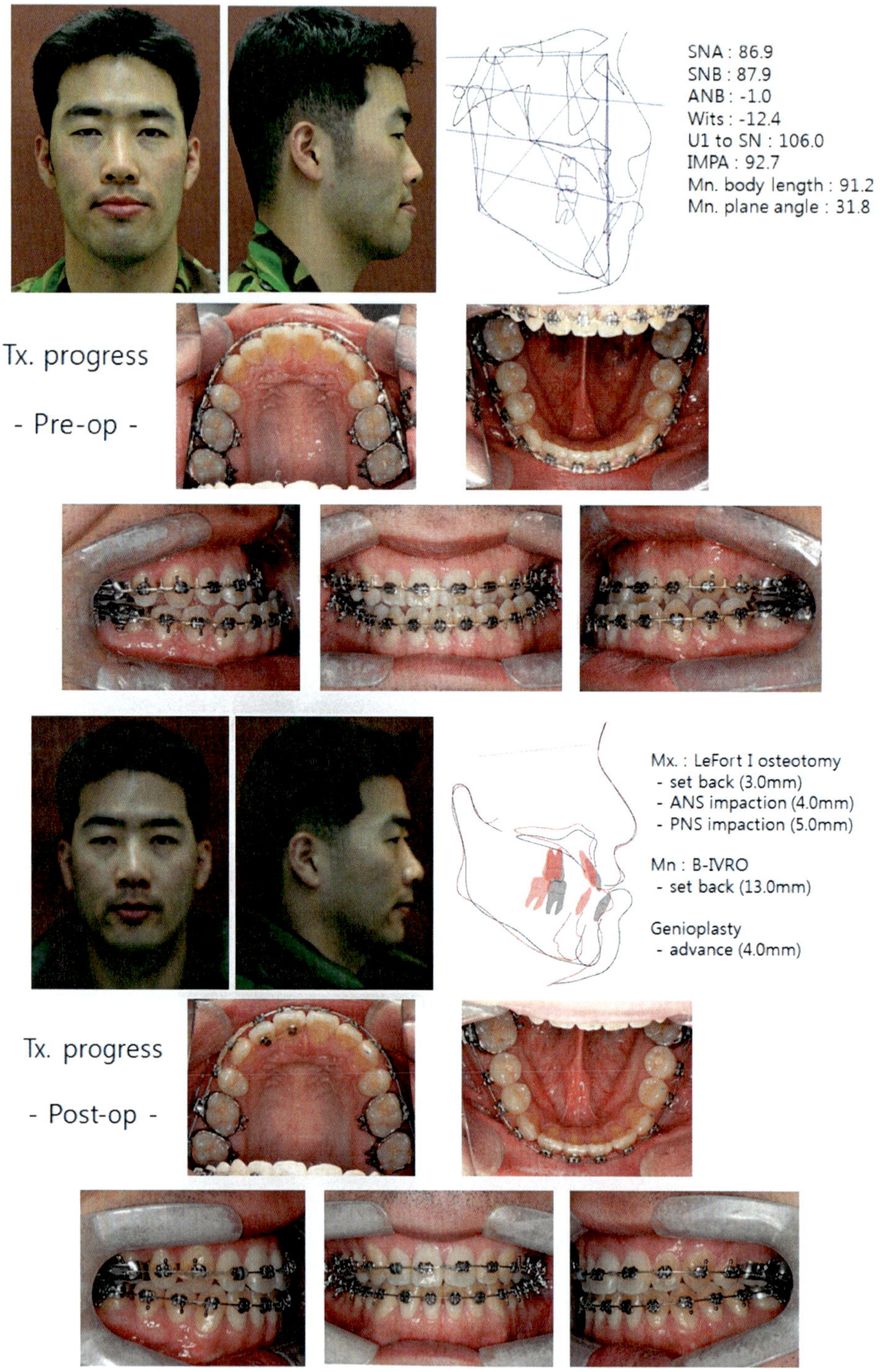

Figure 24: Treatment progress.

Treatment Results and Comments

Figs. **25** and **26** show the results of the treatment. The anterior crossbite was corrected and a satisfactory occlusion was accomplished. An improved concave profile and a reduced anterior facial height were obtained. The dental midline and chin deviation were also corrected. Widening of the nasal base was, however, an unwanted result.

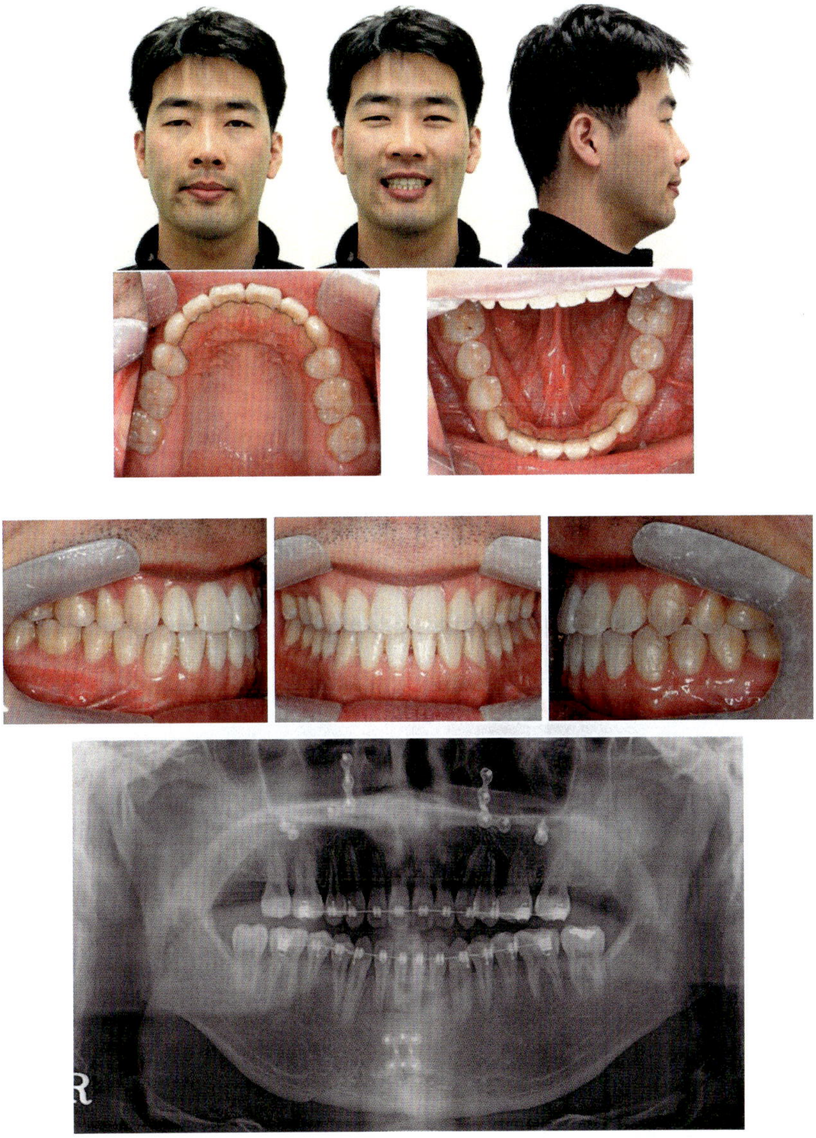

Fig. 25: contd….

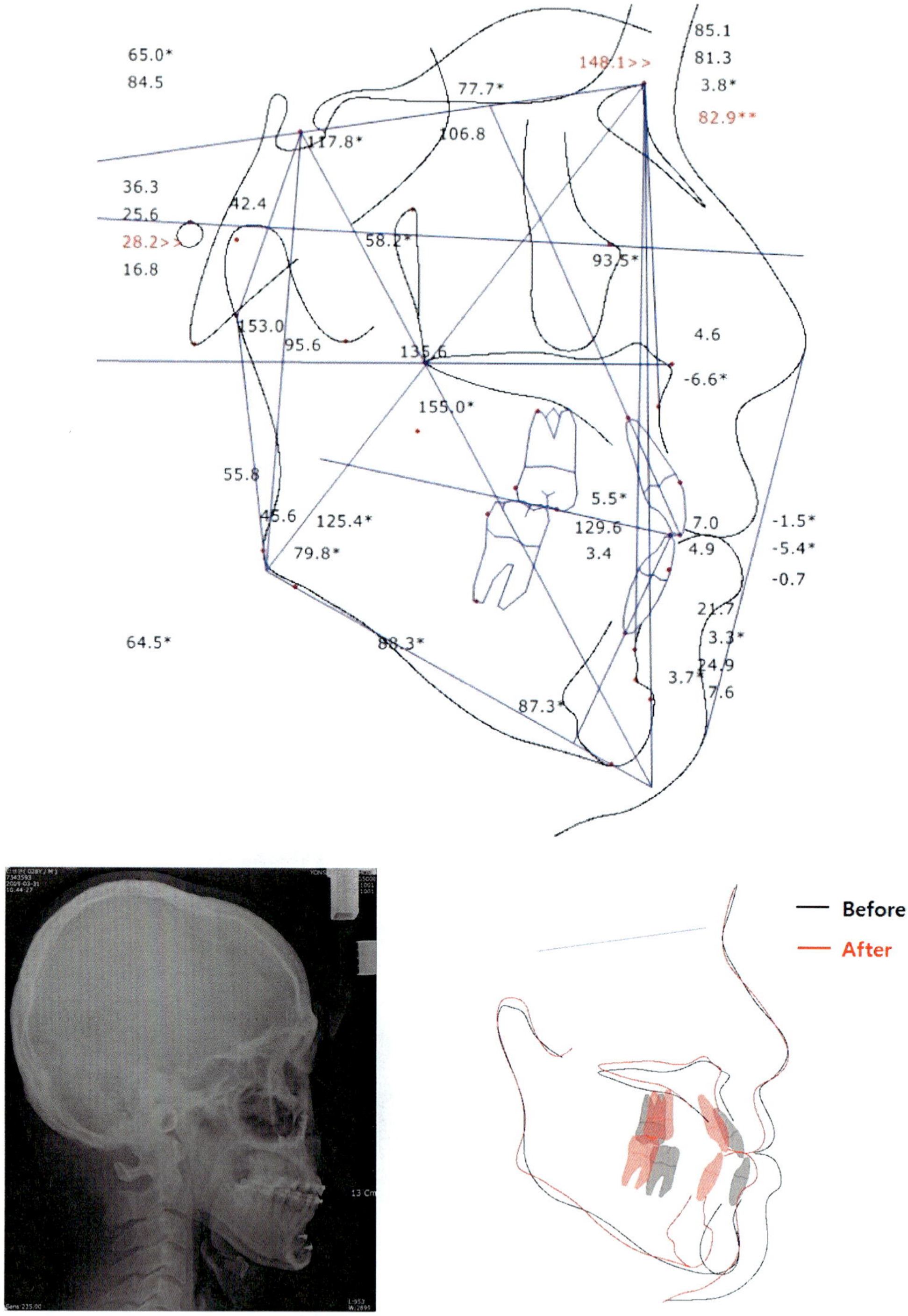

Figure 25: After debonding photos and X-ray.

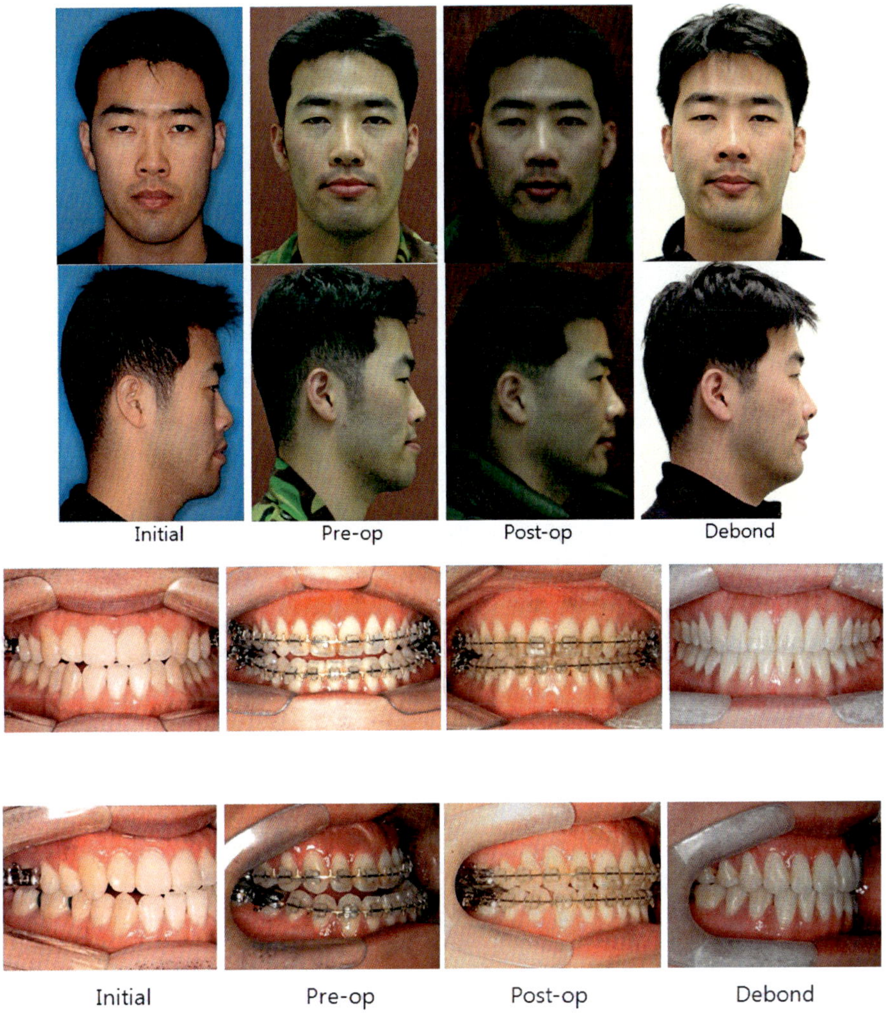

Figure 26: Before and after treatment.

Case 3: Park J S - 49 Years Old, Congenital Missing of #13,23

Diagnosis and Treatment Plan

Fig. **27** shows a woman, aged 49 years, who presented to the Department of Orthodontics with the chief complaint of difficulty in chewing. She had a concave facial profile with a protruded mandible and retruded lips, which gave her an aged profile. Intraoral examination revealed missing upper canines, generalized gingival recession, and prosthetic restoration of the molars She had an anterior openbite and the lower anterior teeth were crowded and in crossbite.

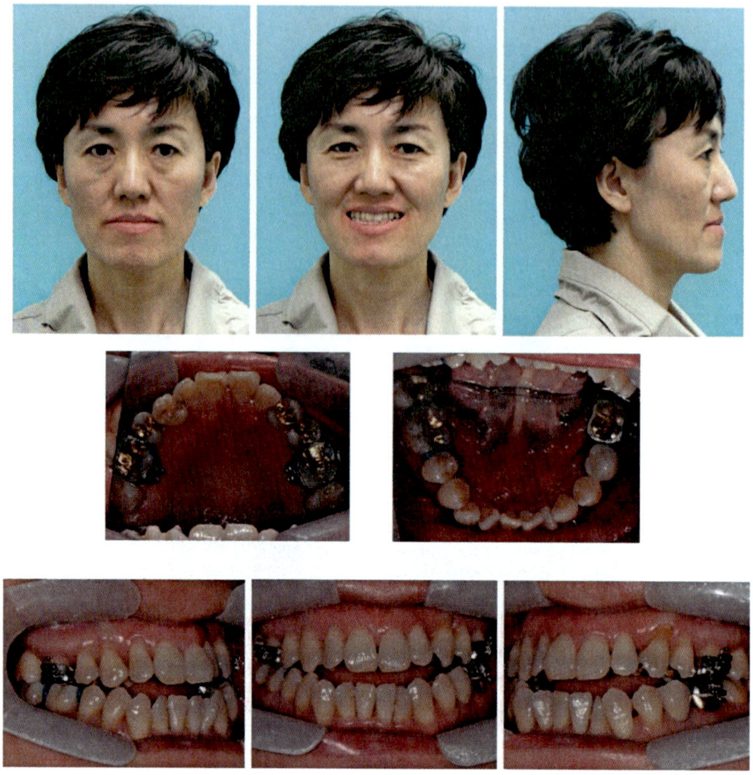

Figure 27: Initial photos.

Cephalometric analysis (Fig. **28**) showed a skeletal Class III relationship with maxillary retrusion and mandibular prognathism (SNA angle: 76.0°, SNB angle: 77.3°, ANB angle: -1.3°, Wits -9.2, mandibular body length 80.7mm). The axial inclinations of the maxillary incisors were within normal limit, but mandibular incisors were lingually inclined.

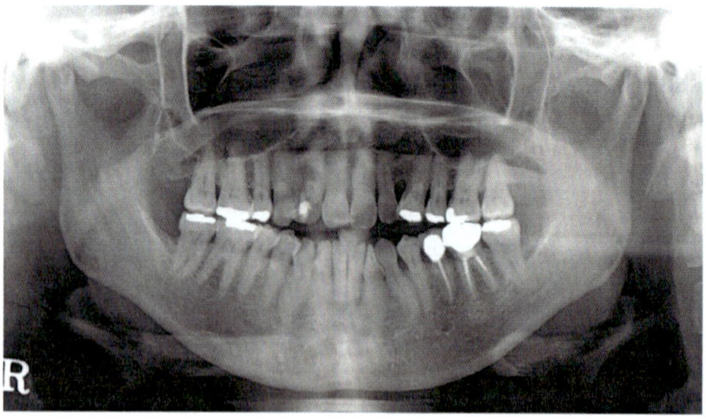

Fig. 28: contd....

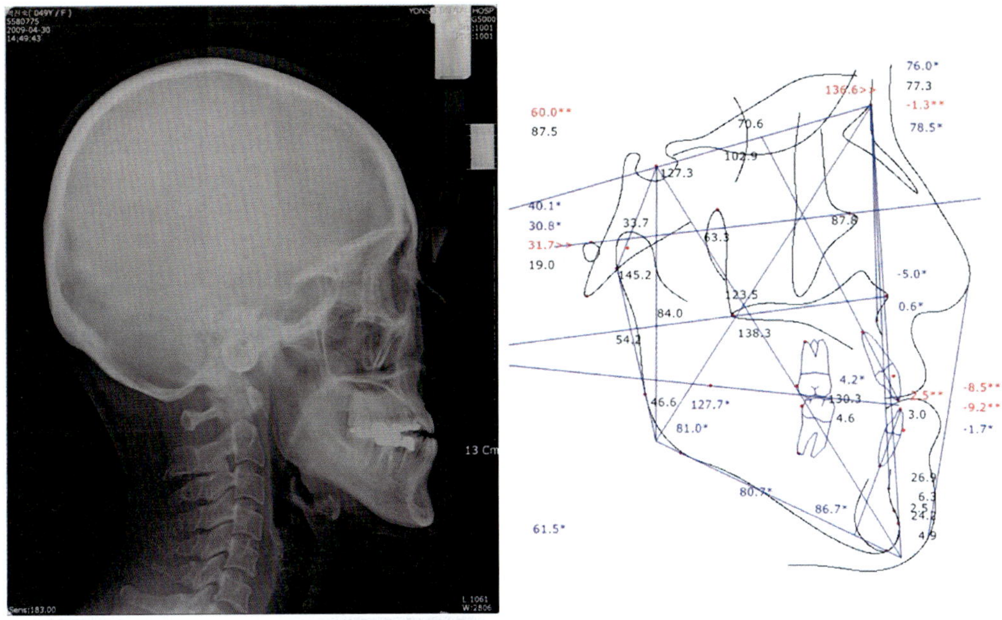

Figure 28: Initial X-ray.

The pre-surgical orthodontic treatment objectives were to substitute maxillary canines (#13 and 23) with the first premolars (#14 and 24), decompensate retroclined lower anterior teeth, and coordinate the upper to the lower arch. A 2-jaw surgery, posterior impaction of maxilla at PNS and set back of mandible, was planned to correct the concave profile (Fig. **27**).

Treatment

Before starting orthodontic treatment, periodontal treatment was performed. To substitute the canine with the 1st premolars, reshaping was done at every visit. Tipping of the lower anterior teeth was corrected by wearing Class II elastics (Fig. **29**). The maxilla was impacted by 7.0mm at PNS with a LeFort 1 osteotomy, and the mandible was set back by 9 mm with an intraoral vertical ramus osteotomy.

Treatment Results and Comments

Figs. **30** and **31** show the results of the treatment. There was no maxillary advancement, because of the mandibular set back sufficiently improved the concave profile, thereby achieving a younger facial appearance. The anterior

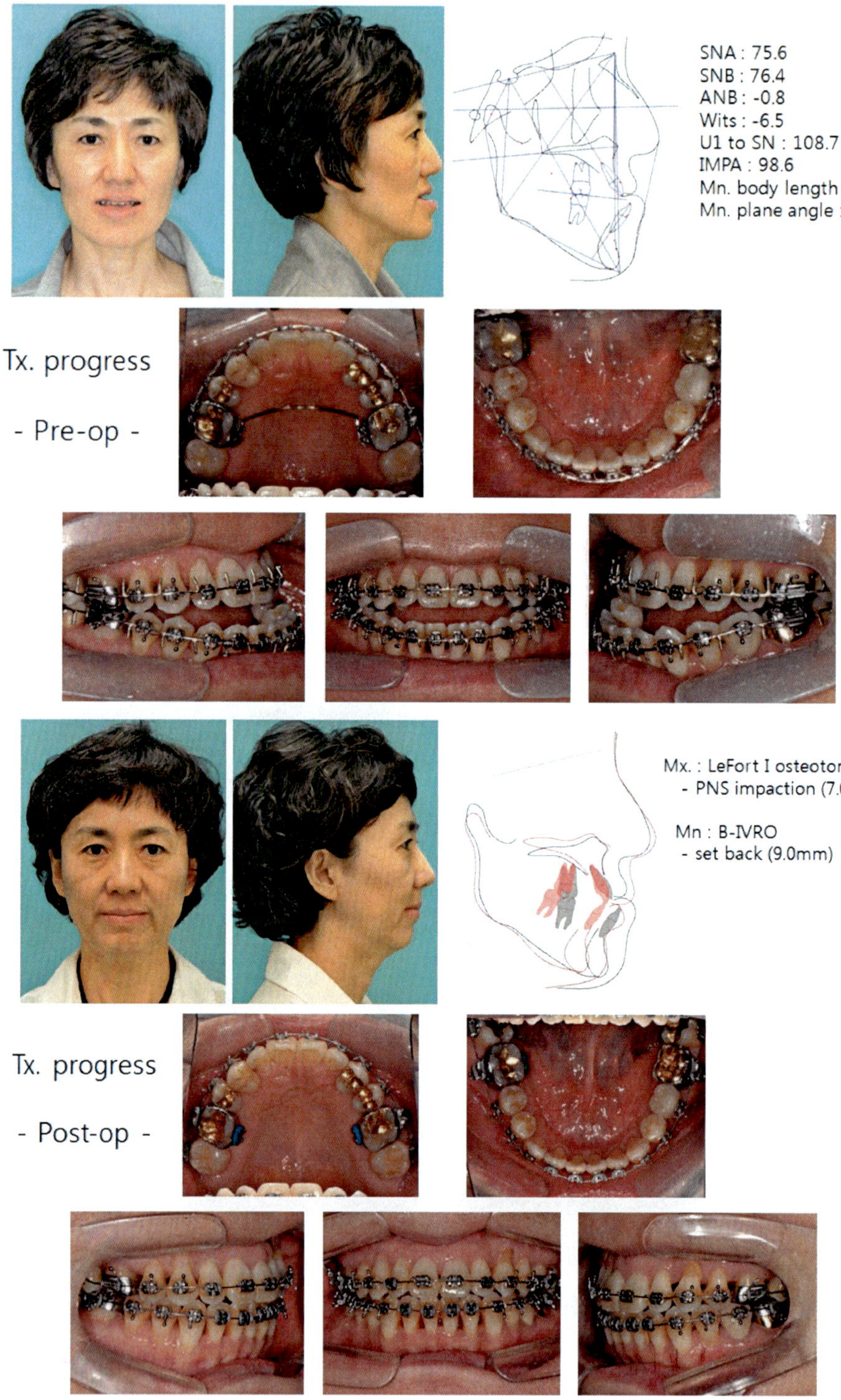

Figure 29: Treatment progress.

openbite and crossbite were improved and the maxillary first premolars settled into a satisfactory occlusion, without interference of the palatal cusps. Black triangles of the lower anterior teeth were reduced by enamel stripping of the incisors. However, the reduction of the mandibular body was excessive and a better result could have been achieved if an advancement genioplasty had been performed as well.

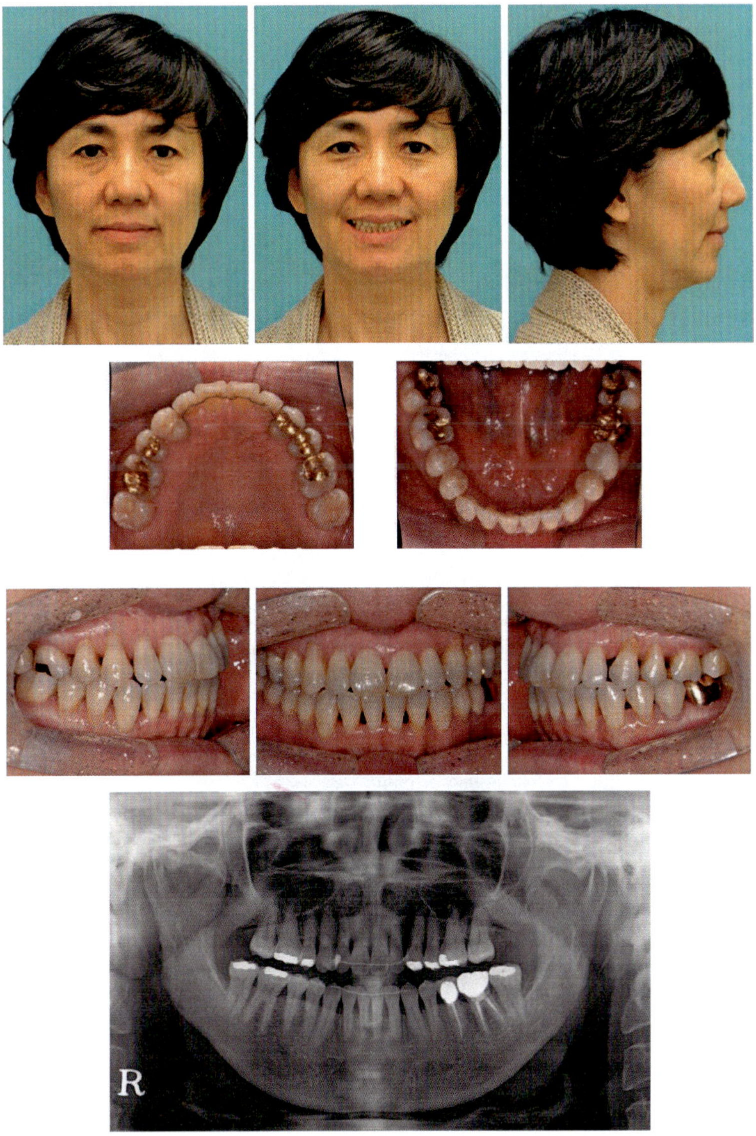

Fig. 30: contd….

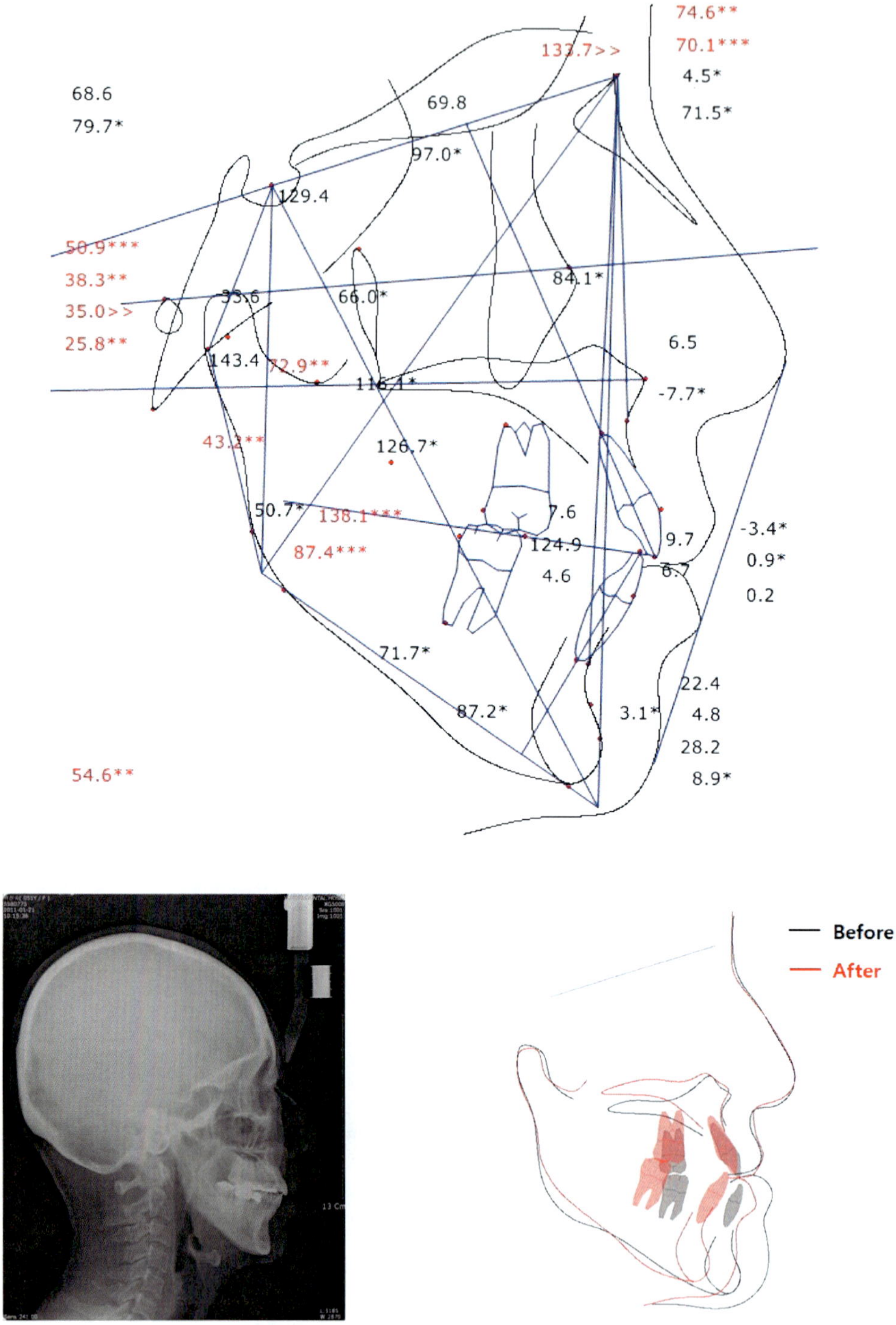

Figure 30: After debonding photos and X-ray.

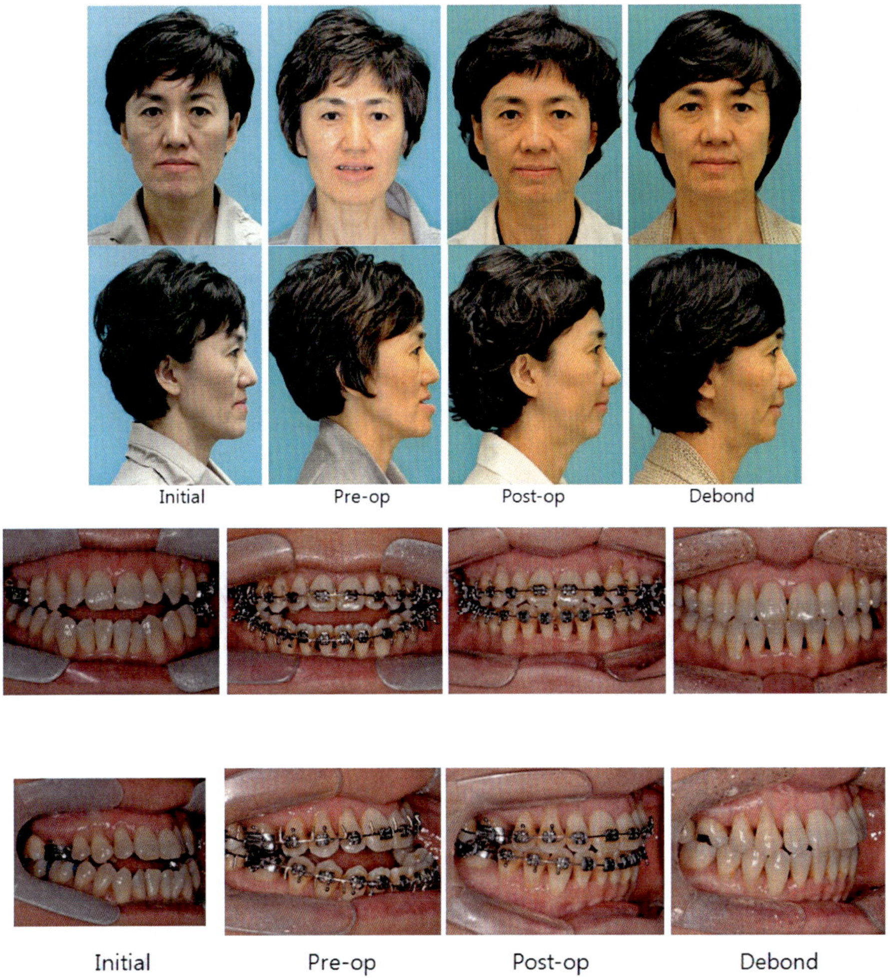

Figure 31: Before and after treatment.

Case 4: Kim T H - Spacing, Mandibular Subapical Osteotomy

Diagnosis and Treatment Plan

Fig. **32** shows a 22 year-old patient who presented to the department with the chief complaint of mandibular protrusion and spacing. Clinically, the patient had a concave facial profile with a protrusive mandible, a retrusive midfacial area, and a retruded upper lip. Intraorally, the patient presented with a diastema between the central incisors and peg shaped upper lateral incisors. In addition, compensation of the upper and lower incisors was noted with spacing. There were bilateral Class III canine and molar relationships as well as anterior and posterior crossbites.

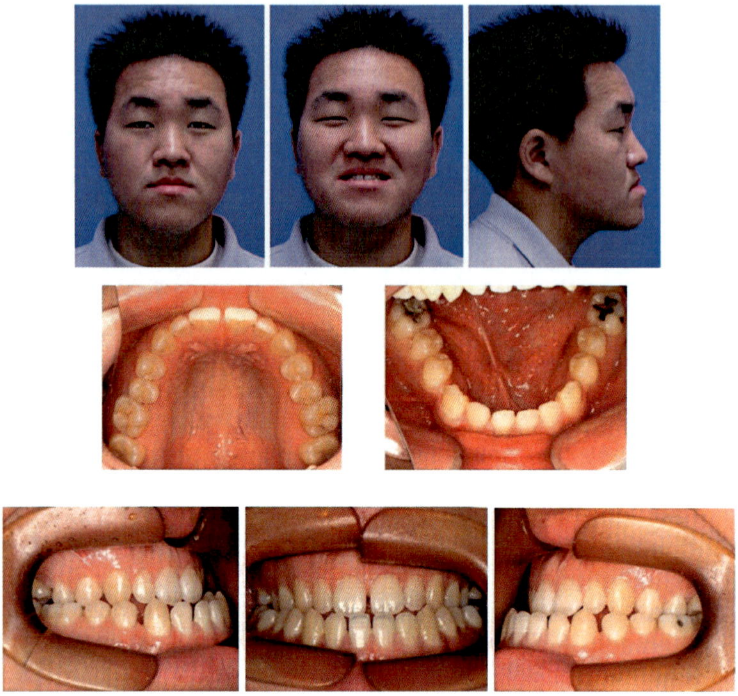

Figure 32: Initial photos.

The cephalometric radiograph and tracing (Fig. **33**) showed a skeletal Class III malocclusion with maxillary deficiency, and mandibular prognathism (SNA angle: 79.2°, SNB angle: 86.5°, ANB angle: -7.3°, Wits -18.1, mandibular body length 87.1mm). The maxillary incisors were proclined (U1 to SN: 112.2°) and the mandibular incisors were retroclined (IMPA: 80.1°), compensating for the skeletal malocclusion. The panoramic radiograph showed generalized alveolar bone loss and short roots of the lower premolars.

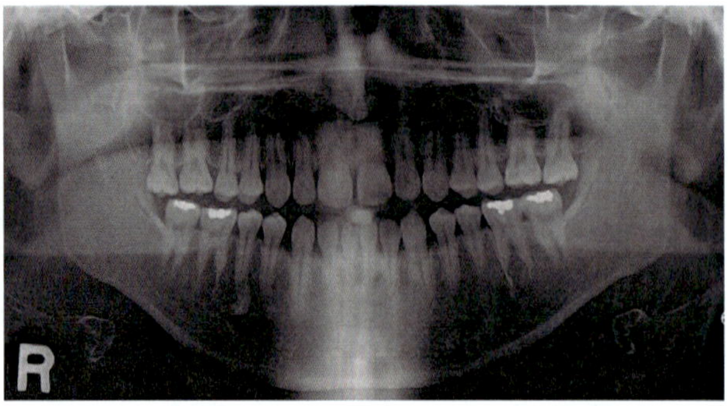

Fig. 33: contd....

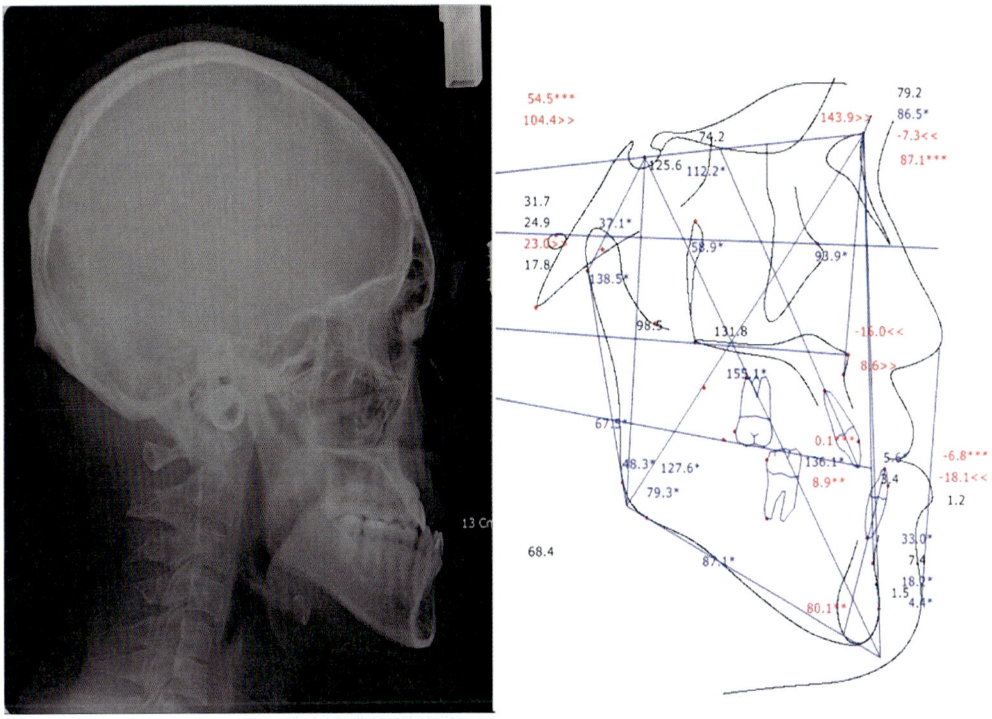

Figure 33: Initial X-ray.

The pre-surgical orthodontic treatment objectives were to close the upper anterior spacing by retraction of incisors and to redistribute space distal to the lower canines (#43 and 33) for an anterior subapical osteotomy. A 2-jaw surgery was planned for posterior impaction and advancement of maxilla, set back of the mandible, and an anterior subapical osteotomy.

Treatment

At pre-surgical orthodontic phase, the upper anterior teeth were tipped lingually by retraction of the anterior teeth (Fig. **34**). The lower anterior teeth were decompensated with Class II elastics and open coil spring, and space was gained on the distal side of teeth #43 and 33 for an anterior subapical osteotomy. The maxilla was advanced 2.0mm and impacted 7.0mm at PNS, with a LeFort 1 osteotomy. Spaces gained between #44-43, 33-34 were closed by setback of the anterior segment with a subapical osteotomy. The mandible was set back 10mm with an intraoral vertical ramus osteotomy.

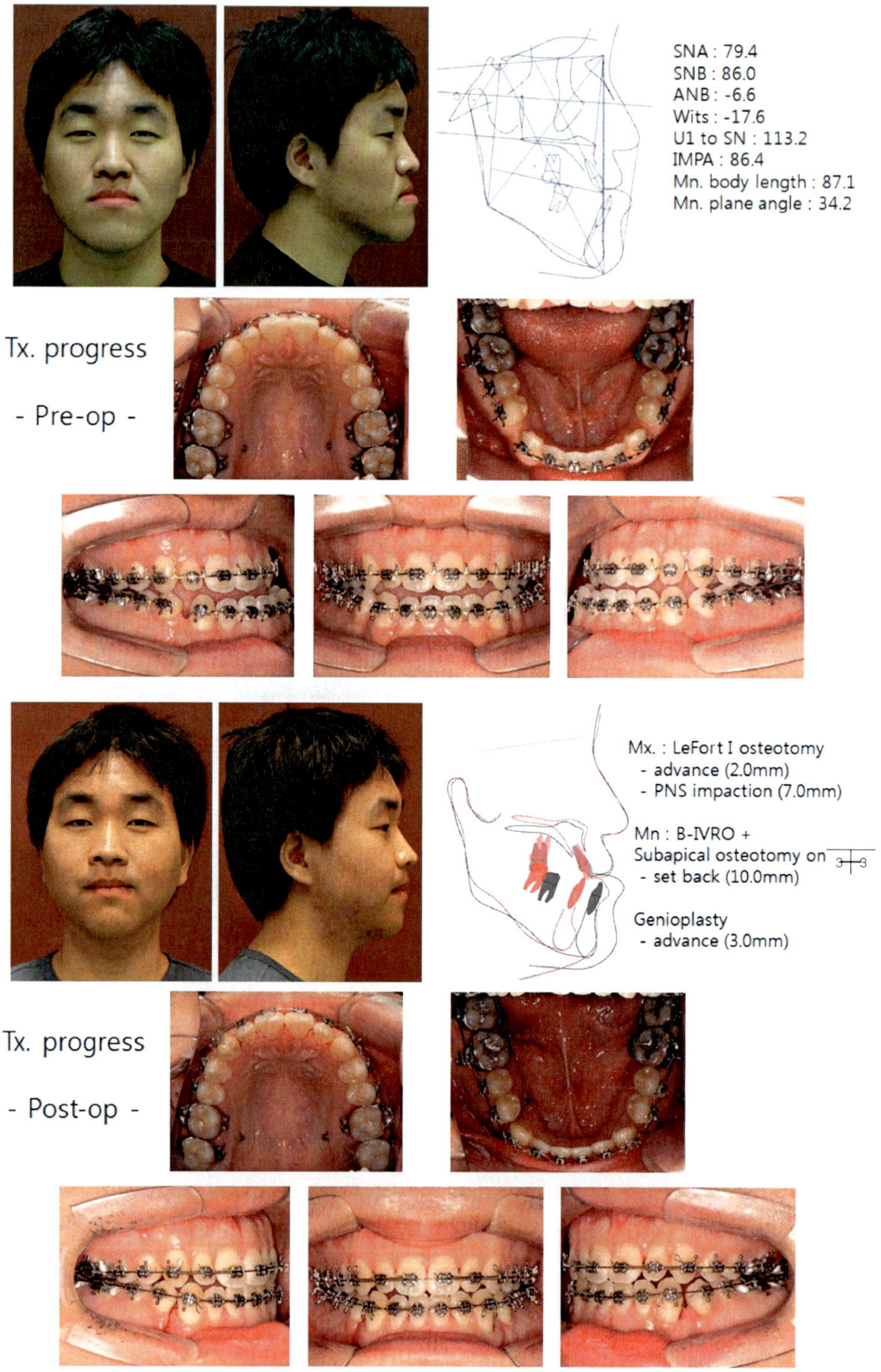

Figure 34: Treatment progress.

Treatment Results and Comments

Figs. **35** and **36** show the results of the treatment. The anterior and posterior crossbites were corrected and a satisfactory occlusion was obtained. The concave profile was much improved. An undesirable sequelae was noted after the subapical osteotomy of the mandible. The patient had hypersensitivity on tooth #44 and 34, which could be a complication of the surgery. Endodontic treatment was planned for these teeth. Also laminates were placed on #12 and #22.

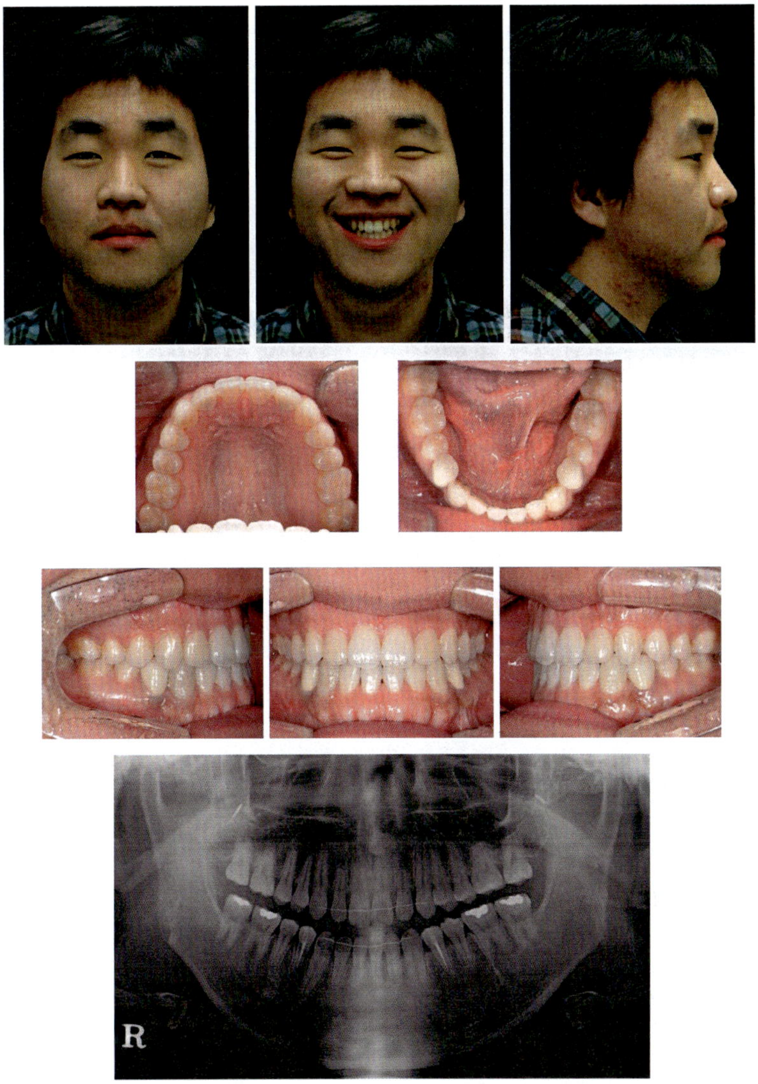

Fig. 35: contd....

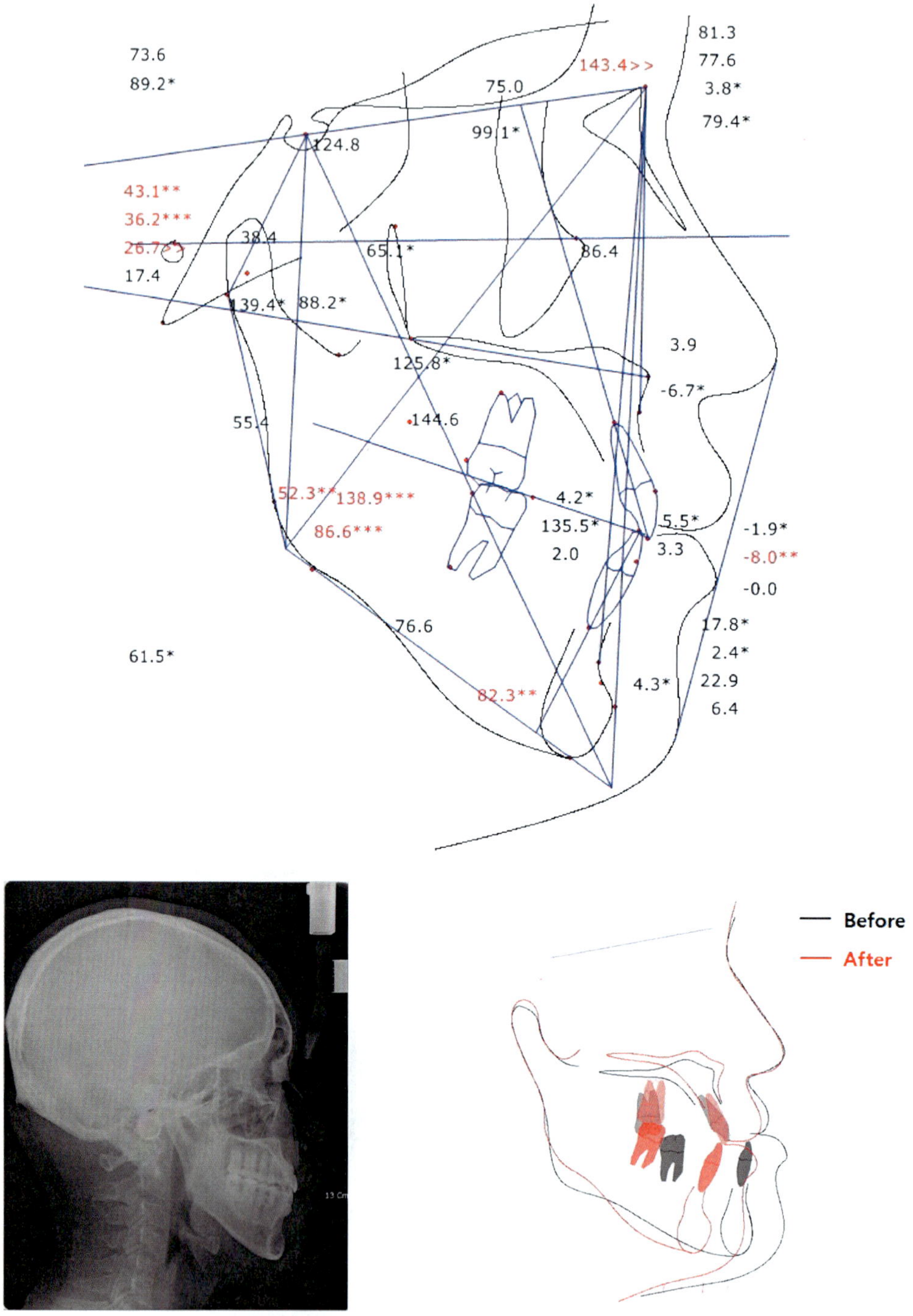

Figure 35: After debonding photos and X-ray.

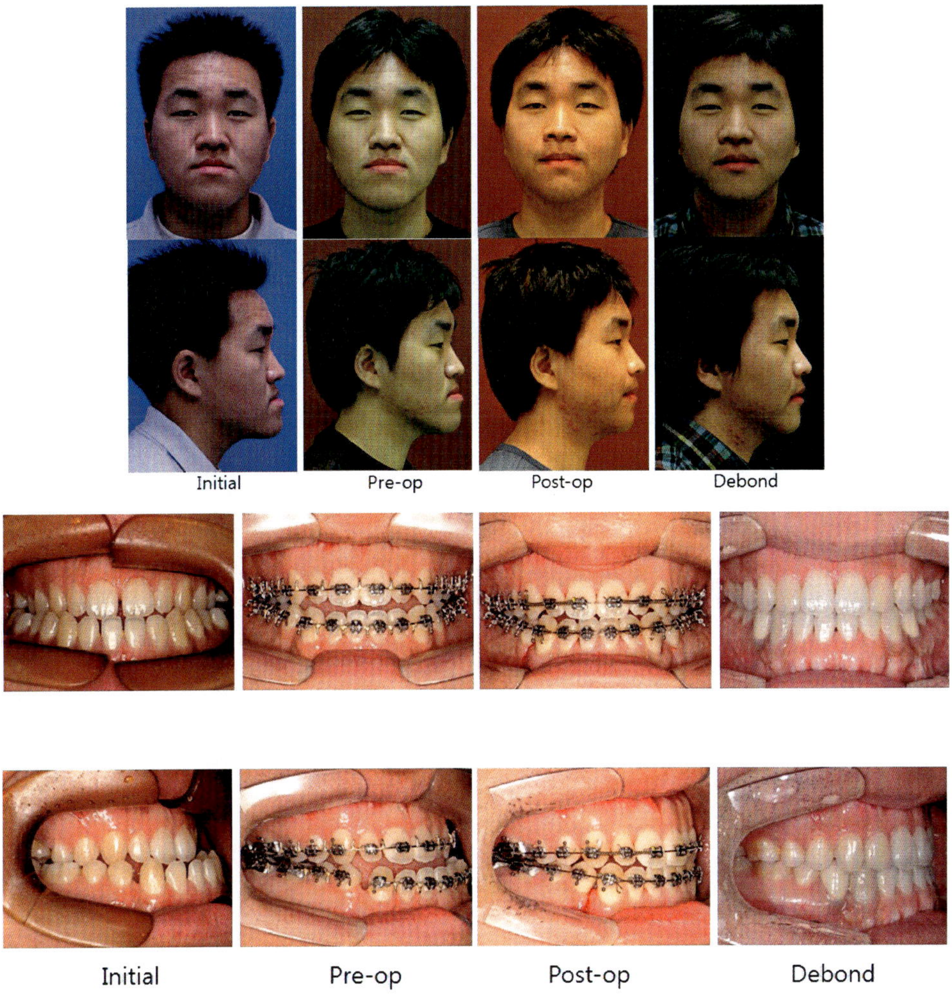

Figure 36: Before and after treatment.

SUMMARY POINTS

- Class III patients with over-developed mandibles are best treated after growth is completed, so that underlying skeletal and dental discrepancies can be corrected with orthognathic surgery.

- In diagnosis and treatment planning for orthognathic surgery, 3-dimensional analysis using CBCT imaging provides more detailed information than 2-dimensional cephalograms.

- Both mandibular condylar and body units appear to contribute to mandibular asymmetry, with the condylar unit playing a more dominant role.

- The 3-dimenisonal soft tissue and hard tissue changes can be quantitatively calculated in the sagittal and frontal dimensions.

- To produce the best results following orthognathic surgery, close interaction between the orthodontist and oral surgeon is needed. Furthermore, well-treated pre-surgical orthodontics simplify the orthognathic surgical treatment plan.

- Recently, demand for a surgery-first approach to achieve a rapid esthetic improvement, is increasing, but appropriate case selection, precise treatment prediction and accurate wafer fabrication are all crucial for avoiding an excessive treatment time and poor results.

ACKNOWLEDGEMENTS

Declared none.

CONFLICT OF INTEREST

The authors confirm that this chapter contents have no conflict of interest.

REFERENCES

[1] Choi, Y. H. (2012), 'The distribution and trend of orthognathic patients – A 10 year study from dental hospital of Yonsei University', Master Thesis,. 2012, University of Yonsei.
[2] Ellis, E., 3RD & McNamara, J. A., JR. (1984), 'Components of adult Class III malocclusion' *J Oral Maxillofac Surg,* 42, 295-305.
[3] Baik, H. S., Han, H. K., Kim, D. J. & Proffit, W. R. (2000), 'Cephalometric characteristics of Korean Class III surgical patients and their relationship to plans for surgical treatment' *Int J Adult Orthodon Orthognath Surg,* 15, 119-28.
[4] Baik, H. S. (2002), 'Limitations in orthopedic treatment and combined surgery in skeletal Class III malocclusion.' *Orthodontics in the 21st century*, Osaka Univ. pp.117-129.
[5] Chung, C. J., Jung, S. & Baik, H. S. (2008), 'Morphological characteristics of the symphyseal region in adult skeletal Class III crossbite and openbite malocclusions' *Angle Orthod,* 78, 38-43.

[6] Park, S. H., Yu, H. S., Kim, K. D., Lee, K. J. & Baik, H. S. (2006), 'A proposal for a new analysis of craniofacial morphology by 3-dimensional computed tomography' *Am J Orthod Dentofacial Orthop,* 129, 600 e23-3.

[7] You, K. H., Lee, K. J., Lee, S. H. & Baik, H. S. (2010), 'Three-dimensional computed tomography analysis of mandibular morphology in patients with facial asymmetry and mandibular prognathism' *Am J Orthod Dentofacial Orthop,* 138, 540 e1-8; discussion 540-1.

[8] Baik, H. S., Lee, H. J. & Lee, K. J. (2006), 'A proposal for soft tissue landmarks for craniofacial analysis using 3-dimensional laser scan imaging' *World J Orthod,* 7, 7-14.

[9] Baik, H. S., Jeon, J. M. & Lee, H. J. (2007), 'Facial soft-tissue analysis of Korean adults with normal occlusion using a 3-dimensional laser scanner' *Am J Orthod Dentofacial Orthop,* 131, 759-66.

[10] Baik, H. S. & Kim, S. Y. (2010), 'Facial soft-tissue changes in skeletal Class III orthognathic surgery patients analyzed with 3-dimensional laser scanning' *Am J Orthod Dentofacial Orthop,* 138, 167-78.

[11] Lee, K. J., Park, Y. C., Park, J. Y. & Hwang, W. S. (2010), 'Miniscrew-assisted nonsurgical palatal expansion before orthognathic surgery for a patient with severe mandibular prognathism' *Am J Orthod Dentofacial Orthop,* 137, 830-9.

[12] Proffit., White, R.P., Sarver, D.M.(2003), *Contemporary Treatment of Dentofacial Deformity* Mosby Inc. 2003, pp. 527-543.

PART IV: CONTEMPORARY APPLIANCES IN TREATMENT OF CLASS III PATIENTS

CHAPTER 11

Designs and Applications of Intraoral Appliances in Class III Malocclusion

Nobuyuki Ishii* **and Ryuzo Kanomi**

Kanomi Orthodontic Office, Himeji, Japan

Abstract: Class III malocclusion results from skeletal disharmony and unfavorable incisor inclination. Early use of intraoral appliances in Class III malocclusion would improve the inclination of retroclined upper incisors and proclined lower incisors. Intraoral appliances used in the upper dental arch include the posterior bite plate containing an anterior spring and the Yanagisawa Class III (YC3) Shield. When using the posterior bite plate, the upper anterior teeth are pushed forward by the force of the spring. The YC3 Shield, developed by M. Yanagisawa, results in forward movement of the upper anterior teeth by tongue pressure. Intraoral appliances used for the lower arch are the inclined bite plate and 2x4 utility archwire. The upper anterior teeth are protracted by the inclined plane of the bite plate, and the lower anterior teeth are retracted by the force of a 2x4 utility archwire. Since the early use of intraoral appliances only improves the inclination and position of the anterior teeth, they are usually used in combination with extraoral protractors in treating early Class III malocclusion. Bone-anchored maxillary protraction (BAMP) was recently developed by H.J. DeClerck and coworkers. BAMP works as an extraoral protractor and provides orthopedic correction. It consists of Class III elastics and two pairs of temporary anchorage devices (TADs). BAMP is a novel intraoral treatment modality for growing patients with Class III malocclusion.

Keywords: Intraoral appliance, Bite plate, YC3 Shield, 2x4 utility arch, BAMP.

INTRODUCTION

Class III malocclusion can result from skeletal disharmony and/or unfavorable inclination of the incisors. Most Class III patients present with both skeletal and dental problems. Skeletal disharmony can be corrected with jaw surgery or an extraoral protractor, depending on the patient's age and severity of the malocclusion. Early use of intraoral appliances in Class III malocclusion helps to

***Address correspondence to Nobuyuki Ishii:** Kanomi Orthodontic Office, 30 Minamiekimae-cho, Himeji 670-0962, Japan; Tel: +81-79-284-2576; Fax: +81-79-284-2584; E-mail: ishii@kanomi-ddsc.or.jp

Peter W. Ngan, Toshi Deguchi and Eugene W. Roberts (Eds)

improve the inclination of the incisors; however, they are usually used in combination with extraoral protractors for simultaneous orthopedic correction.

Intraoral appliances can be divided into two groups: appliances used for the upper and lower dental arches. Examples of the upper intraoral appliances are the posterior bite plate with anterior spring and the Yanagisawa Class III (YC3) Shield. Common lower appliances are the inclined bite plate and 2x4 utility arch-wire. These intraoral appliances improve unfavorable incisor inclination. The upper posterior bite plate, with an anterior spring, as well as the YC3 Shield and the lower inclined bite plate are useful for improving retroclined upper incisors. Likewise, a 2x4 utility archwire is effective for retracting and aligning proclined lower incisors.

APPLIANCES FOR MAXILLARY ARCH

Posterior Bite Plate with Anterior Spring

Fig. **1** is a posterior bite plate with an anterior spring and labial arch (Figs. **2-4**).

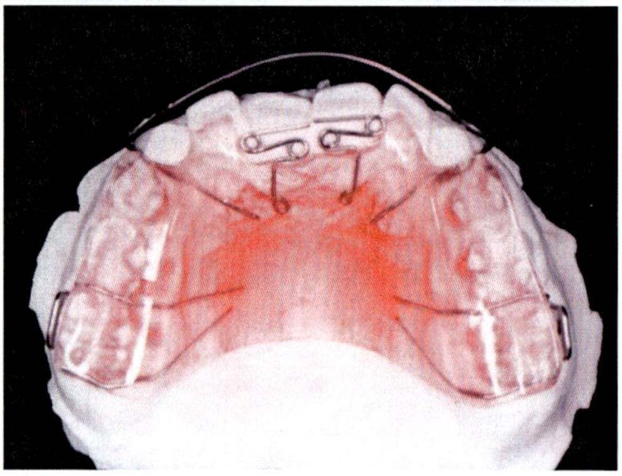

Figure 1: Posterior bite plate with anterior incisal springs.

The bite plate is made of acrylic resin, and the thickness of the posterior bite should be determined by the clearance between the upper and lower incisors (freeway space). The bite opening facilitates anterior cross bite correction by preventing interference of the lower incisors as the upper incisors are advanced. The appliance is usually retained with Adams clasps, and the upper incisors are pushed anteriorly by the activated springs [1, 2, 3]. A labial arch is used to guide the anterior alignment, and it prevents excessive proclination of upper incisors. In addition, the labial arch should be set away from the surface of incisors, with adequate clearance between the labial arch and incisors, to allow forward movement of the upper incisors. The anterior spring and Adams clasps should be adjusted at every appointment. As the anterior crossbite improves, the height of the posterior bite should be reduced gradually at each appointment. The posterior bite should be removed by the end of treatment and the patient should be able to bite with the posterior teeth when the treatment is finished.

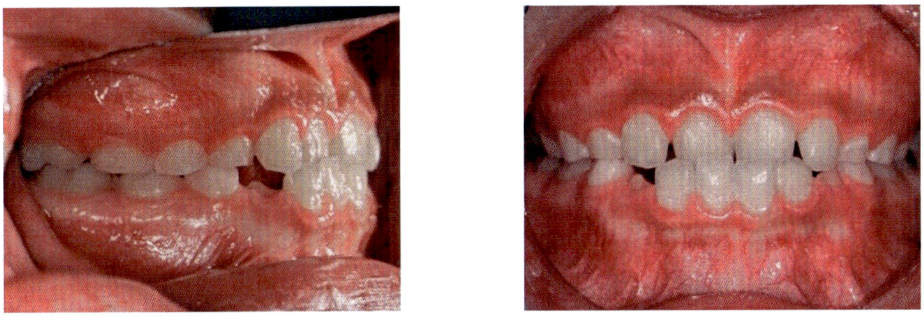

Figure 2: Anterior crossbite before treatment.

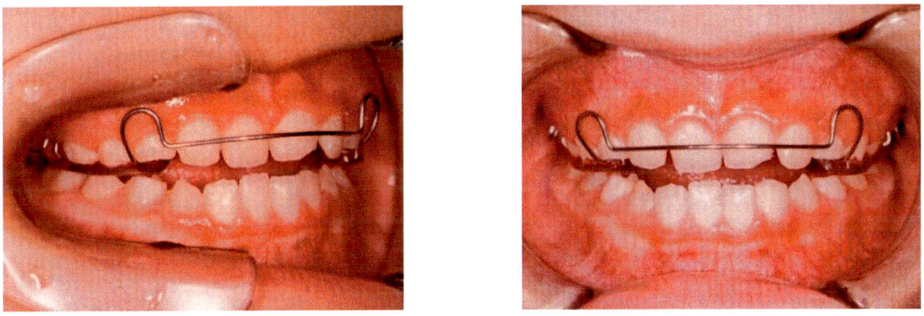

Figure 3: Treatment of anterior crossbite using the posterior bite plate with incisal springs for labial tipping of the maxillary central incisors.

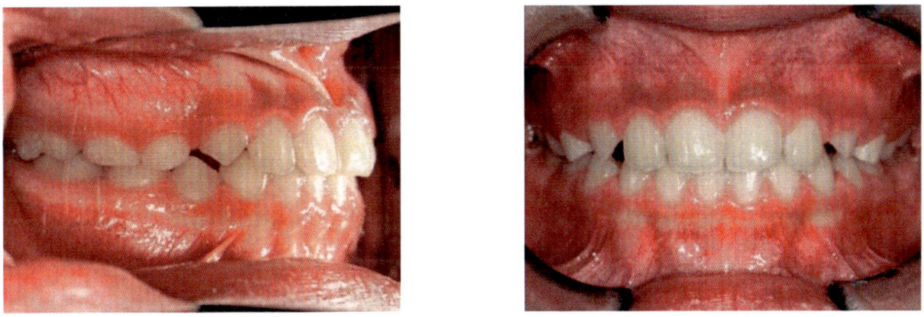

Figure 4: Anterior crossbite after treatment.

Yanagisawa Class III (YC3) Shield

The Yanagisawa Class III (YC3) Shield was developed by M. Yanagisawa (Figs. **5-7**) [4].

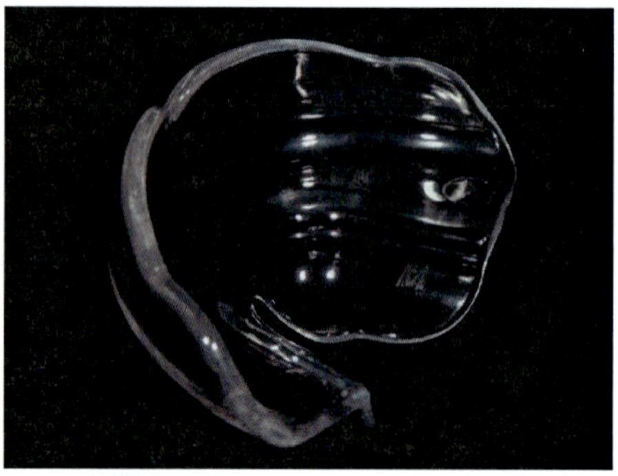

Figure 5: Yanagisawa Class III (YC3) Shield.

According to Yanagisawa [4, 5], the YC3 Shield was developed to elevate the tongue position, which is believed to be a cause for primary anterior crossbite. The YC3 Shield improves the overjet relationship and mandibular position by correcting the axial tooth inclination.

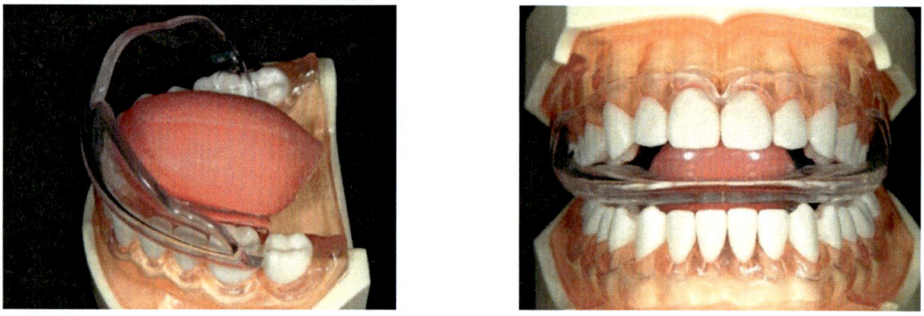

Figure 6: Tongue elevation with the YC3 Shield.

The author [4, 5] also states that the YC3 Shield uses muscular forces (tongue pressure) without applying pressure to the mandible. The YC3 Shield is fitted to the upper dental arch, and the tongue is elevated to the palate; the apex of the tongue is placed behind the upper incisors, and the incisors are pushed forward by the pressure of the tongue. The YC3 Shield corrects not only the dental morphology but also the functional problems, tongue habits and low tongue posture, simultaneously.

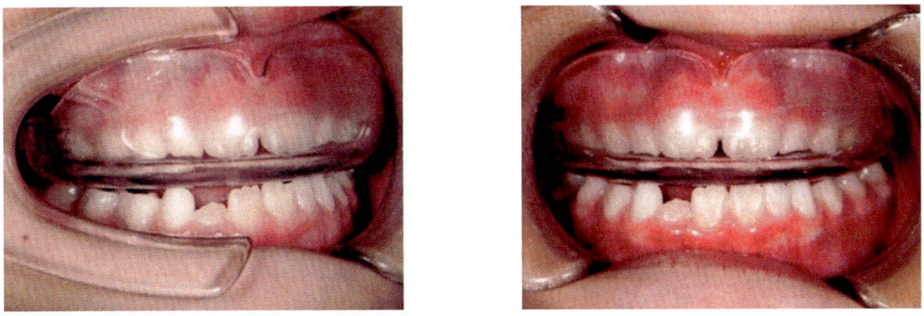

Figure 7: Clinical application of the YC3 Shield.

APPLIANCES FOR THE MANDIBULAR ARCH

Lower Inclined Bite Plate

The lower inclined bite plate consists of a bite plate and an anterior inclined plane. This appliance can be either fixed or removable type, and in some cases, the inclined anterior plane is cemented to the lower incisors [6, 7]. The retroclined upper incisors meet with the lower inclined anterior plane on closure. Maxillary incisors are moved anteriorly by the force of the inclined plane. However, this appliance can be traumatic for the upper incisors; a strong intermittent force is often traumatic. Gentle continuous force is much better for the teeth and periodontal tissues. The lower arch inclined bite plate is cheap, easy to use, and effective, but care must be exercised to prevent trauma to teeth and periodontal tissues. It appears there is no reason for using this appliance instead of the upper bite plate with anterior springs.

Lower 2x4 Utility Archwire

The lower 2x4 utility arch wire (Figs. **8-10**) is a sectional arch. Molar bands with buccal tubes are cemented on the lower permanent molars, and brackets are bonded on the lower incisors. A 0.016 x 0.016 inch stainless steel arch utility wire is contoured and inserted into the molar tubes and incisor brackets. The proclined lower incisors are retracted by the force generated by cinch-back bends on a 2x4 utility archwire [8, 9]. Lingual crown torque is placed in the anterior section of the arch, and tip-back bends are placed anterior to the molars for anchorage. Sometimes, the lower deciduous canines are reduced or extracted to create space in the archform, and an upper bite plate is used simultaneously to create vertical space between the upper and lower incisors. In addition, the 2x4 utility archwire is also applied to the upper arch, and the retroclined upper anterior teeth can be pushed forward in children with Class III malocclusion [9, 10].

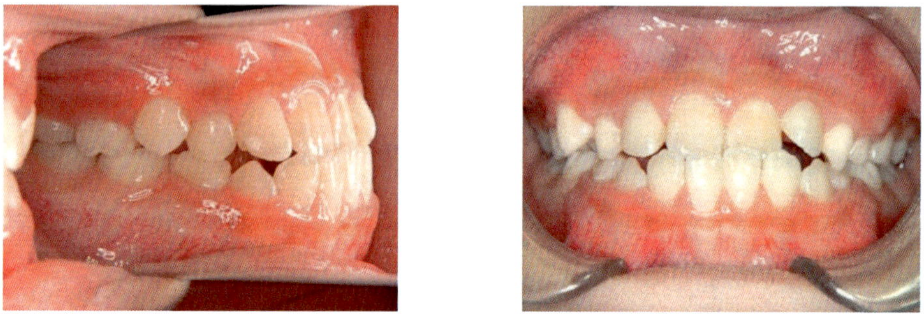

Figure 8: Anterior crossbite before treatment using the lower 2x4 utility arch wire.

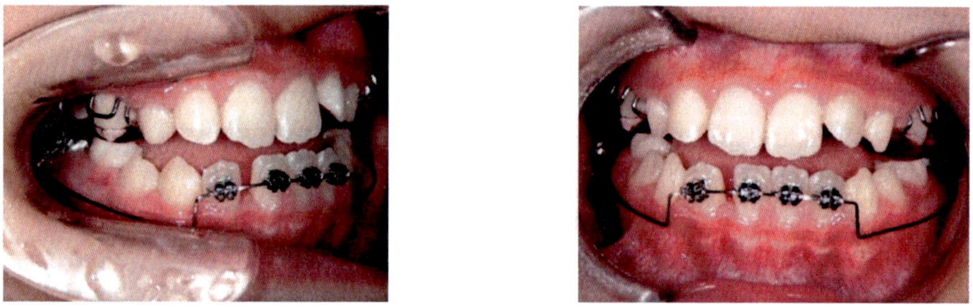

Figure 9: Treatment of anterior crossbite using the lower 2x4 utility arch wire and an upper posterior bite plate.

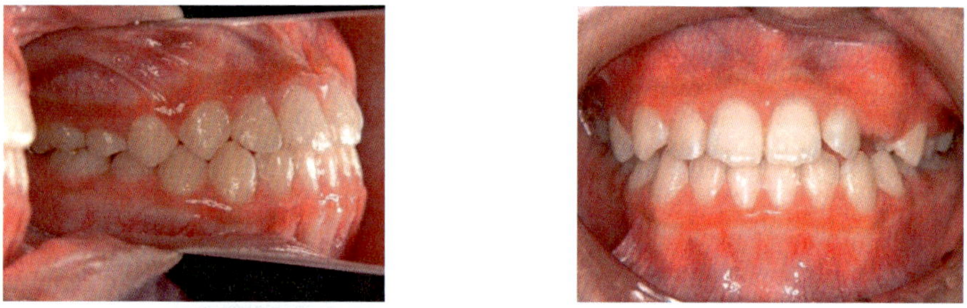

Figure 10: Anterior crossbite after treatment using the lower 2x4 utility arch wire and posterior bite plate.

ORTHOPEDIC CORRECTION

All the intraoral appliances described in this chapter can improve dental and functional problems. Conventional intraoral appliances correct the axis of retroclined upper incisors or proclined lower incisors. However, most children with Class III malocclusions, in the primary dentition, have both dental and skeletal problems. Retrognathic maxilla is a typical skeletal deformity in Class III patients, and an extraoral appliance like a facial mask is usually required to improve the skeletal problems while intraoral appliances are aligning teeth.

Temporary anchorage devices (TADs) have been reported to be effective. Several mini-screws and mini-plates have been developed for absolute anchorage, and most of these devices can be used to correct skeletal deformity while intraoral appliances align the teeth [11-15].

Bone-Anchored Maxillary Protraction (BAMP)

Bone-anchored maxillary protraction (BAMP) was recently developed by H.J. De Clerck and his group [11]. Orthopedic traction is applied to the maxilla with mini-plates; BAMP works as an extraoral protractor and provides orthopedic correction. They used the Bollard Skeletal Anchorage system (Tita-Link, Brussels, Belgium)[12] to improve maxillary deficiencies. The Bollard Skeletal Anchorage devices are inserted into the infrazygomatic crests and canine region in the mandible, and Class III elastics are used for maxillary traction (Fig. **11**) [11, 13, 14, 15].

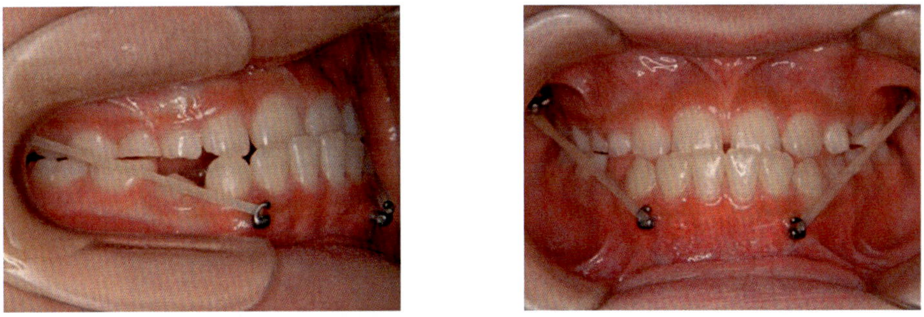

Figure 11: Clinical application of the bone-anchored maxillary protraction (BAMP).

De Clerck stated that titanium miniplates used for anchorage now offer the possibility to apply pure bone-borne orthopedic forces between the maxilla and the mandible for 24 hours per day, avoiding any dentoalveolar compensation [11]. This novel intraoral appliance is completely different from traditional intraoral appliances and can be employed to improve skeletal deficiencies.

SUMMARY

- Early use of intraoral appliances in Class III malocclusion helps to improve the inclination of the retroclined upper incisors and proclined lower incisors.
- Various appliances such as the upper posterior bite plate with anterior springs, the Yanagisawa Class III Shield, the lower inclined bite plane, and the 2x4 utility arches can be used to improve the retroclined upper incisors.
- Intraoral appliances can be used in combination with extraoral protractors to achieve orthopedic treatment. The bone-anchored maxillary protraction (BAMP) works as an extraoral protractor and provides orthopedic correction.

ACKNOWLEDGEMENTS

Declared none.

CONFLICT OF INTEREST

The authors confirm that this chapter content has no conflict of interest.

REFERENCES

[1] Adams P. The design, construction and use of removable orthodontic appliances. 5th ed. Bristol. 1984.

[2] Graber TM, Neuman B. Removable orthodontic appliances. 2nd ed. Saunders. 1984.

[3] Isaacson KG, Muir JD, Reed RT. Removable orthodontic appliances. Butterworth-Heinemann. 2002.

[4] Yanagisawa M. Study of treatment of functional orthodontic appliances in anterior cross-bite (1). J Jpn Orthod Soc. 1985; 44: 734-5.

[5] Onodera K, Niikuni N, Yanagisawa M, Nakajima I. Effects of functional orthodontic appliances in the correction of a primary anterior crossbite--changes in craniofacial morphology and tongue position. Eur J Orthod. 2006; 28: 373-7.

[6] Croll TP, Reisenberger RE. Anterior crossbite correction in the primary dentition using fixed inclined planes. I. Technique and examples. Quintessence Int 1987; 18: 847-53.

[7] Jirgensone I, Liepa A, Abeltins A. Anterior crossbite correction in primary and mixed dentition with removable inclined plane (Bruckl appliance). Stomatologija. 2008; 10: 140-4.

[8] Ricketts RM, Bench RW, Hilgers JJ. Mandibular utility arch. The basic arch in the light progressive technique. Proc Found Orthod Res. 1972: 120-5.

[9] McNamara JA, Brudon WL, Orthodontics and dentofacial orthopedics. Needham Press. 2001.

[10] Dowsing P, Sandler PJ. How to effectively use a 2 x 4 appliance. J Orthod. 2004; 31: 248-58.

[11] De Clerck HJ, Cornelis MA, Cevidanes LH, Heymann GC, Tulloch CJ. Orthopedic traction of the maxilla with miniplates: a new perspective for treatment of midface deficiency. J Oral Maxillofac Surg. 2009; 67: 2123-9.

[12] Cornelis MA, Scheffler NR, Mahy P, Siciliano S, De Clerck HJ, Tulloch JF. Modified miniplates for temporary skeletal anchorage in orthodontics: placement and removal surgeries. J Oral Maxillofac Surg. 2008; 66: 1439-45.

[13] Heymann GC, Cevidanes L, Cornelis M, De Clerck HJ, Tulloch JF. Three-dimensional analysis of maxillary protraction with intermaxillary elastics to miniplates. Am J Orthod Dentofacial Orthop. 2010; 137: 274-84.

[14] De Clerck H, Cevidanes L, Baccetti T. Dentofacial effects of bone-anchored maxillary protraction: a controlled study of consecutively treated Class III patients. Am J Orthod Dentofacial Orthop. 2010; 138: 577-81.

[15] Baccetti T, De Clerck HJ, Cevidanes LH, Franchi L. Morphometric analysis of treatment effects of bone-anchored maxillary protraction in growing Class III patients. Eur J Orthod. 2011; 33: 121-5.

Send Orders for Reprints to reprints@benthamscience.net
Orthodontic Treatment of Class III Malocclusion, 2014, 315-340

CHAPTER 12

Treatment of Class III Malocclusion Using Temporary Anchorage Devices

Young-Chel Park[*] and Yoon Jeong Choi

Department of Orthodentic, Dental College and Dental Hospitals, Yonsei University Seoul, South Korea

Abstract: Class III treatment can be divided into two categories: Orthopedic treatment for developing Class III malocclusions in growing patients and camouflage/surgical treatment for non-growing Class III patients. Recently, several articles have described on the use of temporary anchorage devices (TADs) for protracting the maxilla in developing Class III patients [1, 2]. The application of TADs can maximize the skeletal response of maxillary protraction and minimize the side effects such as dentoalveolar protrusion. TADs can be placed in the inter-proximal alveolar bone, with attachment to a tooth-born protraction device, or can be used directly in the form of a mini-plate for maxillary protraction. In adult patients, Class III malocclusion either is camouflaged by orthodontic tooth movement or is treated in combination with orthognathic surgery. The use of TADs has narrowed the gap between the two types of treatment modalities because it has expanded the range of orthodontic camouflage treatment. In camouflage treatment, a Class III relationship is usually corrected via differential tooth movement of the upper and lower dentition with premolar extraction. In non-extraction treatment, the anterior movement of the upper dentition and/or posterior movement of the lower dentition can be used to correct the Class III relationship. In this chapter, the authors will focus on the anchorage consideration in treatment of Class III malocclusion with extraction of the lower premolars and non-extraction with distalization of the lower dentition. In addition, an adult cleft palate case is presented in which maxillary expansion was reinforced by the use of TADs. The application of TADs for decompensation in Class III surgery cases is also discussed.

Keywords: Class III camouflage treatment, Temporary Anchorage Devices (TADs), Extraction treatment, Non-extraction treatment.

INTRODUCTION

Class III treatments can be divided into the orthopedic approach, which is used for growing patients, and either camouflage treatment or surgical treatment, which is used

***Address correspondence to Young-Chel Park:** Department of Orthodontics, The institute of craniofacial deformity, Dental College and Dental Hospital, Yonsei University, SEO DAI MUN GU, SHIN CHONDONG1234, CPO BOX 8044, Seoul, South Korea; Tel: +82-2-2228-3101; E-mail: ypark@yuhs.ac

Peter W. Ngan, Toshi Deguchi and Eugene W. Roberts (Eds)

for non-growing patients. Recently, the use of protraction of the maxilla by using TADs was reported in growing patients[1, 2]. The application of TADs can maximize the effect of maxillary protraction and minimize side effects such as dentoalveolar protrusion. TADs implanted into interproximal alveolar bone can be attached to a tooth-born protraction device, and it can be used to protract the maxilla directly in the form of a mini-plate.

In adult patients, Class III malocclusion is treated either by orthodontic camouflage or by orthognathic surgery. TADs changed the conventional borderline between the two modalities by expanding the range of the orthodontic camouflage. In the camouflage treatment, the Class III relationship can be corrected by differential tooth movement of the upper and lower dentition with premolar extraction. In non-extraction treatment, the anterior movement of the upper dentition and/or posterior movement of the lower dentition can correct the Class III relationship.

In this chapter, we focus on maximum anchorage in the treatment of lower premolar extraction and distalization of the lower dentition for non-extraction treatment. Additionally, we describe maxillary expansion by using TADs in an adult cleft patient. The application of TADs for decompensation in a Class III surgery patient is also presented.

Anchorage Reinforcement

In the extraction treatment of Class III patients, the canine and molar relationships and the anterior crossbite are corrected by the differential anchorage value of the upper and lower arch. Maximum anchorage is usually required in the mandible, and TADs can be used for this purpose. TADs implanted in the inter-radicular bone are commonly used to retract the anterior teeth that serve as an absolute anchorage.

Several factors should be considered for retraction of the anterior teeth by using a TAD. First, the TAD ensures that the teeth move within the alveolar housing because the teeth, particularly the anterior teeth, are likely to move out of the cortex if full retraction of the anterior teeth occurs without anchorage loss.

Controlled tipping of the anterior teeth would be an alternative if the teeth were expected to be out of the symphysis after full retraction.

Second, the vertical vector of the retraction force should be designed carefully with regard to the occlusal plane cant. If the vertical vector is absent, i.e., the retraction force is parallel to the archwire, the occlusal plane would not be changed. However, when the retraction force has either an intrusive or an extrusive vector, the rotation of the occlusal plane occurs is followed by changes in the anterior facial height and the mandibular position. The change in the occlusal plane can be observed when the 2nd molar was not included the archwire (Fig. **1**).

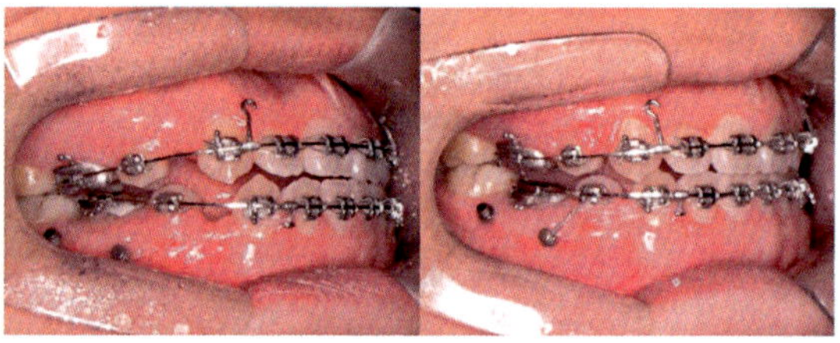

Figure 1: The retraction vector of the mandibular arch from the archwire hook to the TAD was intrusive (left), which resulted in changes in the occlusal plane (right). Note the marginal ridge discrepancy between the 1st and the 2nd molars after space closure (right).

Case 1 (29 years, Female – Fig. 2)

Chief complaint - Lower crowding, edgebite

Problem lists - mild Skeletal Class III

- Missing on #14,24.
- Short root on #21,25,35,45,37,47.
- Class III canine and Class II molar relationships on both sides.
- Edge-to-edge bite.
- Lower anterior crowding.
- Lower dental midline shift to the right (2.5 mm).

Diagnosis - Skeletal Class III with missing on #14,24.

Treatment plans - Extraction of #35,45.

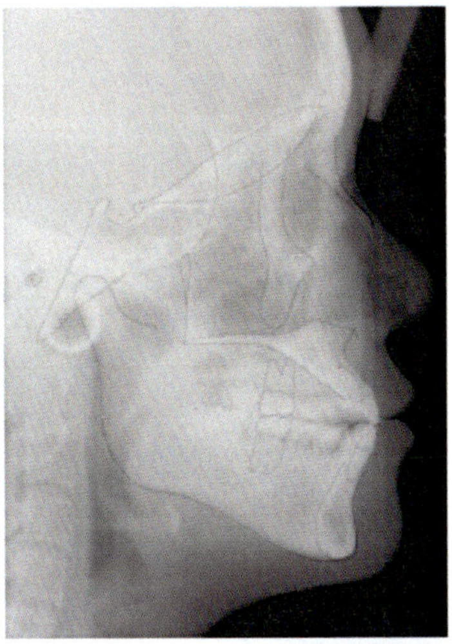

	Initial	Final
SNA (°)	72.8	72.9
SNB (°)	73.4	74.0
ANB (°)	-0.6	-1.1
Wits (mm)	-7.1	-7.3
SN to MP (°)	39.7	38.2
Bjork Sum (°)	399.7	398.2
U1 to SN (°)	104.5	104.0
IMPA (°)	96.2	88.5
U1 to N-Pog (mm)	8.7	8.5
L1 to N-Pog (mm)	7.6	3.1
UL to E-line (mm)	-0.9	-1.6
LL to E-line (mm)	0.4	-3.0

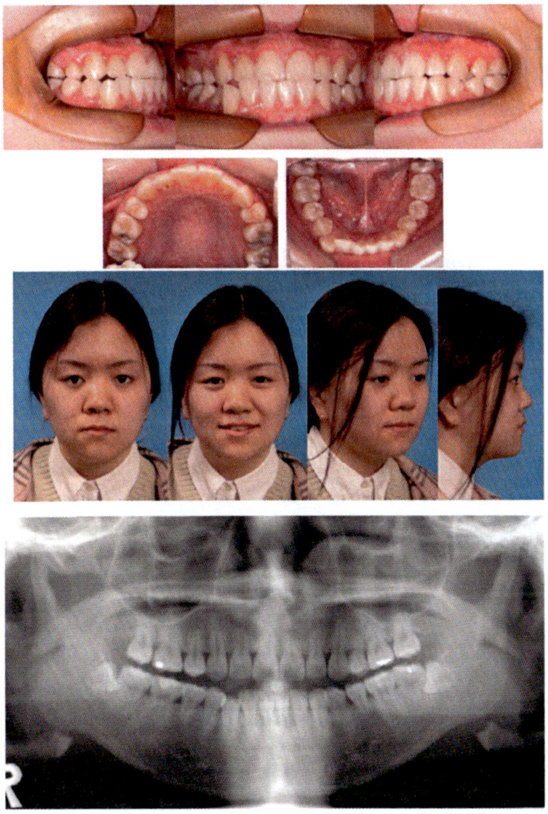

Figure 2-1: Initial photographs and panoramic and lateral cephalometric radiographs.

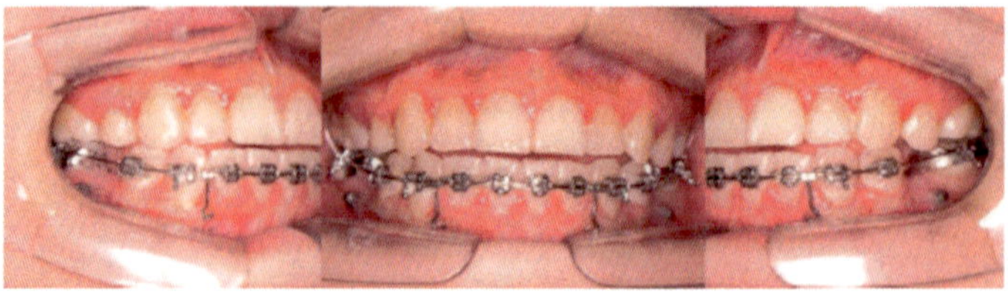

Figure 2-2: During space closure, the retraction forces were applied from the long crimpable hooks to the TADs implanted mesial to the 1st molars. The 2nd premolars were extracted instead of the 1st premolars because of the short root length; therefore, the use of TADs was planned in order to reinforce the anchorage. The archwire was .019x.025 stainless steel (SS), and the retraction vector was parallel to the archwire. A decision was made not to treat the maxillary dentition because the roots were generally short.

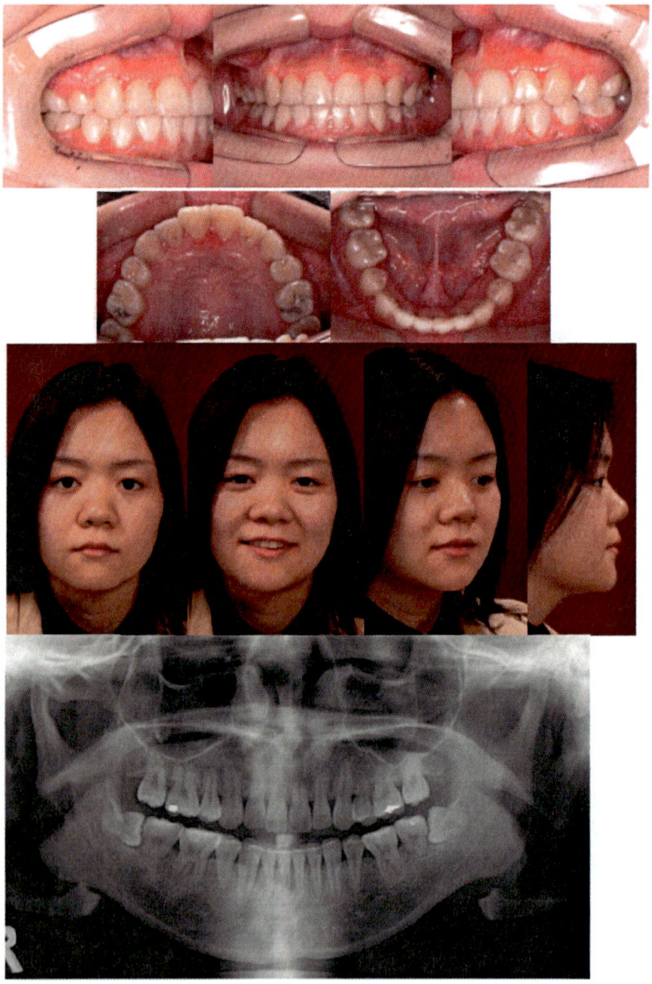

Fig. 2: contd….

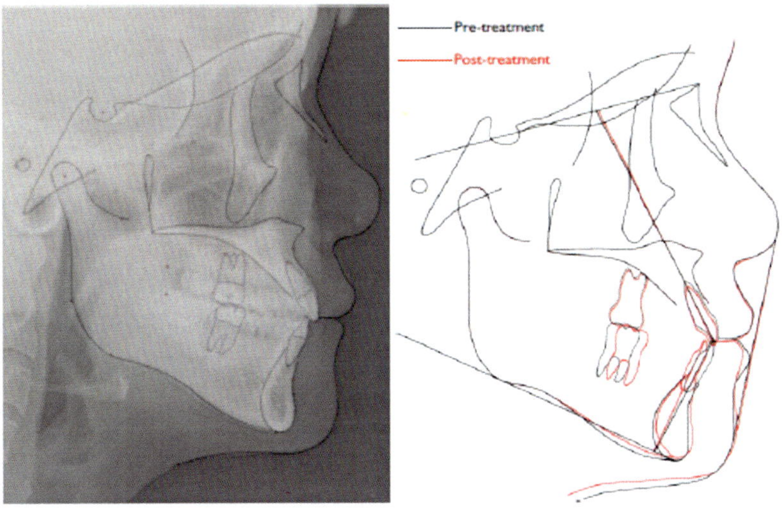

Figure 2-3: Post-treatment records and superimposition of the lateral cephalogram. The lower anterior teeth moved lingually, and a proper overjet and overbite were established. Since the maxillary teeth and the mandibular 2nd molars were not included in the orthodontic treatment, additional root resorption did not occur.

TADs are used either directly or indirectly as a skeletal anchorage. As shown in Fig. **3**, TADS placed between two adjacent roots can be used to place the elastic module and to retract/protract teeth. Under these circumstances, the TAD serves directly as a skeletal anchorage. Sometimes, the TAD can be connected to the adjacent tooth by using a ligature wire (Fig. **3-2**, maxilla) or by the use of resin-wire splinting (Fig. **3-2**, mandible).

Case 2 (19 years, Male – Fig. 3)

Chief complaint - Prognathic chin, lip protrusion

Problem lists - mild Skeletal Class III

- Fused teeth on #32=#33.
- Class III canine molar relationships on both sides
- Anterior crossbite.
- Mild crowding

- Fractured restoration on #14.

Diagnosis - Skeletal Class III with fused teeth on #32=#33.

Treatment plans - Extraction of #14,25,34,44.

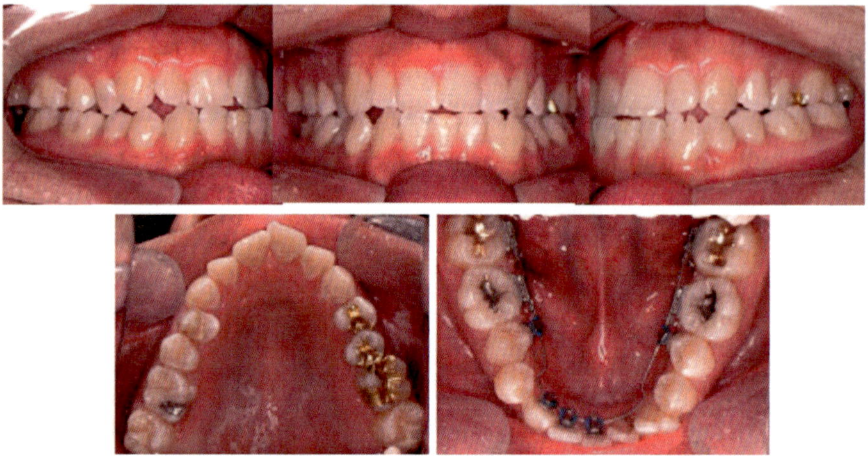

Figure 3-1: Initial intraoral photographs. To correct lip protrusion, #14, 25, 34, and 44 were extracted. Because of the fractured restoration, #14 was selected. Note that #32 and #33 were fused.

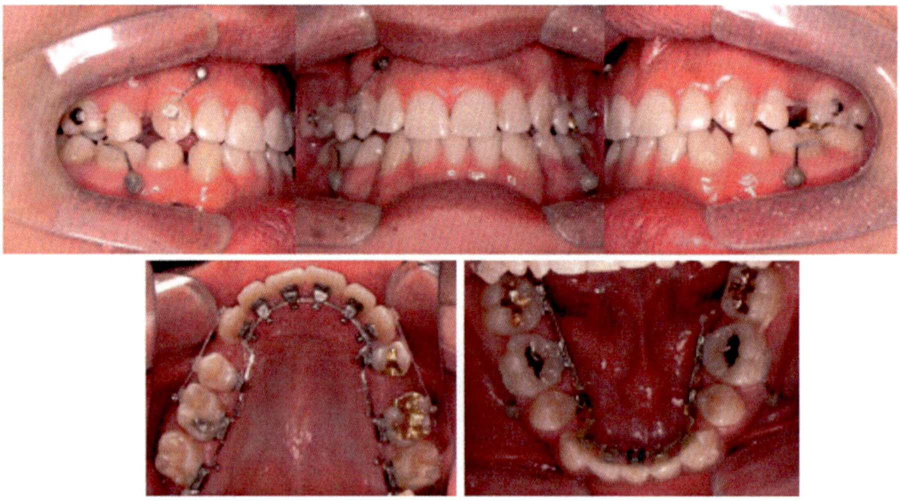

Figure 3-2: During space closure, the TADs in the mandible were bonded to the 1st molars to prevent anchorage loss, and the TAD in the maxilla was connected to the canine with a metal ligature to prevent distal movement of the anterior teeth.

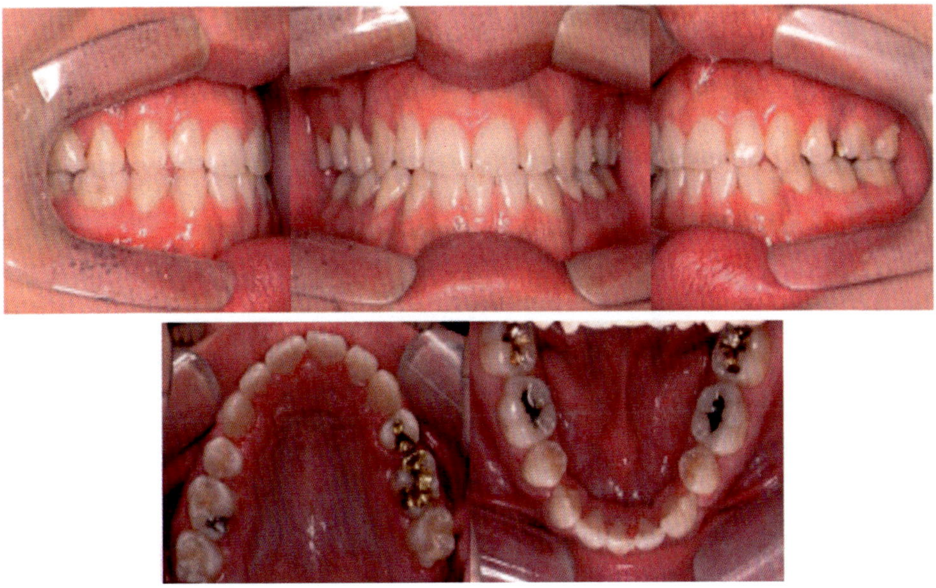

Figure 3-3: Post-treatment intraoral photographs. The posterior teeth in the maxilla were protracted, and the anterior teeth in the mandible were retracted with the aid of TADs.

Case 3 (20 years, Male – Fig. 4)

Chief complaint - Crowding

Problem lists - mild Skeletal Class III

- Congenital missing on #22.
- Class I canine and molar relationships on both sides.
- Anterior crossbite.
- Lower anterior crowding.
- Upper and lower dental midline shift to the left (2.0 mm).

Diagnosis - Skeletal Class III with missing on #22.

Treatment plans - Extraction of #14,44.

Space regaining on #22 and implant.

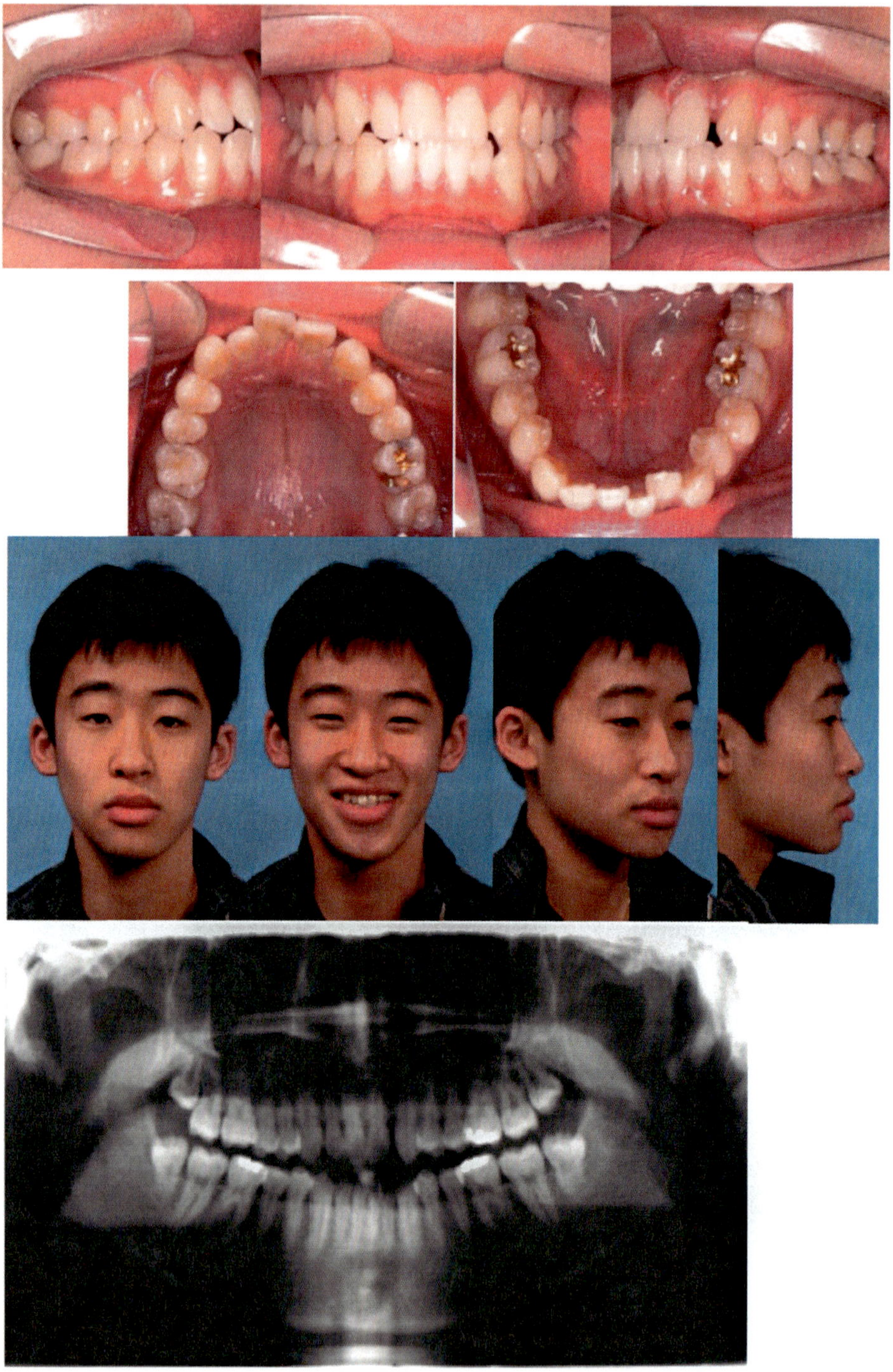

Fig. 4: contd….

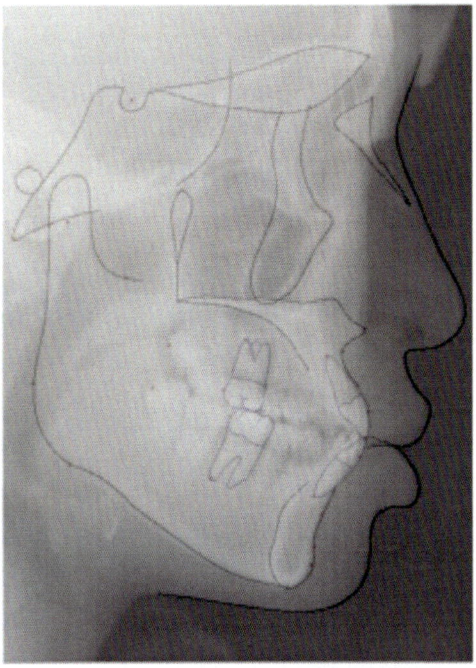

	Initial	Final	Retention
SNA (°)	82.8	82.8	82.9
SNB (°)	82.6	82.9	82.6
ANB (°)	0.2	-0.1	0.3
Wits (mm)	-4.3	-4.6	-5.0
SN to MP (°)	28.9	27.7	28.0
Bjork Sum (°)	388.9	387.7	388.6
U1 to SN (°)	115.9	109.1	111.2
IMPA (°)	103.4	91.4	92.5
U1 to N-Pog (mm)	10.9	8.0	9.0
L1 to N-Pog (mm)	10.6	5.2	6.3
UL to E-line (mm)	1.1	0.9	-1.9
LL to E-line (mm)	4.9	4.2	2.8

Figure 4-1: Initial photographs and panoramic and lateral cephalometric radiographs.

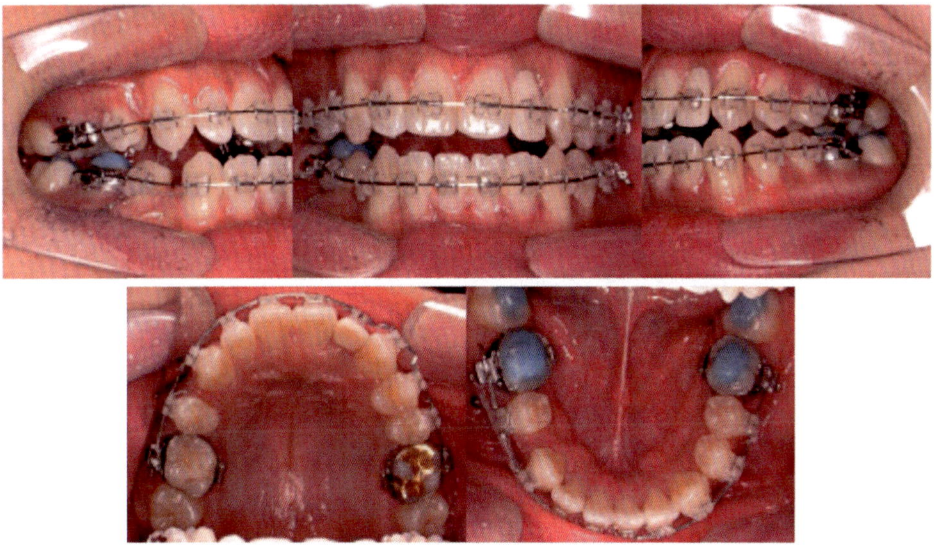

Figure 4-2: During space closure, the TAD was implanted between the lower right 1st molar and the 2nd premolar; subsequently, the TAD was connected to the 2nd premolar to prevent mesial movement. To correct the crossbite, bite resins were temporarily bonded to the occlusal surface of the lower molars.

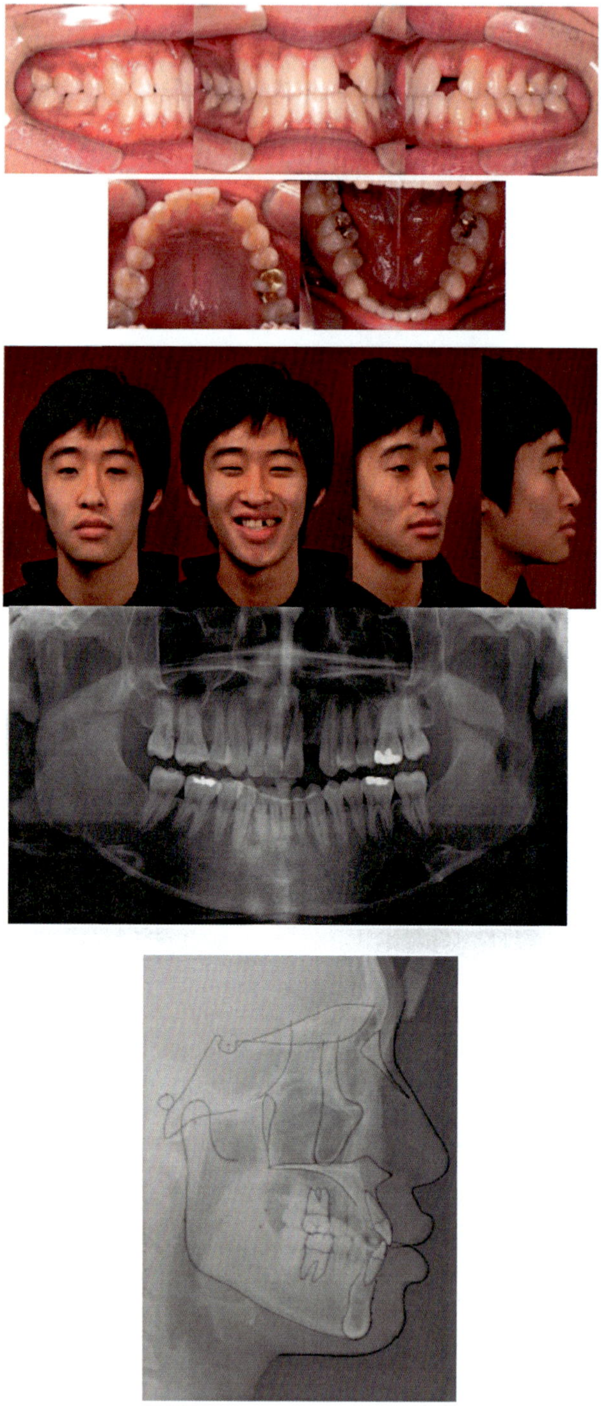

Figure 4-3: Post-treatment records. A space was obtained for the maxillary left lateral incisor, and the upper and the lower dental midlines were coincident with the facial midline.

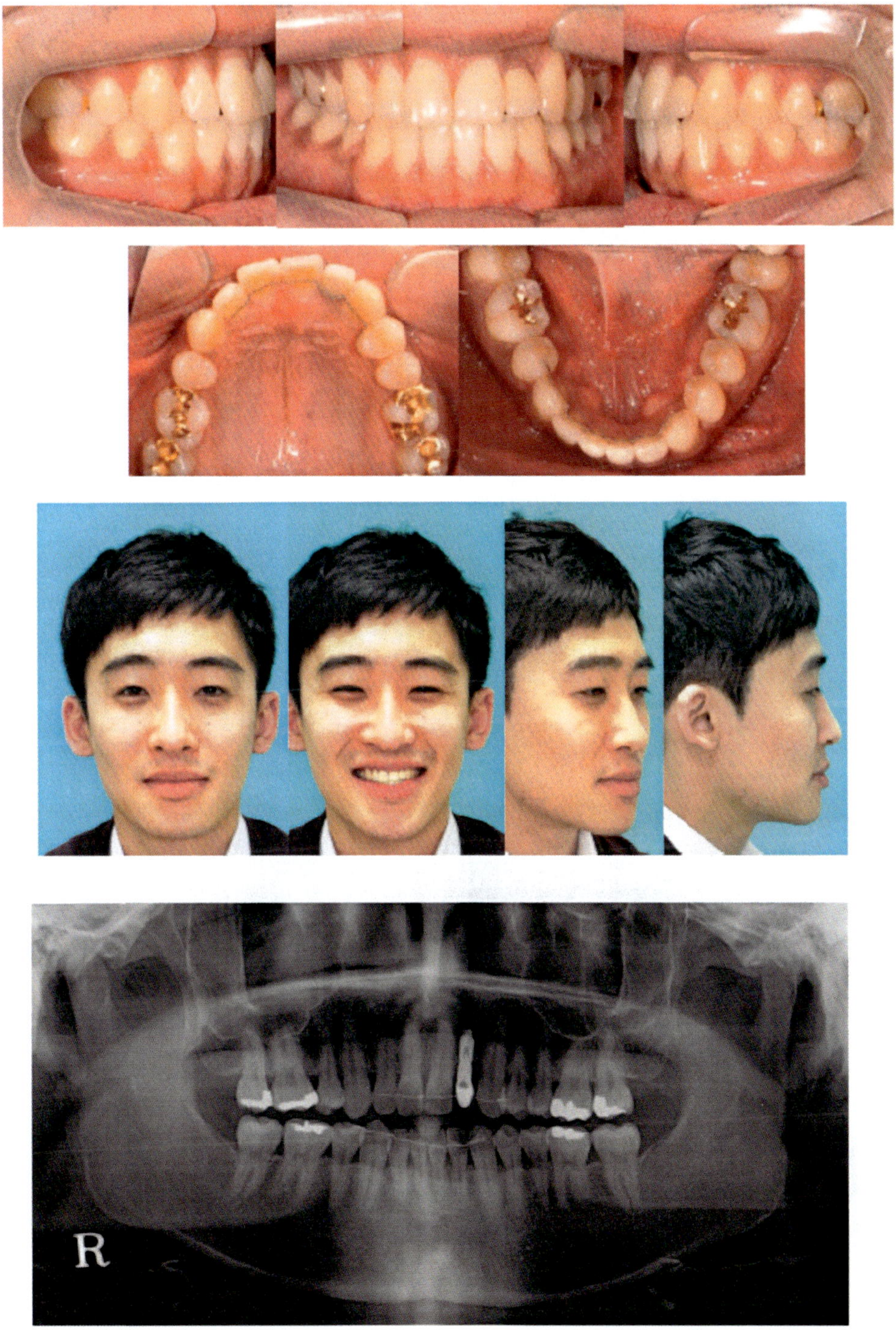

Fig. 4: contd….

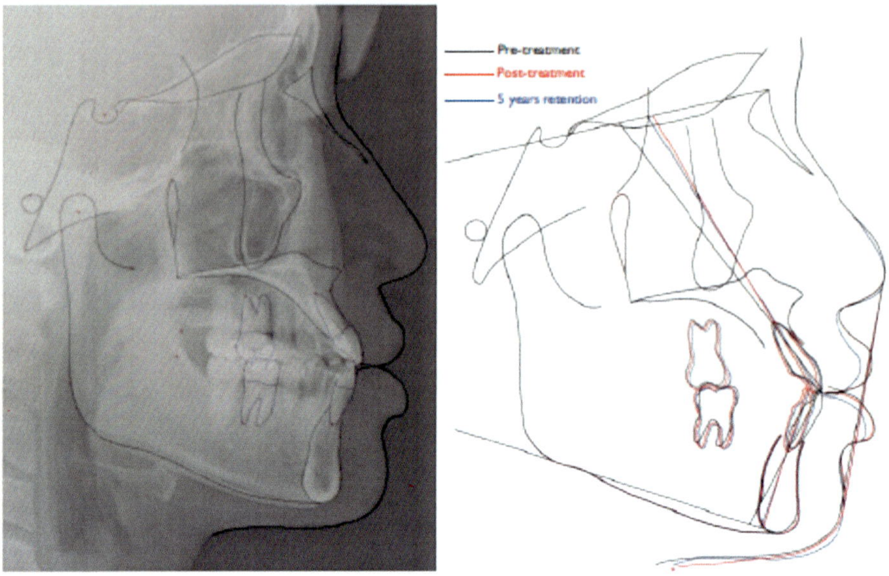

Figure 4-4: 5 years of retention. The maxillary left lateral incisor had been implanted, resulting in satisfactory retention. Although the position of the upper and lower lips showed few changes during treatment, the upper and lower lips were retruded 2.0 mm and 1.4 mm, respectively at 5 years after treatment.

Distalization of the Lower Dentition

TADs can move the entire dentition of the mandible backward to correct Class III relationships. Based on the amount of distalization, either a mini-plate or mini-implant can be used as a skeletal anchorage. As reported by Sugawara *et al.* [3], the mini-plate is capable of moving the entire dentition, regardless of tooth movement, because it is placed below the root apices or in the retromolar area. The mini-implant is an alternative, if a small amount of distalization is planned.

Case 4 (22 years, Male – Fig. 5)

Chief complaint - Anterior crossbite.

Problem lists - mild Skeletal Class III.

- Missing state of four 1st premolars due to previous orthodontic treatment.

- Class III canine and molar relationships on both sides.

- Anterior crossbite.

- Lower anterior spacing.

- Lower dental midline shift to the right (1.0 mm).

Diagnosis - Skeletal Class III with anterior crossbite.

Treatment plans – Total distalization of the lower dentition after extraction of the 3rd molars.

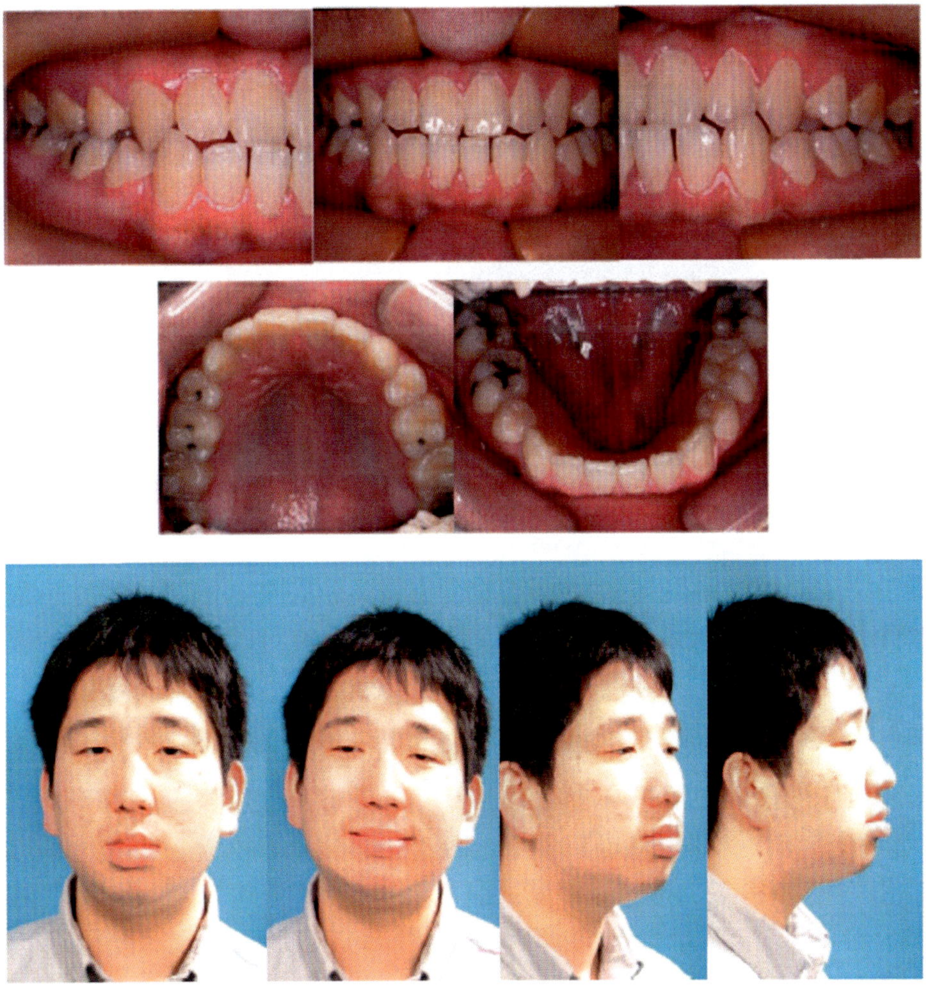

Fig. 5: contd....

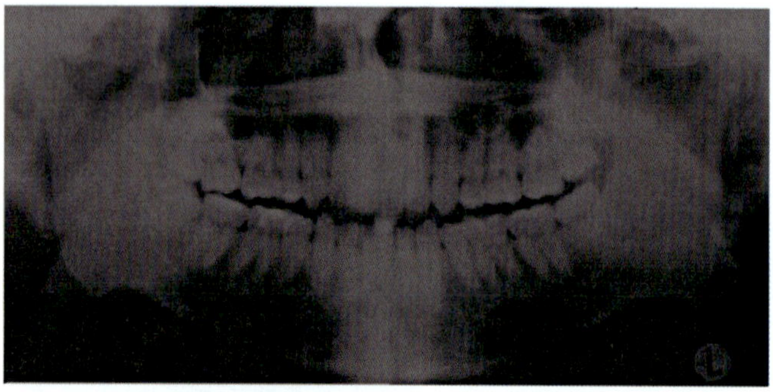

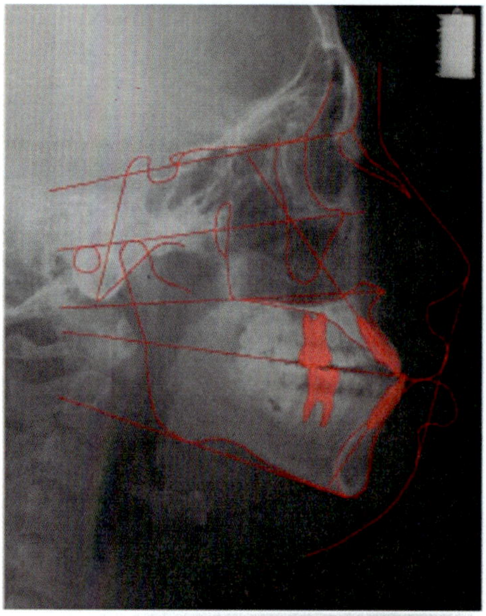

	Initial	Final
SNA (°)	81.6	82.3
SNB (°)	80.3	80.8
ANB (°)	1.3	1.5
Wits (mm)	-6.3	-4.4
SN to MP (°)	31.5	31.8
Bjork Sum (°)	391.5	391.8
U1 to SN (°)	110.3	111.3
IMPA (°)	106.5	95.3
U1 to N-Pog (mm)	12.8	12.8
L1 to N-Pog (mm)	14.8	9.4
UL to E-line (mm)	1.2	1.8
LL to E-line (mm)	8.9	8.0

Figure 5-1: Initial photographs and panoramic and lateral cephalometric radiographs.

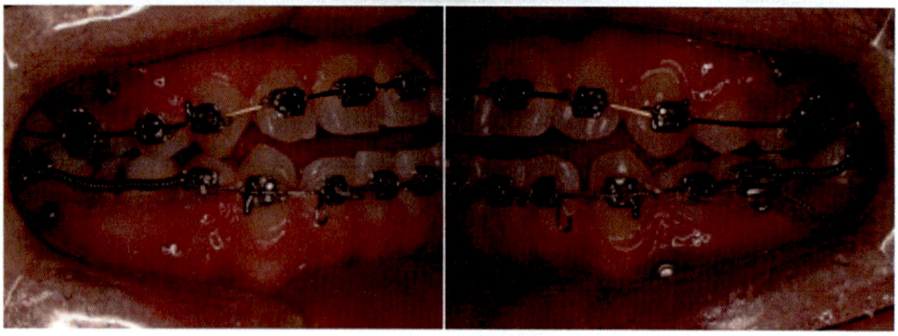

Figure 5-2: During total distalization of the lower arch, the mesial movement of the anterior teeth was prevented by the TADs between the lower 1st and 2nd molars. The 2nd molars were distalized with an open-coil spring, and the elastic module cancelled out the counteracting force.

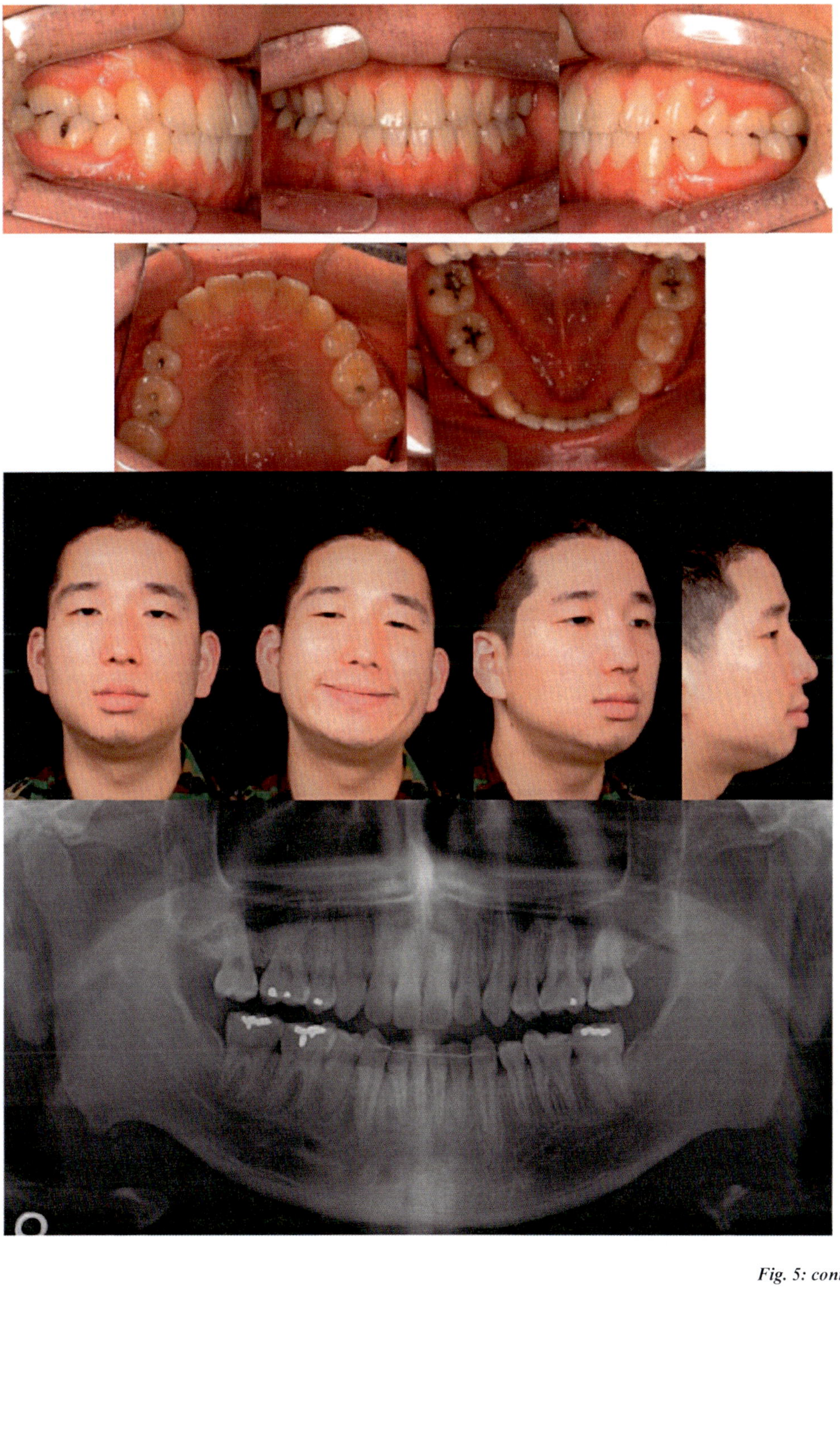

Fig. 5: contd….

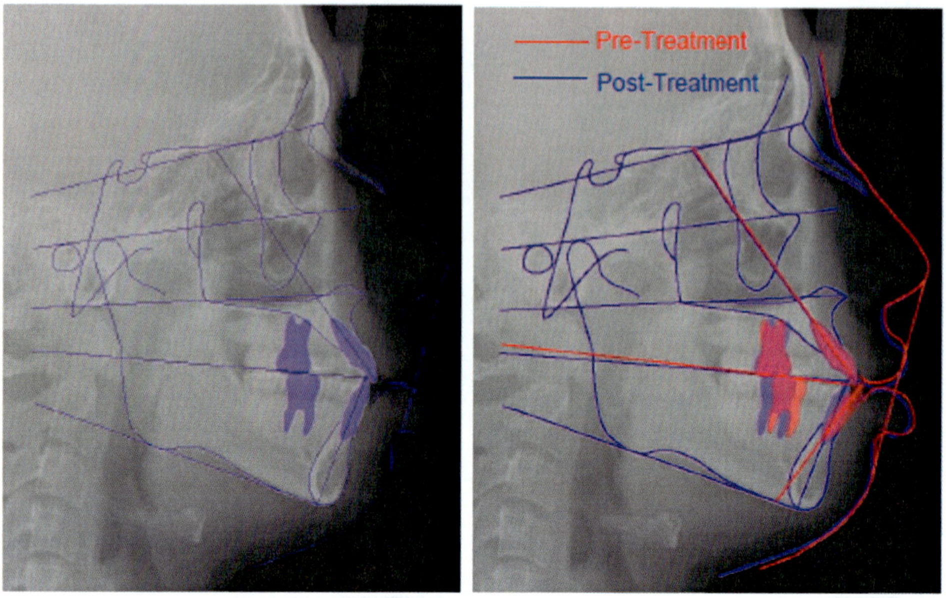

Figure 5-3: Post-treatment records and the superimposition of lateral cephalograms. The mandibular arch was distalized 2.5 mm, and a Class I molar relationship and proper overjet were established.

Maxillary Expansion in Adult Patients

Maxillary expansion is a challenging issue in non-growing patients. Previously, surgically assisted rapid maxillary expansion (RME) was the only solution for the constricted maxilla. However, TADs have been used for this purpose recently. Hyrax-type-RME can be combined with TADs implanted in the palate, and the achievement of maxillary orthopedic expansion by using this technique has been reported [4]. The miniscrew-assisted RME expands the maxilla sufficiently with minimal tipping of the buccal segment.

Maxillary constriction owing to the scar tissue in the palate is commonly observed in cleft palate patients who received palatal surgery in their youth. The constricted maxilla should be expanded for arch coordination, and the miniscrew-assisted RME can be a good alternative.

Case 5 (19 years, Male – Fig. 6)

Chief complaint - Crowding, anterior crossbite.

Problem lists - unilateral cleft lip and palate with scar tissue in the palate.

- Mild Skeletal Class III.
- Congenital missing state of #12,22.
- Class I on right and Class II on left canine and molar relationships.
- Anterior crossbite.
- Transverse discrepancy in the canine and the premolar areas.
- Lower anterior crowding.

Diagnosis - Skeletal Class III with unilateral cleft lip and palate congenital missing of #12,22.

Treatment plans - Maxillary expansion with miniscrew-assisted fan-type RME with extracton of #34,44 reshaping of #13,33.

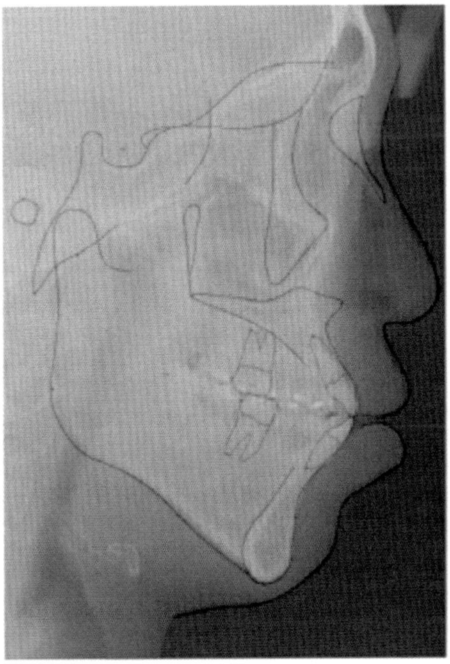

	Initial	Final
SNA (°)	69.5	69.6
SNB (°)	69.6	69.7
ANB (°)	-0.1	-0.1
Wits (mm)	-3.4	-5.7
SN to MP (°)	47.8	47.4
Bjork Sum (°)	407.8	407.4
U1 to SN (°)	105.8	96.2
IMPA (°)	96.8	85.0
U1 to N-Pog (mm)	12.4	8.6
L1 to N-Pog (mm)	12.3	5.5
UL to E-line (mm)	3.7	1.6
LL to E-line (mm)	9.6	3.3

Fig. 6: contd....

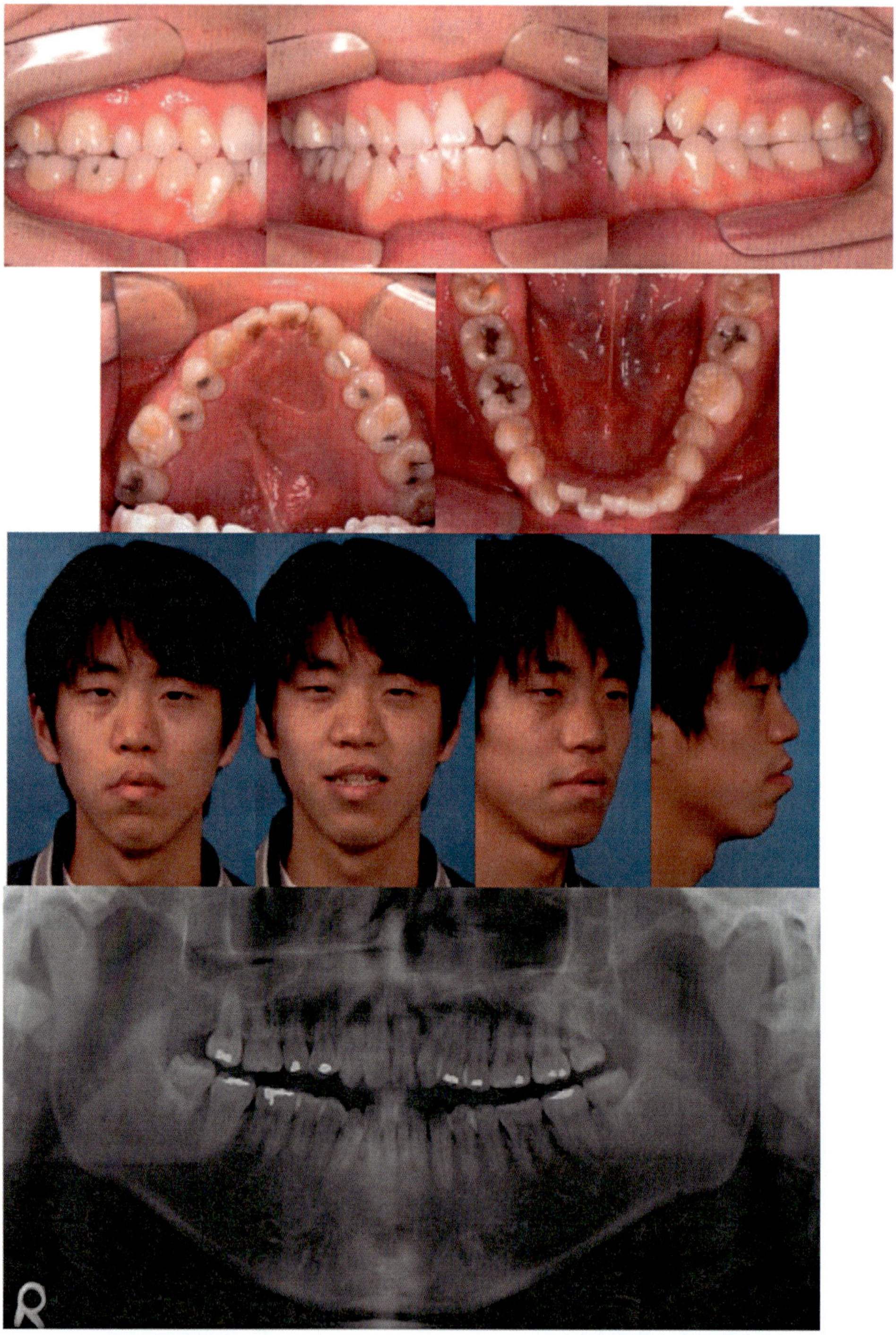

Figure 6-1: Initial photographs and panoramic and lateral cephalometric radiographs.

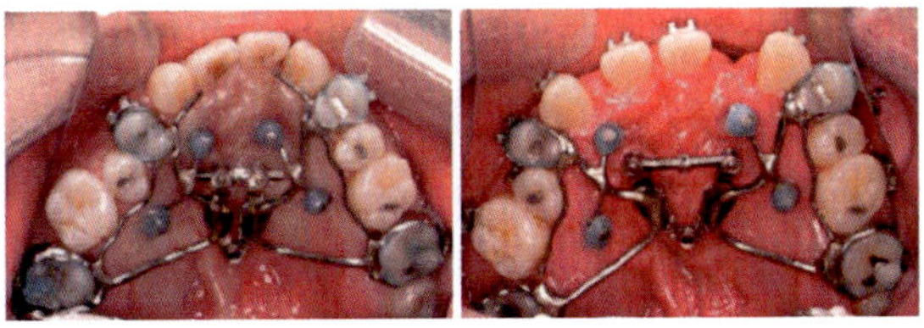

Figure 6-2: Miniscrew-assisted rapid maxillary expansion (RME). A fan-type RME was placed to resolve the transverse discrepancy in the canine and the premolar areas. Four miniscrews were implanted into the palatal slope and were connected to the extension arms of the RME with resin bonding material (left). The patient was instructed to turn the screw every day, and maxillary expansion was noted after 2 months (right). However, the total amount of turning was not certain because the patient did not turn the screw everyday. After 4 months of retention, the RME was removed and a fixed appliance was bonded in the upper and lower arches.

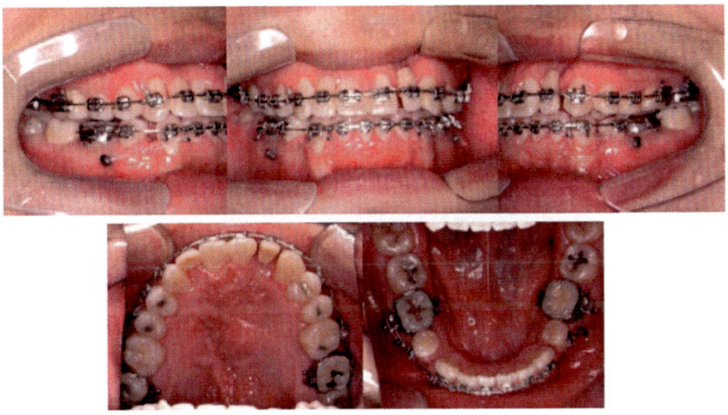

Figure 6-3: After bonding the fixed appliances, the two lower 1st premolars were extracted and the pontics between the central incisor and canine were placed for esthetic reasons. TADs were implanted in the mesial alveolar bone of the lower 1st molars for the purpose of retracting the anterior teeth.

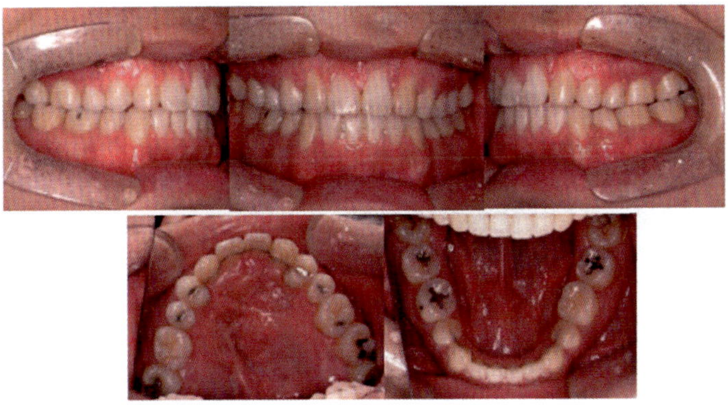

Fig. 6: contd....

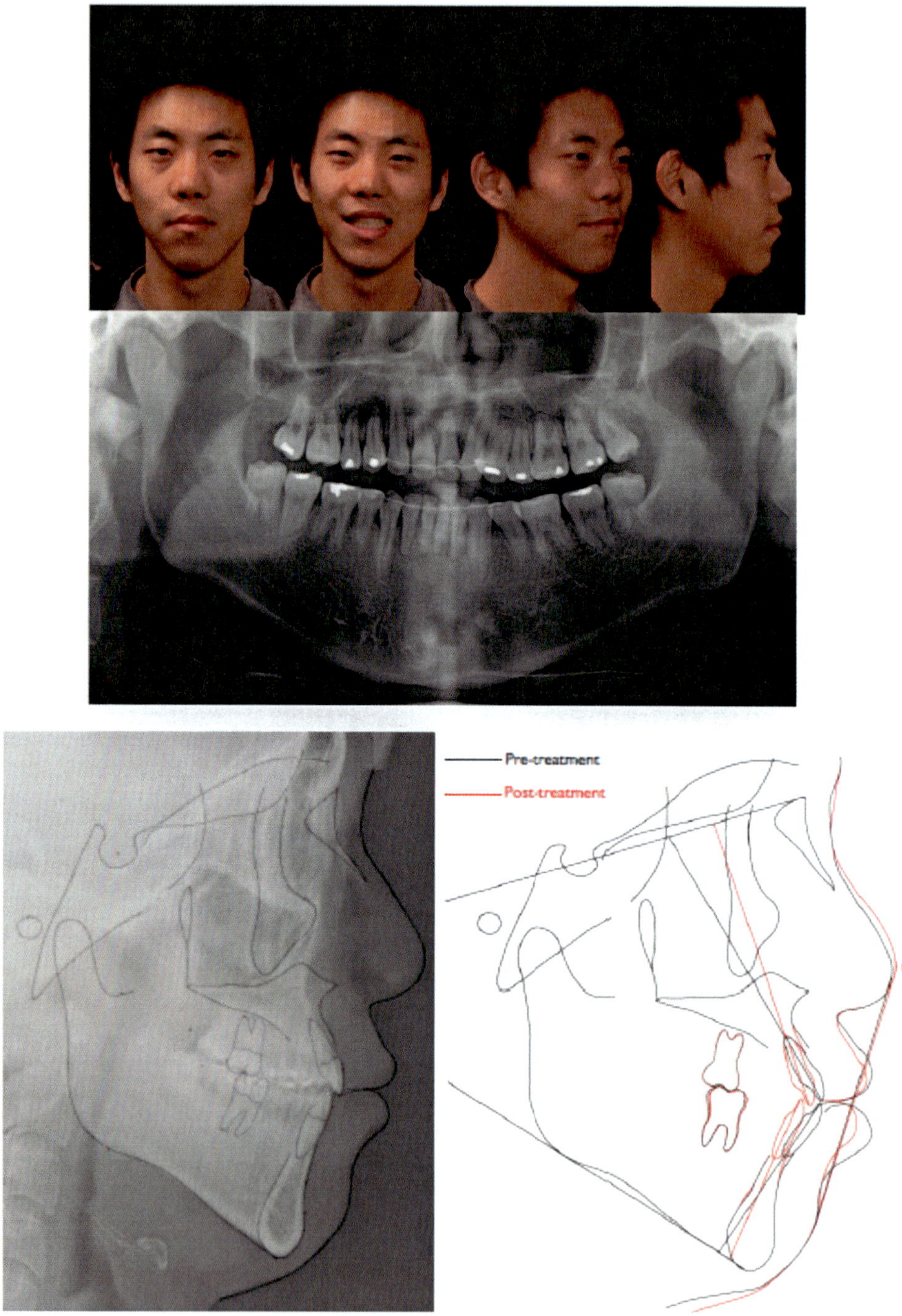

Figure 6-4: Post-treatment records and the superimposition of lateral cephalograms. (continued) The maxillary canines were substituted for the missing lateral incisors, and a proper buccal overjet was established by expanding the maxillary arch.

Efficient Decompensation Treatment in Class III Surgery Patients

In Class III surgery patients, the upper and lower teeth show dental compensation. The lower anterior teeth are tipped lingually, and this should be de-compensated during the pre-surgical orthodontic treatment. When lower anterior crowding exists, relief of crowding can decompensate the lingual-tipped incisors. However, if spacing exists in the lower arch, labial flaring for decompensation creates more space. In this situation, anterior segmental surgery or an implant after space re-distribution can be considered.

Total protraction is possible by using TADs for total distalization of the lower dentition. The elastic module from the distal hook to the mesial TAD delivers the protraction force to the total dentition. Controlled tipping should be used for labial movement of the lower anterior teeth to prevent or reduce the possibility of gingival recession.

Case 6 (18 years, Female – Fig. 7)

Chief complaint - Mandibular prognathism.

Problem lists - Skeletal Class III.

- Facial asymmetry.
- Class III canine and molar relationships on both sides.
- Anterior crossbite.
- Linguoversion of lower anterior teeth (IMPA: 69.5°).
- Lower anterior spacing.

Diagnosis - Skeletal Class III with facial asymmetry.

Treatment plans - Non-extraction 2 jaw surgery with proclination of lower dentition for decompensation using TADs.

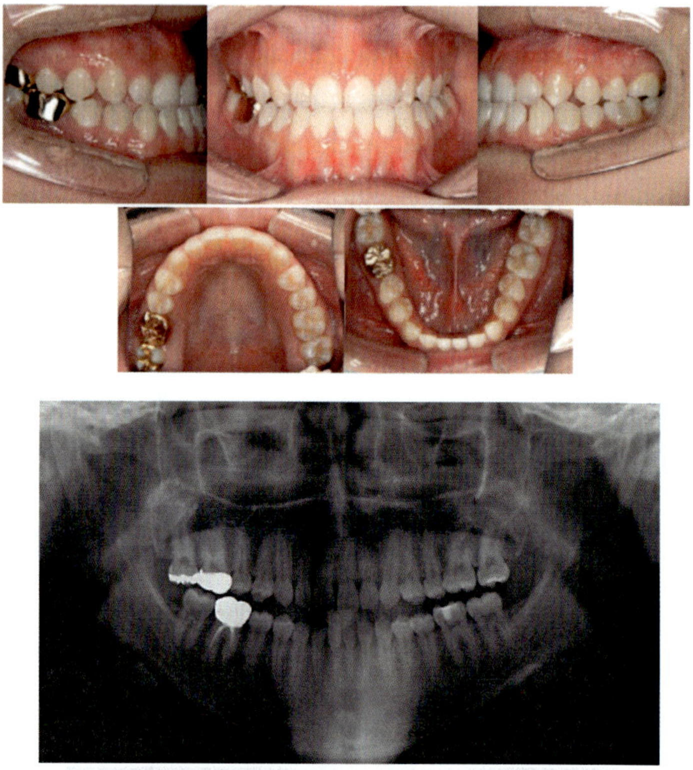

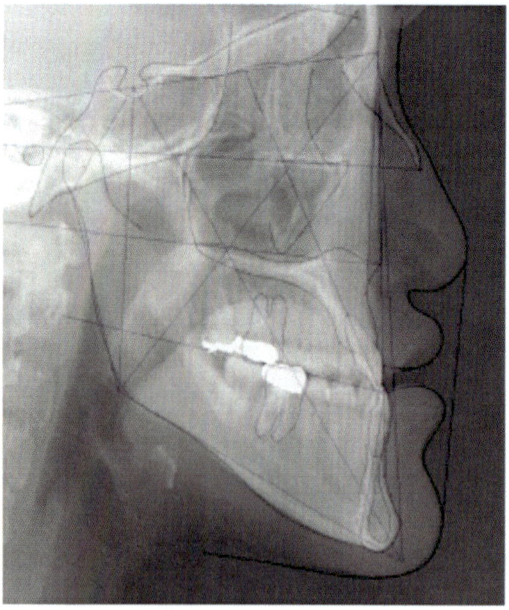

	Initial	Pre-op
SNA (°)	79.7	80.2
SNB (°)	83.5	83.8
ANB (°)	-3.8	-3.6
Wits (mm)	-16.3	-13.8
SN to MP (°)	37.8	36.9
Bjork Sum (°)	397.8	396.9
U1 to SN (°)	105.9	107.1
IMPA (°)	69.7	79.1
U1 to N-Pog (mm)	4.0	4.1
L1 to N-Pog (mm)	2.6	4.8
UL to E-line (mm)	-4.5	-5.6
LL to E-line (mm)	-2.0	-0.4

Figure 7-1: Initial photographs and panoramic and lateral cephalometric radiographs.

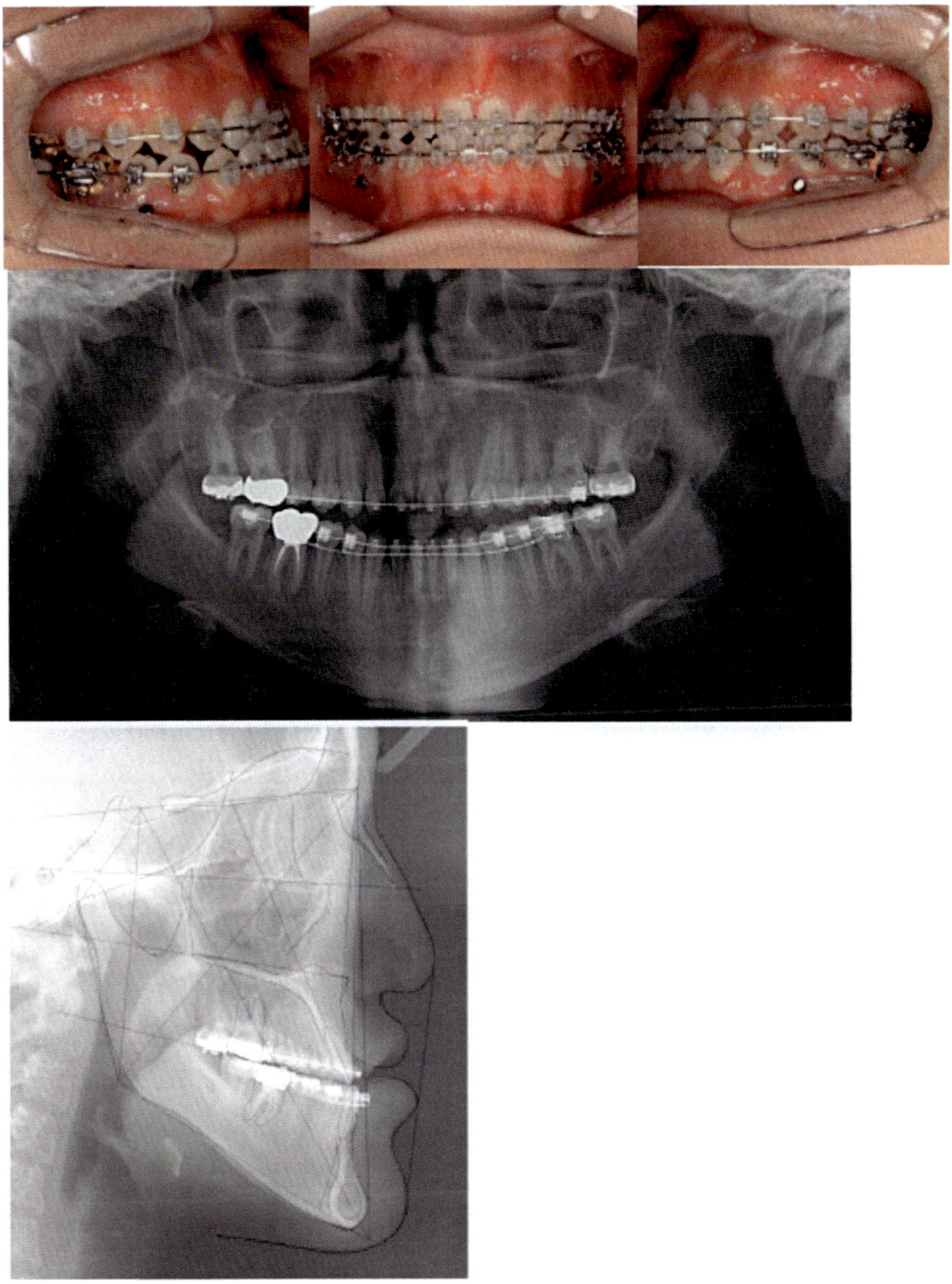

Figure 7-2: Intraoral photographs obtained during mandibular protraction (top) and panoramic and lateral cephalometric radiographs obtained after pre-surgical orthodontic treatment (middle and bottom). The mandibular arch was protracted from the long crimpable hook attached the distal archwire of the 1st molar tube to the TADs between the 1st and 2nd premolars. Note the increase in the anterior crossbite.

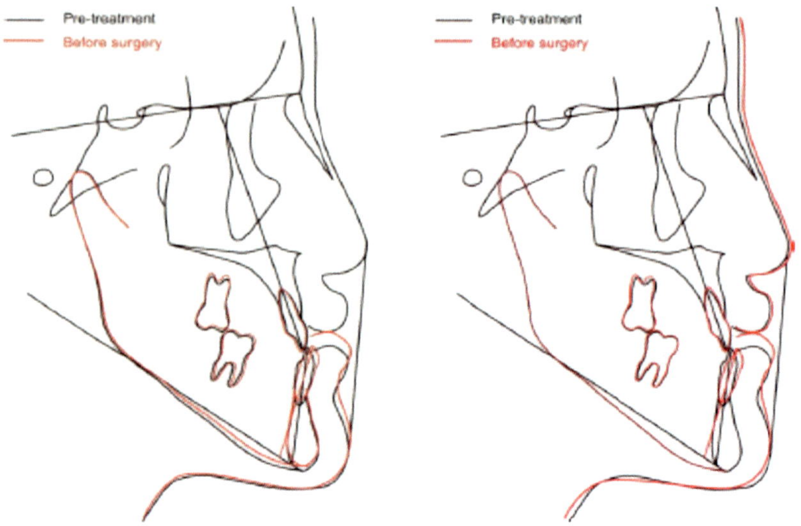

Figure 7-3: Superimposition of the lateral cephalograms. The lower incisal edge moved labially after pre-surgical orthodontic treatment. Left, cranial base superimposition; right, mandibular superimposition; white outline, initial; gray outline, immediately before surgery.

CONCLUSIONS

The application of TADs has changed the conventional approach of Class III treatment. The range of orthodontic camouflage has been expanded, and the quality of treatment has been improved. The stability of TADs in the mandible is lower compared to that in the maxilla [5], however, the success of the Class III treatment when using a TAD depends on the stability of the TADs. Therefore, Class III malocclusion can be treated successfully with various applications of TADs.

ACKNOWLEDGEMENTS

Declared none.

CONFLICT OF INTEREST

The authors confirm that this chapter contents have no conflict of interest.

REFERENCES

[1] Lee JS, Kim JK, Park YC, Vanarsdall RL Jr. Applications of orthodntic mini-implants. Hanover Park: Quintessence Pub; 2007.

[2] Cha BK, Choi DS, Ngan P, Jost-Brinkmann PG, Kim SM, Jang IS. Maxillary protraction with miniplates providing skeletal anchorage in a growing Class III patient. Am J Orthod Dentofacial Orthop 2011;139:99-112.

[3] Sugawara J, Daimaruya T, Umemori M, Nagasaka H, Takahashi I, Kawamura H, Mitani H. Distal movement of mandibular molars in adult patients with the skeletal anchorage system. Am J Orthod Dentofacial Orthop 2004;125:130-8.

[4] Lee KJ, Park YC, Park JY, Hwang WS. Miniscrew-assisted nonsurgical palatal expansion before orthognathic surgery for a patient with severe mandibular prognathism. Am J Orthod Dentofacial Orthop 2010;137:830-9.

[5] Park HS, Jeong SH, Kwon OW. Factors affecting the clinical success of screw implants used as orthodontic anchorage. Am J Orthod Dentofacial Orthop 2006;130:18-25.

Orthodontic Treatment of Class III Malocclusion, **2014, 341-417**

CHAPTER 13

Class III Treatment with Lingual Orthodontics

Toshiaki Hiro*

Hiro Orthodontic Clinic, Nagano, Japan

Abstract: Lingual Orthodontics is believed to require long treatment time and the results are usually unsatisfactory. However, Lingual Orthodontics has a lot of advantages that are not seen with Labial Orthodontics. In this chapter, the author will illustrate with cases that Lingual Orthodontics can be very effective in treating Class III cases due to the ease in tipping back mandibular molars. In addition, the author will demonstrate that tooth movement in Lingual Orthodontics is quite different from Labial Orthodontics. Quite often, cases that require orthognathic surgery with Labial Orthodontics may be done non-surgically if Lingual Orthodontics is used.

Keywords: Lingual Orthodontics, Skeletal Class III malocclusions, Anterior crossbite, Non-surgical treatment, Backward rotation of the mandible.

INTRODUCTION

Patients with skeletal Class III problems are usually addressed during mixed or early permanent dentition by orthodontic/orthopedic treatment [1]. However, patients who did not benefit from early orthodontic/orthopedic treatment may still have severe jaw discrepancies in their adulthood. These adult patients are usually treated by orthognathic surgery [2-4]. Japanese patients tend to have higher incidence of Class III malocclusion compare with other nations [5]. Therefore, mandibular set back procedure is rather popular because orthognathic surgery is often covered by national insurance. Although sagittal split ramus osteotomy (SSRO) is the preferred procedure for mandibular setback [6-8], the number of cases treated by two jaw surgery is gradually increasing [9] since the introduction of the Le Fort I maxillary procedure in combination with the SSRO in treatment of mandibular prognathism [10].

***Address correspondence to Toshiaki Hiro:** 1, 1658-23 Hirooka-Nomura, Shiojiri, Nagano, Japan, 3990702 2; Tel: 81-263-54-6622 3; Fax: 81-263-54-6740 4; E-mail: T.Hiro@mienai.com

Peter W. Ngan, Toshi Deguchi and Eugene W. Roberts (Eds)

Lingual Orthodontic is commonly used in the treatment of adult orthodontic patients [11]. One may be assumed that more of these patients will need surgical procedure to resolve the skeletal discrepancies. However, the percentage of surgical orthodontic cases in the author's office is less than 0.1%. This is remarkably low compared with other medical institutions that reported the frequency around 10-20% [12, 13]. The reason is that the author is making an effort to practice without surgery because the treatment results may be compromised by a third party [14-16]. In addition, tooth movement in Lingual Orthodontics is different from that of Labial Orthodontics. The brackets are bonded on the lingual surface so that teeth tend to tip lingually [17-19] when intrusion force is applied. Lingual Orthodontics is believed to require longer treatment time and resulted in less satisfactory results compare with Labial Orthodontics. However, the author believes that excellent results can be obtained with proper mechanics as demonstrated by a sample of cases presented below.

Case 1

The patient was a 24y-8m-old female presented to the clinic with a chief complaint of an anterior crossbite (Figs. **1A-Q**). An initial examination showed a symmetrical face in the frontal view. In lateral view, the lower lip was slightly protruded. However, the profile was almost as good as the Japanese standard (Fig. **1A**). The intraoral view revealed an Angle Class I molar relationship on both sides in spite of the severe anterior crossbite (Fig. **1B**). This is because the upper right second bicuspid was blocked out palatally, and the upper left second bicuspid was missing. The upper lateral incisor to lateral incisor and the lower canine to canine were in anterior crossbite. The canine relationship was 3 mm Class III on the right side and 6 mm Class III on the left side. The upper right central and lateral incisors were treated with prostheses. The panoramic radiograph showed that the lower third molars were horizontally impacted on both sides. The upper left second bicuspid was impacted (Fig. **1C**). No root resorption or periodontal problems were noted on the periapical radiographs (Fig. **1D**). The lateral cephalometric analysis showed a normal skeletal anteroposterior relationship with SNA = 82.3°, SNB = 80.4° and ANB = 1.9°. The position of the upper incisors were good. The lower incisors were protruded and proclined (Fig. **1E**, Table **1**).

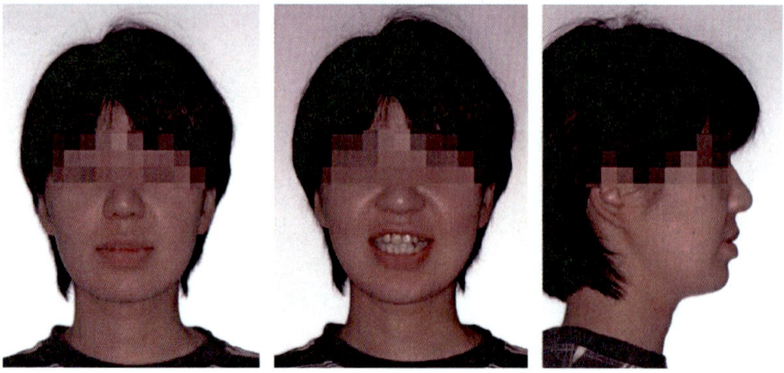

Figure 1A: Case 1: Pre-treatment facial photographs.

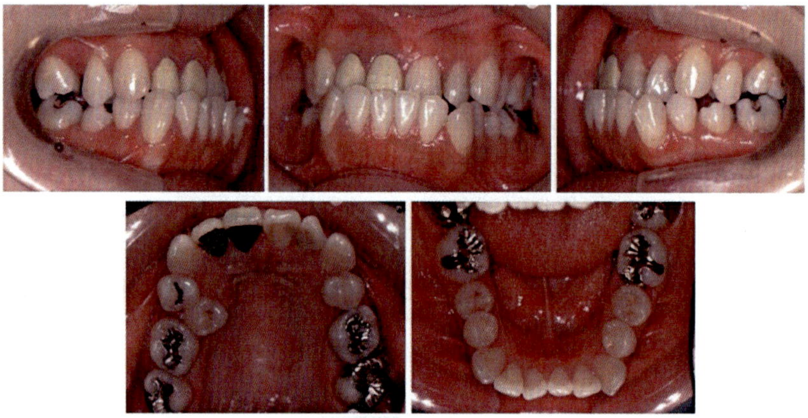

Figure 1B: Case 1: Pre-treatment intra-oral photographs.

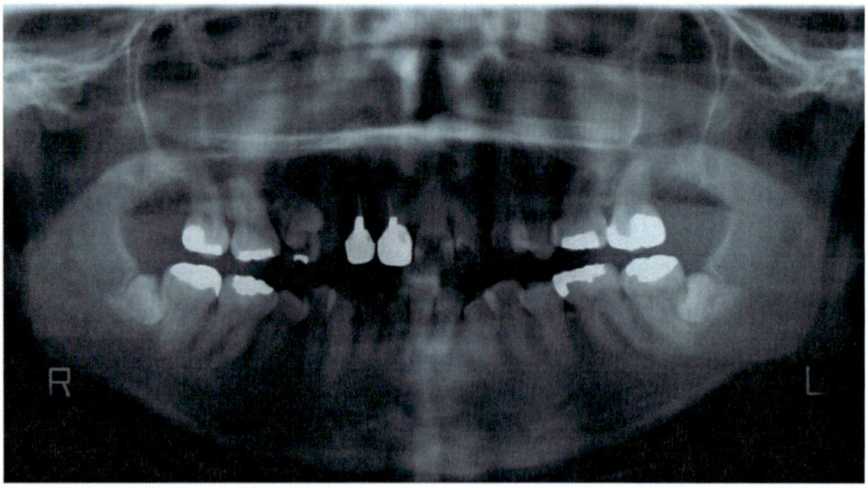

Figure 1C: Case 1: Pre-treatment panoramic radiograph.

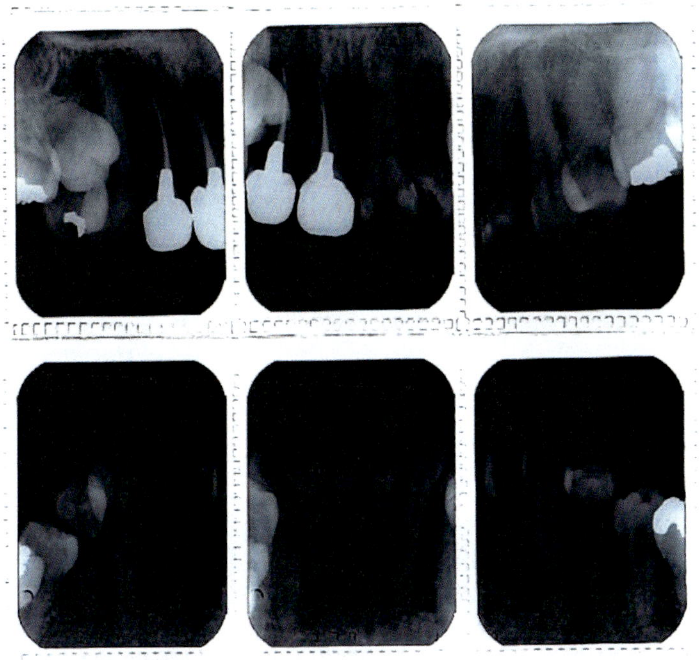

Figure 1D: Case 1: Pre-treatment dental radiographs.

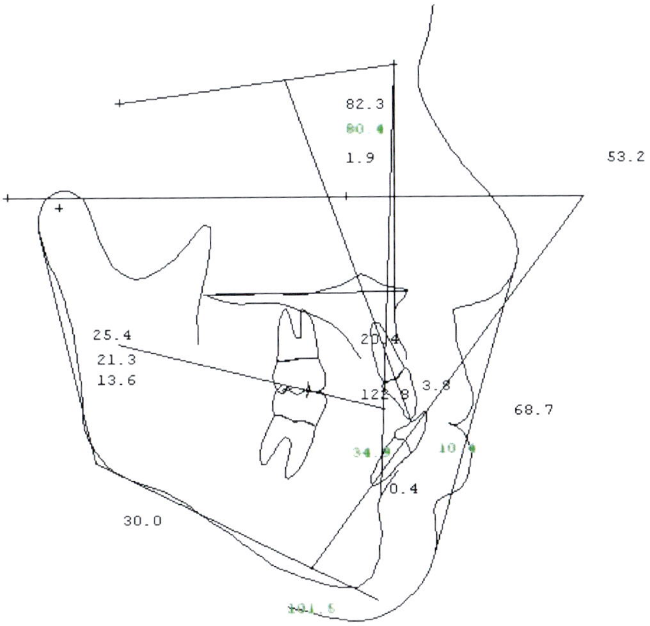

Figure 1E: Case 1: Pre-treatment cephalometric tracing.

Table 1: Case 1: Pre-treatment cephalometric analysis.

Factor	Mean	S.D.	Wn1	Wn2	Wn3
SNA	80.0	3.0	82.3		
SNB	77.0	3.0	80.4		
ANB	3.0	2.0	1.9		
MX1 -NA	4.0	3.0	3.8		
MX1 -NA Angle	23.0	6.0	20.4		
Md1 -NB	5.0	3.0	10.4		
Md1 -NB Angle	26.0	6.0	34.9		
PO - NB	2.0	1.8	0.4		
Occlusal Plane - SN	18.0	3.5	21.3		
GO-GN-SN	34.0	4.5	30.0		
Interincisor Angle	128.0	6.0	122.8		
Wits Appraisal	1.1	1.9	-7.9		
calculated ANB	3.0	2.0	3.8		
FMA	25.0	6.0	25.4		
FMIA	65.0	6.0	53.2		
IMPA	90.0	6.0	101.5		
Occulusal Plane - FH			13.6		
Z Angle			68.7		

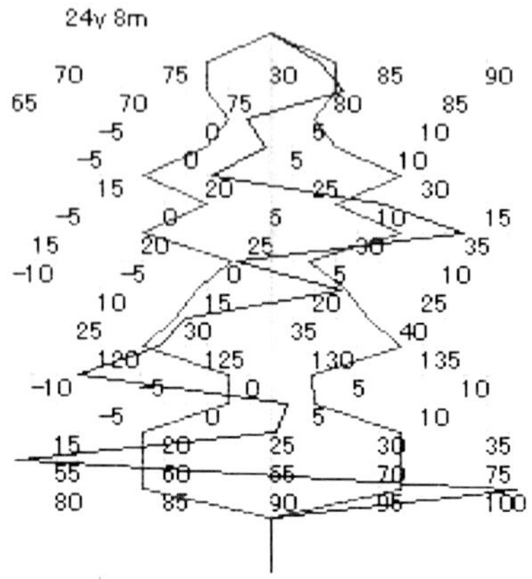

Diagnosis

1. Angle Class I molar relationship.
2. Skeletal Class I (ANB of 1.9 °) anteroposterior jaw relationship.
3. Anterior crossbite.
4. Proclined lower incisors.
5. Arch length discrepancy: Upper: -6.0mm, Lower: -6.0mm.
6. Missing upper left 2nd bicuspid.
7. Bolton analysis: 77.38/89.09 %.

Treatment Objectives

1. Correct anterior crossbite.
2. Retraction and upright lower incisors.
3. Align upper and lower arches.
4. Establish Class I canine relationship.

5. Improve molar occlusion.

Treatment Plan

1. Extract upper right second bicuspid, lower right second and left first bicuspid.

2. Non-surgical treatment.

3. Leveling of upper and lower arch.

4. Space closing of upper and lower arch.

5. Detailing and finishing.

Treatment Progress

After extraction of the bicuspids, the treatment was started with the Kurz Lingual Appliance. Figs. **1F** showed the intra-oral photographs during treatment. The author normally uses sliding mechanics for space consolidation. However, the loop mechanics was used in this case. Fig. **1G** shows the patient 2 months in treatment with upper .014 Ni-Ti and lower .016x.022 TMA archwires. Fig. **1H** shows the patient 5 months in treatment with upper .018 Ni-Ti and lower .016x.022 TMA closing arch archwires. Class II elastics were worn from the lower first molar to the upper canine only on the right side. Fig. **1I** shows the patient 7 months in treatment with upper .016x.022 TMA and lower .017x.025 TMA archwires without vertical loops. Fig. **1J** shows patient 14 months in treatment with upper .018x.025 S.S. and lower .017x.025 TMA archwires for final detailing and finishing. Elastic chains were worn from second molars to second molars on both arches in order to obtain tight contacts.

Treatment Results

Excellent facial and dental esthetics was obtained. Class I canine and molar relationships were established. The anterior crossbite was corrected (Figs. **1K** and **L**). The treatment time was 26 months. Post-treatment panoramic radiograph showed good root paralleling (Fig. **1M**). The horizontally impacted third molars were extracted. Periapical radiographs showed root resorption was minimal

(Fig. **1N**). After removal of the upper and lower appliances, fixed lingual retainers were bonded on both arches. Figs. **1O** and **P** show patient 35 months after treatment. Superimposition of pre- and post-treatment radiographs showed a backward rotation of the mandible. Upper incisors were moved labially and lower incisors were up righted and retracted (Fig. **1Q**, Table **2**).

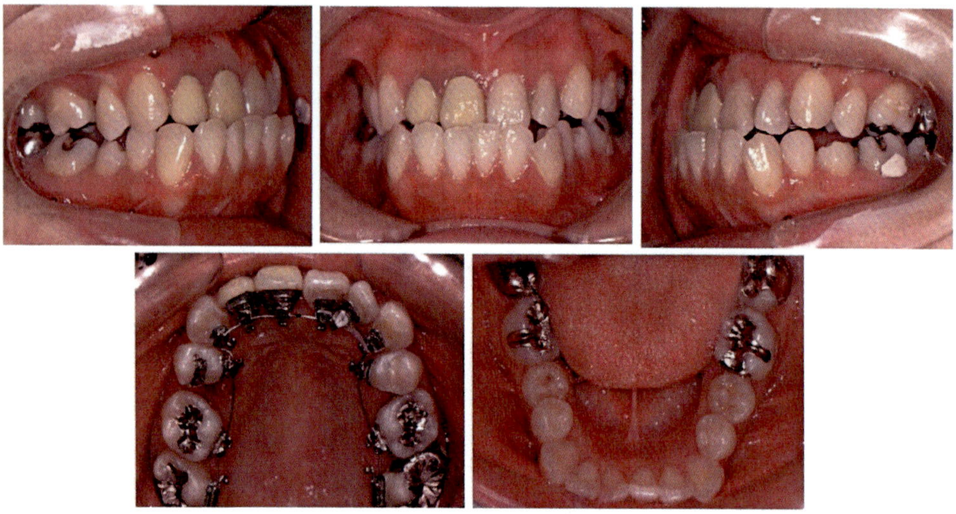

Figure 1F: Case 1: Intra-oral photographs after brackets were bonded to upper arch.

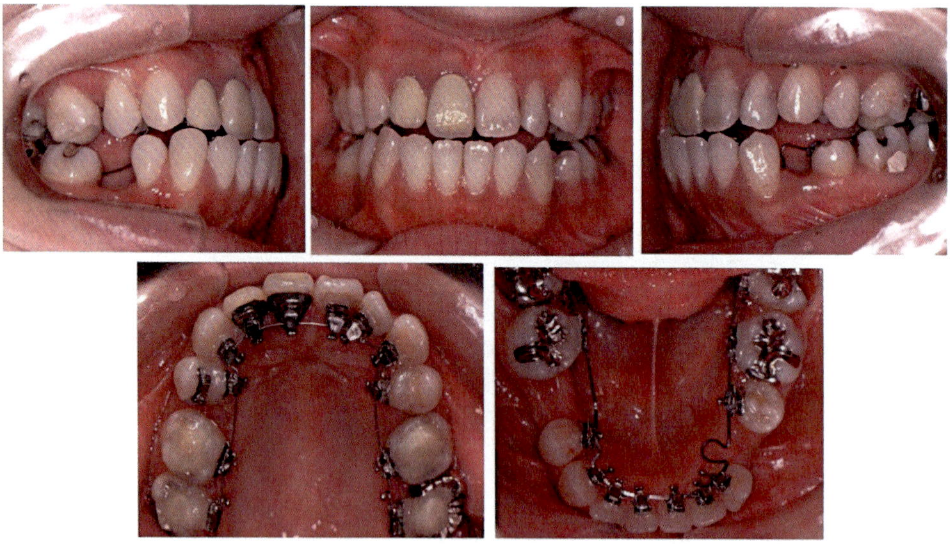

Figure 1G: Case 1: Intra-oral photographs taken at 2 month into the treatment. The arch wires were .014 Ni-Ti in the upper arch and .016x.022 beta-titanium with closing loop in the lower arch.

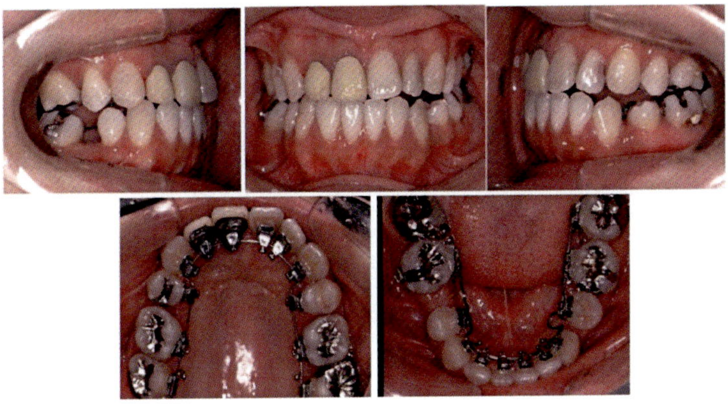

Figure 1H: Case 1: Intra-oral photographs at 5 months into the treatment. The arch wires were .018 Ni-Ti in the upper arch and .016x.02 TMA closing arch in the lower arch.

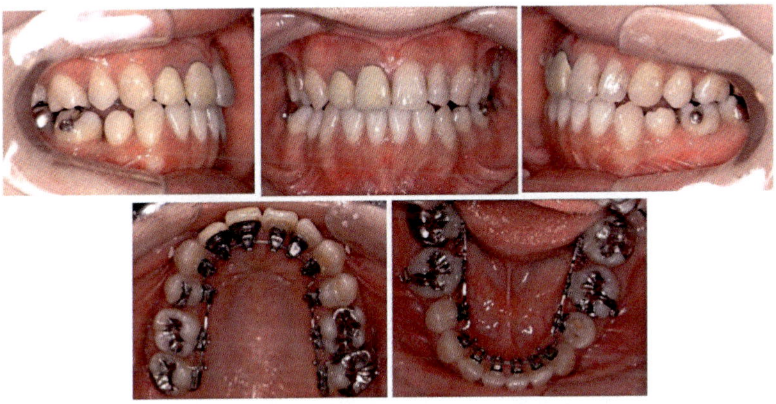

Figure 1I: Case 1: Intra-oral photographs at 7 months into the treatment. The arch wires were .016x.022 TMA in the upper arch and .017x.025 TMA in the lower arch.

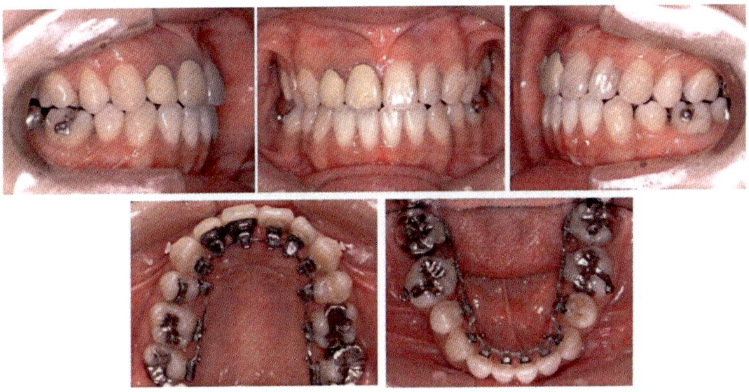

Figure 1J: Case 1: Intra-oral photographs at 14 months into the treatment. The arch wires were .018x.025 S.S. in the upper arch and .017x.025 TMA in the lower arch.

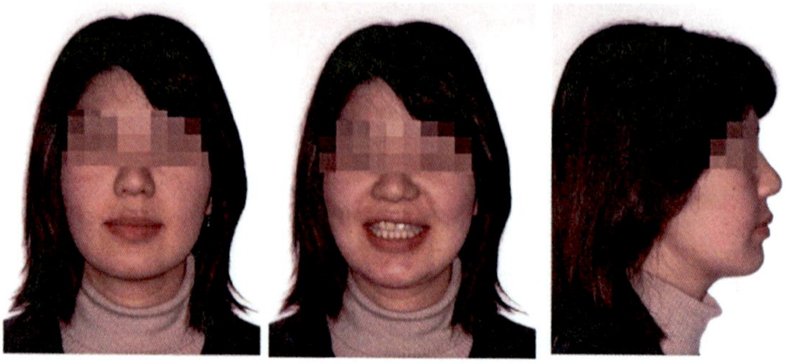

Figure 1K: Case 1: Post-treatment facial photographs showing improved facial profile.

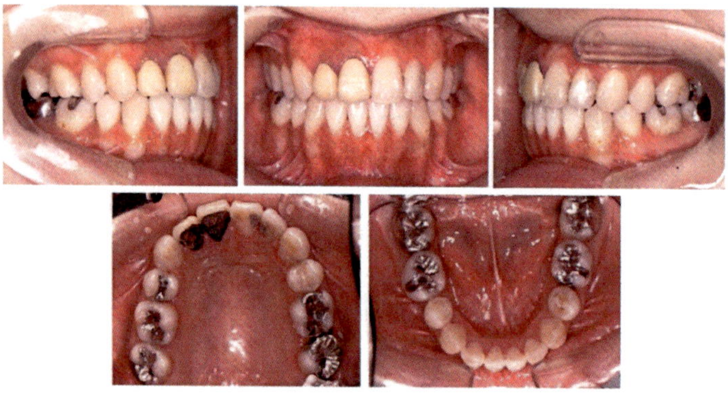

Figure 1L: Case 1: Post-treatment intra-oral photographs.

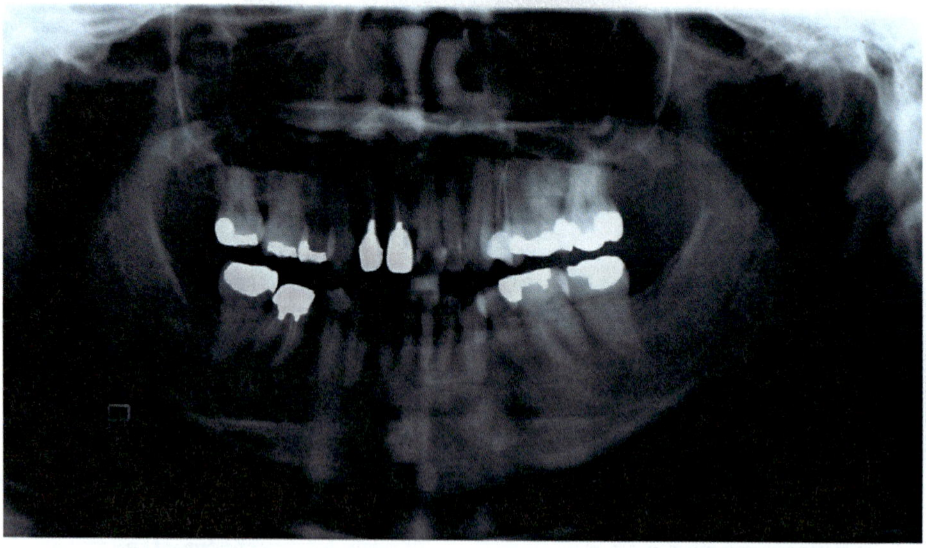

Figure 1M: Case 1: Post-treatment panorama radiograph showing good root paralleling and extracted lower third molars.

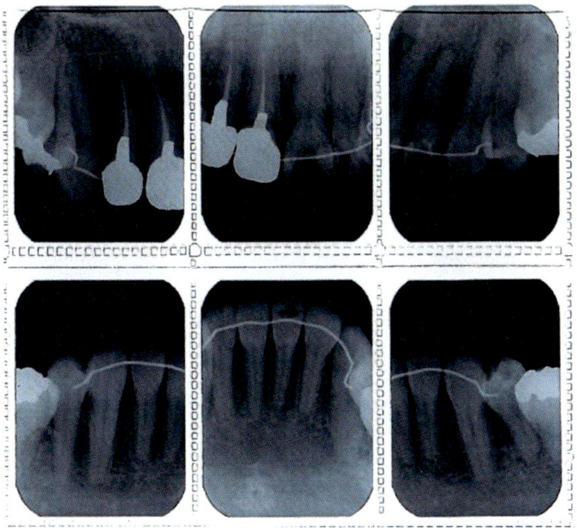

Figure 1N: Case 1: Post-treatment dental radiograph showing minimal root resorption.

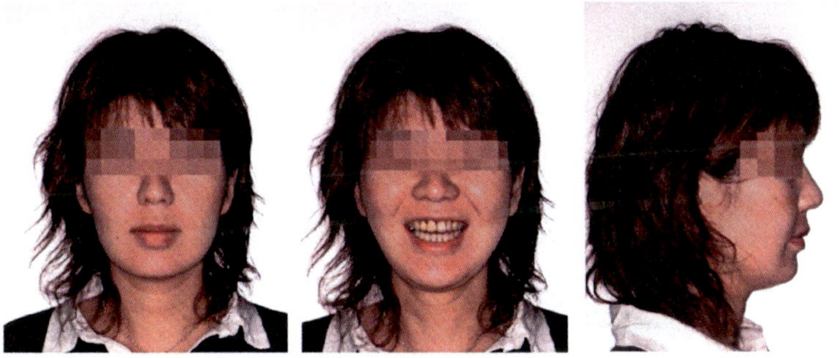

Figure 1O: Case 1: Facial photographs 35 months after completion of the treatment.

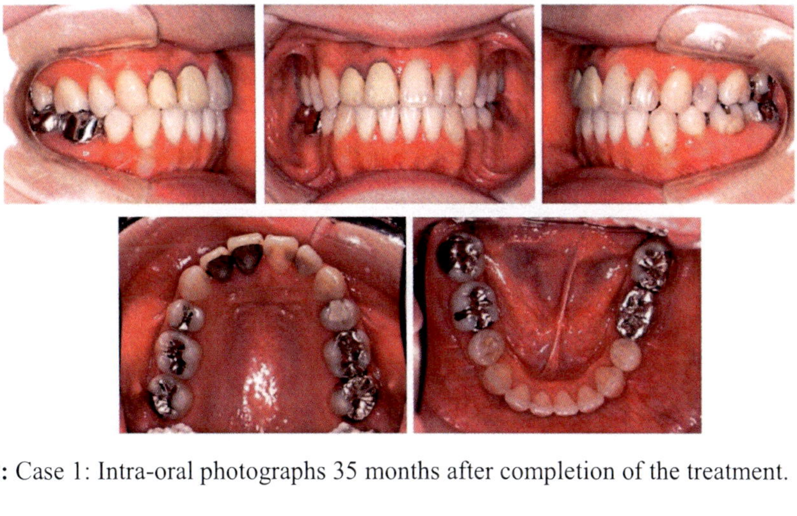

Figure 1P: Case 1: Intra-oral photographs 35 months after completion of the treatment.

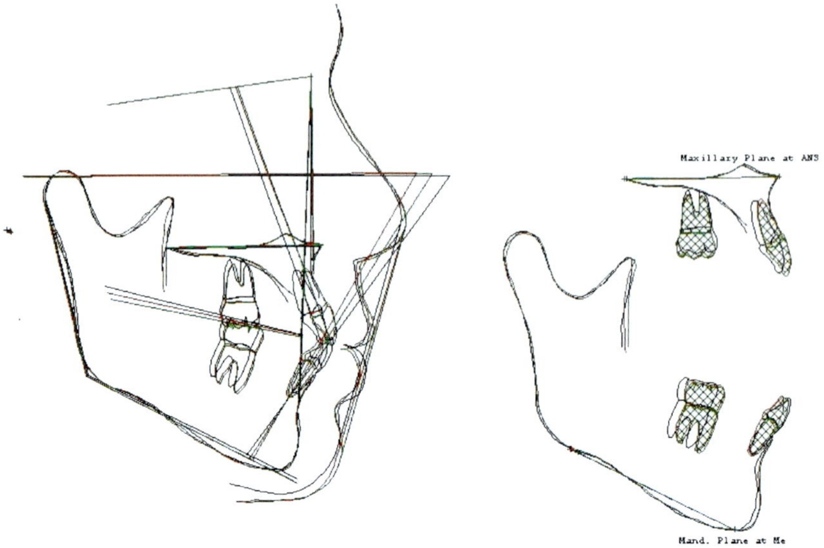

Figure 1Q: Case 1: Superimpositions of cephalometric tracings before and after treatment, and after retention.

Table 2: Case 1: Pre-treatment, post-treatment and after retention cephalometric analysis.

Factor	Mean	S.D.	Win1	Win2	Win3
SNA	80.0	3.0	82.3	83.1	83.4
SNB	77.0	3.0	80.4	80.2	80.4
ANB	3.0	2.0	1.9	2.9	3.0
Mx1 –NA	4.0	3.0	3.8	5.8	5.8
Mx1 –NA Angle	23.0	6.0	20.4	20.7	19.8
Md1 –NB	5.0	3.0	10.4	7.2	8.4
Md1 –NB Angle	26.0	6.0	34.9	28.4	31.4
PO – NB	2.0	1.8	0.4	–0.0	0.5
Occlusal Plane – SN	18.0	3.5	21.3	19.6	18.6
GO–GN–SN	34.0	4.5	30.0	32.8	32.4
Interincisor Angle	128.0	6.0	122.8	128.1	125.8
Wits Appraisal	1.1	1.9	–7.9	–6.0	–4.7
calculated ANB	3.0	2.0	3.8	4.7	4.7
FMA	25.0	6.0	25.4	26.3	26.4
FMIA	65.0	6.0	53.2	59.1	56.2
IMPA	90.0	6.0	101.5	94.6	97.4
Occulusal Plane – FH			13.6	12.3	11.4
Z Angle			68.7	74.3	74.8

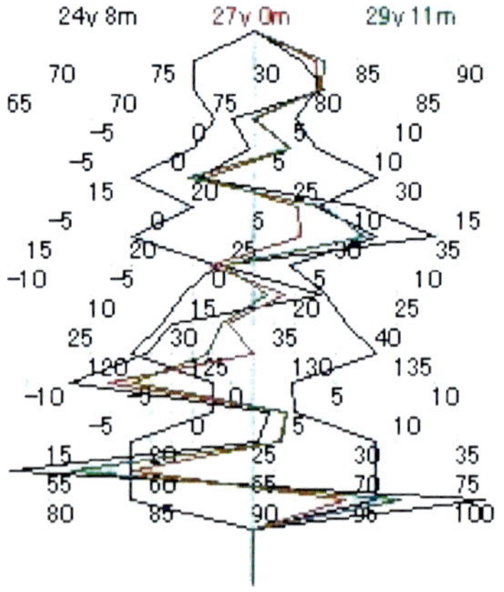

Case 2

The patient was a 32y-3m-old female visited the author's clinic with a chief complaint of anterior crossbite. The front view showed symmetrical face. The lateral view shows the lower lip was slightly protruded (Fig. **2A**). The intraoral view reveals an anterior crossbite. The upper right central incisor was prosthetically restored. In spite of the severe anterior crossbite, the molar relation was 2 mm Angle Class II on the right side and 7 mm on left side (Fig. **2B**). The third molars were present only on the upper right quadrant. The upper right central incisor and lower right first molar had root canal treatment. No abnormal findings were seen on the panoramic radiograph (Fig. **2C**). No root resorption or periodontal problems were seen on the dental radiograph (Fig. **2D**). The head of the mandibular condyles was round, and the TM joint space was normal (Fig. **2E**). Cephalometric analysis showed a skeletal Class III anteroposterior jaw relationship with SNA=68.5°, SNB=72.5° and ANB= -4.0°. The distance and the angle of upper incisors to NA showed that the upper incisors were protruded and labially inclined due to retrognathia of the maxilla (Fig. **2F**, Table **3**).

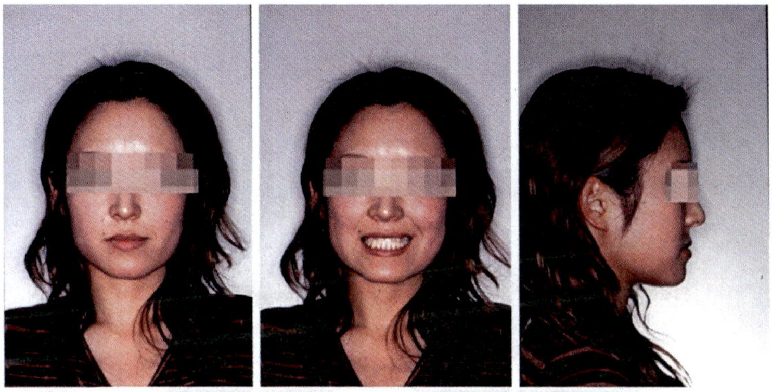

Figure 2A: Case 2: Pre-treatment facial photographs.

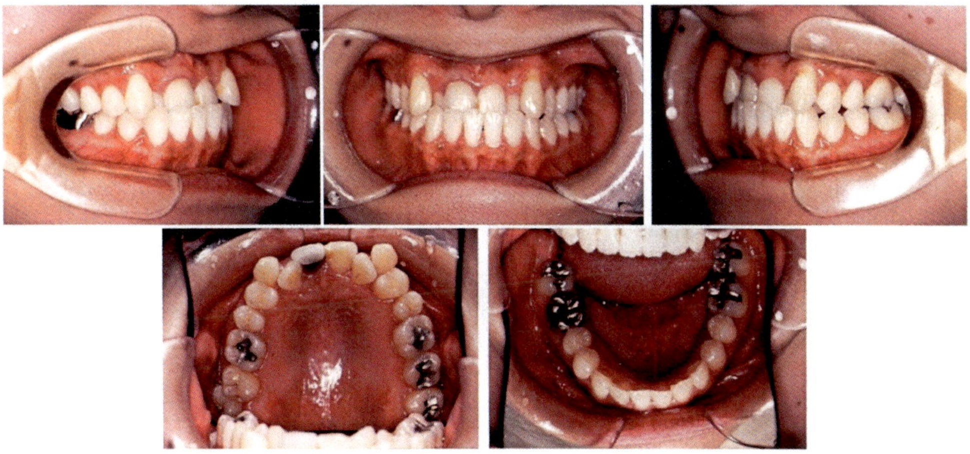

Figure 2B: Case 2: Pre-treatment intra-oral photographs.

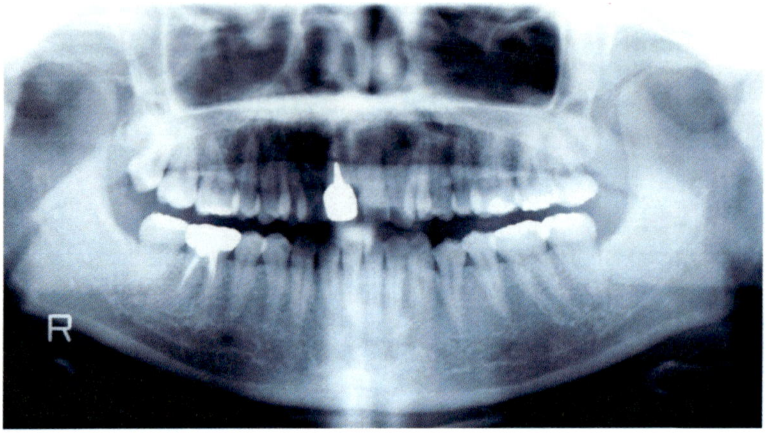

Figure 2C: Case 2: Pre-treatment panorama radiograph.

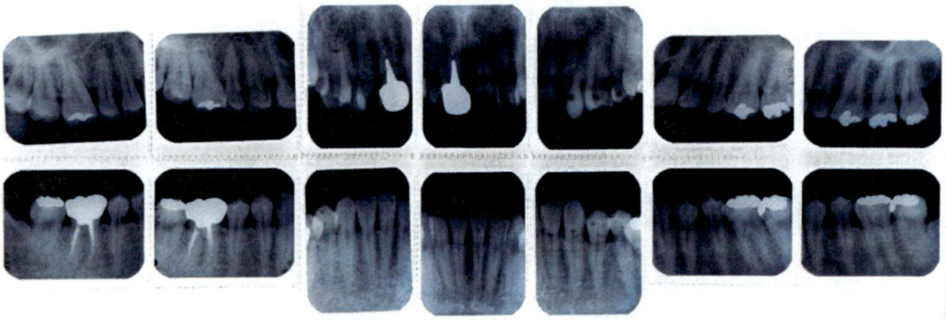

Figure 2D: Case 2: Pre-treatment dental radiographs.

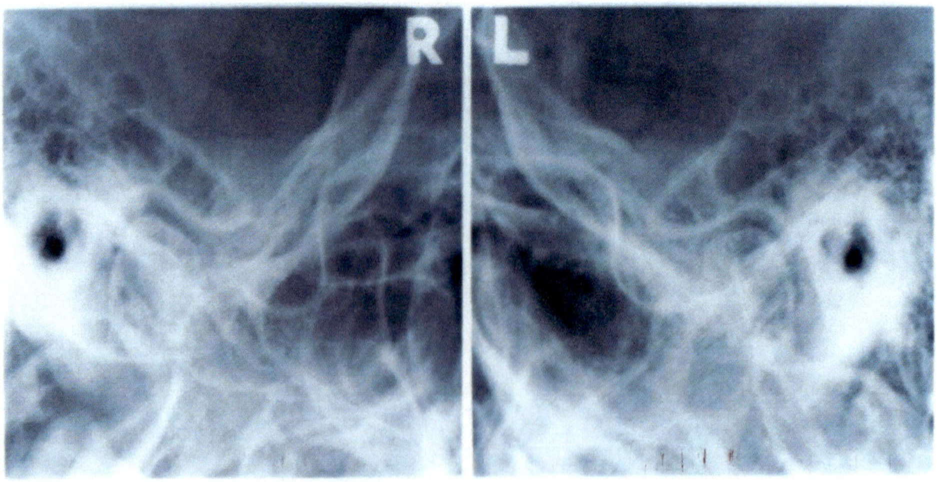

Figure 2E: Case 2: Pre-treatment TMJ radiographs.

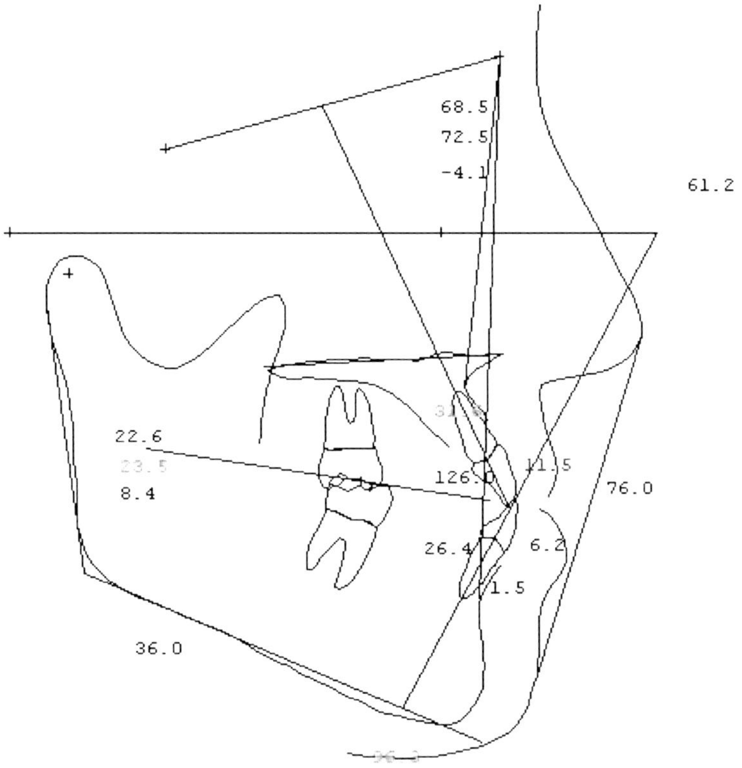

Figure 2F: Case 2: Pre-treatment cephalometric tracing.

Table 3: Case 2: Pre-treatment cephalometric analysis.

Factor	Mean	S.D.	Wn1	Wn2	Wn3
SNA	80.0	3.0	68.5		
SNB	77.0	3.0	72.5		
ANB	3.0	2.0	-4.1		
Mx1-NA	4.0	3.0	11.5		
Mx1-NA Angle	23.0	6.0	31.6		
Md1-NB	5.0	3.0	6.2		
Md1-NB Angle	26.0	6.0	26.4		
PO - NB	2.0	1.8	1.5		
Occlusal Plane - SN	18.0	3.5	23.5		
GO-GN-SN	34.0	4.5	36.0		
Interincisor Angle	128.0	6.0	126.0		
Wits Appraisal	1.1	1.9	-9.4		
calculated ANB	3.0	2.0	-0.6		
FMA	25.0	6.0	22.6		
FMIA	65.0	6.0	61.2		
IMPA	90.0	6.0	96.3		
Occulusal Plane - FH			8.4		
Z Angle			76.0		

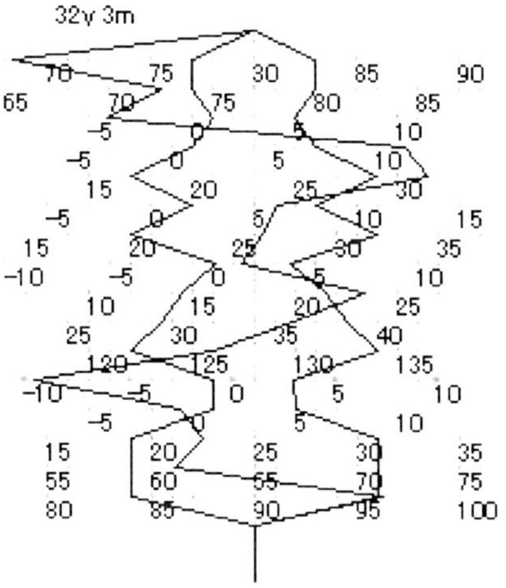

Diagnosis

1. Class II molar relationship (2 mm on the right, 7 mm on the left).

2. Class III skeletal anteroposterior jaw relationship (ANB -4.0^{o}).

3. Anterior cross bite.

4. Upper midline 5mm shift to right.

6. Arch length discrepancy: Upper: -9.5 mm, Lower: 0 mm.

Treatment Objectives

1. Correct anterior cross bite.

2. Establish stable molar occlusion.

3. Class II finish on the left side.

Treatment Plan

1. Extract upper left first bicuspid.

2. Non-surgical treatment.

4. Correct anterior crossbite.

5. Correct maxillary midline.

6. Class II molar finish on the left side.

Treatment Progress

After extraction of the upper left first bicuspid, treatment was started with placement of the mini lingual orthodontics fixed appliance. At first, brackets were bonded on the upper arch together with an initial .012 NiTi archwire. Upper left canine was preliminary retracted with elastic chain (Fig. **2G**). After 2 months, brackets were bonded on the lower arch. Upper left canine was retracted, gaining space for upper right canine with open coil spring (Fig. **2H**). Upper and lower rectangular arch wires were used for final detailing (Figs. **2I** and **J**).

Treatment Results

Excellent result was obtained with 25 months of treatment. The lower lip was retracted to obtain a better profile. The upper midline was coincident with the lower midline. Class I molar and canine relationship was established on the right side and Class II on the left side. Adequate overjet and overbite were obtained (Figs. **2K** and **L**). Post-treatment panoramic radiograph showed good root paralleling. Upper right 3rd molar was not extracted and placed under observation (Fig. **2M**). Dental radiograph showed root resorption was minimal (Fig. **2N**). Compare with pre-treatment records, no significant changes were seen with the TM joint (Fig. **2O**). Figs. **2P** and **Q** showed the stable occlusion 37 months after treatment. Superimpositions of the pre- and post-treatment radiographs showed improvement of ANB with backward rotation of the mandible. Upper incisors were slightly proclined with treatment. Lower molars and incisors were uprighted (Fig. **2R**, Table **4**).

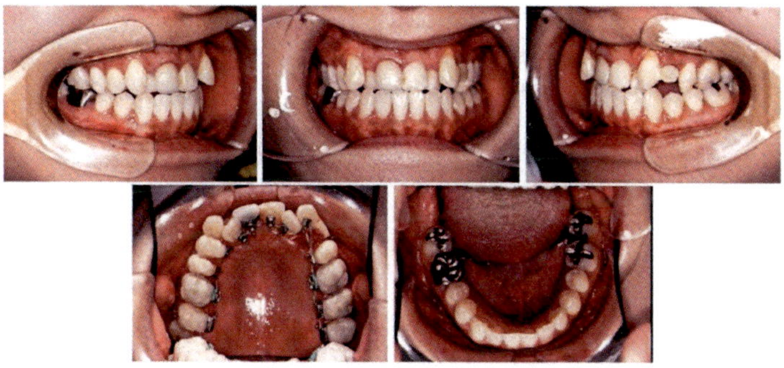

Figure 2G: Case 2: Intra-oral photographs taken after brackets were bonded on the upper arch. The arch wires were .012 Ni-Ti in the upper and lower arches. Upper left canine was preliminary retracted with elastic chain.

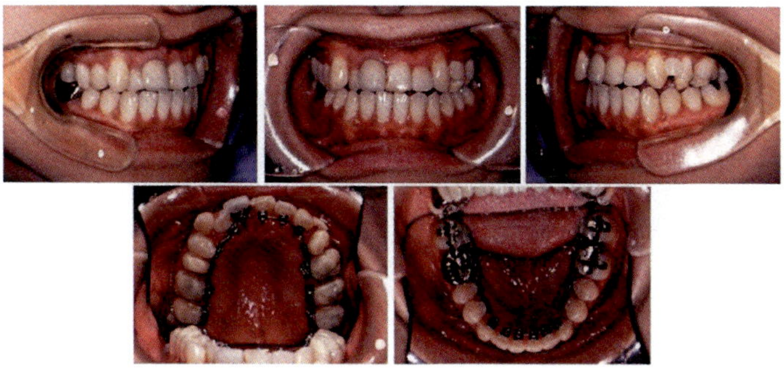

Figure 2H: Case 2: Intra-oral photographs 2 months into treatment showing space gaining with coil spring in the upper right canine.

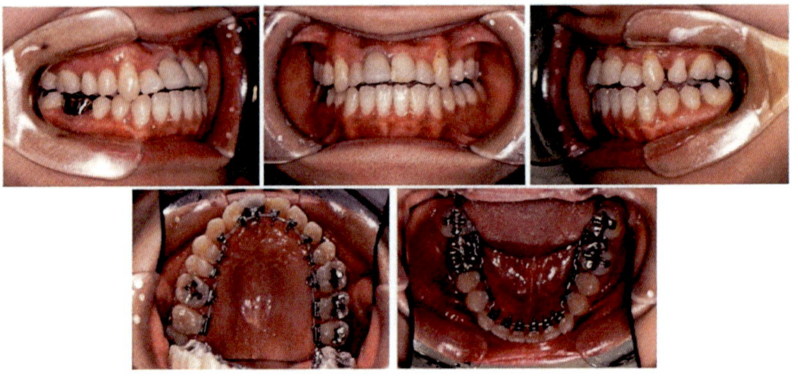

Figure 2I: Case 2: Intra-oral photographs 7 months into treatment. The arch wires were .016 TMA in the upper arch and .0175x.0175 TMA in the lower arch.

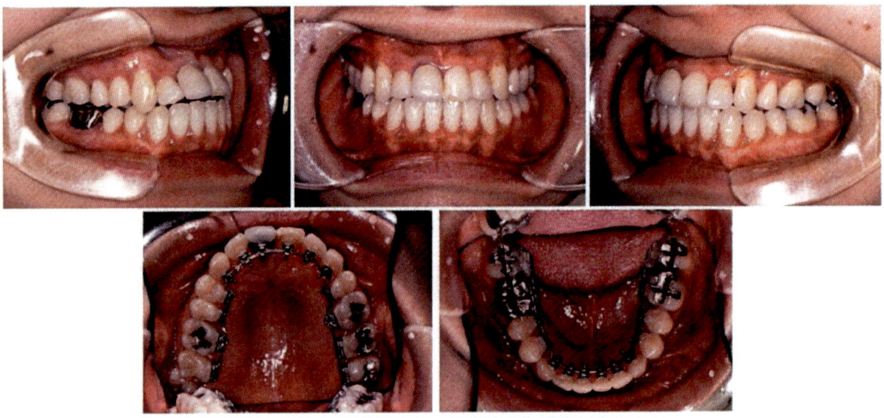

Figure 2J: Case 2: Intra-oral photographs 15 months into treatment. The arch wires were .016x.022 TMA in the upper arch and .016x.022 TMA in the lower arch. Midline elastic was worn from the right upper lateral incisor to the left lower canine.

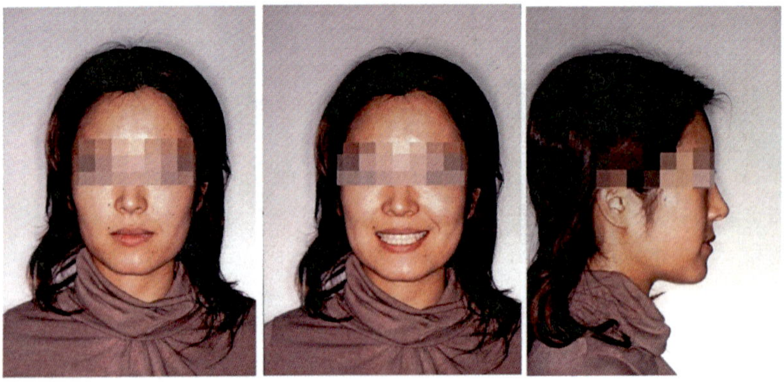

Figure 2K: Case 2: Post-treatment facial photographs.

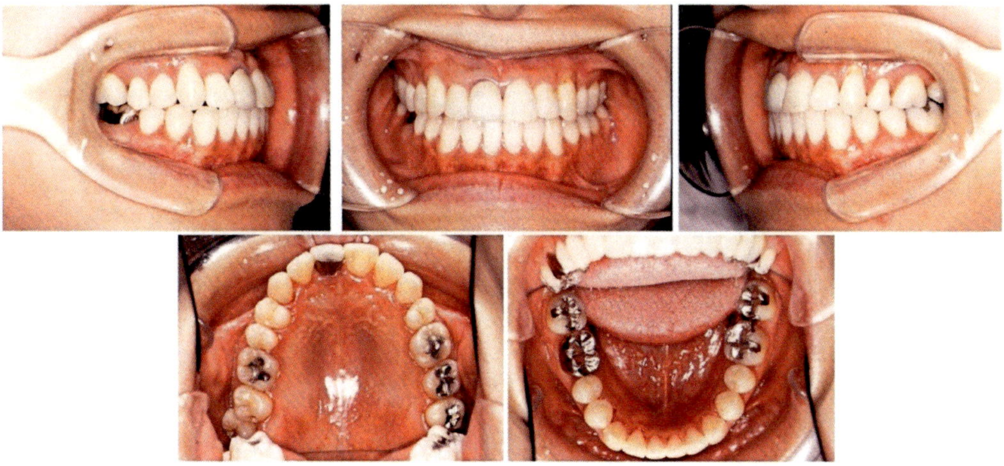

Figure 2L: Case 2: Post-treatment intraoral photographs.

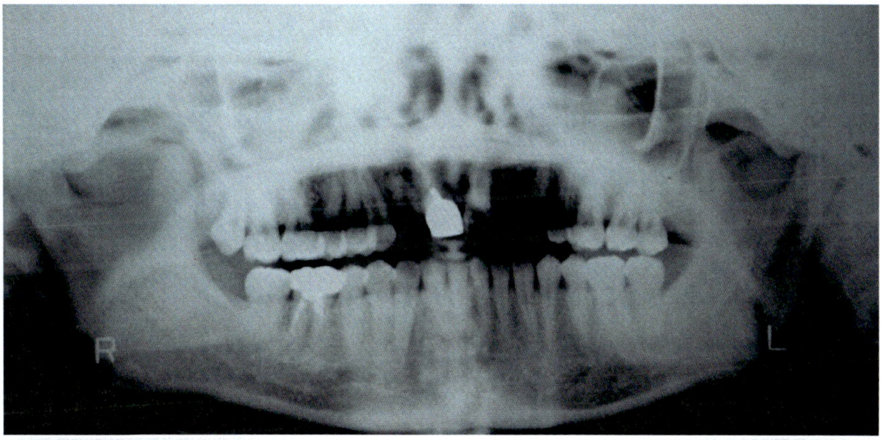

Figure 2M: Case 2: Post-treatment panorama radiograph.

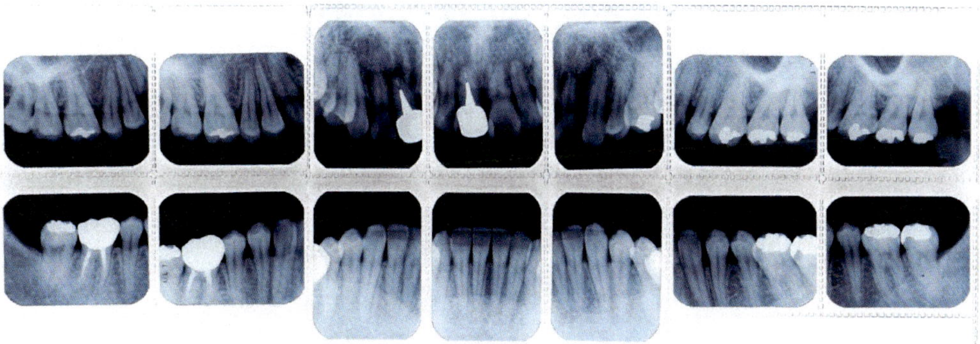

Figure 2N: Case 2: Post-treatment dental radiograph.

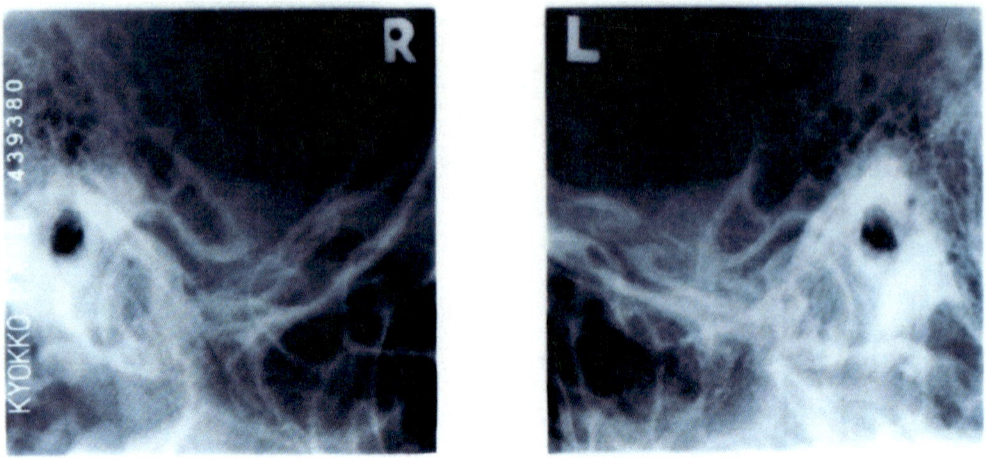

Figure 2O: Case 2: Post-treatment TMJ radiographs.

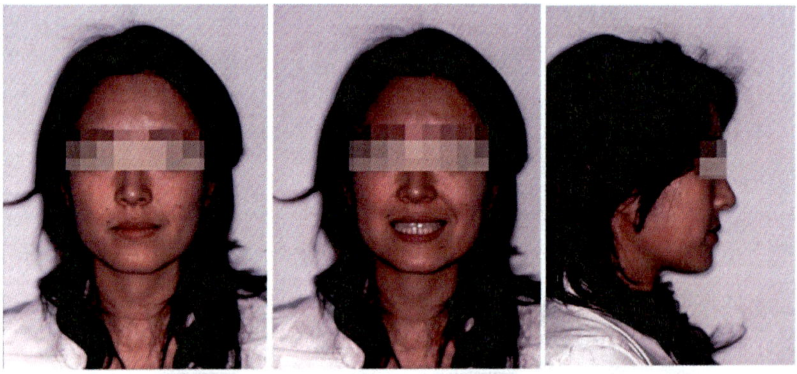

Figure 2P: Case 2: Facial photographs 37 months after completion of the treatment.

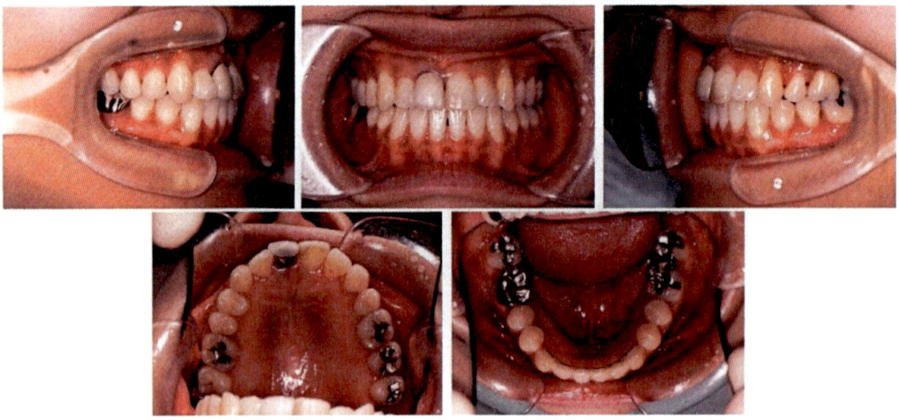

Figure 2Q: Case 2: Intra-oral photographs 37 months after completion of the treatment.

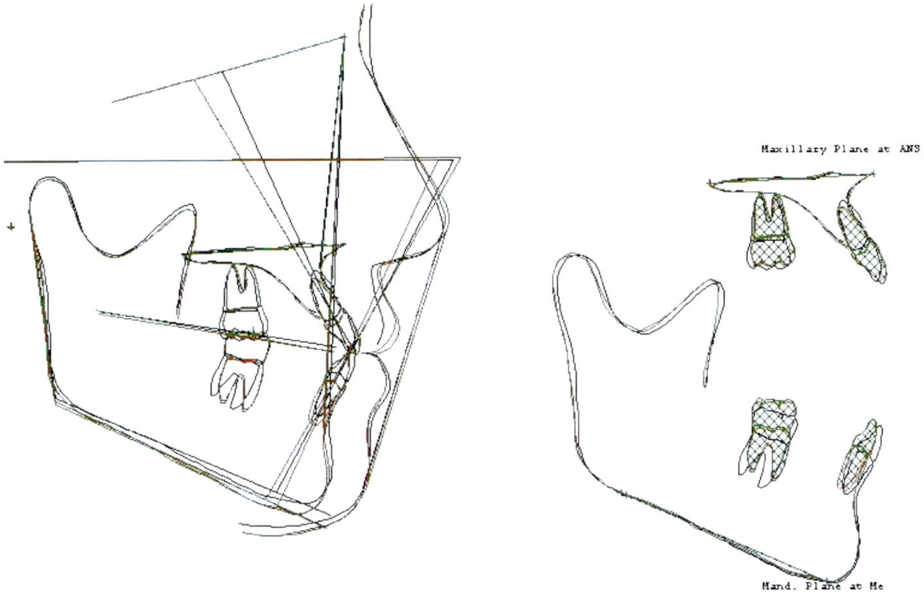

Figure 2R: Case 2: Superimpositions of cephalogram tracings before and after treatment, and after retention.

Table 4: Case 2: Pre-treatment, post-treatment and after retention cephalometric analysis.

Factor	Mean	S.D.	Wn1	Wn2	Wn3
SNA	80.0	3.0	68.5	68.8	68.9
SNB	77.0	3.0	72.5	71.6	71.8
ANB	3.0	2.0	−4.1	−2.8	−2.9
Mx1 −NA	4.0	3.0	11.5	12.9	12.9
Mx1 −NA Angle	23.0	6.0	31.6	37.5	37.5
Md1 −NB	5.0	3.0	6.2	5.8	5.9
Md1 −NB Angle	26.0	6.0	26.4	22.2	27.2
PO − NB	2.0	1.8	1.5	2.1	2.3
Occlusal Plane − SN	18.0	3.5	23.5	24.0	24.7
GO-GN-SN	34.0	4.5	36.0	36.9	36.8
Interincisor Angle	128.0	6.0	126.0	123.1	118.2
Wits Appraisal	1.1	1.9	−9.4	−7.4	−8.3
calculated ANB	3.0	2.0	−0.6	−0.2	−0.2
FMA	25.0	6.0	22.6	24.8	24.5
FMIA	65.0	6.0	61.2	64.4	59.3
IMPA	90.0	6.0	96.3	90.8	96.2
Occulusal Plane − FH			8.4	9.0	10.0
Z Angle			76.0	78.5	78.0

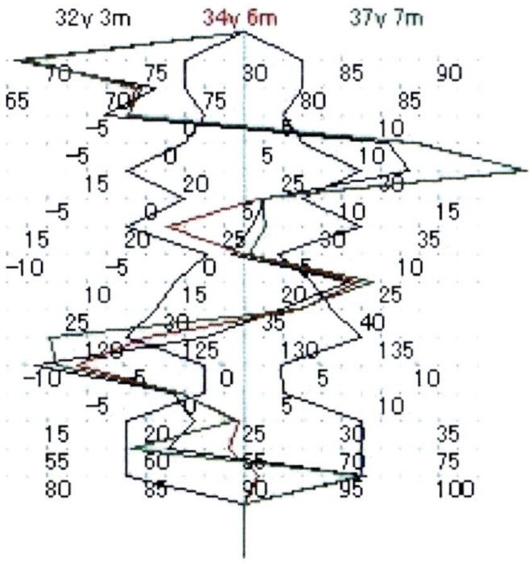

Case 3

The patient was a 47y 10m old female who visited the author's clinic with a chief complaint of an anterior crossbite. The frontal view showed a symmetrical face.

The lateral view showed a concave profile (Fig. **3A**). The molar relationship was Class I on both sides. The upper and lower incisors were slightly crowded with an anterior crossbite (Fig. **3B**). No abnormal findings were found on the panoramic radiograph (Fig. **3C**). The upper incisors root length was short with a 1:1 crown: root ratio (Fig. **3D**). The shape of the mandibular condyle heads was round, located in the center of fossa (Fig. **3E**). Lateral cephalometric analysis showed a Class III skeletal anteroposterior jaw relationship with SNA= 80.7°, SNB=83.8° and ANB= -3.1°. Over closure of mandible was observed. Upper incisors were labial inclined and lower Incisors were lingual inclined (Fig. **3F**, Table **5**).

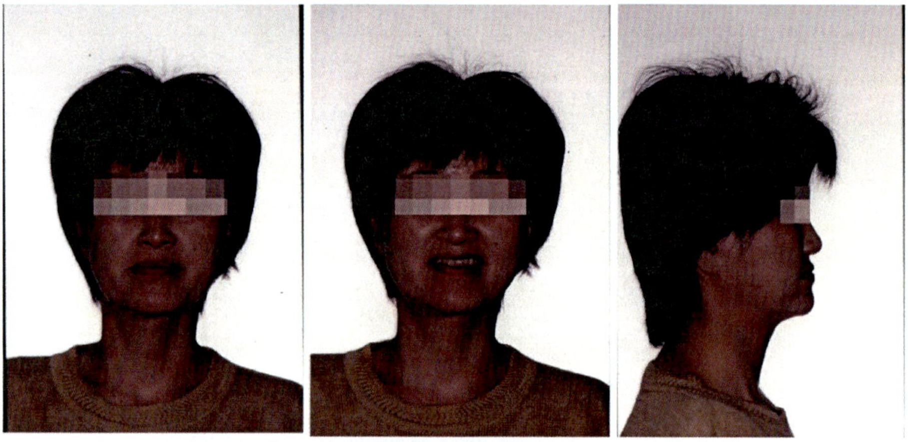

Figure 3A: Case 3: Pre-treatment facial photographs.

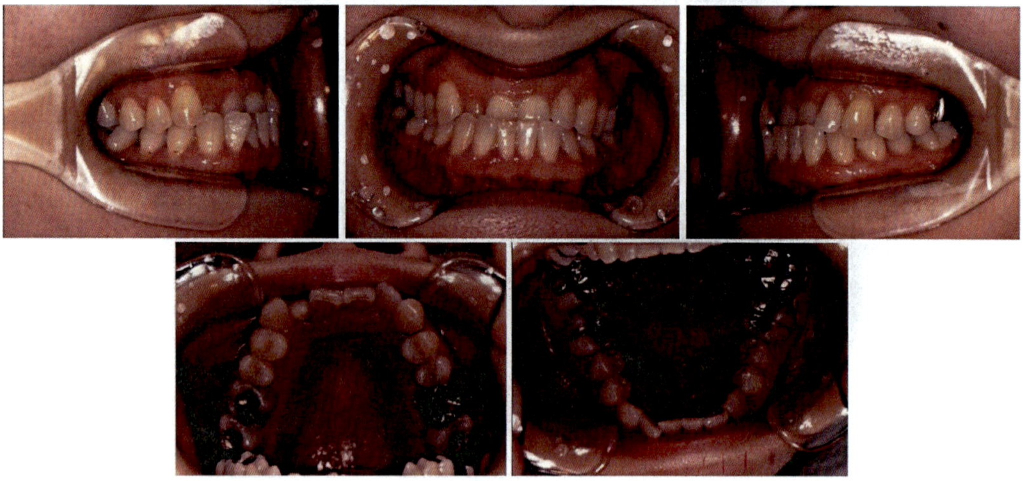

Figure 3B: Case 3: Pre-treatment intra-oral photographs.

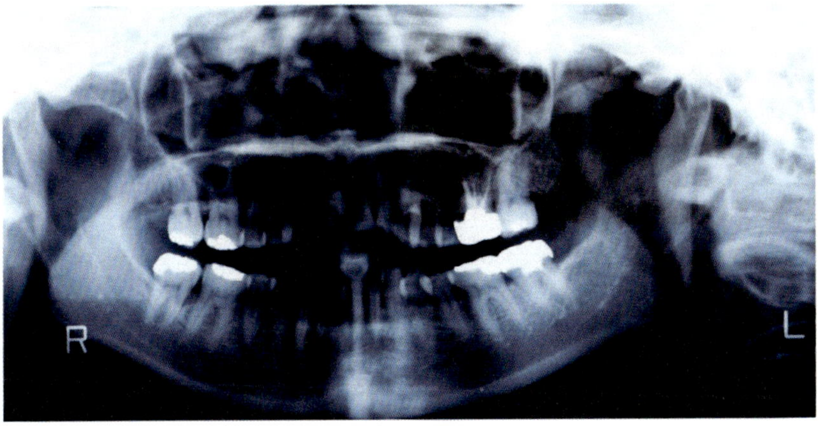

Figure 3C: Case 3C: Pre-treatment panoramic radiograph.

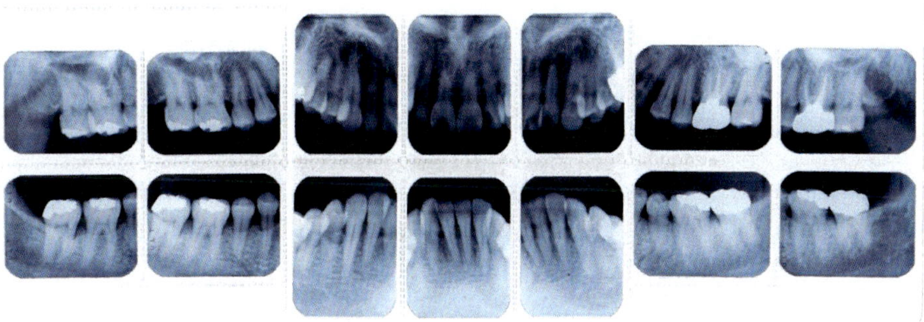

Figure 3D: Case 3: Pre-treatment dental radiographs.

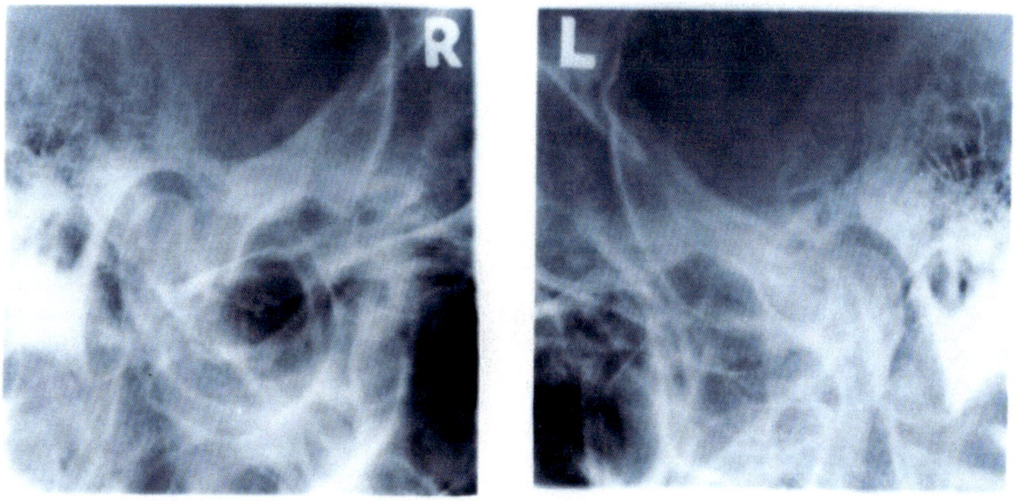

Figure 3E: Case 3: Pre-treatment TMJ radiographs.

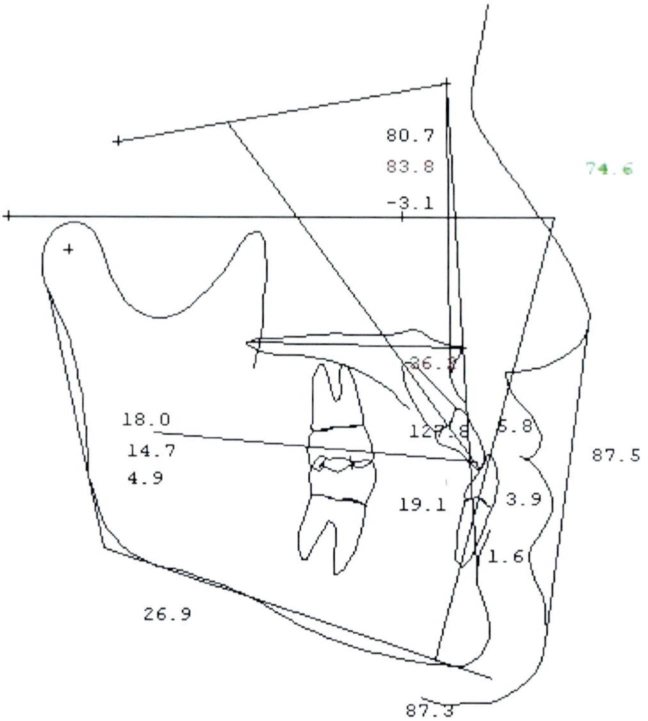

Figure 3F: Case 3: Pre-treatment cephalometric tracing.

Table 5: Case 3: Pre-treatment cephalometric analysis.

Factor	Mean	S.D.	Wn1	Wn2	Wn3
SNA	80.0	3.0	80.7		
SNB	77.0	3.0	83.8		
ANB	3.0	2.0	-3.1		
Mx1 -NA	4.0	3.0	5.8		
Mx1 -NA Angle	23.0	6.0	36.2		
Md1 -NB	5.0	3.0	3.9		
Md1 -NB Angle	26.0	6.0	19.1		
PO - NB	2.0	1.8	1.6		
Occlusal Plane - SN	18.0	3.5	14.7		
GO-GN-SN	34.0	4.5	26.9		
Interincisor Angle	128.0	6.0	127.8		
Wts Appraisal	1.1	1.9	-11.5		
calculated ANB	3.0	2.0	2.5		
FMA	25.0	6.0	18.0		
FMIA	65.0	6.0	74.6		
IMPA	90.0	6.0	87.3		
Occulusal Plane - FH			4.9		
Z Angle			87.5		

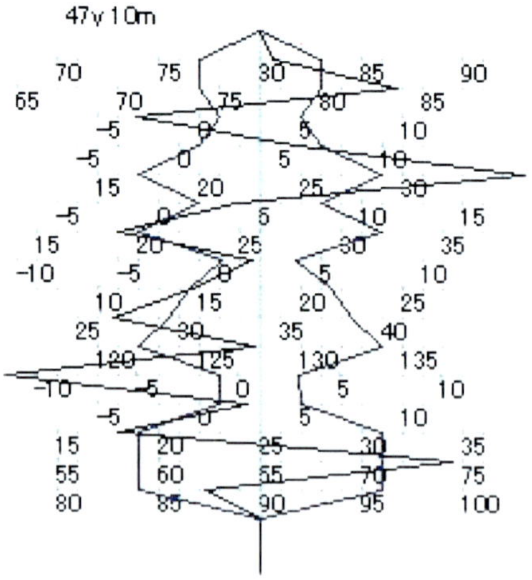

Diagnosis

1. Class I molar relationship.
2. Class III skeletal anteroposterior jaw relationship (ANB -3.1°).
3. Anterior crossbite.
4. Arch length discrepancy: Upper: -2.0 mm, Lower: -2.0 mm.

Treatment Objectives

1. Correction of anterior cross bite.
2. Improvement of jaw relationship with backward rotation of mandible.
3. Improvement of upper and lower crowding.
4. Improvement of profile, if possible.

Treatment Plan

1. Non-extraction.
2. Non-surgical treatment.
3. Improvement of anterior crossbite with a backward rotation of the mandible.

Treatment Progress

Treatment was started with the Kurz Lingual Appliance. When brackets were bonded on the upper arch, a sandwich technique (resin build up) was used in order to make bite- jumping easier. Because of crowding, a few brackets were temporally bonded at the beginning of the treatment (Fig. **3G**). Brackets were then bonded on the lower arch. The archwires were .012 NiTi on the upper and lower arches (Fig. **3H**). Fig. **3I** shows the intraoral photographs at 7 months in treatment with .0175x.0175 TMA upper and lower archwires.

Treatment Results

Excellent results were obtained with canines and molars in Class I relationship (Figs. **3J** and **K**). Treatment was completed in 23 months. Post-treatment panorama radiograph showed good root paralleling (Fig. **3L**). Dental radiograph showed no root resorption (Fig. **3M**). The position and the shape of mandibular condyle heads were not changed with treatment (Fig. **3N**). Figs. **3O** and **P** show the patient 36 months after treatment stable and excellent occlusion. Superimposition of the pre- and post-treatment radiographs showed no further backward rotation of the mandible. The correction of the anterior crossbite was accomplished with proclination of the upper incisors and retraction of the lower molars (Fig. **3Q**, Table **6**).

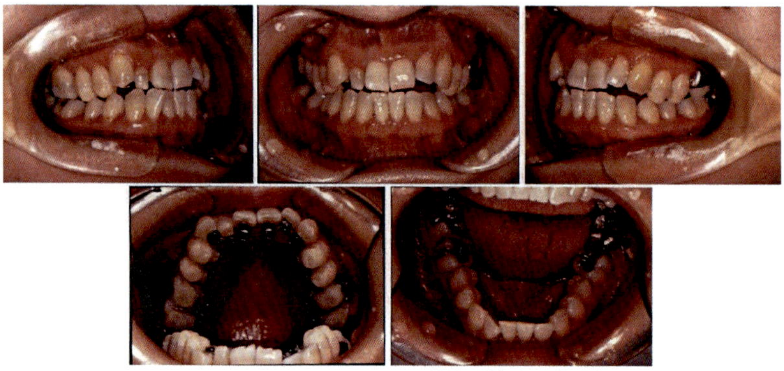

Figure 3G: Case 3: Intra-oral photographs after brackets were bonded on the upper arch. In order to avoid interference between the upper incisors and lower brackets, resin build up was made on upper molars.

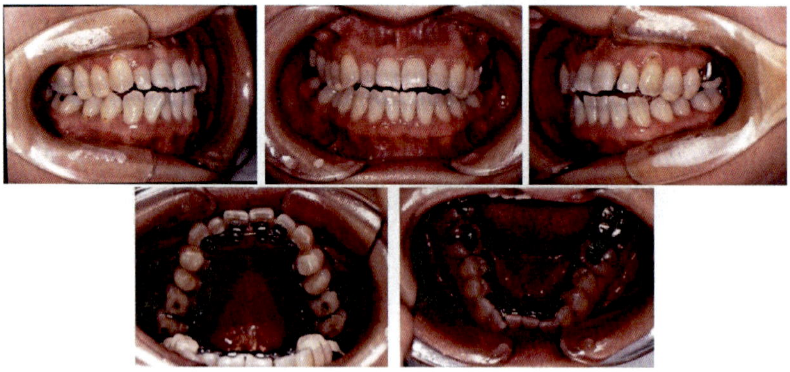

Figure 3H: Case 3: Intra-oral photographs 1 month into treatment. Brackets were bonded on the lower arch. The arch wires used were .012 Ni-Ti in the upper arch and .012 Ni-Ti in the lower arch.

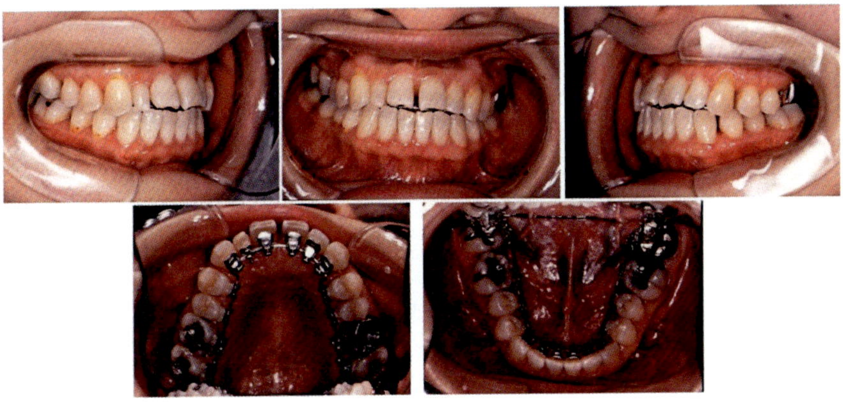

Figure 3I: Case 3: Intra-oral photographs 7 months into treatment. The arch wires used were .0175x.0175 TMA in the upper arch and .0175x.0175 TMA in the lower arch.

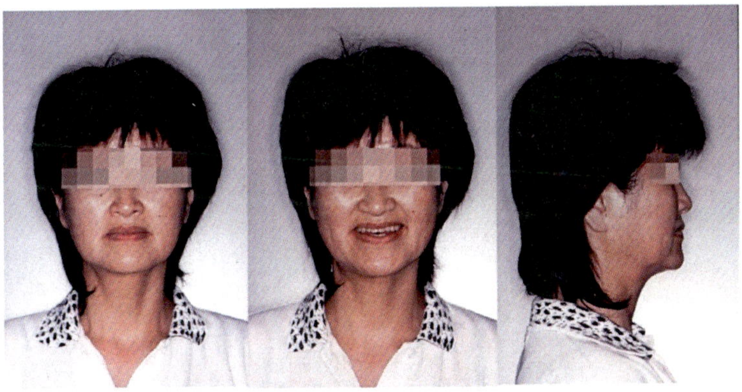

Figure 3J: Case 3: Post-treatment facial photographs.

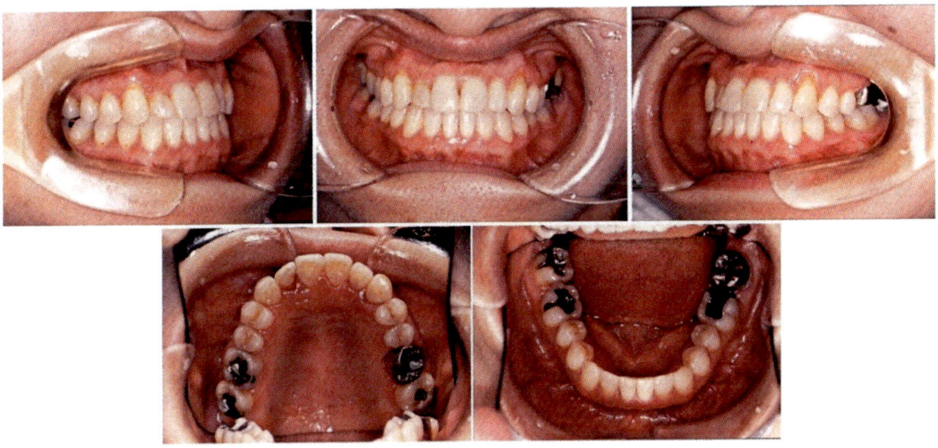

Figure 3K: Case 3: Post-treatment intra-oral photographs.

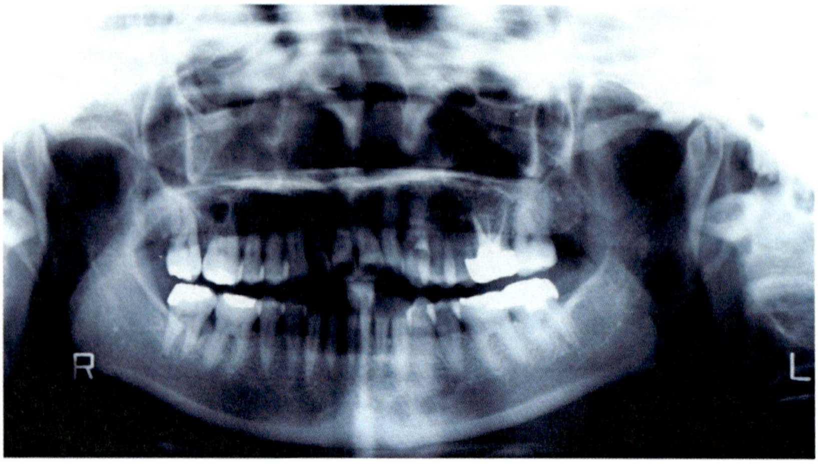

Figure 3L: Case 3: Post-treatment panorama radiograph.

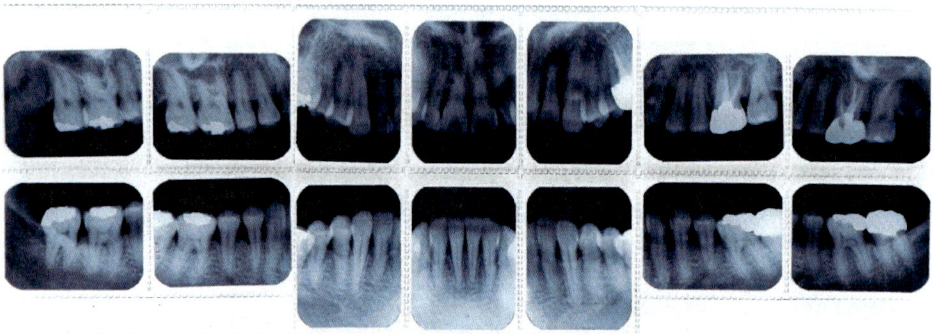

Figure 3M: Case 3: Post-treatment dental radiographs.

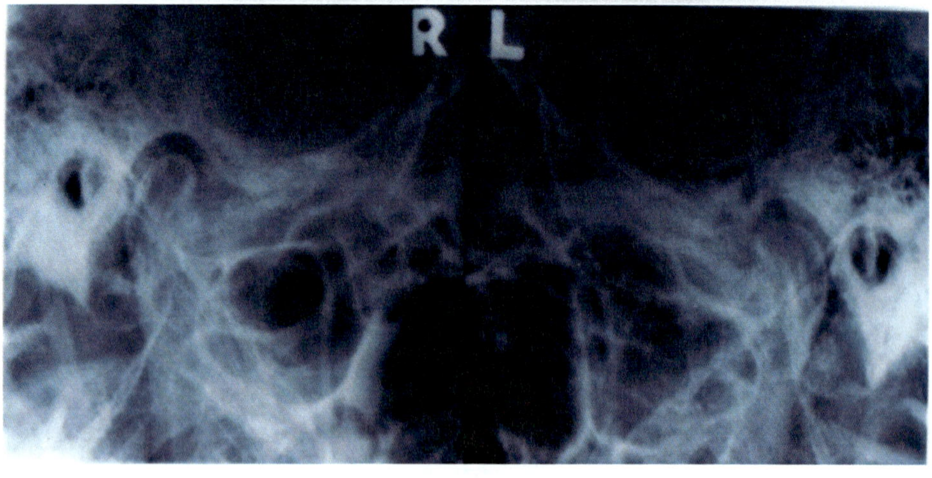

Figure 3N: Case 3: Post-treatment TMJ radiographs.

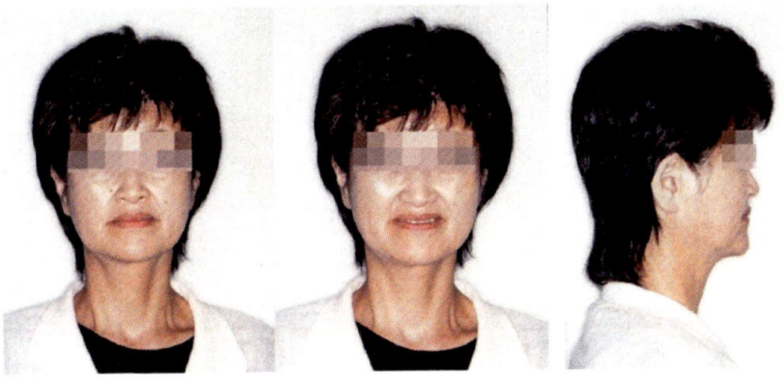

Figure 3O: Case 3: Facial photographs 36 months after completion of the treatment.

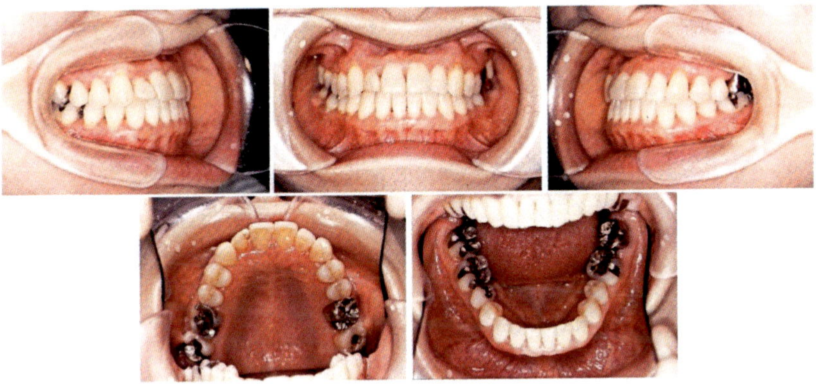

Figure 3P: Case 3: Intra-oral photographs 36 months after completion of the treatment.

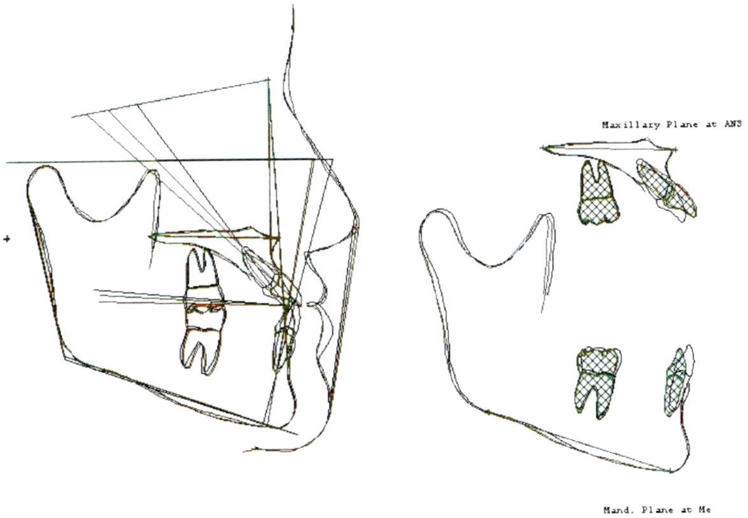

Figure 3Q: Case 3: Superimpositions of cephalogram tracings before and after treatment, and after retention.

Table 6: Case 3: Pre-treatment, post-treatment and after retention cephalometric analysis.

Factor	Mean	S.D.	Win1	Win2	Win3
SNA	80.0	3.0	80.7	80.4	80.9
SNB	77.0	3.0	83.8	83.7	83.9
ANB	3.0	2.0	-3.1	-3.2	-3.1
Mx1-NA	4.0	3.0	5.8	9.7	9.3
Mx1-NA Angle	23.0	6.0	36.2	44.5	47.7
Md1-NB	5.0	3.0	3.9	1.5	1.5
Md1-NB Angle	26.0	6.0	19.1	13.6	14.3
PO - NB	2.0	1.8	1.6	1.8	1.9
Occlusal Plane - SN	18.0	3.5	14.7	11.6	13.4
GO-GN-SN	34.0	4.5	26.9	27.0	26.6
Interincisor Angle	128.0	6.0	127.8	125.2	121.0
Wits Appraisal	1.1	1.9	-11.5	-8.4	-11.0
calculated ANB	3.0	2.0	2.5	2.4	2.5
FMA	25.0	6.0	18.0	18.6	18.6
FMIA	65.0	6.0	74.6	79.8	79.3
IMPA	90.0	6.0	87.3	81.6	82.1
Occulusal Plane - FH			4.9	1.9	3.7
Z Angle			87.5	93.2	91.8

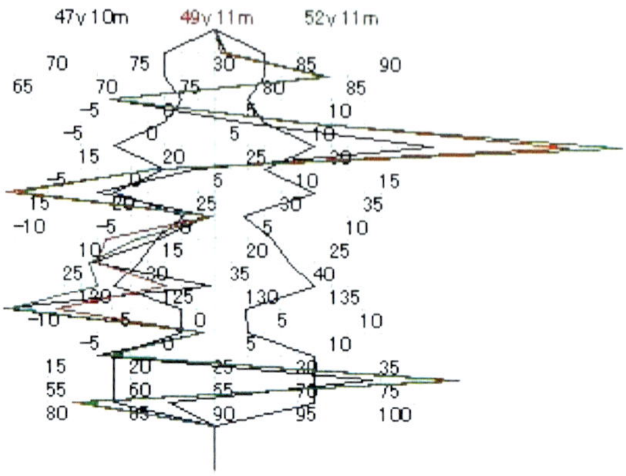

Case 4

The patient was a 33y-7m-old female who visited the author's clinic with a chief complaint of an anterior crossbite. The frontal view showed a symmetrical face but large mandible. The lateral view showed an orthognathic profile (Fig. **4A**). The intraoral view showed molars were 2 mm Class III on both sides (Fig. **4B**). The panoramic radiograph showed horizontally impacted lower third molars (Fig. **4C**). No abnormal findings such as root resorption or periodontal problems were found on the periapical radiographs (Fig. **4D**). The shape of mandibular condyle heads was round, located in the center of the fossa (Fig. **4E**). Lateral cephalometric analysis showed a Class III skeletal anteroposterior jaw relationship with SNA= 82.6°, SNB= 84.7° and ANB= -2.1° (Fig. **4F**, Table **7**).

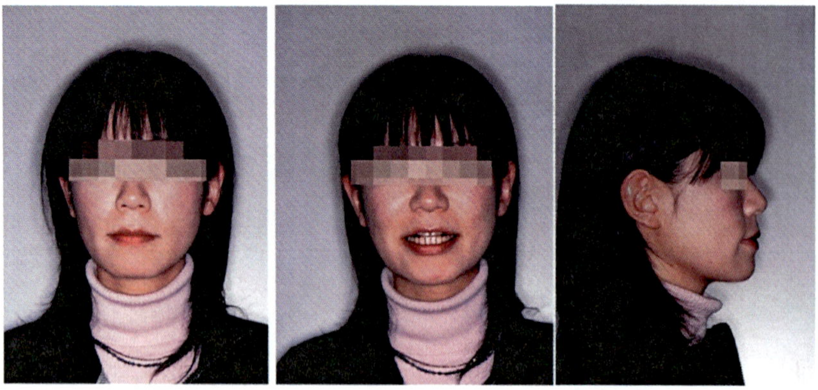

Figure 4A: Case 4: Pre-treatment facial photographs.

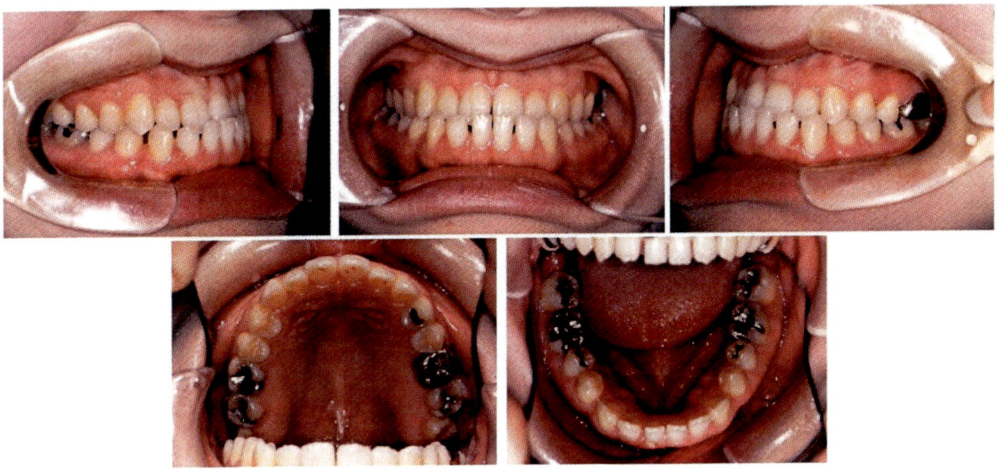

Figure 4B: Case 4: Pre-treatment intra-oral photographs.

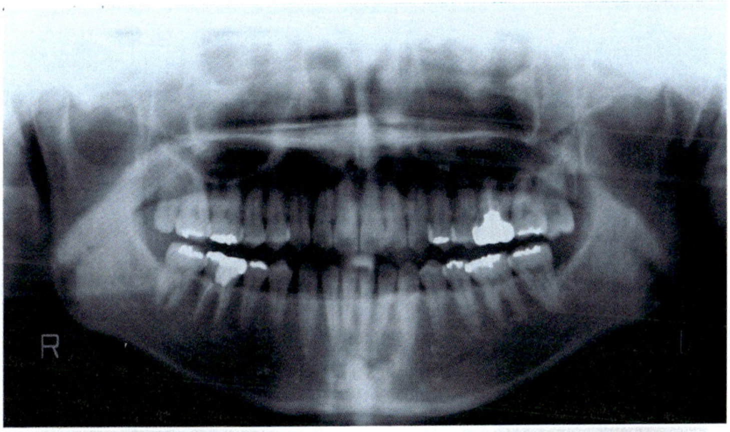

Figure 4C: Case 4: Pre-treatment panorama radiograph.

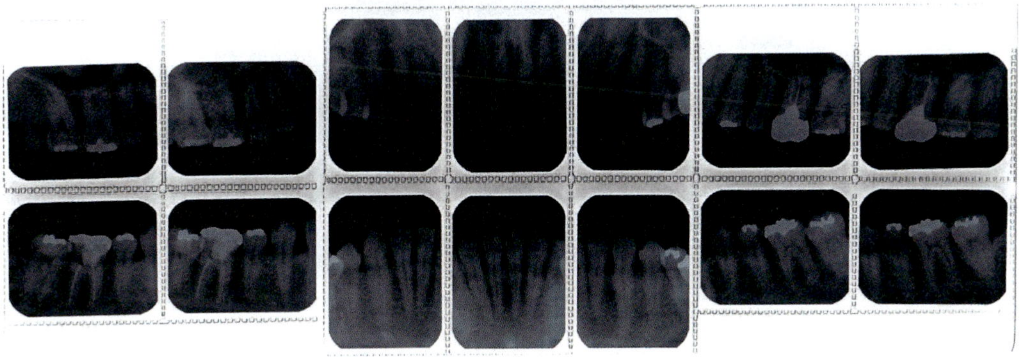

Figure 4D: Case 4: Pre-treatment dental radiographs.

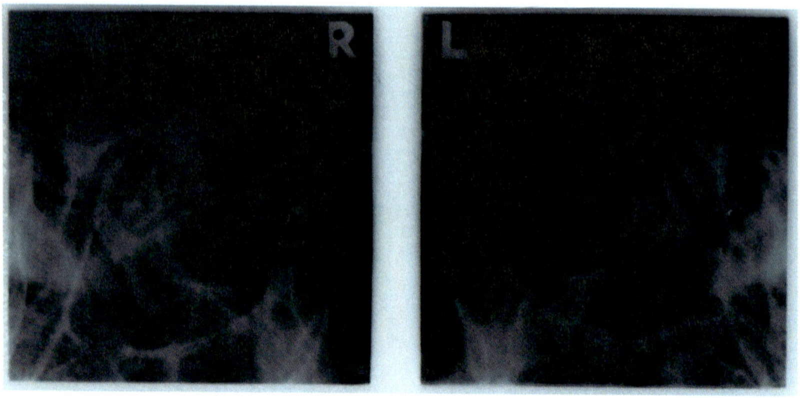

Figure 4E: Case 4: Pre-treatment TMJ radiographs.

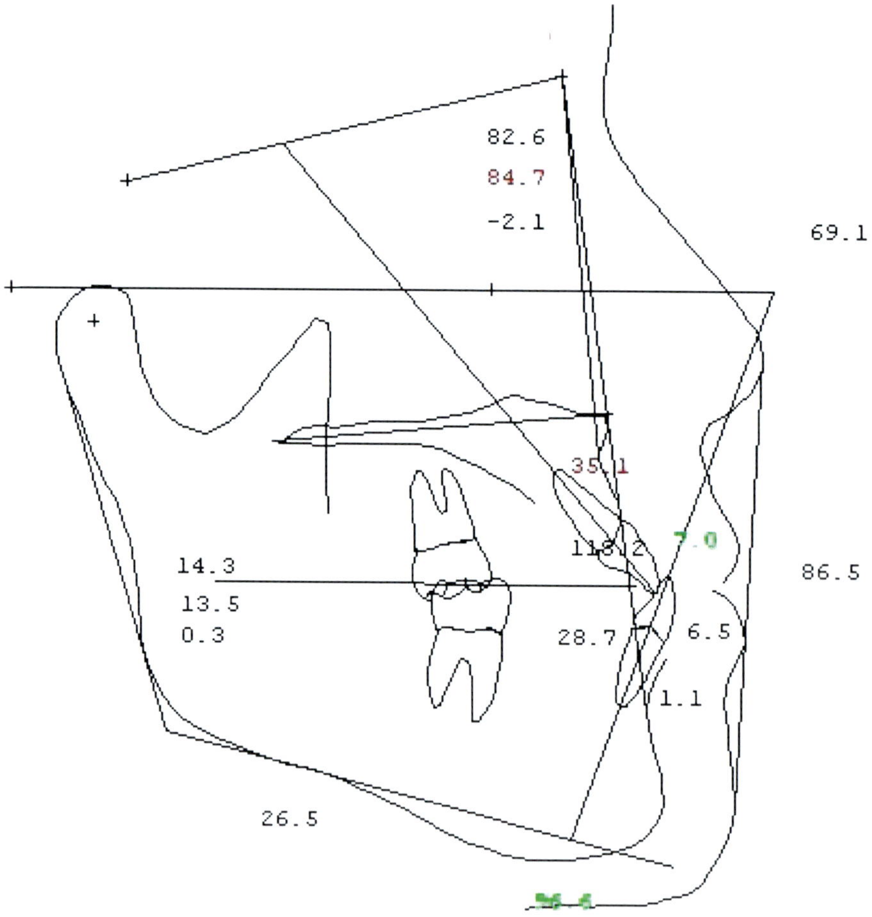

Figure 4F: Case 4: Pre-treatment cephalometric tracing.

Table 7: Case 4: Pre-treatment cephalometric analysis.

Factor	Mean	S.D.	Win1	Win2	Win3
SNA	80.0	3.0	82.6		
SNB	77.0	3.0	84.7		
ANB	3.0	2.0	−2.1		
Mx1-NA	4.0	3.0	7.0		
Mx1-NA Angle	23.0	6.0	35.1		
Md1-NB	5.0	3.0	6.5		
Md1-NB Angle	26.0	6.0	28.7		
PO - NB	2.0	1.8	1.1		
Occlusal Plane - SN	18.0	3.5	13.5		
GO-GN-SN	34.0	4.5	26.5		
Interincisor Angle	128.0	6.0	118.2		
Wits Appraisal	1.1	1.9	−9.0		
calculated ANB	3.0	2.0	3.2		
FMA	25.0	6.0	14.3		
FMIA	65.0	6.0	69.1		
IMPA	90.0	6.0	96.6		
Occulusal Plane - FH			0.3		
Z Angle			86.5		

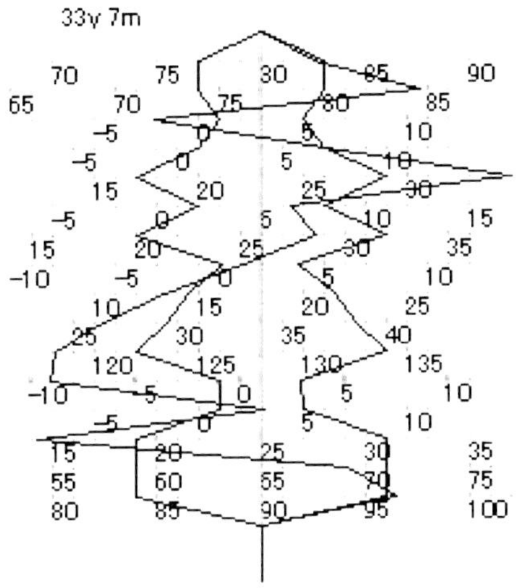

Diagnosis

1. Class III molar relationship (2 mm on each side).
2. Skeletal Class III anteroposterior jaw relationship (ANB -2.1°).
3. Anterior crossbite.
4. Spacing in the lower arch.
5. Arch length discrepancy: Upper: -2.0 mm, Lower: +3.0 mm.

Treatment Objectives

1. Correction of anterior crossbite.
2. Close space in the lower arch.
3. Backward rotation of the mandible.

Treatment Plan

1. Non-extraction treatment.
2. Non-surgical treatment.

3. Correction of anterior cross bite.

4. Class III mechanics.

Treatment Progress

Treatment was started with Lingual Appliance with an initial archwire .012 NiTi on the upper arch (Fig. **4G**). Brackets were bonded on the lower arch the next month with .016 Beta-Ti archwire was given on the upper arch and .012 NiTi on the lower arch (Fig. **4H**). Fig. **4I** showed patient 9 months in treatment. The anterior crossbite was corrected with .017x.025 Beta-Titanium archwires on both arches. Fig. **4J** shows patient 18 months in treatment with Class III elastics worn from upper canine to lower canine on both sides.

Treatment Results

Excellent results were obtained in 21 months of treatment (Figs. **4K** and **L**). Post-treatment panoramic radiograph showed good root paralleling (Fig. **4M**). Periapical radiographs showed minimal root resorption (Fig. **4N**). The position and shape of mandibular condylar head were not changed with treatment (Fig. **4O**). Figs. **4P** and **Q** showed patient 45 months after treatment with stable and excellent occlusion. Superimposition of pre- and post- treatment radiographs showed backward rotation of mandible, retraction and upright of lower incisors and correction of the anterior crossbite (Fig. **4R**, Table **8**).

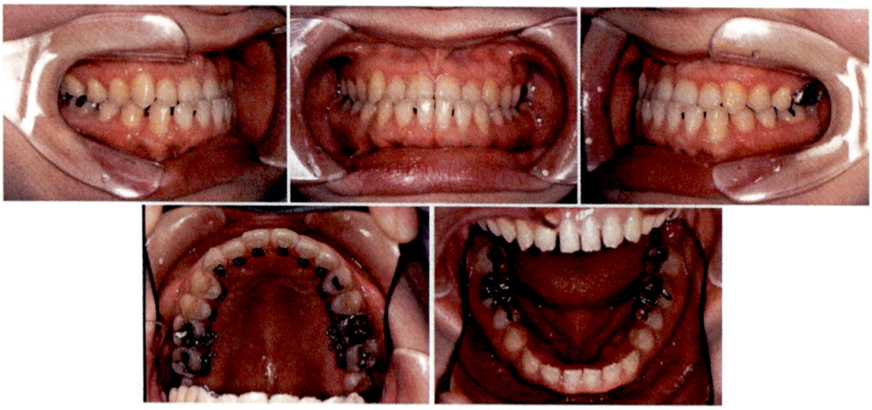

Figure 4G: Case 4: Intra-oral photographs after brackets were bonded on the Upper arch. The arch wire was .012 Ni-Ti.

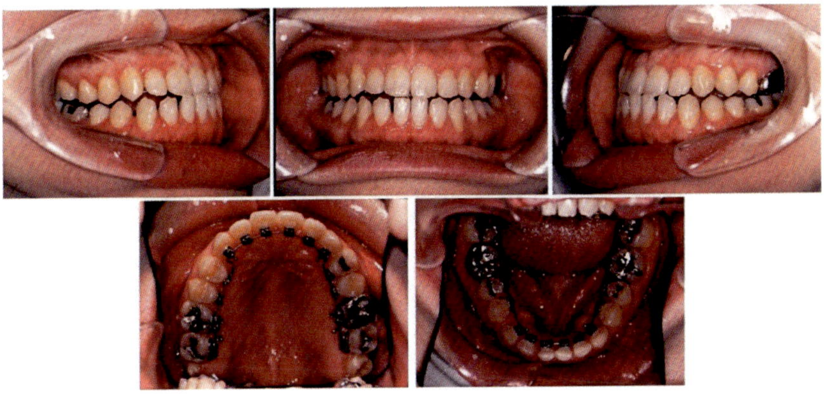

Figure 4H: Case 4: Intra-oral photographs 1 month into treatment. Brackets were bonded on the lower arch. The arch wires used were .016 beta-titanium in the upper arch and .012 Ni-Ti in the lower arch.

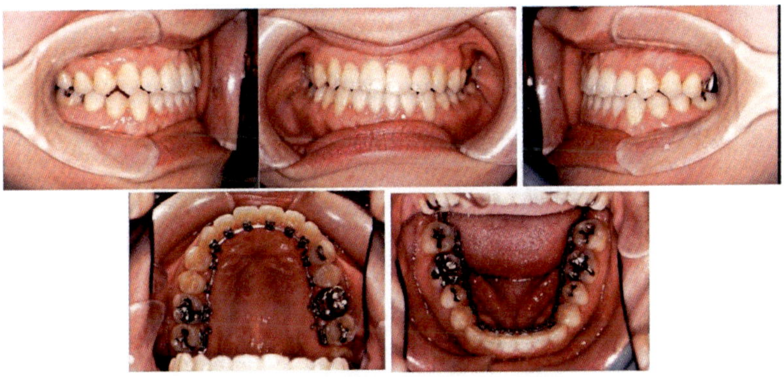

Figure 4I: Case 4: Intra-oral pictures 9 months into treatment. The arch wires used were .017x.025 beta-titanium in the upper and lower arches.

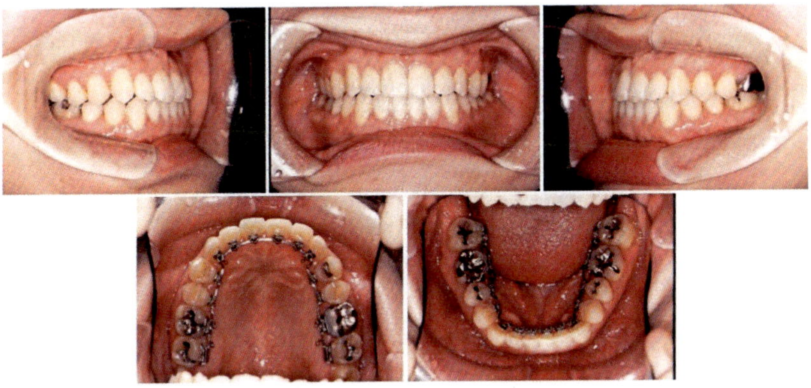

Figure 4J: Case 4: Intra-oral pictures 18 months into treatment. Class III elastics were worn from upper canine to lower canine on both sides.

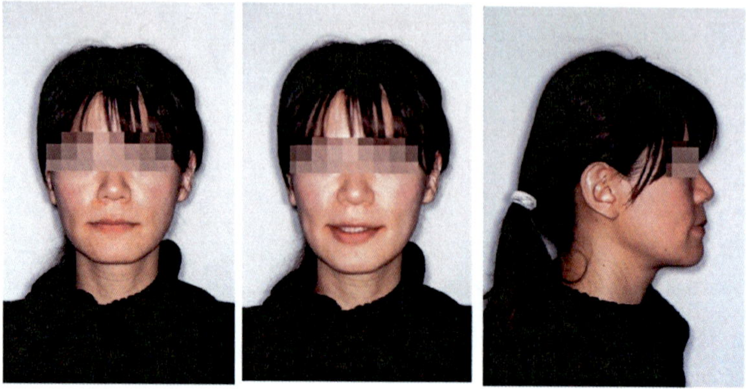

Figure 4K: Case 4: Post-treatment facial photographs.

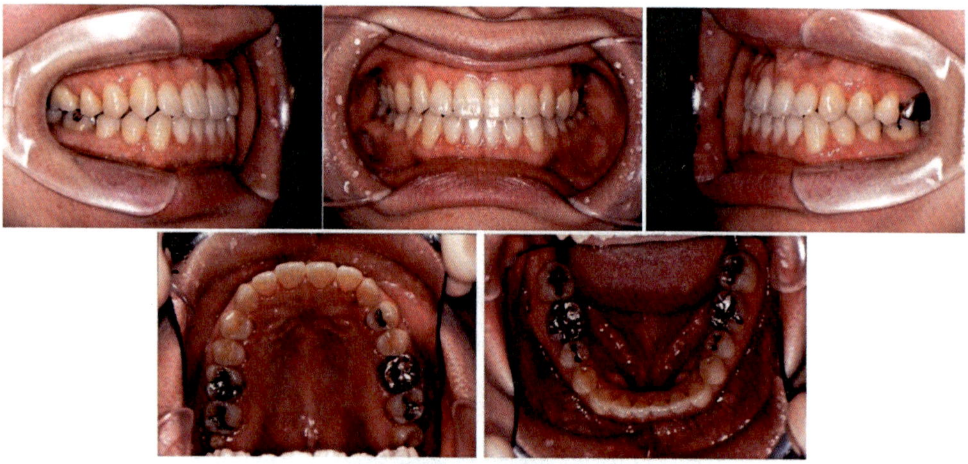

Figure 4L: Case 4: Post-treatment intra-oral photographs.

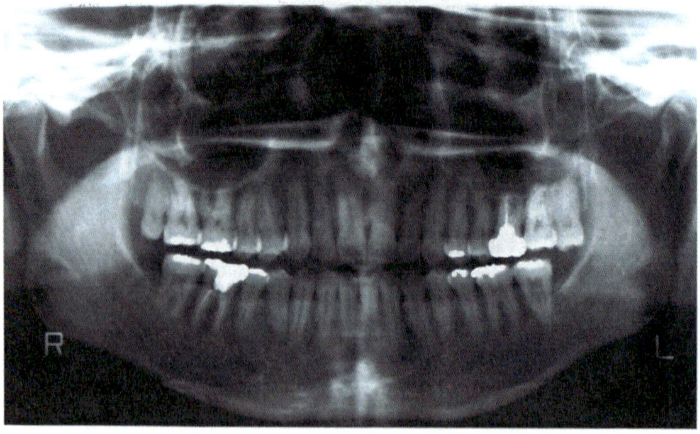

Figure 4M: Case 4: Post-treatment panoramic radiograph.

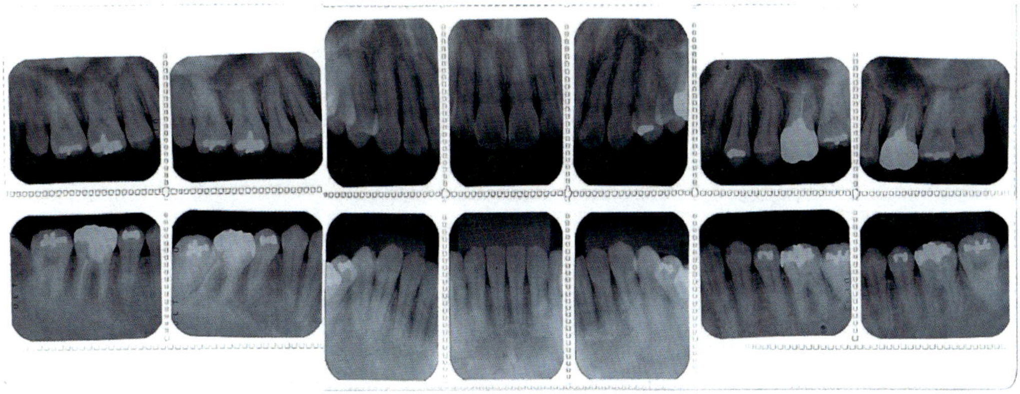

Figure 4N: Case 4: Post-treatment dental radiograph.

Figure 4O: Case 4: Post-treatment TMJ radiograph.

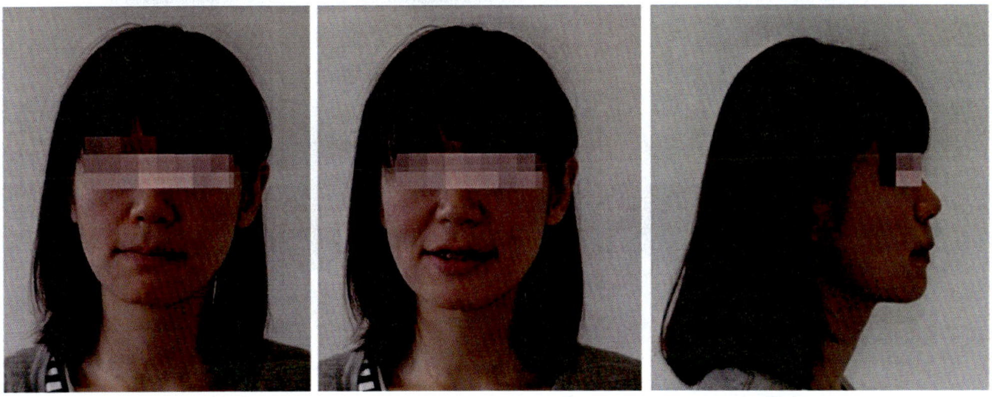

Figure 4P: Case 4: Facial photographs 45 months after completion of the treatment.

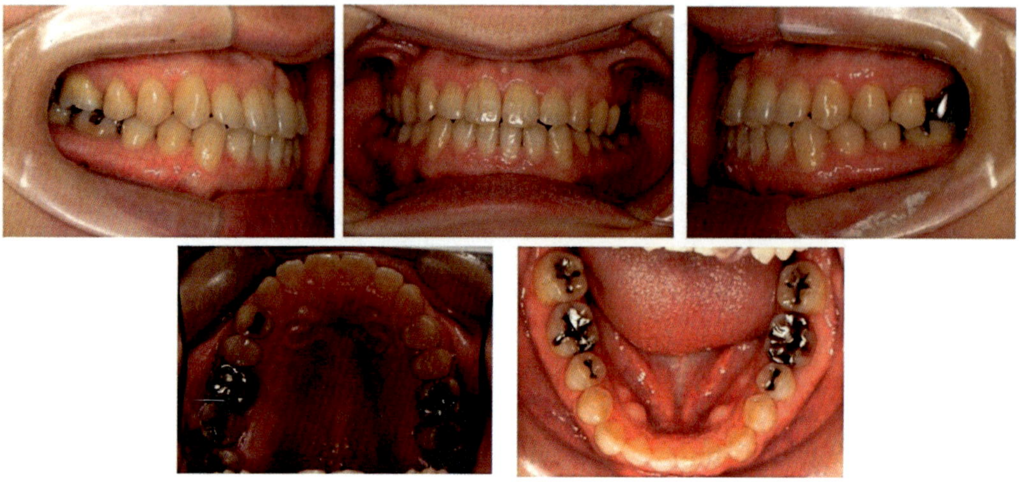

Figure 4Q: Case 4: Intra-oral photographs 45 months after completion of the treatment.

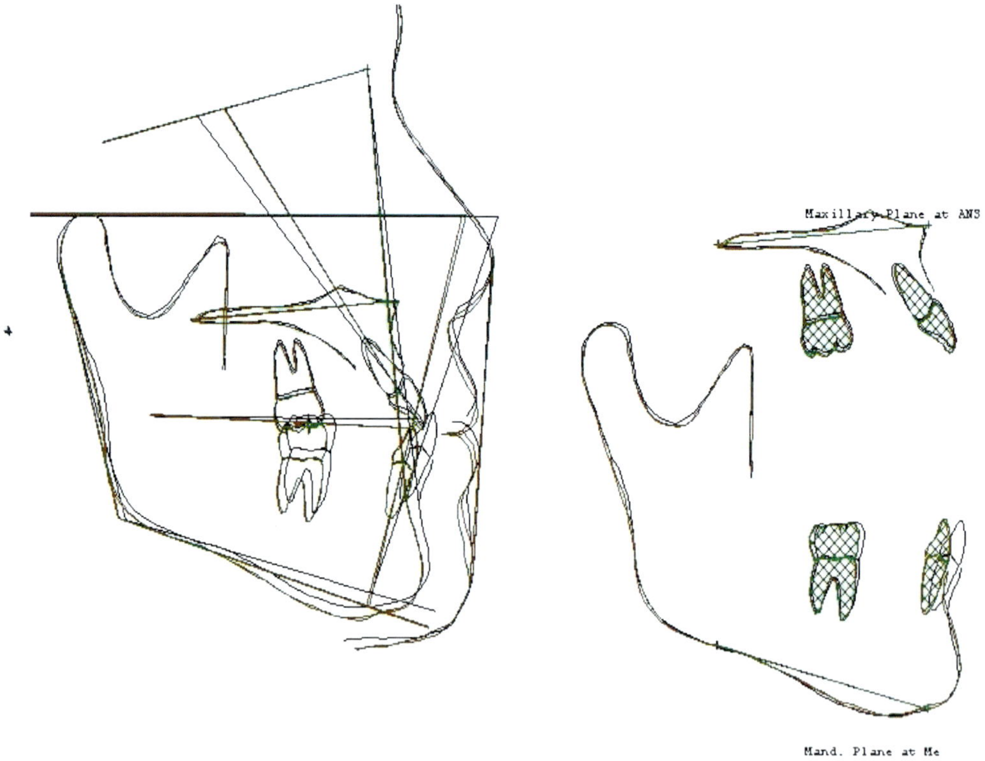

Figure 4R: Case 4: Superimpositions of cephalogram tracings before and after treatment, and after retention.

Table 8: Case 4: Pre-treatment, post-treatment and after retention cephalometric analysis.

Factor	Mean	S.D.	Win1	Win2	Win3
SNA	80.0	3.0	82.6	82.6	82.6
SNB	77.0	3.0	84.7	83.1	82.8
ANB	3.0	2.0	-2.1	-0.4	-0.2
Mx1-NA	4.0	3.0	7.0	6.4	6.3
Mx1-NA Angle	23.0	6.0	35.1	30.1	30.0
Md1-NB	5.0	3.0	6.5	2.9	3.6
Md1-NB Angle	26.0	6.0	28.7	21.3	22.1
PO - NB	2.0	1.8	1.1	2.2	2.8
Occlusal Plane - SN	18.0	3.5	13.5	15.6	15.5
GO-GN-SN	34.0	4.5	26.5	28.2	28.1
Interincisor Angle	128.0	6.0	118.2	129.0	128.1
Wits Appraisal	1.1	1.9	-9.0	-8.2	-7.7
calculated ANB	3.0	2.0	3.2	3.5	3.5
FMA	25.0	6.0	14.3	16.6	16.9
FMIA	65.0	6.0	69.1	75.0	74.0
IMPA	90.0	6.0	96.6	88.4	89.1
Occulusal Plane - FH			0.3	2.3	2.3
Z Angle			86.5	88.1	86.9

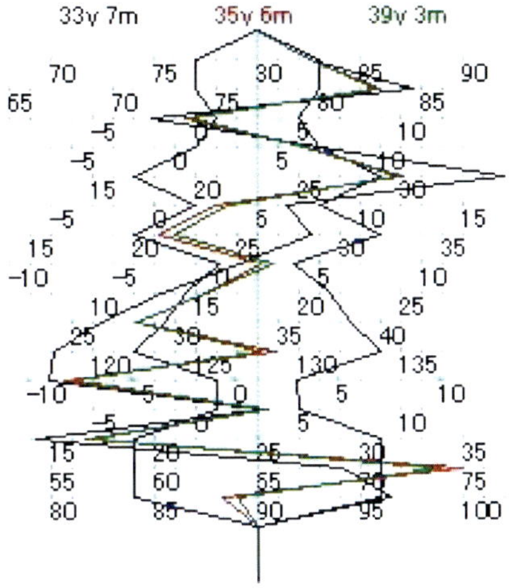

Case 5

The patient was a 30y-0m-old female who visited the author's clinic with a chief complaint of an anterior crossbite and upper anterior crowding. The frontal view showed a symmetrical face and the lateral view showed a concave profile (Fig. **5A**). The intraoral view showed molar relationship was 8 mm Class III on the right side and 7mm Class III on left side (Fig. **5B**). No abnormal findings were found on the panoramic or periapical radiographs (Figs. **5C** and **D**). The shape of mandibular condylar heads was round, located in the center of fossa (Fig. **5E**). The lateral cephalometric analysis showed a Class III skeletal anteroposterior jaw relationship with SNA= 75.0°, SNB= 78.7° and ANB= -3.7° (Fig. **5F**, Table **9**).

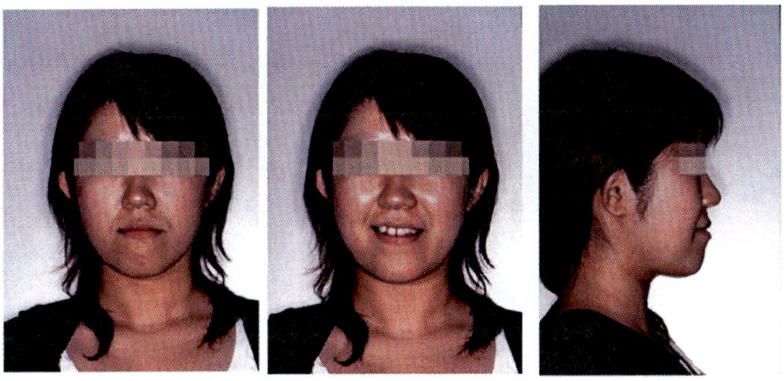

Figure 5A: Case 5: Pre-treatment facial photographs.

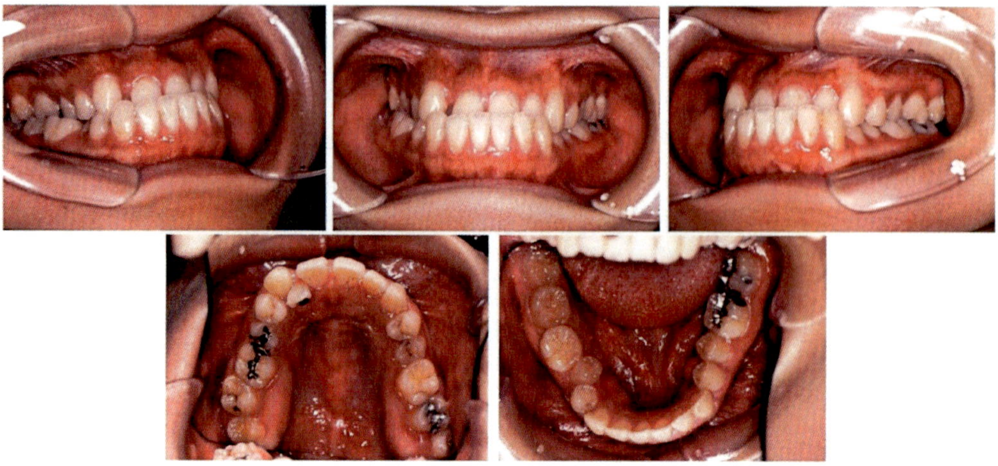

Figure 5B: Case 5. Pre-treatment intra-oral photographs.

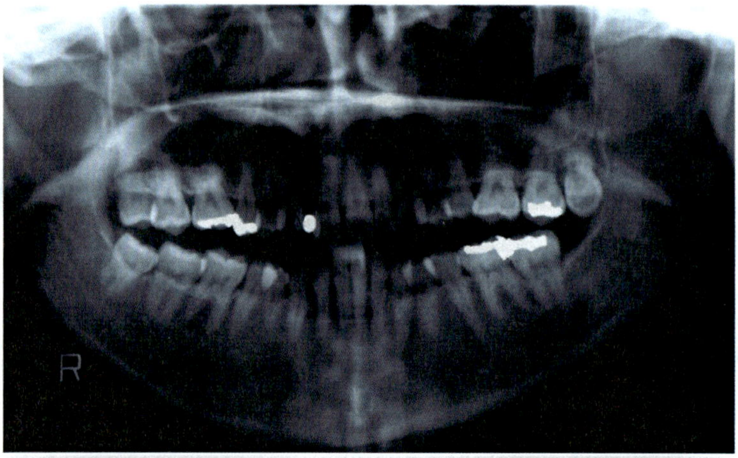

Figure 5C: Case 5: Pre-treatment panoramic radiograph.

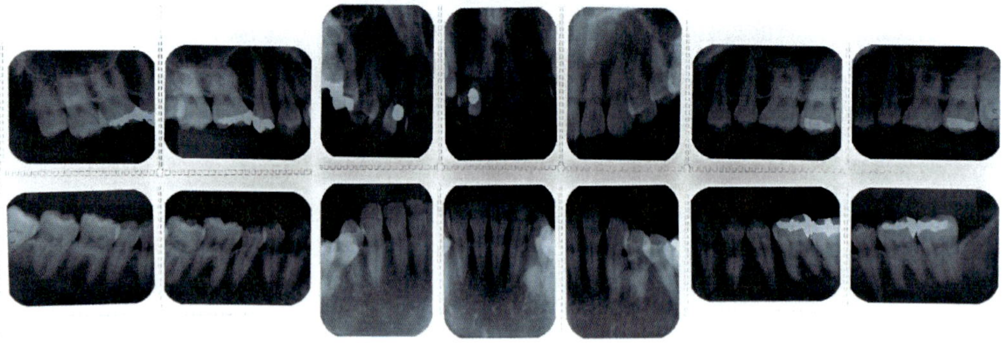

Figure 5D: Case 5: Pre-treatment dental radiographs.

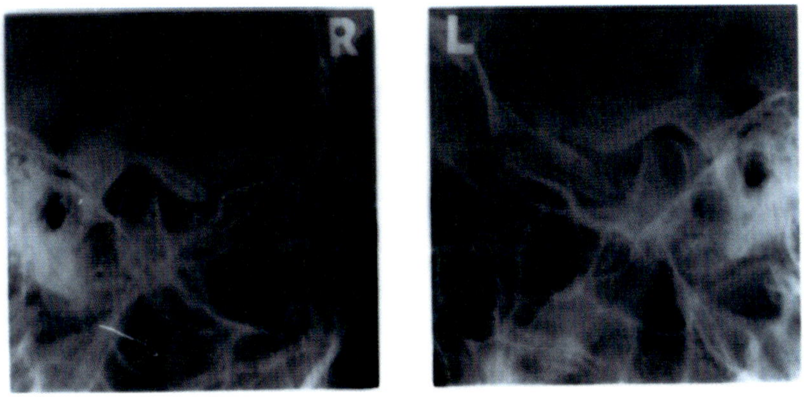

Figure 5E: Case 5: Pre-treatment TMJ radiographs.

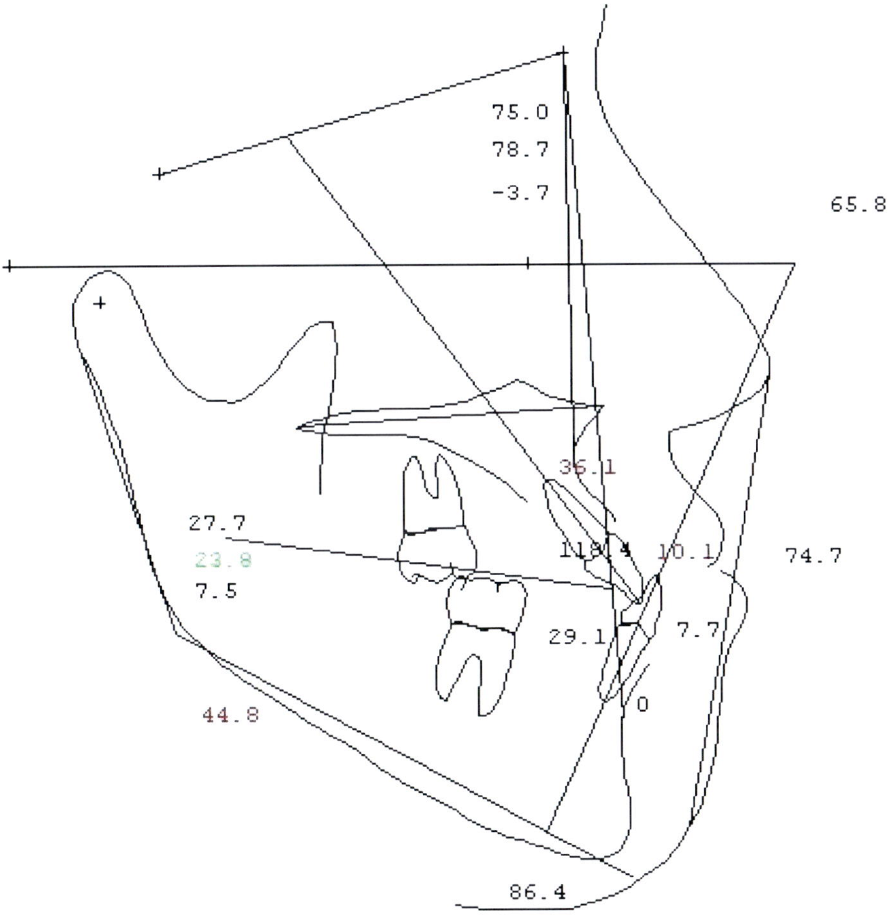

Figure 5F: Case 5: Pre-treatment cephalometric tracing.

Table 9: Case 5: Pre-treatment Cephalometric analysis.

Factor	Mean	S.D.	Wn1	Wn2	Wn3
SNA	80.0	3.0	75.0		
SNB	77.0	3.0	78.7		
ANB	3.0	2.0	-3.7		
Mx1-NA	4.0	3.0	10.1		
Mx1-NA Angle	23.0	6.0	36.1		
Md1-NB	5.0	3.0	7.7		
Md1-NB Angle	26.0	6.0	29.1		
PO - NB	2.0	1.8	-0.5		
Occlusal Plane - SN	18.0	3.5	23.8		
GO-GN-SN	34.0	4.5	44.8		
Interincisor Angle	128.0	6.0	118.4		
Wts Appraisal	1.1	1.9	-16.0		
calculated ANB	3.0	2.0	3.8		
FMA	25.0	6.0	27.7		
FMIA	65.0	6.0	65.8		
IMPA	90.0	6.0	86.4		
Occulusal Plane - FH			7.5		
Z Angle			74.7		

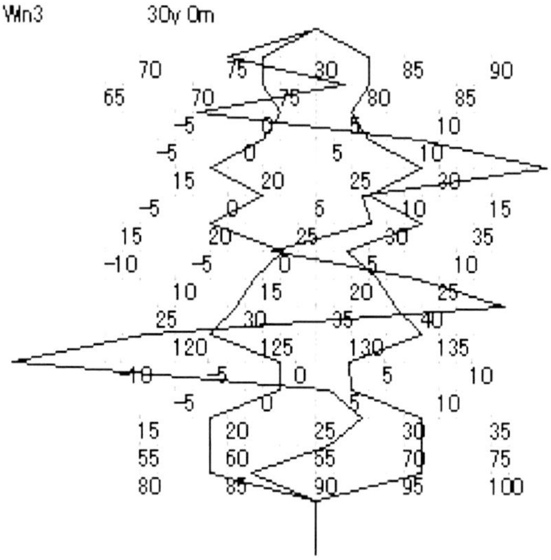

Diagnosis

1. Class III molar relationship (right: 8 mm, left: 7mm).

2. Skeletal III anteroposterior jaw relationship (ANB -3.7°).

3. Anterior crossbite.

5. Upper right lateral incisor erupted palatally.

6. Arch length discrepancy: Upper: -5.0mm, Lower: -1.0mm.

Treatment Objectives

1. Establish Class I molar relationship.

2. Improve skeletal jaw relationship and minimize mandibular backward rotation.

3. Gain adequate overjet & overbite.

4. Correct crowding in the upper arch.

Treatment Plan

1. Non-extraction
2. Non-surgical treatment
3. Leveling of upper and lower arch
2. Correct crowding in the upper arch
3. Upright lower molars to obtain Class I molar relationship

Treatment Progress

Treatment was started with author's original mini lingual brackets. Brackets were bonded on the upper arch first and then lower arch in the next month (Fig. **5G** and **H**). After 4 months, .0175x.0175 Beta-Titanium archwires were placed on both arches, Class III elastics were worn from upper 1st molar to lower canine on both sides. Vertical loops were made between upper canine and 1st bicuspids in order to improve the anterior crossbite. After 15 months of treatment, .017x.025 Beta-Titanium were placed on the upper arch and .0175x.0175 Beta-Titanium on the lower arch (Fig. **5I**). Class III elastics were worn from upper 1st molar to lower canine on both side (Figs. **5J**).

Treatment Results

Excellent result was obtained with Class I molar relationship on both sides (Figs. **5K** and **L**). Treatment time was 32 months. Post-treatment panoramic radiograph showed good root paralleling (Fig. **5M**). Periapical radiograph showed no root resorption (Fig. **5N**). The position and shape of the mandibular condyle heads were not changed with the treatment (Fig. **5O**). Figs. **5P** and **Q** showed patient after 36 months of treatment with excellent and stable occlusion. Superimposition of the pre- and post-treatment radiographs showed backward rotation of the mandible. The lower molars were uprighted and the jaw relationship was improved. (Fig. **5R**, Table **10**).

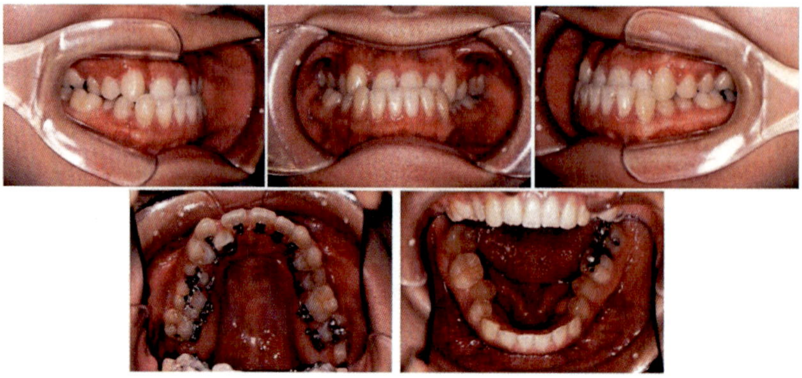

Figure 5G: Case 5: Intra-oral photographs taken after brackets were bonded on the upper arch. The arch wire used was .012 Ni-Ti.

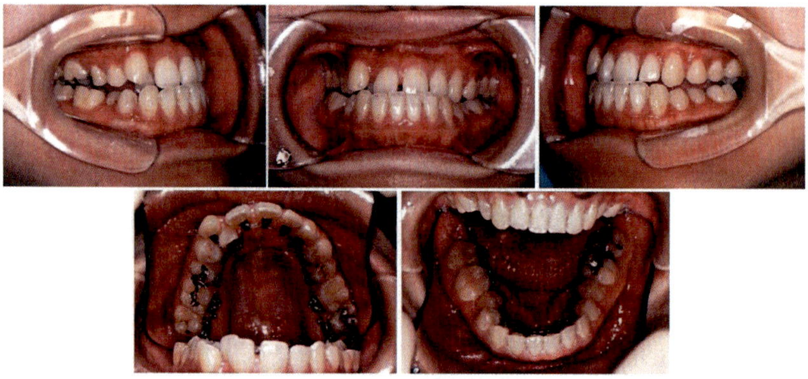

Figure 5H: Case 5: Intra-oral photographs 1 month into treatment. Brackets were bonded on the lower arch. Arch wires used were .012 Ni-Ti on the upper and lower arches.

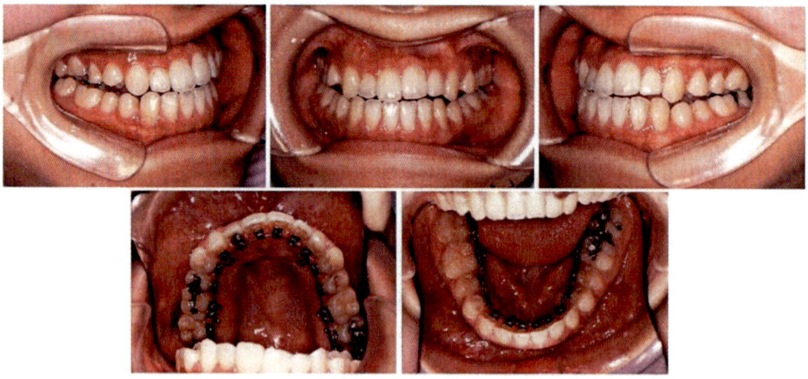

Figure 5I: Case 5: Intra-oral photographs 4 months into treatment. Arch wires used were .0175x.0175 beta-titanium on both arches. Class III elastics were worn from the upper first molar to the lower canine on the right and left sides.

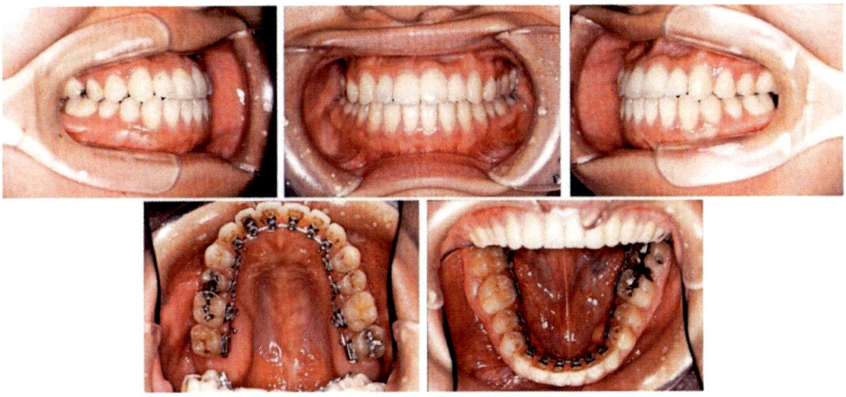

Figure 5J: Case 5: Intra-oral photographs 15 months into treatment. The arch wires used were .017x.025 beta-titanium on the upper arch and .0175x.0175 beta-titanium on the lower arch. Class III elastics were worn from the upper first molar to the lower canine on both sides.

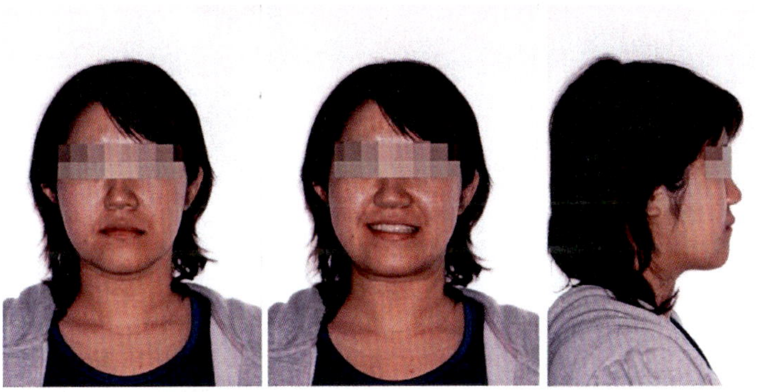

Figure 5K: Case 5: Post-treatment facial photographs.

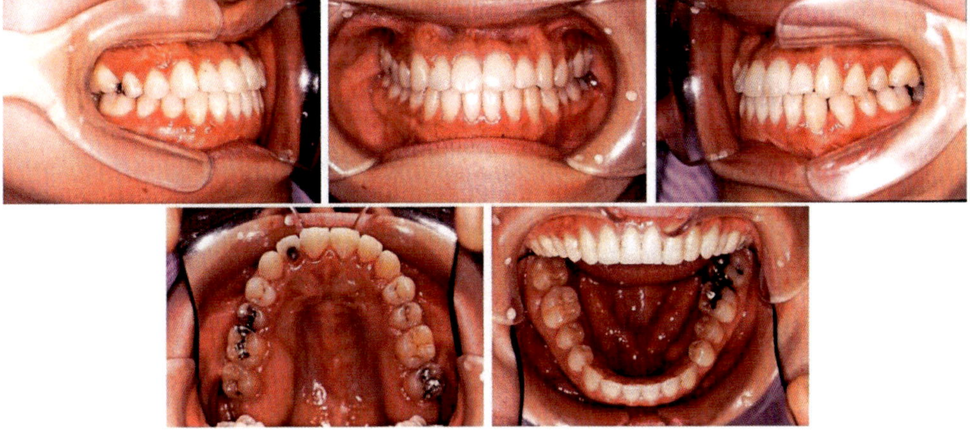

Figure 5L: Case 5: Post-treatment intra-oral photographs.

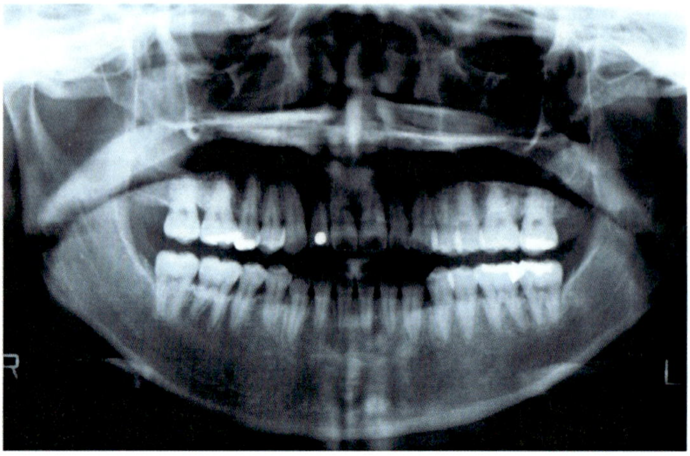

Figure 5M: Case 5: Post-treatment panoramic radiograph.

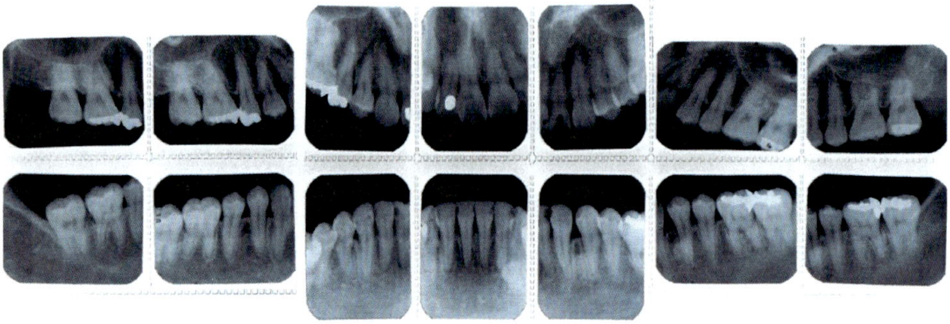

Figure 5N: Case 5: Post-treatment dental radiographs.

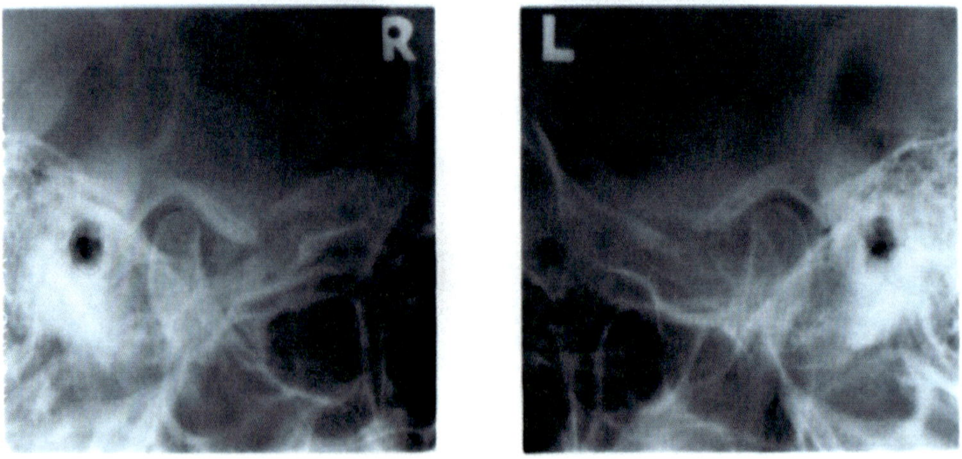

Figure 5O: Case 5: Post-treatment TMJ radiographs.

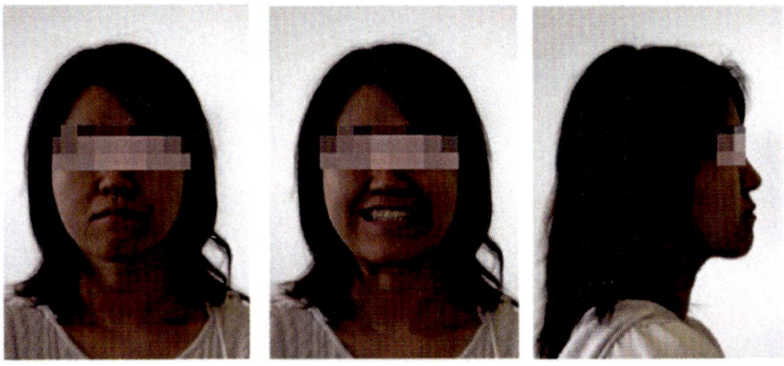

Figure 5P: Case 5: Facial photographs 3 year and 2 months after completion of the treatment.

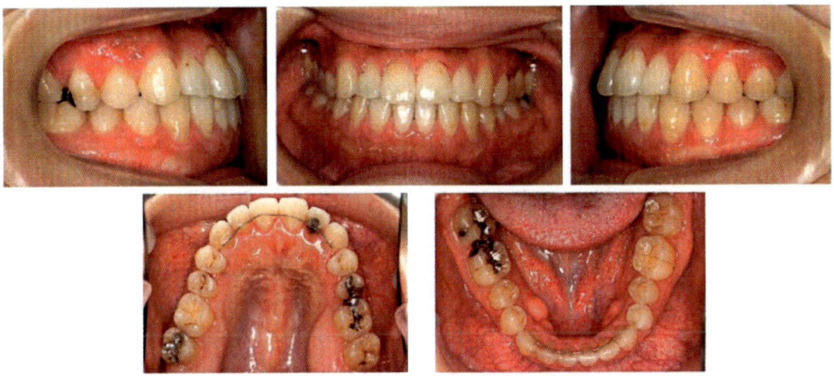

Figure 5Q: Case 5: Intra-oral photographs 3 years and 2 months after completion of the treatment.

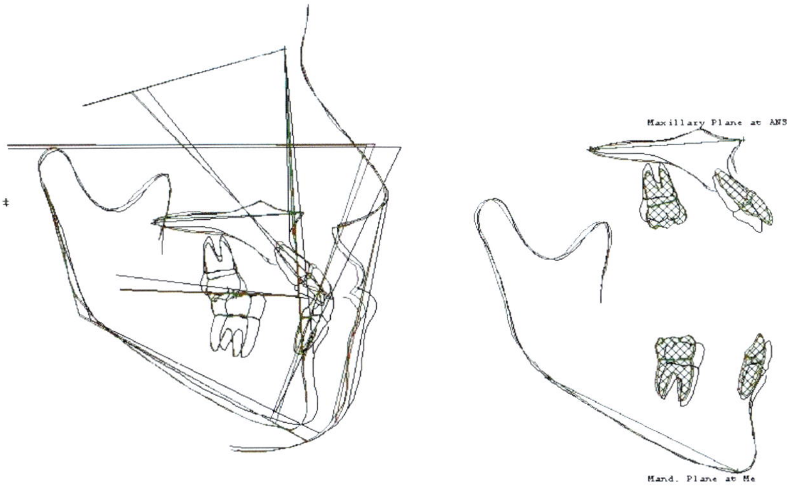

Figure 5R: Case 5: Superimpositions of cephalogram tracings before and after treatment, and after retention.

Table 10: Pre-treatment, post-treatment and after retention cephalometric analysis.

Factor	Mean	S.D.	Wn1	Wn2	Wn3
SNA	80.0	3.0	75.0	75.8	75.9
SNB	77.0	3.0	78.7	76.9	76.7
ANB	3.0	2.0	−3.7	−1.1	−0.8
Mx1 -NA	4.0	3.0	10.1	11.1	11.8
Mx1 -NA Angle	23.0	6.0	36.1	40.8	40.0
Md1 -NB	5.0	3.0	7.7	6.2	6.2
Md1 -NB Angle	26.0	6.0	29.1	23.0	20.3
PO - NB	2.0	1.8	−0.5	−0.4	0.0
Occlusal Plane - SN	18.0	3.5	23.8	18.5	18.5
GO-GN-SN	34.0	4.5	44.8	47.3	47.5
Interincisor Angle	128.0	6.0	118.4	117.4	120.5
Wits Appraisal	1.1	1.9	−16.0	−8.2	−6.9
calculated ANB	3.0	2.0	3.8	4.6	4.7
FMA	25.0	6.0	27.7	30.5	29.7
FMIA	65.0	6.0	65.8	70.2	73.0
IMPA	90.0	6.0	86.4	79.3	77.3
Occulusal Plane - FH			7.5	2.2	1.9
Z Angle			74.7	76.6	73.7

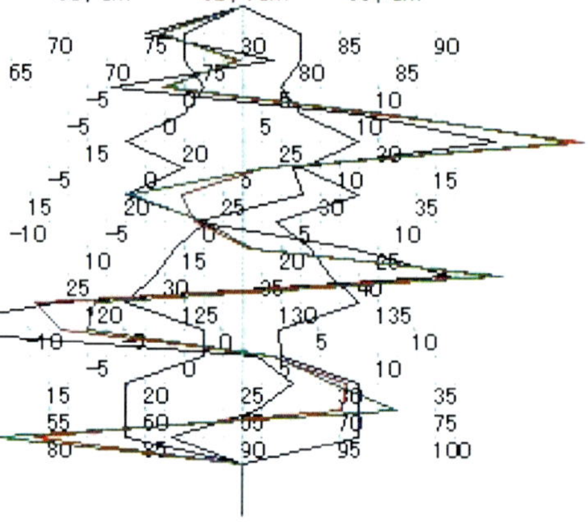

Case 6

The patient was a 43y-5m-old female who visited the author's clinic with a chief complaint of an anterior crossbite. The frontal view showed a symmetrical face and the lateral view showed a concave profile (Fig. **6A**). The intraoral view showed the molar relationship was 4 mm Class III on the right side and Class I on the left side (Fig. **6B**). No abnormal findings were found on the panoramic and periapical radiographs (Figs. **6C** and **D**). The shape of mandibular condylar heads was slightly flattened on both sides, located in the center of fossa (Fig. **6E**). The lateral cephalometric analysis showed a Class III skeletal anteroposterior jaw relationship with a SNA=85.7°, SNB=84.2° and ANB=1.5°. The upper and lower incisors were proclined (Fig. **6F**, Table **11**).

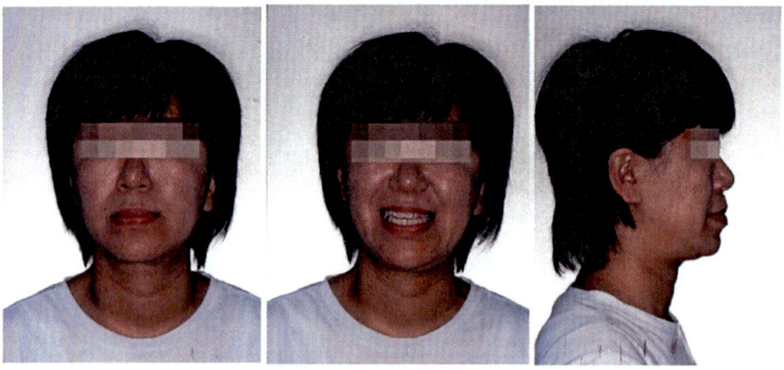

Figure 6A: Case 6: Pre-treatment facial photographs.

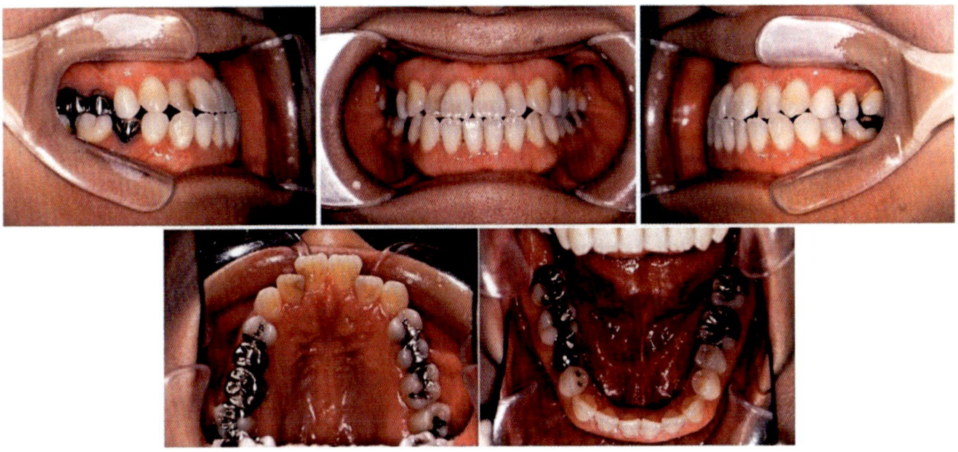

Figure 6B: Case 6: Pre-treatment intra-oral photographs.

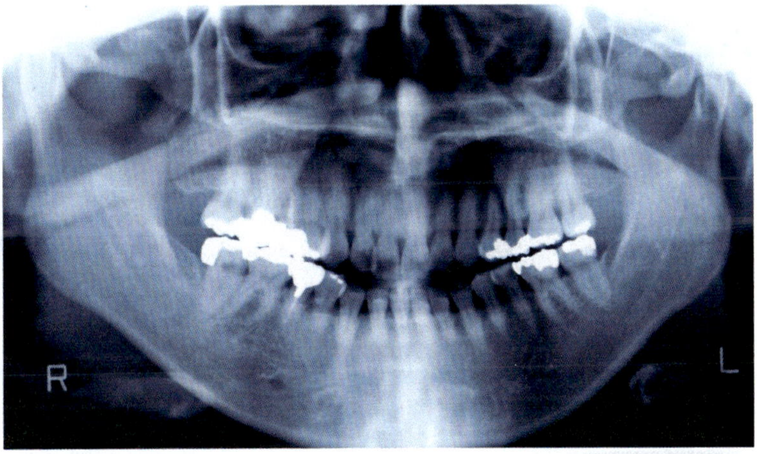

Figure 6C: Case 6: Pre-treatment panoramic radiograph.

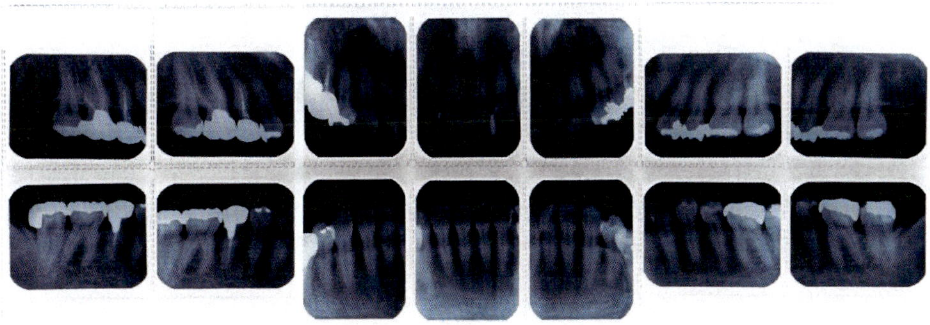

Figure 6D: Case 6: Pre-treatment dental radiographs.

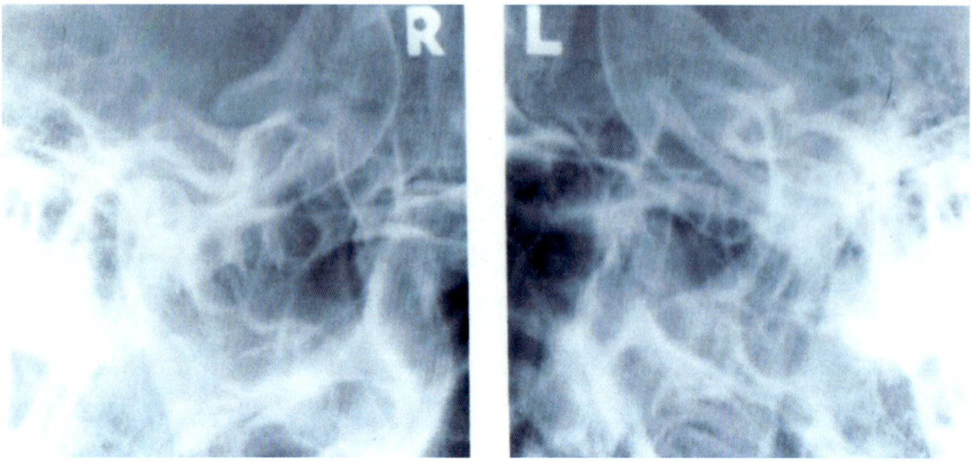

Figure 6E: Case 6: Pre-treatment TMJ radiographs.

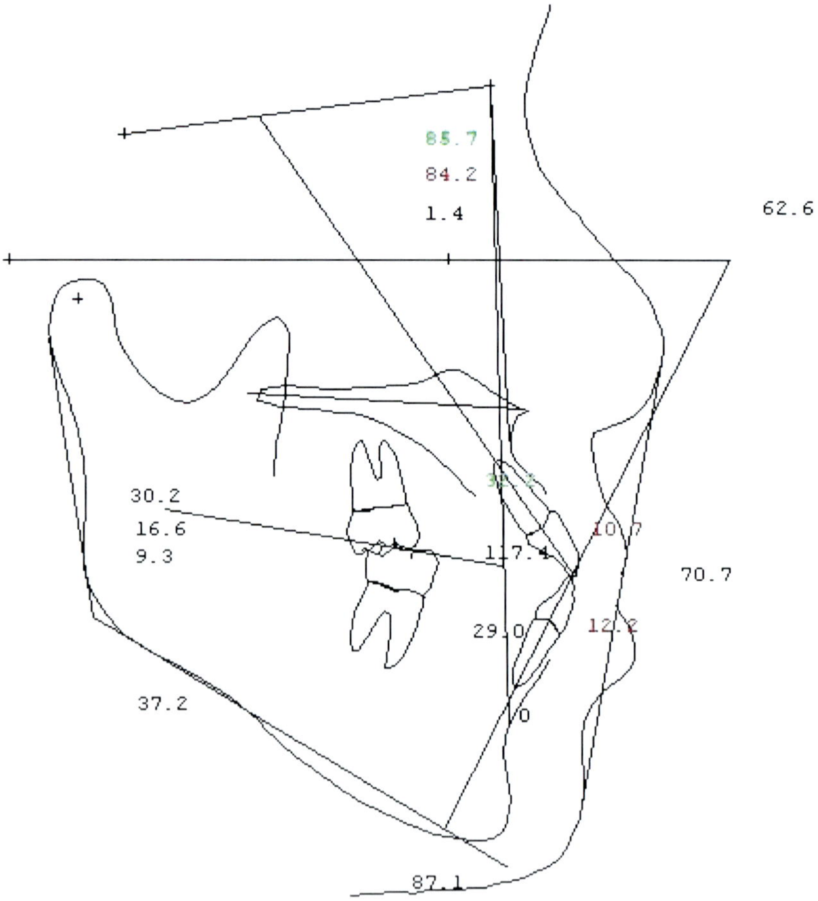

Figure 6F: Case 6: Pre-treatment cephalometric tracing.

Table 11: Case 6: Pre-treatment Cephalometric analysis.

Factor	Mean	S.D.	Wn1	Wn2	Wn3
SNA	80.0	3.0	85.7		
SNB	77.0	3.0	84.2		
ANB	3.0	2.0	1.4		
Mx1-NA	4.0	3.0	10.7		
Mx1-NA Angle	23.0	6.0	32.2		
Md1-NB	5.0	3.0	12.2		
Md1-NB Angle	26.0	6.0	29.0		
PO - NB	2.0	1.8	-0.4		
Occlusal Plane - SN	18.0	3.5	16.6		
GO-GN-SN	34.0	4.5	37.2		
Interincisor Angle	128.0	6.0	117.4		
Wits Appraisal	1.1	1.9	-8.8		
calculated ANB	3.0	2.0	6.5		
FMA	25.0	6.0	30.2		
FMIA	65.0	6.0	62.6		
IMPA	90.0	6.0	87.1		
Occulusal Plane - FH			9.3		
Z Angle			70.7		

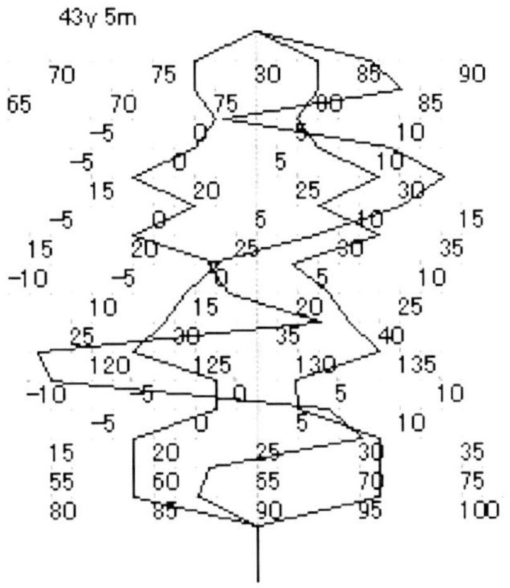

Diagnosis

1. Angle Class III subdivision (3mm class III in right)
2. Lower midline 3mm shift to left
3. Skeletal Class III anteroposterior jaw relationship (ANB 1.9°)
4. Anterior crossbite of lateral incisors on both sides
5. Arch length discrepancy: Upper: -2.0 mm, Lower: 0 mm

Treatment Objectives

1. Improvement of upper lateral incisors' cross bite
2. Improvement of anterior cross bite and mid line
3. Improvement of jaw relationship with backward rotation of mandible

Treatment Plan

1. Extraction of lower right second bicuspid
2. Non-surgical treatment

3. Correct upper lateral incisors in anterior crossbite

4. Correct midline discrepancy

5. Finish Class III on the right side

Treatment Progress

After extraction of the lower right second bicuspid, treatment was started with author's original mini lingual brackets. At first, the brackets were bonded on the lower arch with an initial .012 NiTi archwire (Fig. **6G**). After 3 months of treatment, brackets were bonded on the upper arch with a .012 NiTi arch and a .0175x.0175 Beta-Ti archwire. Fig. **6H** shows the patient 18 month in treatment with .0175x.0175 TMA archwires on both arches. Lower space consolidation was completed with sliding mechanics (Fig. **6I**).

Treatment Results

Excellent result was obtained in 23 months with Class III molar relationship on the right side (Figs. **6J** and **K**). Post-treatment panoramic radiograph showed good root paralleling (Fig. **6L**). Periapical radiograph showed minimal root resorption in the lower anteriors (Fig. **6M**). No significant changes were noted in the position and the shape of mandibular condylar head (Fig. **6N**). Figs. **6O** and **P** showed patient 36 months after treatment with excellent and stable occlusion. Superimposition of the pre- and post-treatment radiographs showed slight backward rotation of mandible (Fig. **6Q**, Table **12**).

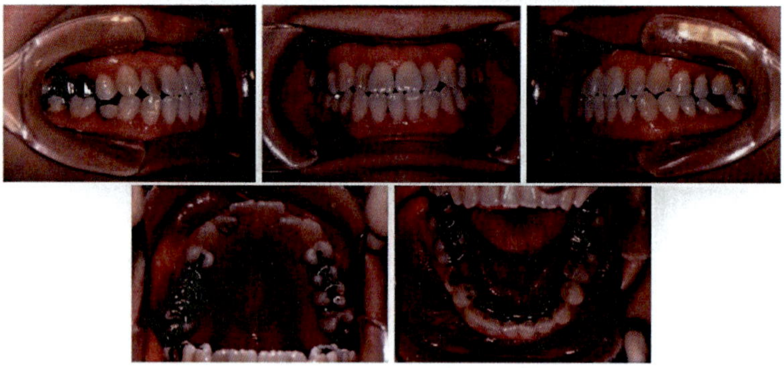

Figure 6G: Case 6: Intra-oral photographs taken after brackets were bonded on the upper arch. Arch wire used was .012 Ni-Ti.

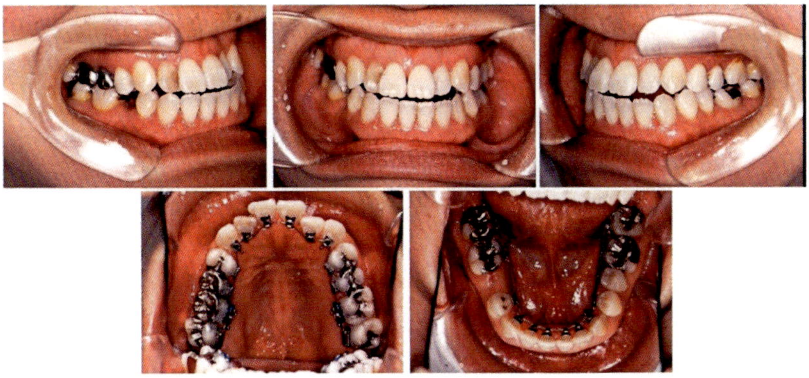

Figure 6H: Case 6: Intra-oral photographs 3 month into treatment. Brackets were bonded on the lower arch. The arch wires used were .012 Ni-Ti on the upper arch and .0175x.0175 beta-titanium on the lower arch.

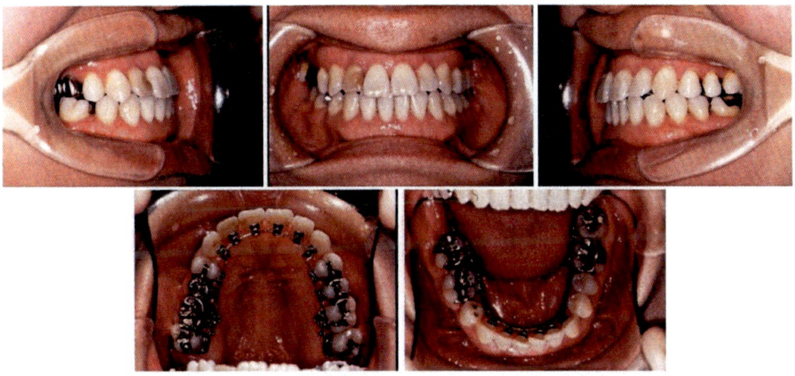

Figure 6I: Case 6: Intra-oral photographs 18 month into treatment. Arch wires used were .0175x.0175 TMA on both arches. Lower space consolidation was done with sliding mechanics.

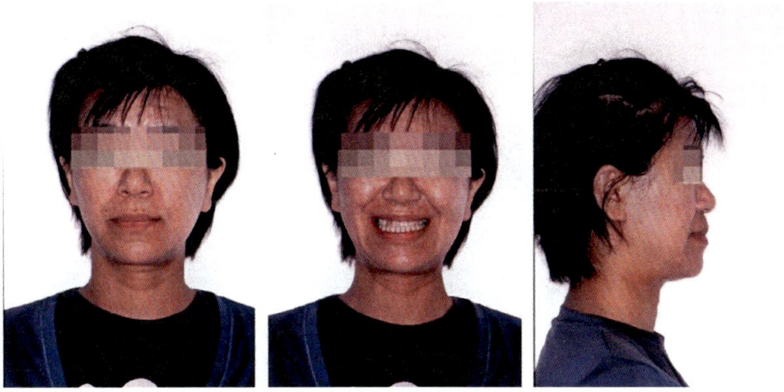

Figure 6J: Case 6: Post-treatment facial photographs.

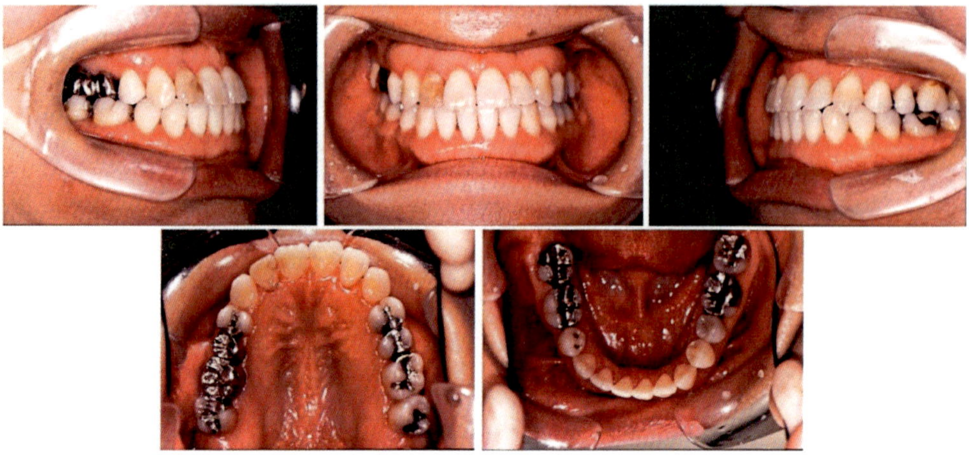

Figure 6K: Case 6: Post-treatment intra-oral photographs.

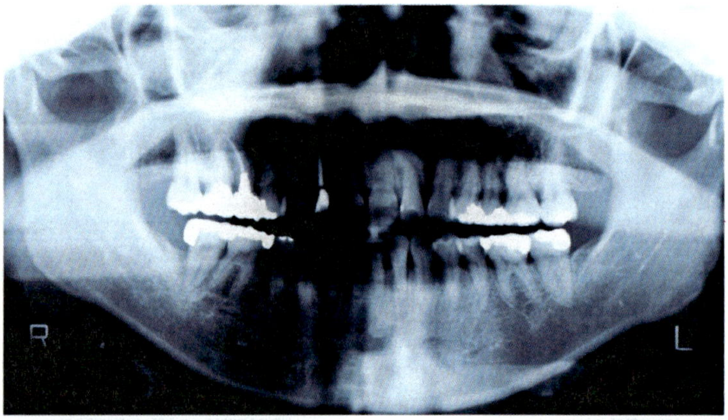

Figure 6L: Case 6: Post-treatment panoramic radiograph.

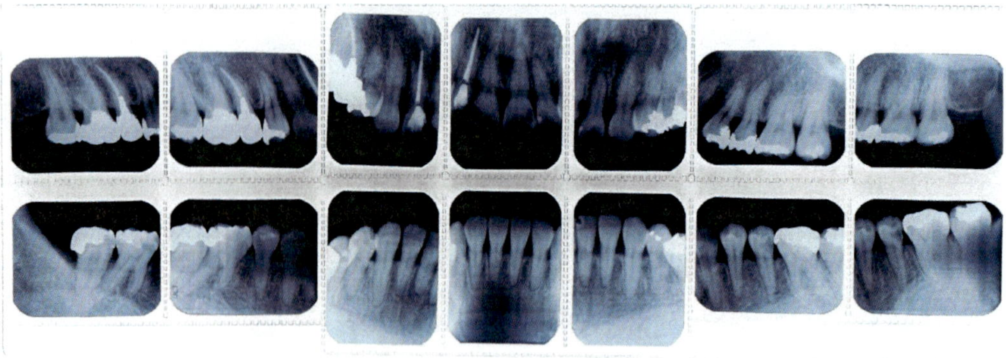

Figure 6M: Case 6: Post-treatment dental radiograph showing minimal root resorption in the lower anteriors.

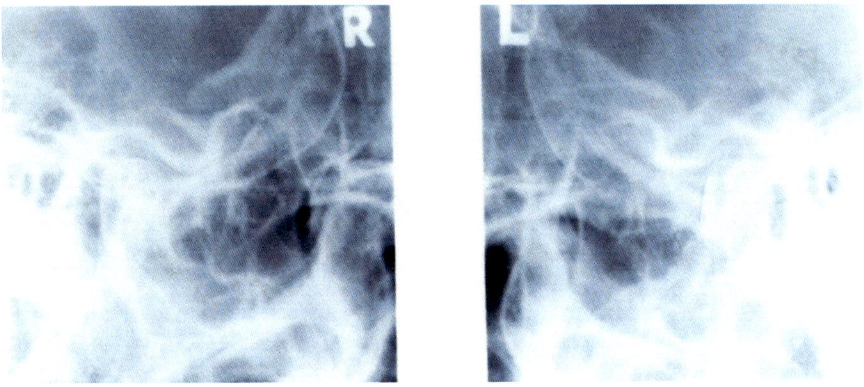

Figure 6N: Case 6: Post-treatment TMJ radiographs.

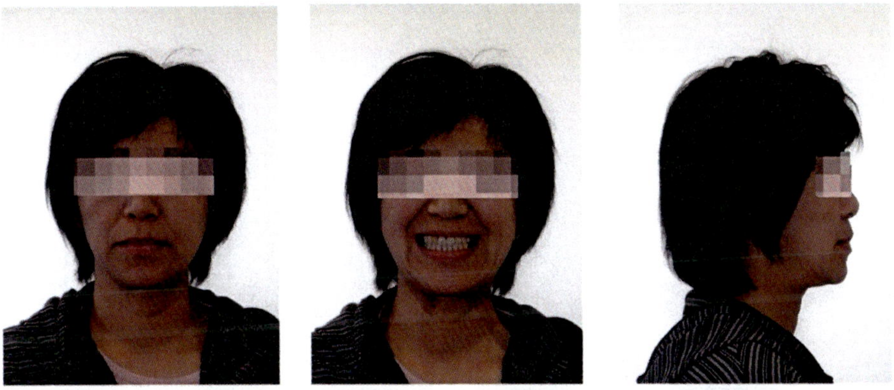

Figure 6O: Case 6: Facial photographs 3 year after completion of the treatment.

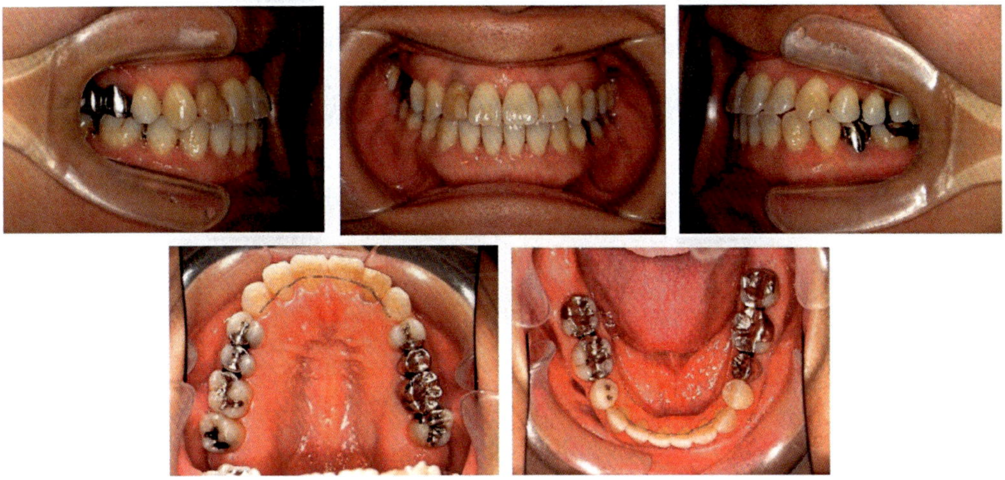

Figure 6P: Case 6: Intra-oral photographs 3 year after completion of the treatment.

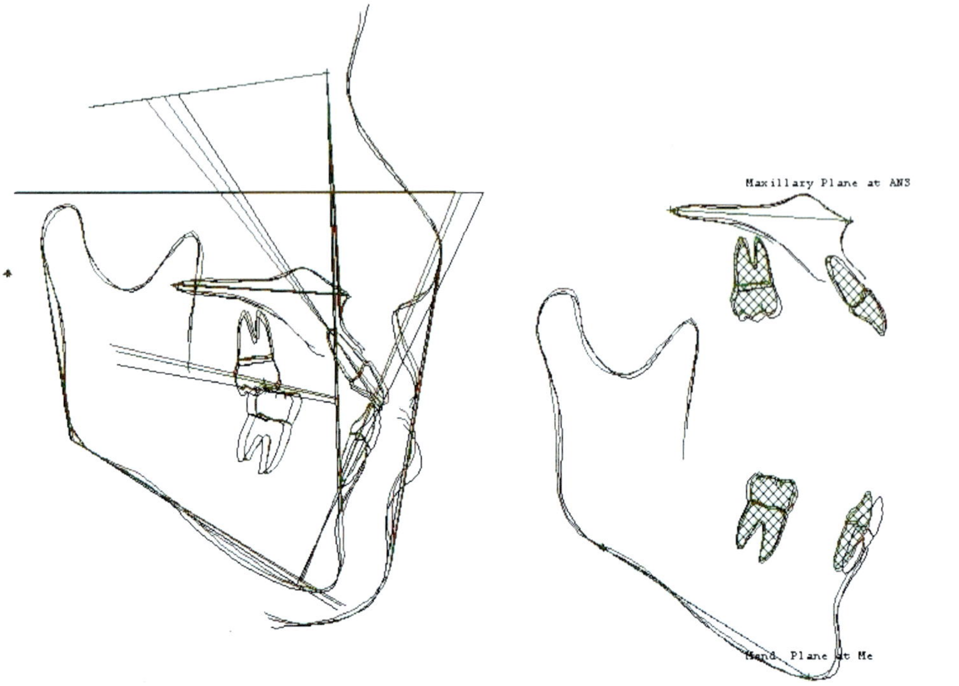

Figure 6Q: Case 6: Superimpositions of cephalogram tracings before and after treatment, and after retention.

Table 12: Case 6: Pre-treatment, post-treatment and after retention cephalometric analysis.

Factor	Mean	S.D.	Wn1	Wn2	Wn3
SNA	80.0	3.0	85.7	86.1	86.4
SNB	77.0	3.0	84.2	84.9	84.6
ANB	3.0	2.0	1.4	1.1	1.7
Mx1-NA	4.0	3.0	10.7	11.7	9.9
Mx1-NA Angle	23.0	6.0	32.2	37.5	33.9
Md1-NB	5.0	3.0	12.2	9.4	10.0
Md1-NB Angle	26.0	6.0	29.0	25.3	26.1
PO - NB	2.0	1.8	-0.4	0.2	-0.5
Occlusal Plane - SN	18.0	3.5	16.6	19.5	18.4
GO-GN-SN	34.0	4.5	37.2	34.1	35.3
Interincisor Angle	128.0	6.0	117.4	116.0	118.2
Wits Appraisal	1.1	1.9	-8.8	-14.3	-11.6
calculated ANB	3.0	2.0	6.5	6.1	6.4
FMA	25.0	6.0	30.2	28.9	29.5
FMIA	65.0	6.0	62.6	67.0	66.0
IMPA	90.0	6.0	87.1	84.1	84.5
Occulusal Plane - FH			9.3	12.0	10.9
Z Angle			70.7	77.9	80.0

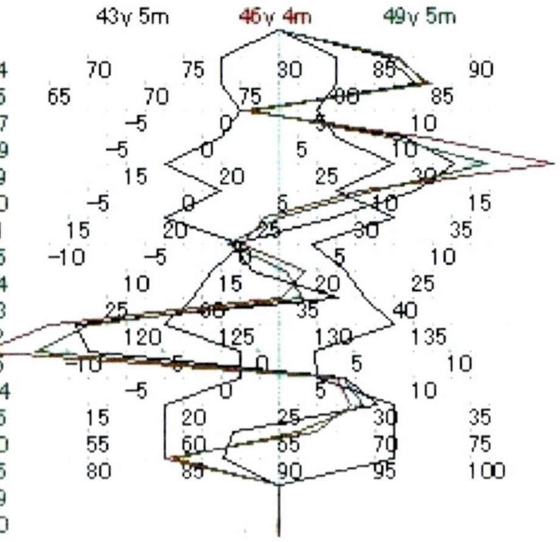

Case 7

The patient was a 25y-9m-old female who visited the author's clinic with a chief complaint of an anterior crossbite. The frontal view showed a symmetrical but large mandible and the lateral view showed a concave profile (Fig. **7A**). The intraoral view showed the molar relationship was 6mm Class III on the right side and 5mm on the left side (Fig. **7B**). No abnormal findings were found on the panoramic and periapical radiographs (Figs. **7C** and **D**). The upper third molars were impacted and the lower third molars were missing. The shape of mandibular condylar heads was round and located in the center of the fossa (Fig. **7E**). The lateral cephalometric analysis showed a Class III skeletal anteroposterior jaw relationship with SNA=82.9°, SNB=84.1° and ANB= -1.2° (Fig. **7F**, Table **13**). The patient had a history of orthodontic treatment when she was a teenager but the dentist could not improve her crossbite. The patient also visited a University hospital for another opinion. She was told that she needs orthognathic surgery to correct the malocclusion and she declined the treatment. She did not have any orthodontic treatment until she found out that she can be treated non-surgically with lingual orthodontics in the author's clinic.

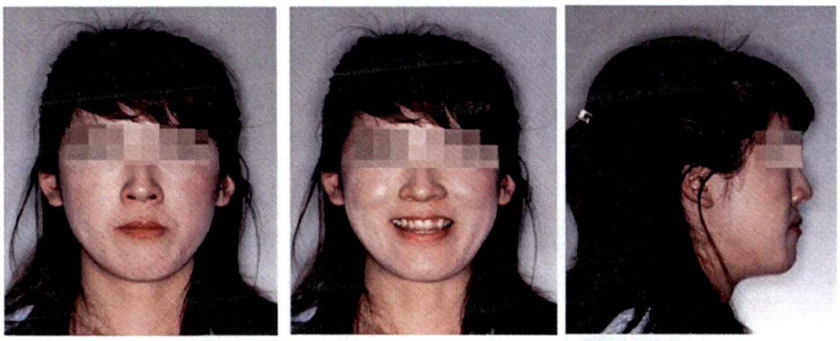

Figure 7A: Case 7: Pre-treatment facial photographs.

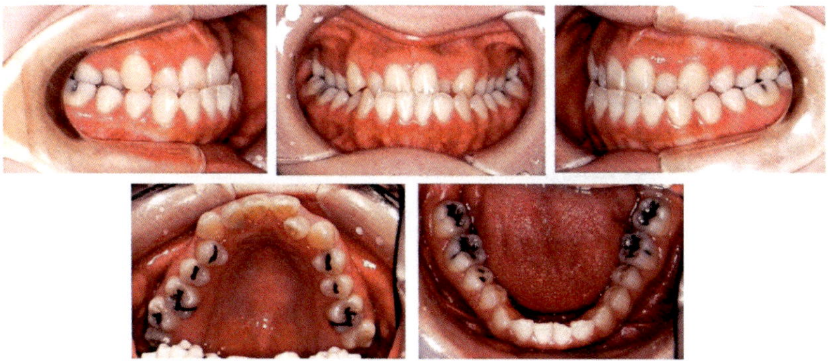

Figure 7B: Case 7: Pre-treatment intra-oral photographs.

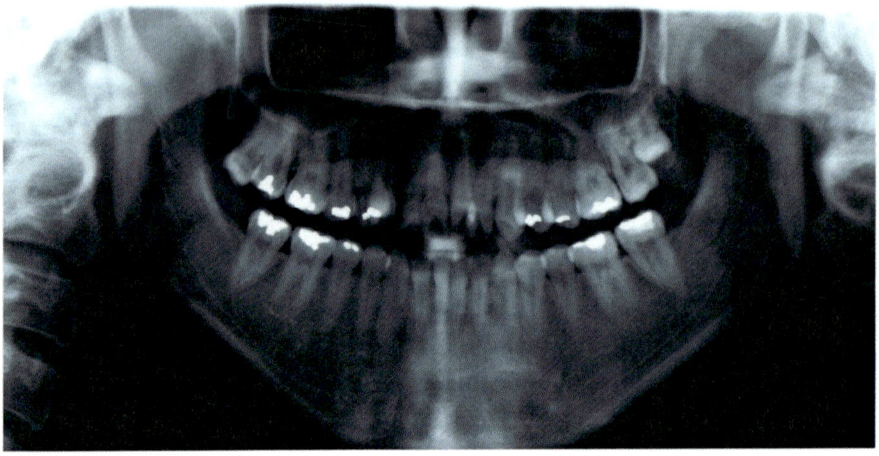

Figure 7C: Case 7: Pre-treatment panoramic radiograph.

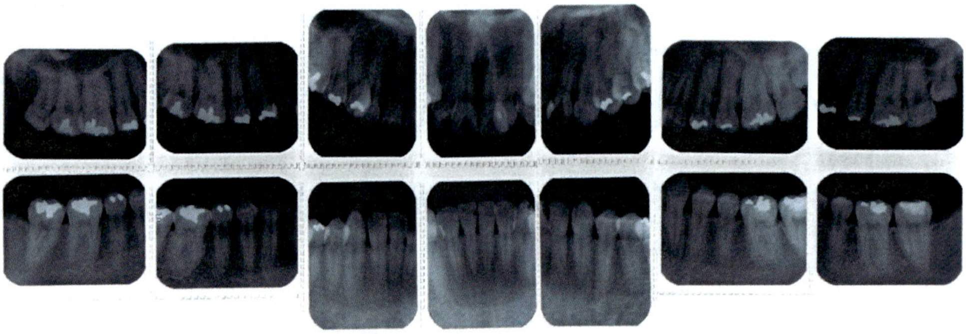

Figure 7D: Case 7: Pre-treatment dental radiographs.

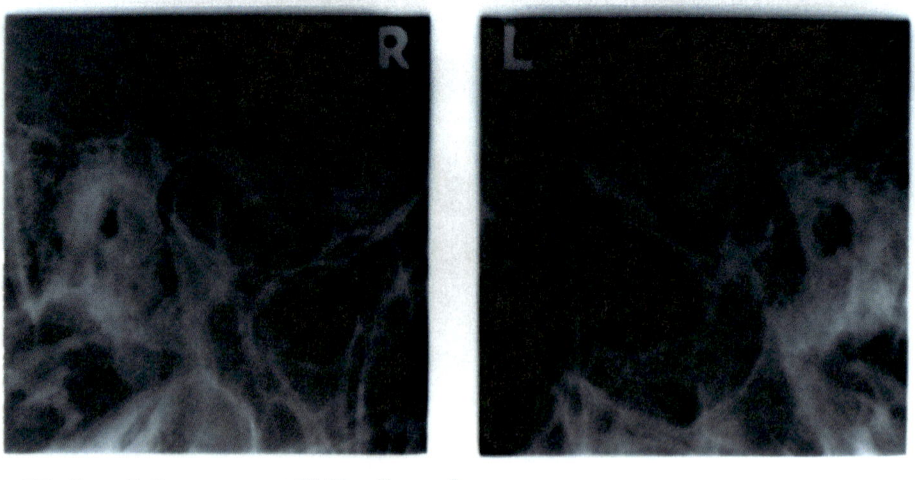

Figure 7E: Case 7: Pre-treatment TMJ radiographs.

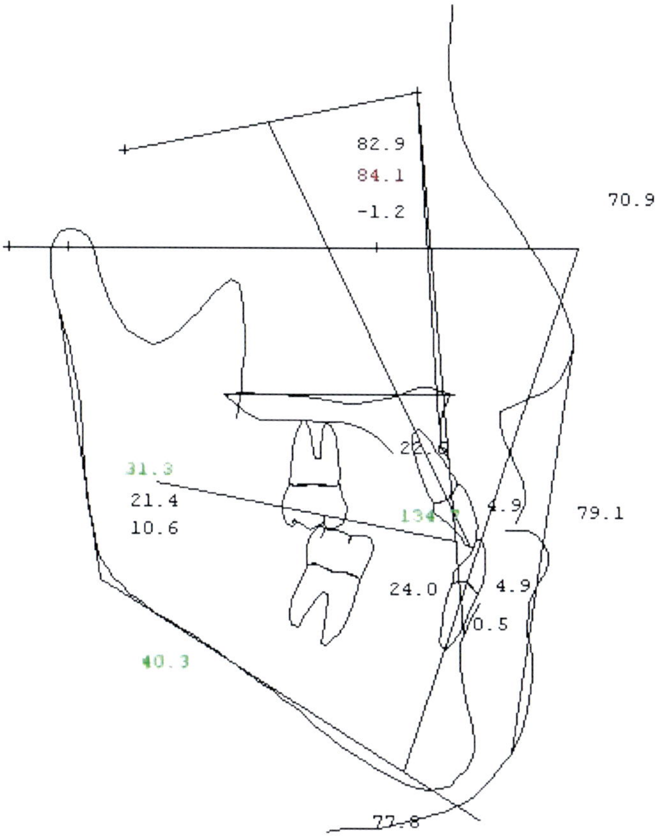

Figure 7F: Case 7: Pre-treatment cephalometric tracing.

Table 13: Case 7: Pre-treatment cephalometric analysis.

Factor	Mean	S.D.	Wn1	Wn2	Wn3
SNA	80.0	3.0	82.9		
SNB	77.0	3.0	84.1		
ANB	3.0	2.0	-1.2		
Mx1-NA	4.0	3.0	4.9		
Mx1-NA Angle	23.0	6.0	22.6		
Md1-NB	5.0	3.0	4.9		
Md1-NB Angle	26.0	6.0	24.0		
PO - NB	2.0	1.8	0.5		
Occlusal Plane - SN	18.0	3.5	21.4		
GO-GN-SN	34.0	4.5	40.3		
Interincisor Angle	128.0	6.0	134.7		
Wits Appraisal	1.1	1.9	-15.1		
calculated ANB	3.0	2.0	6.0		
FMA	25.0	6.0	31.3		
FMIA	65.0	6.0	70.9		
IMPA	90.0	6.0	77.8		
Occulusal Plane - FH			10.6		
Z Angle			79.1		

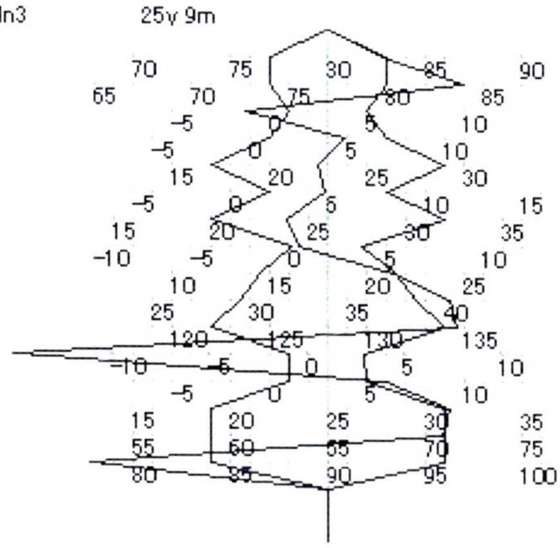

Diagnosis

1. Class III molar relationship (6mm in right, 5mm in left).
2. Skeletal III anteroposterior jaw relationship (ANB -1.2^{o}).
3. Mandibular protrusion (large mandible).
4. Anterior crossbite.
5. Constricted upper arch.
6. Arch length discrepancy: Upper: -1.0mm, Lower: +1.0mm.
7. Bolton analysis: 81.30/89.92%.

Treatment Objectives

1. Correct anterior crossbite.
2. Expand upper arch.
3. Backward rotation of the mandible to improve anteroposterior skeletal relationship.
4. Establish Class I molar relationship.

Treatment Plan

1. Non-extraction treatment.
2. Non-surgical treatment.
3. Expansion of upper arch.
4. Correction of anterior crossbite.
5. Upright lower molars to obtain Class I molar relationship.

Treatment Progress

Treatment was started with the placement of the mini-lingual orthodontic brackets. They were bonded on the upper and lower arches at the same time together with .012 NiTi on both arches (Fig. **7G**). After 2 months of treatment, a .016 thermal activate archwire was placed in the upper arch and a .012 NiTi archwire on the lower arch (Fig. **7H**). After 10 months of treatment, expansion of upper arch was done with a .0175x.0175 Beta-Titanium archwire on the upper arch and a .016x.022 S.S. on the lower arch. In order to improve the midline, Class III elastics were worn from the upper second bicuspids to lower canine only on right side (Fig. **7I**). At that time, patient was pregnant and treatment was re-initiated after the birth of her child. Fig. **7J** showed the intraoral photographs at 30 months in treatment with finishing and detailing.

Treatment Results

Excellent result was obtained in 39 months with Class I molar relationship (Figs. **7K** and **L**). Post-treatment panoramic radiograph showed good root paralleling (Fig. **7M**). Periapical radiograph showed no root resorption (Fig. **7N**). The position and shape of mandibular condylar heads were not changed with treatment (Fig. **7O**). Figs. **7P** and **Q** showed patient 31 months after treatment with excellent and stable results. Superimposition of the pre- and post-treatment radiographs showed backward rotation of the mandible which helped in improving the anteroposterior skeletal relationship (Fig. **7R**, Table **14**).

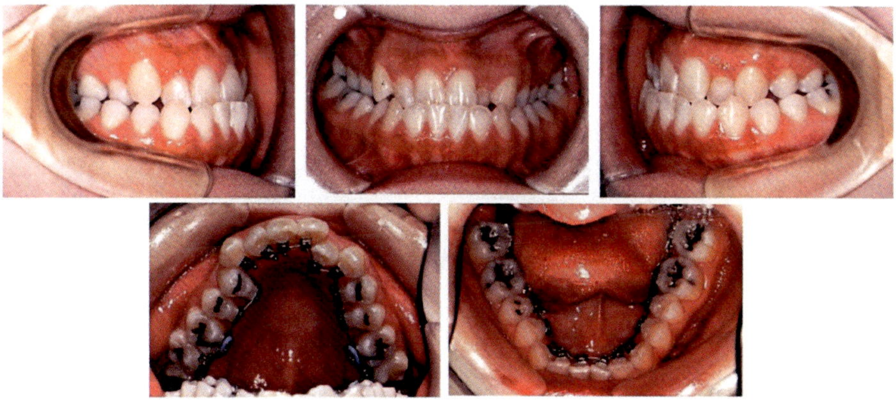

Figure 7G: Case 7: Intra-oral photographs taken after treatment brackets were bonded on the upper and lower arches. The arch wires used were .012 Ni-Ti in both arches.

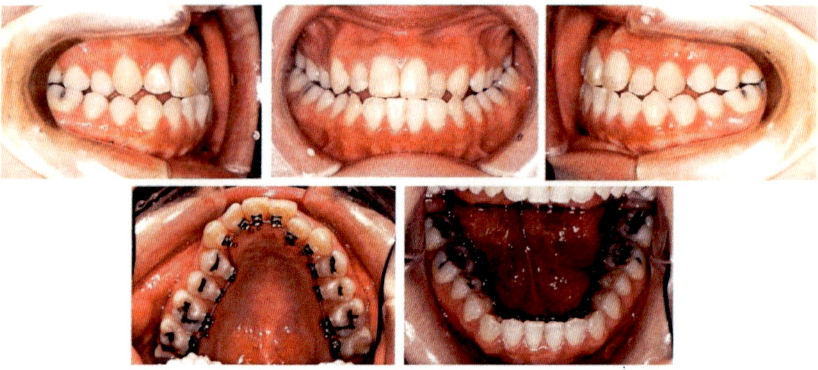

Figure 7H: Case 7: Intra-oral photographs 2 months into treatment. Arch wires used were .016 thermal activate on the upper arch and. 012 Ni-Ti on the lower arch.

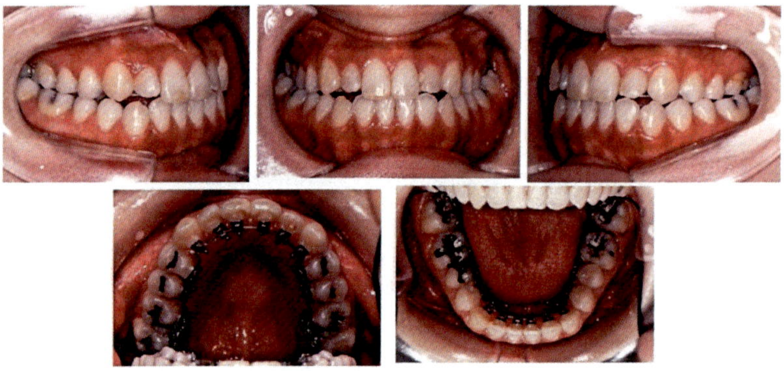

Figure 7I: Case 7: Intra-oral photographs 10 months into treatment. The arch wires used were .0175x.0175 beta-titanium on the upper arch and .016x.022 SS on the lower arch. In order to improve the midline shift, Class III elastics were worn from the upper second bicuspids to the lower canine only on the right side.

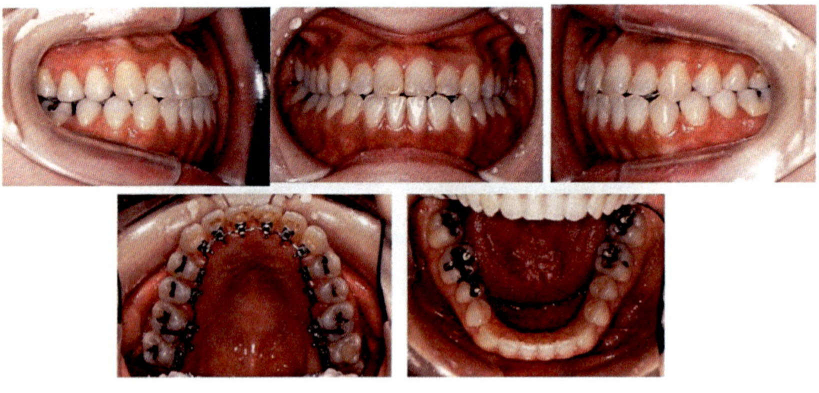

Figure 7J: Case 7: Intra-oral photographs 30 months into treatment. The arch wires used were .0175x.0175 beta-titanium on the upper arch and .017x.025 beta-titanium on the lower arch.

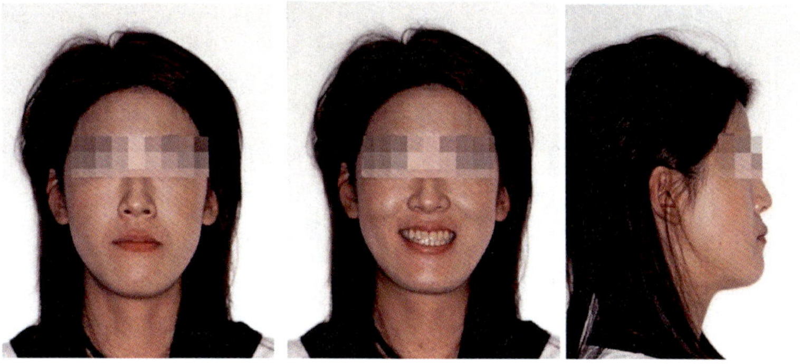

Figure 7K: Case 7: Post-treatment facial photographs.

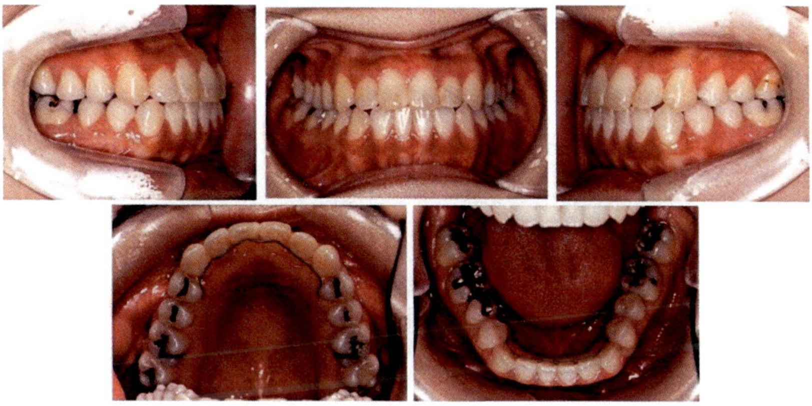

Figure 7L: Case 7: Post-treatment intra-oral photographs taken at 39 months due to pregnancy during treatment.

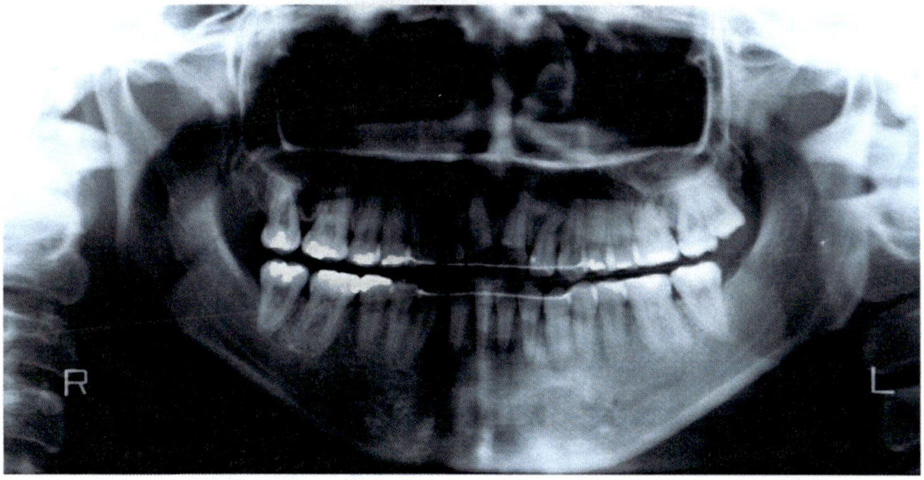

Figure 7M: Case 7: Post-treatment panoramic radiograph.

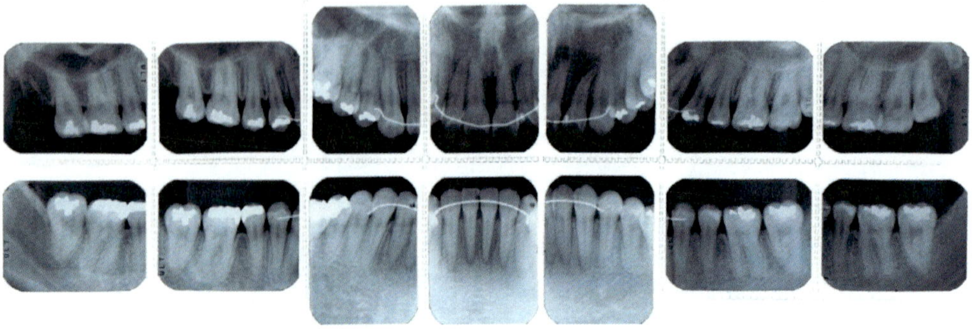

Figure 7N: Case 7: Post-treatment dental radiographs.

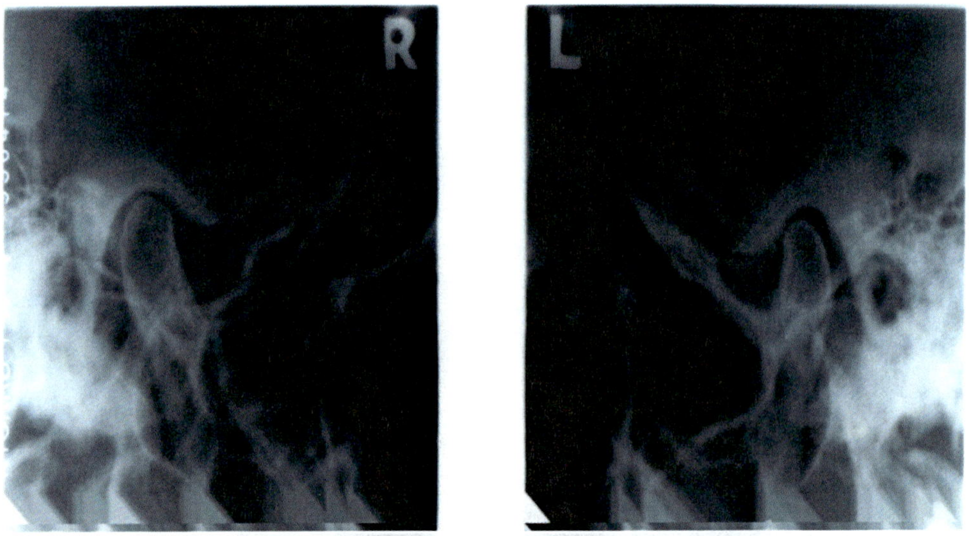

Figure 7O: Case 7: Post-treatment TMJ radiographs.

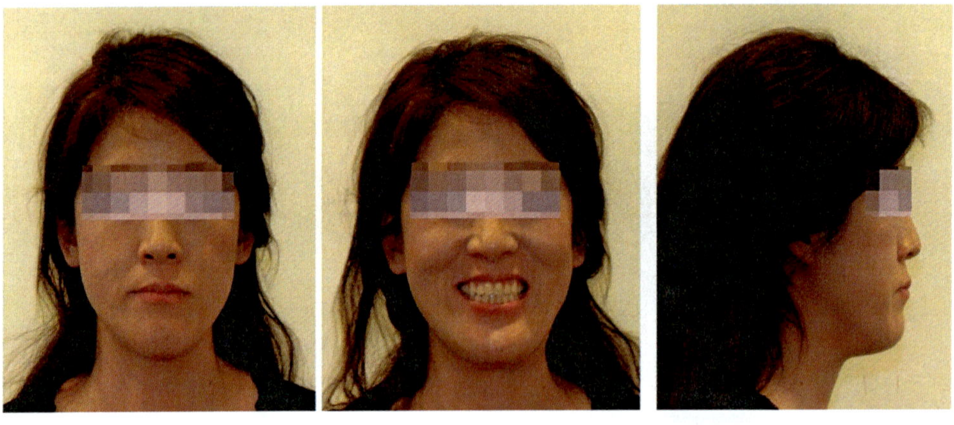

Figure 7P: Case 7: Facial photographs 31 months after completion of the treatment.

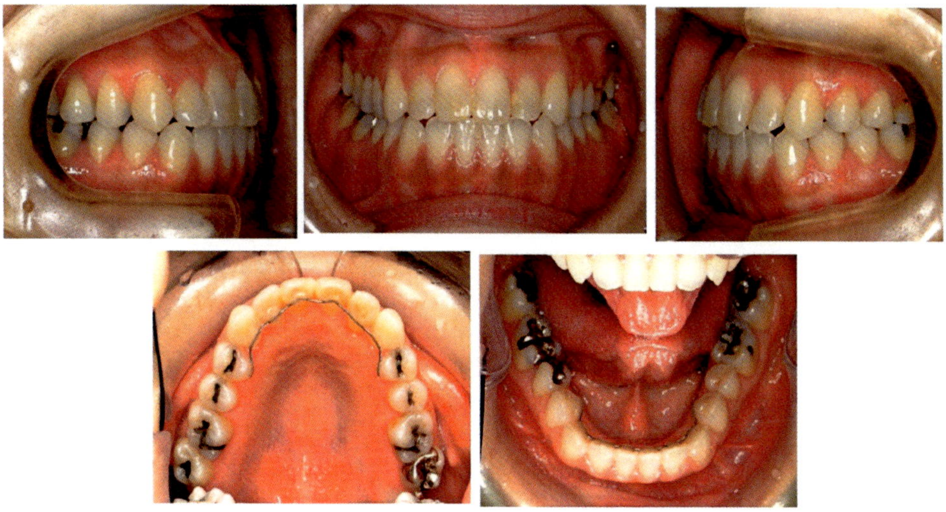

Figure 7Q: Case 7: Intra-oral photographs 31 months after completion of the treatment.

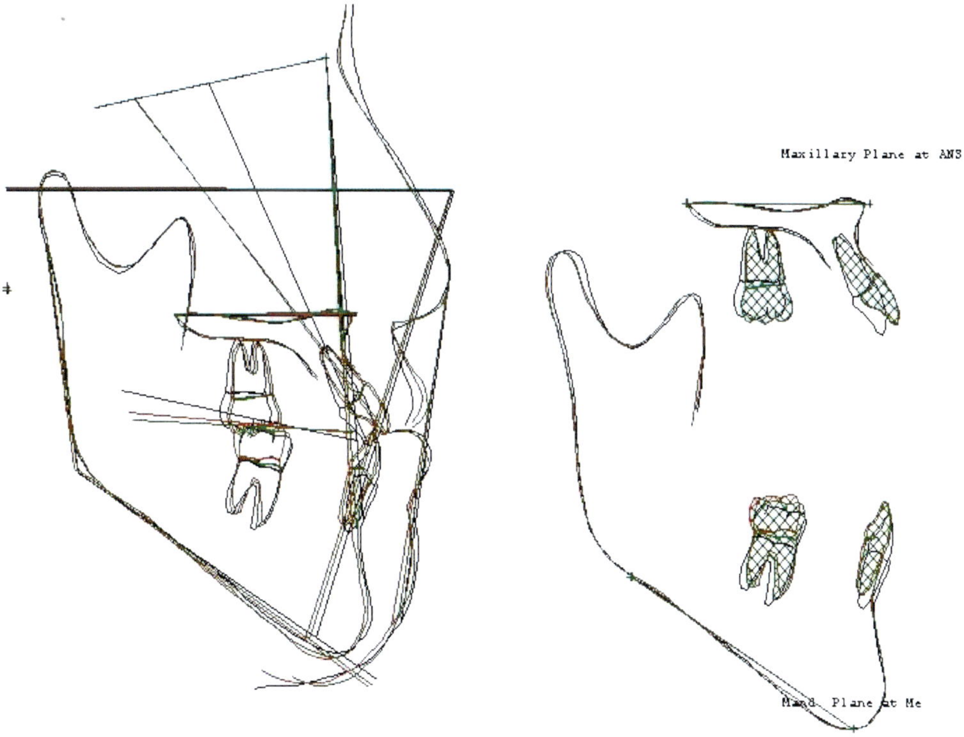

Figure 7R: Case 7: Superimpositions of cephalometric tracings before and after treatment, and after retention.

Table 14: Pre-treatment, post-treatment and after retention cephalometric analysis.

Factor	Mean	S.D.	Wn1	Wn2	Wn3
SNA	80.0	3.0	82.9	82.1	82.6
SNB	77.0	3.0	84.1	82.6	83.0
ANB	3.0	2.0	−1.2	−0.5	−0.4
Mx1-NA	4.0	3.0	4.9	10.1	10.0
Mx1-NA Angle	23.0	6.0	22.6	37.0	37.0
Md1-NB	5.0	3.0	4.9	6.2	6.2
Md1-NB Angle	26.0	6.0	24.0	23.4	23.4
PO - NB	2.0	1.8	0.5	1.7	1.8
Occlusal Plane - SN	18.0	3.5	21.4	15.2	13.4
GO-GN-SN	34.0	4.5	40.3	42.7	42.5
Interincisor Angle	128.0	6.0	134.7	120.1	120.0
Wits Appraisal	1.1	1.9	−15.1	−8.0	−6.0
calculated ANB	3.0	2.0	6.0	6.2	6.4
FMA	25.0	6.0	31.3	33.3	33.0
FMIA	65.0	6.0	70.9	70.1	70.2
IMPA	90.0	6.0	77.8	76.7	76.8
Occulusal Plane - FH			10.6	4.2	2.8
Z Angle			79.1	75.7	78.9

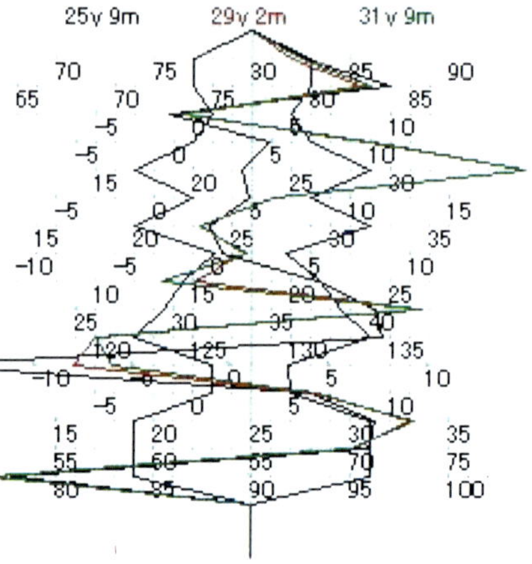

Case 8

The patient was a 33y-2m-old female who visited the author's clinic with a chief complaint of an anterior crossbite. The frontal view showed symmetrical face and lateral view showed a concave profile (Fig. **8A**). The intraoral view showed molar relationship was Class III on both sides (Fig. **8B**). No abnormal findings were found on the panoramic and periapical radiographs (Fig. **8C** and **D**). Mandibular condylar heads were round and located in the center of the fossa (Fig. **8E**). The cephalometric analysis showed a Class III skeletal anteroposterior jaw relationship with a small maxilla, SNA=78.8°, slightly large mandible, SNB=78.4°, and an ANB=0.4° (Fig. **8F**, Table **15**).

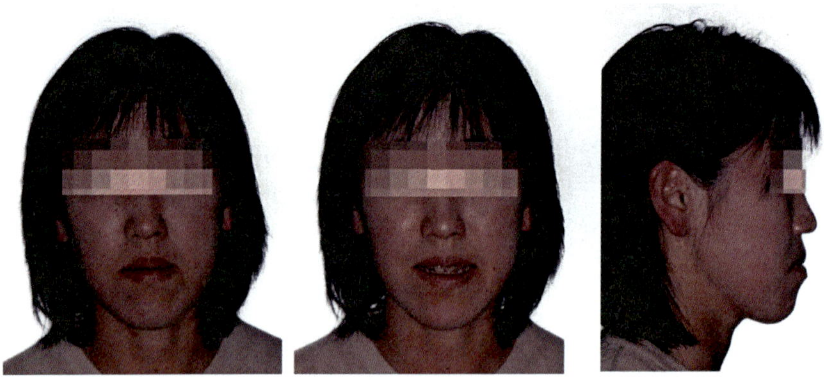

Figure 8A: Case 8: Pre-treatment facial photographs.

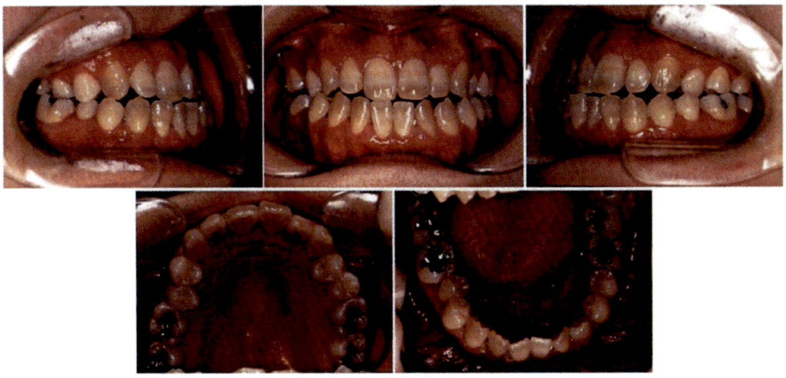

Figure 8B: Case 8: Pre-treatment intra-oral photographs.

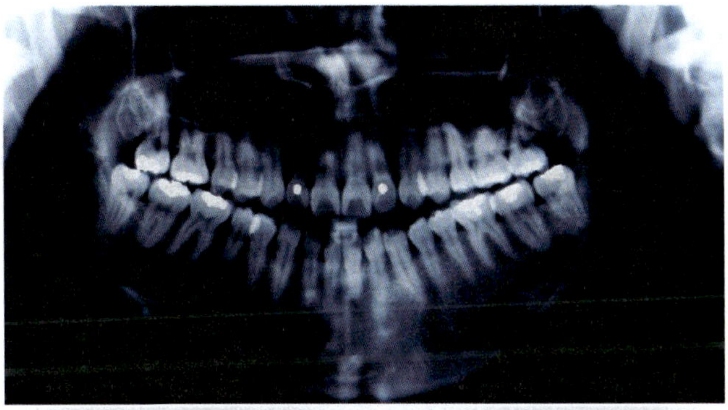

Figure 8C: Case 8: Pre-treatment panorama radiograph.

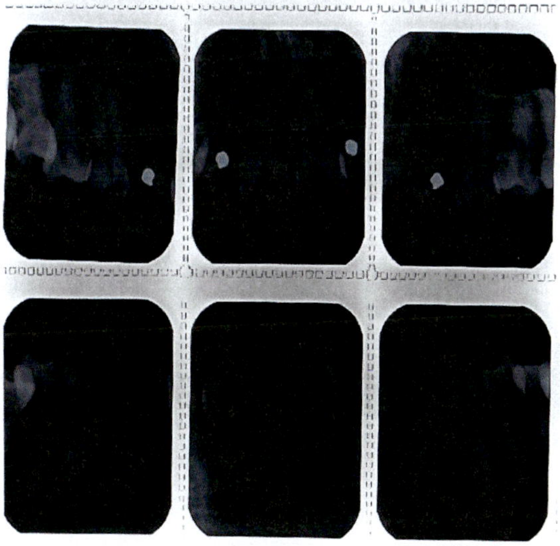

Figure 8D: Case 8: Pre-treatment dental radiographs.

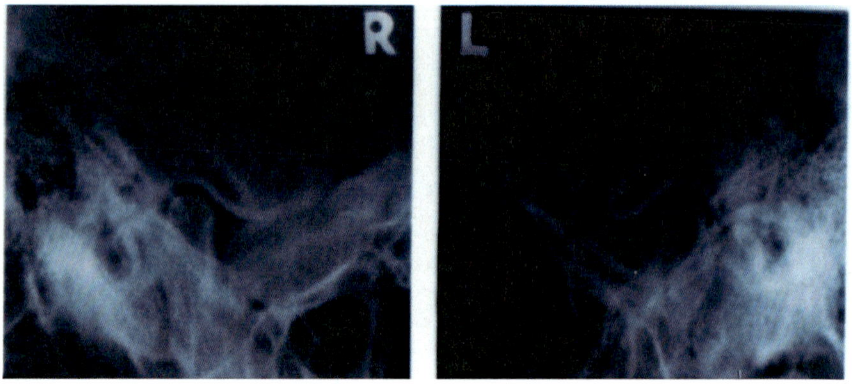

Figure 8E: Case 8: Pre-treatment TMJ radiograph.

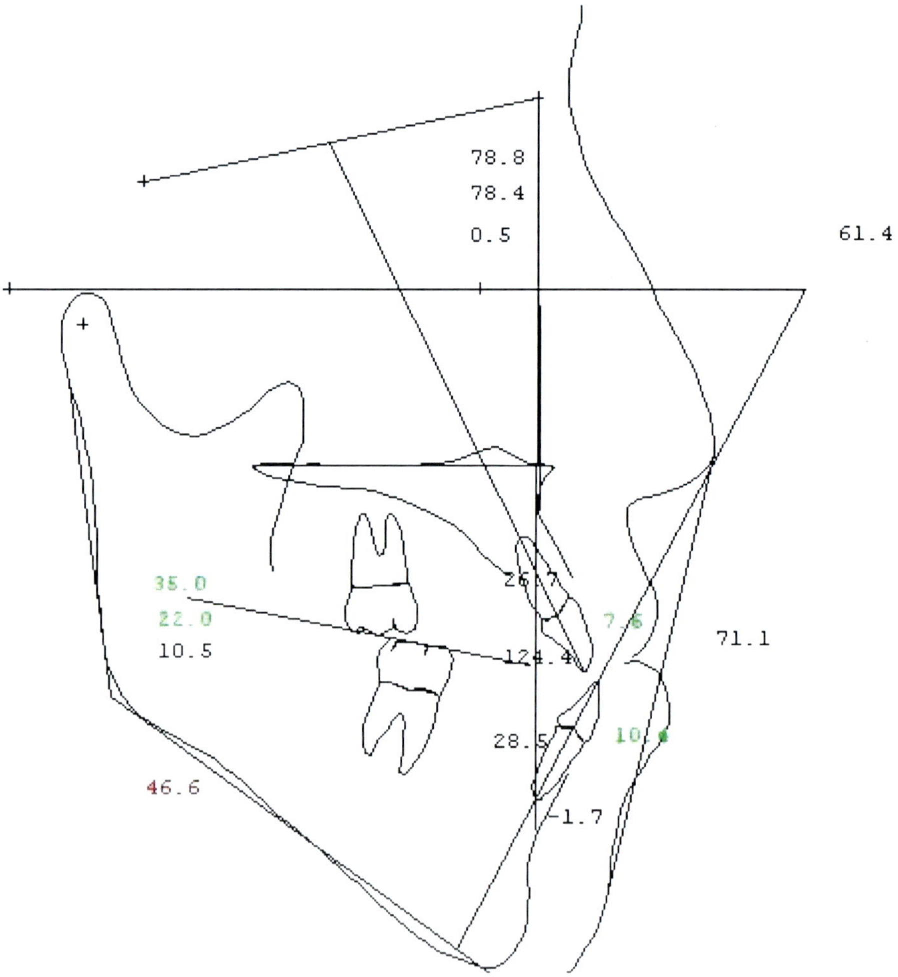

Figure 8F: Case 8: Pre-treatment cephalometric tracing.

Table 15: Case 8: Pre-treatment Cephalometric analysis.

Factor	Mean	S.D.	Wn1	Wn2	Wn3
SNA	80.0	3.0	78.8		
SNB	77.0	3.0	78.4		
ANB	3.0	2.0	0.5		
Mx1-NA	4.0	3.0	7.6		
Mx1-NA Angle	23.0	6.0	26.7		
Md1-NB	5.0	3.0	10.4		
Md1-NB Angle	26.0	6.0	28.5		
PO - NB	2.0	1.8	-1.7		
Occlusal Plane - SN	18.0	3.5	22.0		
GO-GN-SN	34.0	4.5	46.6		
Interincisor Angle	128.0	6.0	124.4		
Wits Appraisal	1.1	1.9	-9.1		
calculated ANB	3.0	2.0	5.7		
FMA	25.0	6.0	35.0		
FMIA	65.0	6.0	61.4		
IMPA	90.0	6.0	83.6		
Occulusal Plane - FH			10.5		
Z Angle			71.1		

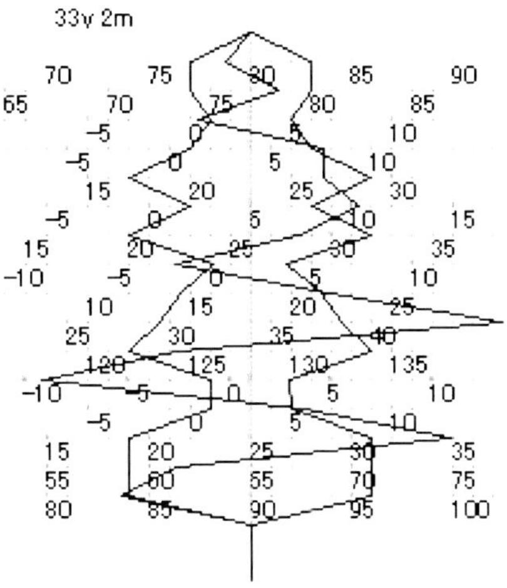

Diagnosis

1. Class III molar relationship (6mm on the right, 7mm on the left)

2. Skeletal Class III anteroposterior jaw relationship (ANB 0.4°)

3. Anterior crossbite

4. Lingual inclination of the lower incisors

5. Arch length discrepancy: Upper: 0mm, Lower: -3.0mm

6. Bolton analysis: 77.69/92.22%

Treatment Objectives

1. Retraction of lower incisors

2. Correction of under bite

3. Expansion of upper arch and contraction of lower arch

Treatment Plan

1. Non-surgical treatment

2. Extraction of the lower second bicuspids on both sides

3. Retraction of the lower incisors and correction of the anterior cross bite

4. Expansion in the upper arch and constriction of the lower arch

Treatment Progress

Treatment was started with the placement of the Kurz Lingual Appliance. Fig. **8G** shows the intraoral photographs of patient at 2 months in treatment, brackets were bonded on both arches. Figs. **8H** and **I** show patient 16 months in treatment with sliding mechanics to close space. Fig. **8J** shows patient 27 months in treatment with finishing and detailing .0175x.0175 TMA archwires on upper and lower arches.

Treatment Results

Excellent results were obtained in 41 months without surgery (Figs. **K** and **L**). Post-treatment panoramic radiograph showed good root paralleling (Fig. **8M**). Periapical radiographs showed no root resorption (Fig. **8N**). The position and shape of the mandibular condylar head was not changed with treatment (Fig. **8O**). Figs. **8P** and **Q** showed patient 40 months after treatment with excellent and stable occlusion. Superimposition of the pre- and post-treatment radiographs showed minimal backward rotation of mandible. The anterior crossbite was corrected with the retraction of the lower incisors (Fig. **8R**, Table **16**).

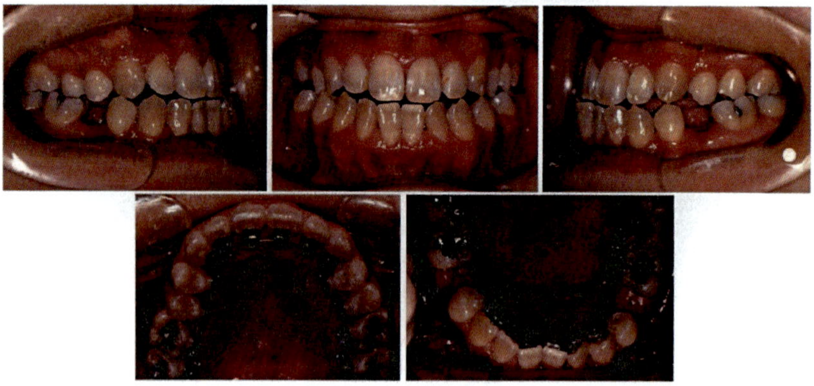

Figure 8G: Case 8: Intra-oral photographs 2 months into treatment. Brackets were bonded on both arches. The arch wires used were .014 Ni-Ti on the upper and lower arches.

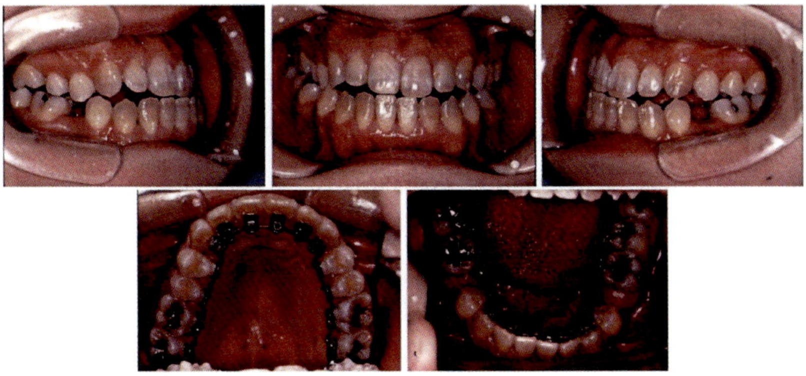

Figure 8H: Case 8. Intraoral photographs 8 months in treatment.

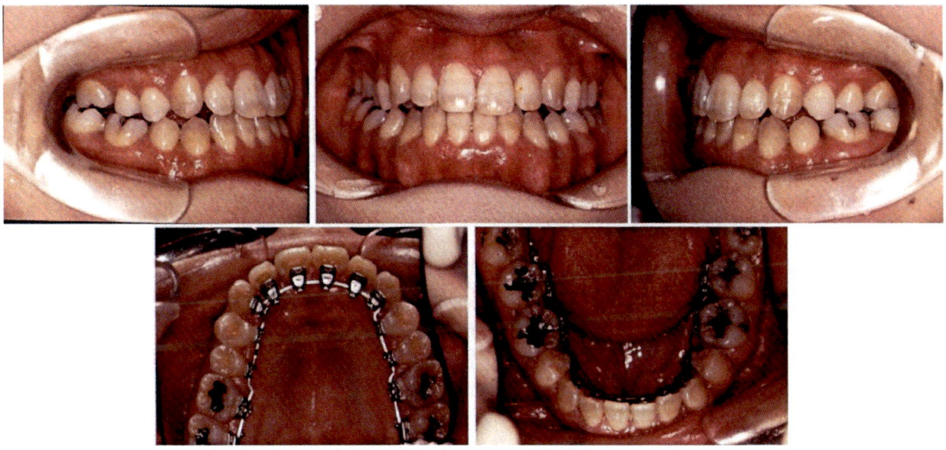

Figure 8I: Case 8: Intraoral photographs 26 months in treatment showing sliding mechanics to close space and improve overbite.

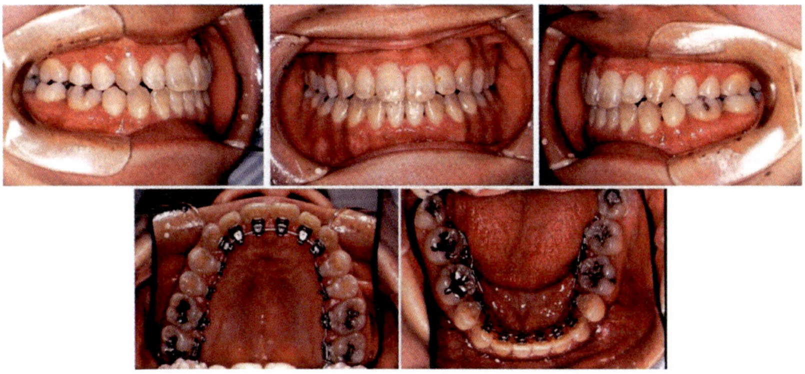

Figure 8J: Case 8: Intraoral photographs 27 months in treatment showing finishing and detailing with .0175x.0175 TMA archwires on upper and lower arches.

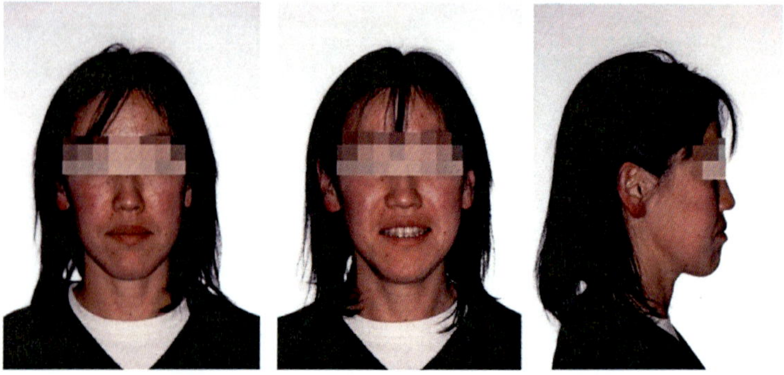

Figure 8K: Case 8. Facial photographs after completion of treatment.

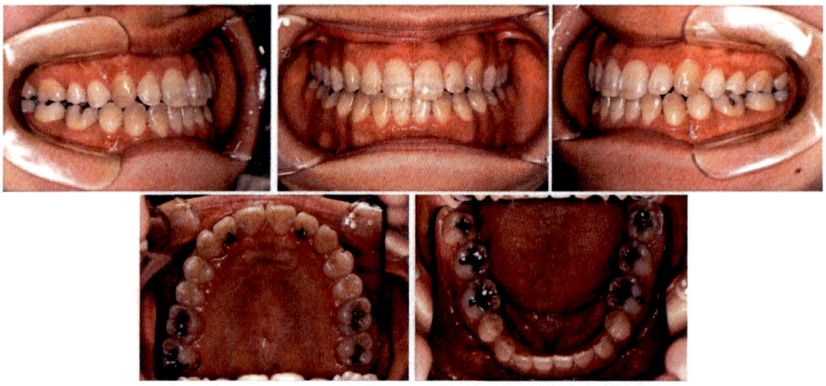

Figure 8L: Case 8: Intraoral photographs after completion of treatment.

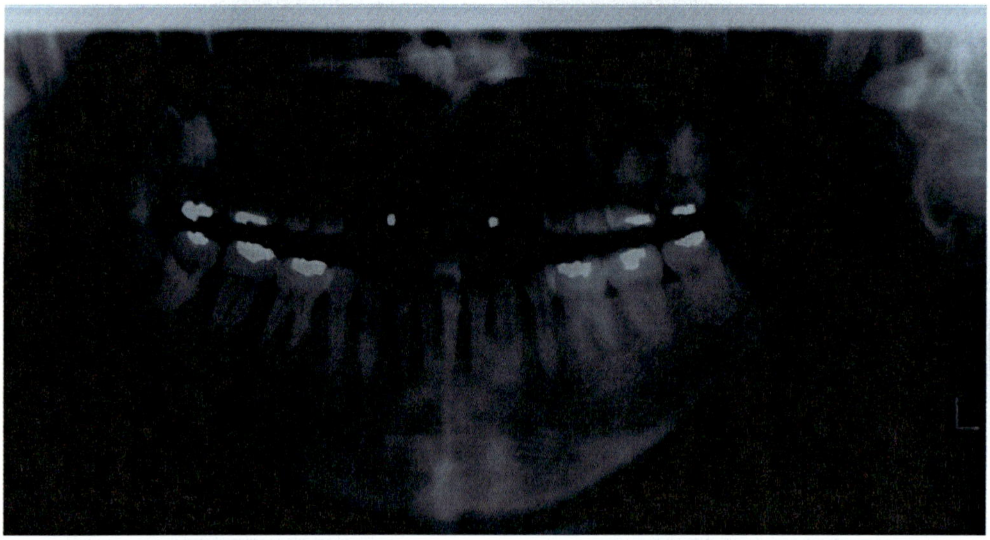

Figure 8M: Case 8: Panoramic radiograph after completion of treatment.

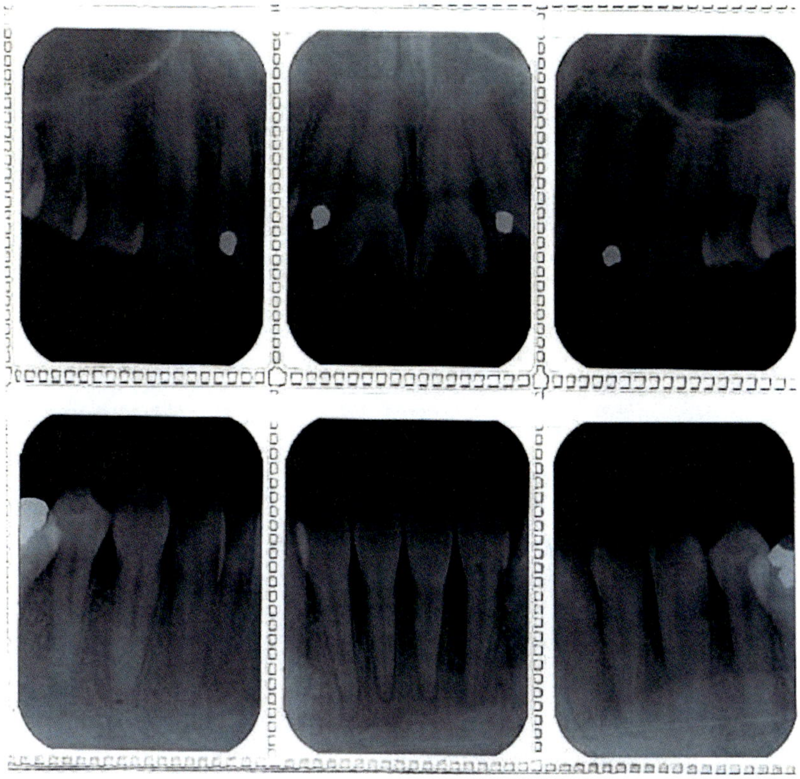

Figure 8N: Case 8: Intraoral radiographs after completion of treatment.

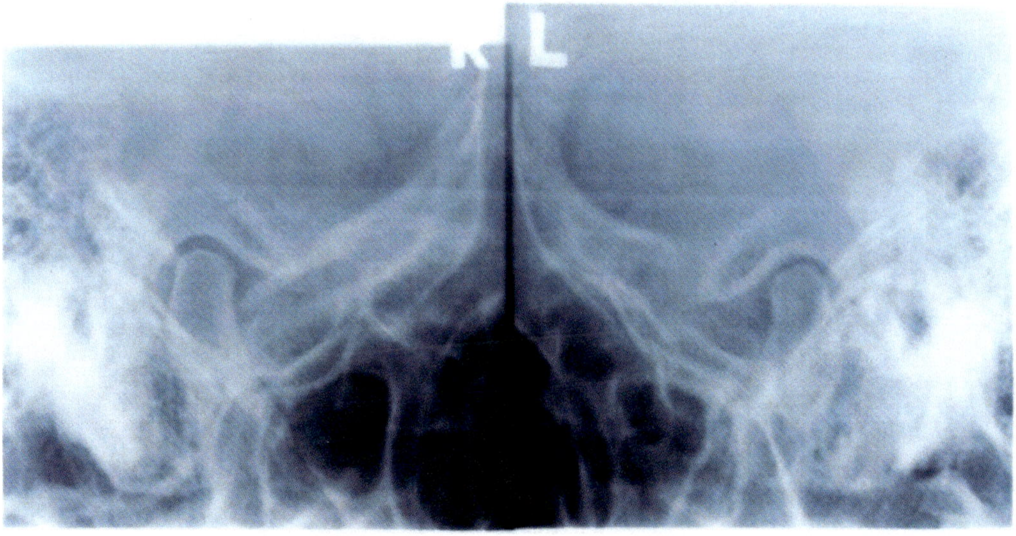

Figure 8O: Case 8: TMJ radiographs after completion of treatment.

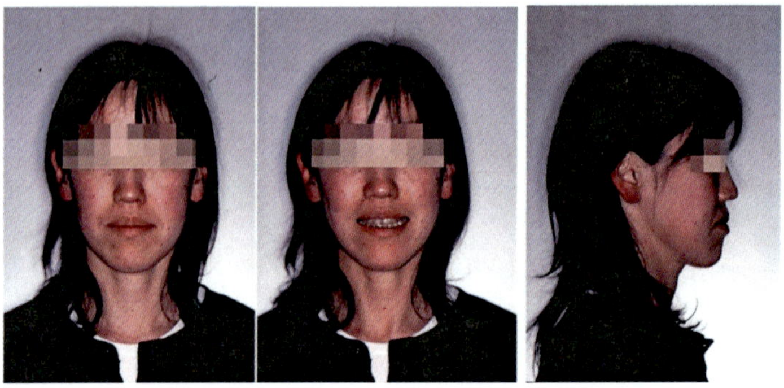

Figure 8P: Case 8: Facial photographs 40 months after completion of treatment.

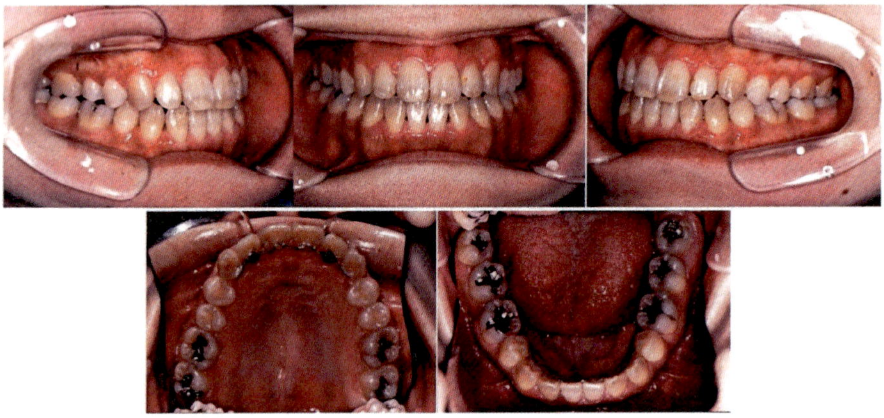

Figure 8Q: Case 8: Intra-oral photographs 40 months after completion of the treatment.

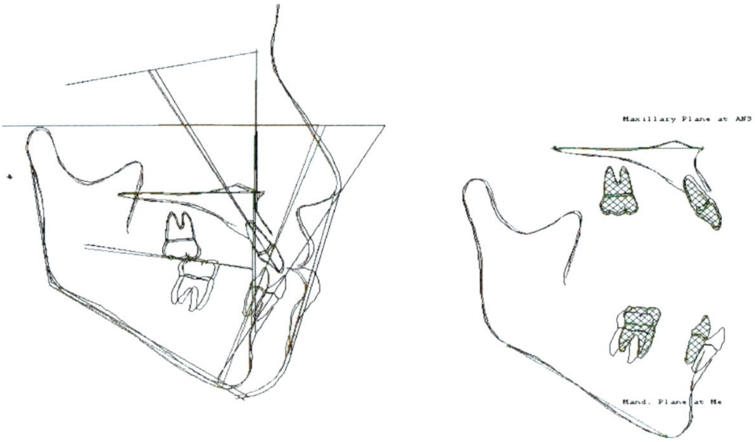

Figure 8R: Superimpositions of cephalometric tracings before and after treatment, and after retention.

Table 16:

Factor	Mean	S.D.	Wn1	Wn2	Wn3
SNA	80.0	3.0	78.8	78.7	78.0
SNB	77.0	3.0	78.4	77.6	77.7
ANB	3.0	2.0	0.5	1.0	0.3
Mx1-NA	4.0	3.0	7.6	8.6	9.7
Mx1-NA Angle	23.0	6.0	26.7	28.1	29.0
Md1-NB	5.0	3.0	10.4	4.8	4.6
Md1-NB Angle	26.0	6.0	28.5	16.1	18.3
PO - NB	2.0	1.8	-1.7	-1.4	-1.4
Occlusal Plane - SN	18.0	3.5	22.0	21.1	20.0
GO-GN-SN	34.0	4.5	46.6	46.8	46.7
Interincisor Angle	128.0	6.0	124.4	134.7	132.4
Wits Appraisal	1.1	1.9	-9.1	-7.1	-6.1
calculated ANB	3.0	2.0	5.7	5.7	5.4
FMA	25.0	6.0	35.0	35.6	35.3
FMIA	65.0	6.0	61.4	72.9	70.8
IMPA	90.0	6.0	83.6	71.5	73.9
Occulusal Plane - FH			10.5	9.7	8.5
Z Angle			71.1	76.4	78.0

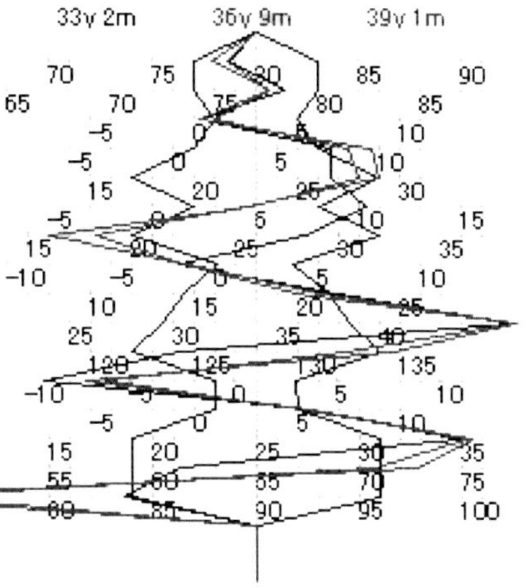

DISCUSSIONS

Surgical orthodontic treatment is usually indicated for moderate to severe skeletal Class III malocclusions. However, there are reports in the literature that these cases can also be treated without surgery [20-26]. Class III jaw relationship can be improved by clockwise rotation of mandible. This can be achieved by the following objectives:

1. Tip back of the lower molars.

2. Lingual movement and extrusion of lower incisors.

3. Extrusion of the upper molars.

4. Counterclockwise rotation of the occlusal plane with a resultant clockwise rotation of the mandible.

The above cases showed that the first two objectives can easier be achieved with the help of lingual orthodontics. This is because tooth movement is different with lingual appliances. When intrusion force is applied on the lingual surface of the incisors, the incisors usually tip lingually. The center of resistance is located on lingual surface of the teeth. The lingual tipping force will be transmitted to the distally adjacent teeth, resulting in uprighting of the posterior molars. Therefore, diagnosis is different for lingual compared to labial fixed appliances [18]. In the author's experience, the bicuspid extractions that are frequently required for labial appliance treatment are not necessary for the lingual appliance. There are additional advantages for treatment of Class III patients because of low tongue posture and aberrant physiologic pressure [27, 28]. Improving abnormal tongue pressure is a key to success in Class III treatment. In lingual orthodontics, the brackets bonded on the lingual surface of the incisors helps in correcting low tongue posture or tongue thrusting.

SUMMARY POINTS

- Lingual orthodontics can be very effective in Class III treatment due to the ease in tipping back the lower molars.
- Tooth movement in lingual orthodontics is quite different from abial appliances.
- Often cases that require orthognathic surgery with labial orthodontics may be treated without surgery if lingual orthodontics is used.
- Lingual brackets are effective for improving low tongue posture or tongue thrusting.
- Lingual orthodontics can be used for efficient treatment of all types of malocclusion, including severe Class III patients.

ACKNOWLEDGEMENTS

Declared none.

CONFLICT OF INTEREST

The authors confirm that this chapter contents have no conflict of interest.

REFERENCES

[1] Sugawara J, Mitani H, *et al.* Facial growth of skeletal Class III malocclusion and the effects, limitations, and long-term dentofacial adaptations to chin cap therapy. Semin Orthod 1997;3:244-254.

[2] Sorihashi Y, Stephens CD, *et al.* An inference modeling of sagittal jaw-base relationships based on cephalometry: part II. Am J Orthod Dentofac Orthop 2000;117: 303-311.
[3] Takada K, Sorihashi Y, *et al.* An inference modeling of human visual judgement of sagittal jaw-base relationships based on cephalometry: part 1. Am J Orthod Dentofac Orthop 2000;117:140-7.
[4] Takaharu K, Tatsuo K, *et al.* Hard and soft tissue changes following orthognathic surgery in mandibular prognathic patients with open bite: Comparison between two jaw surgery and one jaw surgery. Jpn J Jaw Deform 2005;15:105-113.
[5] El-Mangoury NH and Mostafa YA. Epdemiologio panorama of Occlusion, Angle Orthod 1990; 60:207-214.
[6] Tadaharu K, Chikara Saito, *et al.* Treatment of jaw deformity. A nation wide surgery of the situation in Japan. Jpn J Jaw Deform 2008;18:237-250.
[7] Izumi Yoshihisa, Kazuhisa Soejima, *et al.* Clinical Outcome of Orthognathic Surgery for the Last 10 Years in the Department of Oral and Maxillofacial Surgery, Miyazaki University Hospital. Jpn J Jaw Deform 2010;20(4):292-296.
[8] Eiko Kishimoto, Youhei Usui, *et al.* Clinical statistical investigation of patients with jaw deformity. Orthod Waves-Jpn Ed 2010;69(2):118-125.
[9] Tuyoshi Suzuki, Tatsuo Kawamoto, *et al.* Clinical Statistical Analysis of Treatment for Jaw Deformities in the Section of Maxillofacial Orthognathics, Department of Orthodontics, Tokyo Medical and Dental University Dental School Hospital, during the Past 30 Years. Jpn J Jaw Deform 2010;20(3):220-227.
[10] Ryohei Kitamura, Tatsuo Kawamoto, *et al.* Dento-facial Changes following a Combination of Le Fort I with Horseshoe Osteotomy and a Bilateral Sagittal Split Ramus Osteotomy for Mandibular Prognathism. Jpn J Jaw Deform 2010;20(3):211-219.
[11] Toru Inami, Ichiro Aizawa, *et al.* Part 3, Diagnosis; Treatment planning and Evaluation of Lingual Bracket Orthodontic Technique; Lingual bracket orthodontic technique, Ishiyaku. 2009;Tokyo:31-77.
[12] Yoshimitsu Oguri, Kazuo Naganuma, *et al.* Clinical Survey of Surgical-orthodontics Cases Treated in the Past Decade at the Orthodontic Department, Niigata University Medical and Dental Hospital. Jpn J Jaw Deform 2010;20:297-304.
[13] Kyoko Hanji, Takuya Fujiwara, *et al.* Investigation of Jaw-Deformity Patients over 10 year in the Department of Orthodontics, Aichi-gakuin University Hospital. Jpn J Jaw Deform 2010;20(4):267-274.
[14] Junichi Noike, Takeshi Shimizu, *et al.* A Survey of Sagittal Split Ramus Osteotomy in the Nagano Red Cross Hospital. Jpn J Jaw Deform 2010;20(4):275-282.
[15] Toshio Sugahara, Mori Yoshihide, *et al.* Skeletal relapse following sagittal split osteotomy for correction of mandibular prognathism postural change of the hyoid bone and skeletal relapse. J Jpn Oral Surg 1992;38:1558-1563.
[16] Tatsuo Kawamoto, Nobuyoshi Motohashi, *et al.* Dentofacial following orthognathic surgery in seven mandibular prognathic patients with open bite and mandibular asymmetry. Jpn J Jaw Deform 1995;5:53-63.
[17] Hitoshi Koyata. Chapter 8, Biomechanics of Lingual Orthodontics, Esthetic Orthodontics 2nd Edition, Quitessence, 2003, Tokyo, 44-60.
[18] Toshiaki Hiro. Preparation for the new generation of Lingual Orthodontics -Six keys to success with Lingual Straight Wire Appliance-, J Lingual Orthodontics 2002;2(2):29-47.

[19] Toru Inami, Ichiro Aizawa, *et al.* Lingual bracket orthodontic technique, Part 4, Biomechanics of Lingual Bracket Orthodontic Technique, Ishiyaku, 2009, Tokyo, 79-107.

[20] Toshiaki Hiro. Presentation de huit cas d'orthodontie linguale soumis en vue de l'examen de l'European Board of Orthodontists. J International Orthodontics 2008;1:53-132.

[21] Akiko Sakai, Seiji Haraguchi, *et al.* Orthodontic camouflage of a late adolescent patient with Class III malocclusion. Orthodontic Waves 2006;65:127-133.

[22] Hiroshi Kamioka, Noriko Shiraga, *et al.* Camouflage treatment using implant anchorage in a skeletal Class III patient. Orthodontic Waves 2009;68:171-177.

[23] Maeda Yoshihiko, Hashimoto Fumio, *et al.* Camouflage orthodontic treatment of an adult skeletal Class III patient with anterior/lateral crossbite and severe crowding. Orthodontic Waves 2005;64:75-80.

[24] Costa pinho TM, Ustrell Torrent JM, Correia pinto JGR, orthodontic camouflage in the case of a skeletal class III malocclusion. World J Orthod 2004;5:213-23.

[25] Sugawara J, Daimaruya T. *et al.* Distal movement of mandibular molars in adult patients with the skeletal anchorage system. Am J Orthod Dentofac Orthop 2004;125: 130-138.

[26] For JN. An American Board of Orthodontics case report. A non-surgical and non-extraction approach in the treatment of a skeletal and dental Class I malocclusion in a growing patient. Am J Orthod Dentofac Orthop 1990;98:470-475.

[27] Serkan Görgülü, Deniz Sağdıç,*et al.* Tongue movements in patients with skeletal Class III malocclusions evaluated with real-time balanced turbo field echo cine magnetic resonance imaging, Am J Orthod Dentofac Orthop 2011;139(5):e405-e414.

[28] Chie Sakakura, Tadao Fukui, *et al.* A Feature of the Deglutition Muscle Activity Form in Patients with Mandibular Prognathism. Jpn J Jaw Deform 2010;20(4):238-291.

PART V: TREATMENT OF CLASS III PATIENTS WITH CRANIOFACIAL ANOMALIES

CHAPTER 14

Class III Treatment for Patients with Cleft Lip and Palate

Takashi Yamashiro[1,*] and Seiji Iida[2]

[1]Department of Orthodontics, Graduate School of Medicine, Dentistry and Pharmaceutical Sciences Okayama University Okayama, Japan and [2]Department of Oral and Maxillofacial Surgery, Graduate School of Medicine, Dentistry and Pharmaceutical Sciences Okayama University, Okayama, Japan

Abstract: Class III malocclusion and midfacial retrusion are major problems in patients with cleft lip and palate (CLP) because maxillary growth is compromised by postsurgical scar contraction. As well as dental problems, these patients also suffer from multiple functional problems, such as suckling, swallowing, speech, and hearing problems. Successful management of patients with CLP requires a multidisciplinary approach. In contrast to conventional Class III treatment, treating cleft palate patients requires attention to multiple functional problems during orthodontic treatment. CLP patients often have multiple, complex problems that require coordinated and comprehensive treatment. Although major progress had been made towards the effective treatment of dentofacial complications, the diversity of approaches to cleft treatment remains great. Furthermore, there is insufficient clinical data about cleft palate treatment to establish an evidence-base for treatment of CLP. A European intercenter comparative study of treatment outcomes in CLP patients provided a methodology for comparing practices, highlighted the potential for wider collaboration including opportunities to promote clinical trials, and encouraged intercenter comparisons. In this chapter, the authors will discuss the problems of cleft palate patients and the implications for their orthodontic and orthognathic management. The findings obtained from recent intercenter comparative studies will also be presented.

Keywords: Cleft lip and palate, Velopharyngeal dysfunction, Bone graft, Maxillary protraction, Maxillary distraction, Orthognathic surgery.

INTRODUCTION

Class III malocclusion and midfacial retrusion are major problems in patients with cleft lip and palate (CLP) due to poor growth caused by postsurgical scar

***Address correspondence to Takashi Yamashiro:** Department of Orthodontics and Dentofacial Orthopedics, Graduate School of Dentistry, Osaka University, 1-8 Yamada-Oka, Suita, Osaka 565-0871, Japan; Tel: +81-6-6879-2958; Fax: +81-6-6879-2960; Email: yamashiro@dent.osaka-u.ac.jp

Peter W. Ngan, Toshi Deguchi and Eugene W. Roberts (Eds)

contraction [1-3]. As well as dental problems, CLP patients suffer multiple functional problems, such as suckling, swallowing, speech, and hearing problems. The ideal treatment for such patients involves a multidisciplinary specialist team including orthodontists, surgeons, dentists, language therapists, audiologists, and/or hearing specialists [4, 5]; *i.e.*, the successful management of patients with cleft lip/palate requires a multidisciplinary approach [4, 5]. In contrast to conventional class III treatment, cleft palate patients require attention to be focused on multiple functional problems during orthodontic treatment. Since orthodontists are involved in both dental and craniofacial development they should recognize that cleft palate patients require coordinated and comprehensive treatment. In particular, cleft lip palate patients have speech difficulties due to their impaired velopharyngeal function, *e.g.*, CLP patients suffer from nasal voice resonance and various types of articulation disorders. Orthodontists have to understand how orthodontic treatment affects speech problems and treatment. In this chapter, we discuss the problems of cleft palate patients including the speech problems they suffer during orthodontic and orthognathic treatment. We focus on the following clinical topics: 1) lateral expansion and bone grafting, 2) maxillary protraction, and 3) surgical treatment including distraction osteogenesis.

Major progress has been made on the treatment of dentofacial complications. However, the diversity of approaches to cleft treatment remains great. There is insufficient clinical evidence about approaches to cleft palate treatment to establish an evidence-base for CLP management. In 1992, the landmark Eurocleft study [6-10] clearly established the value of intercenter collaboration for carrying out assessments of treatment outcomes using retrospective data. Such studies allow for the objective and unbiased discrimination of the favorable and unfavorable effects of various clinical management protocols. Similar approaches were also taken in the Dutchcleft [11] and Americleft [12-16] studies to establish standard treatments and treatment sequences for CLP patients [11-16]. These intercenter comparative studies of treatment outcomes in CLP patients have highlighted the potential of wider collaboration, including opportunities to promote clinical trials and encouraged intercenter comparisons. They have also reported various important findings, which we will discuss below.

The Anatomy of Cleft Lip and Palate Patients

Patients with a history of unilateral CLP generally present with a variable degree of midfacial deficiency in the anteroposterior dimension and a class III malocclusion [4, 17]. The upper jaw is unable to keep up with the normal growth of the lower jaw because of postsurgical scar contraction and anatomical anomalies [4, 18]. The stripping of the periosteum results in fibrosis, especially around the pterygopalatine-tuberosity sutures, which adversely affects the patient's facial profile and dental occlusion [19]. Thus, maxillary hypoplasia and class III malocclusion become more marked during the patient's adolescence, and a concave skeletal profile develops with aging [20, 21]. In bilateral CLP patients, the premaxilla is prominent initially, but evolves into midface deficiency later in life [18, 20, 22].

The mandible in cleft lip and palate patients is also the subject of controversy. Cleft patients display a shorter mandibular ramus and body length. These patients also show significant backward and downward rotation of the mandible, which leads to a more posterior position of point B and a greater ANB angle [23]. It has been shown that cleft lip and palate patients tend to be mouth breathers due to nasal airway impairment, and such oral breathing results in an increase in lower face height and posterior rotation of the mandible [24, 25]. Such mandibular retrusion can occasionally mask a maxillary deficiency, and patients with this condition tend to show a bimaxillary retrognathic facial profile [21, 26, 27].

In addition, surgical procedures, involving mucoperiosteal denudation of the bone and ossification of the palate, lead to maxillary deficiency. The absence of palatal sutures results in maxillary dental and skeletal arch constriction in cleft patients, which often results in posterior crossbites [28-32].

These inhibitory effects of scar formation resulting in dental arch constriction were confirmed by animal studies [33-35]. Transverse growth of the alveolar bone is initially inhibited by wound contraction immediately after palatal surgery. It is subsequently arrested by scar tissue contraction over areas of previously denuded bone [36]. Posterior crossbites become worse in the permanent dentition, and significant arch asymmetry and maxillary dental midline deviations are all common characteristics of unilateral clefts [18]. These problems appear to be related to the proximity and amount of scarring that is adjacent to the alveolar ridge, which results in lingual deflection of the erupting permanent dentition, thereby aggravating the initial segment collapse [33, 37]. The severity of maxillary dental arch constriction is also closely related to the scar tissue distribution over the hard palate [38].

Velopharyngeal Function in Cleft Palate Patients

Velopharyngeal function is an important component of speech, and patients with cleft palate or submucous cleft are at risk of articulation problems, due to impaired velopharyngeal function [39, 40]. In CLP patients, the muscles of the palate are separated and do not form a sling across the back of the soft palate. Such problems are treated surgically, but the palate often remains too short to reach the back of the throat and achieve complete closure between the mouth and nose during speech [41]. Velopharyngeal insufficiency causes hypernasality and the nasal emission of air during the production of non-nasal sounds (Fig. **1**), consequently reducing the intelligibility of speech. Such problems are treated by speech-aid prostheses or surgery to improve velopharyngeal closure [42, 43].

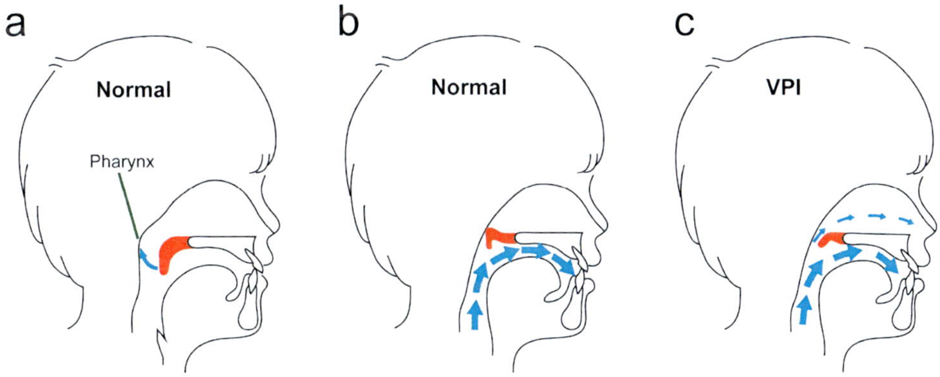

Figure 1: The velum moves in a superior and posterior direction to contact the posterior and lateral pharyngeal walls during closure (a and b). When the velum fails to close the nasopharvnx, air and phonation escape through the nose during speech, resulting in hypernasality (c).

The use of speech-aid prosthesis, such as palatal lift prosthesis (PLP) or bulb-attached palatal lift prosthesis (bulb-PLP), is one of several strategies used to improve hypernasality and speech intelligibility (Fig. **2**). Several studies on the clinical effects of these prostheses have reported that they can correct hypernasality and also stimulate velopharyngeal function, to the extent that some patients can permanently discard the prosthesis [44]. A recent paper showed that the wearing of a speech aid reduces levator muscle fatigue, which is consequently involved in the activation of physiologic velopharyngeal closure [45].

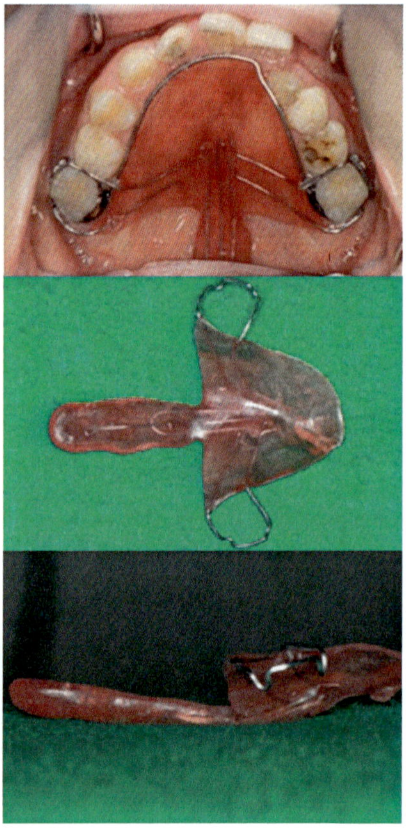

Figure 2: Speech-Aid Prostheses can elevate the velum and fill the residual velopharyngeal gap.

Lateral Expansion and Bone Graft

An osseous cleft results in serious disruption of the dentition and collapse of the alveolar segments. During the transition from deciduous to mixed dentition, the discrepancies increase between the size of the maxillary and mandibular dental arches [1, 36]. Cleft lip and palate patients suffer osseous defects of the alveolus. Bone grafting of these defects improves facial esthetics and dental function [46]. Bone grafting provides continuity to the alveolar ridge, allowing canines to erupt and adjacent teeth to drift into near ideal positions [5] (Fig. **3**). CLP patients often display flattening and widening of the alar base, and bone grafting also improves these problems.

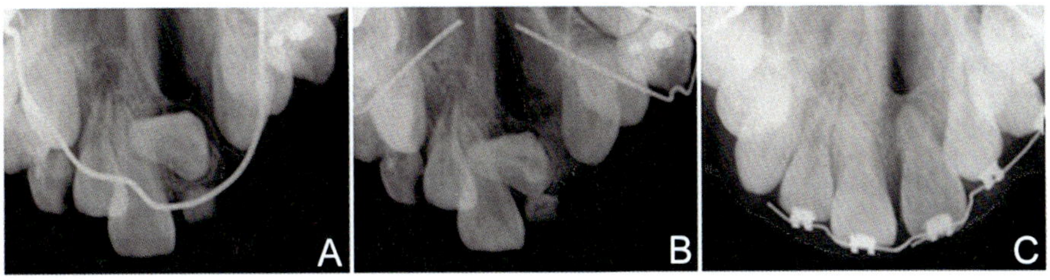

Figure 3: Bone grafting provides continuity to the alveolar bone, allowing the canines to erupt. (a) Occlusal radiography, age 9, just prior to a bone graft. (b) Age10 just after the graft procedure, showing bone fill-in at the cleft site. (c) Age 14, near the completion of orthodontic treatment.

Orthodontics in conjunction with bone grafting focuses on alignment of teeth within individual arches and lateral and anterior expansion of the arch. Developing a favorable arch form and eliminating crossbites improves dental function and esthetics [5, 47]. Posterior crossbites are usually corrected using palatal expanders, such as the Hyrax and Quad Helix. If a crossbite is limited to the anterior buccal segment, a fan type expander might be indicated to obtain differential expansion, *e.g.*, more anterior than posterior [47] (Fig. **4**). The selection of an expansion appliance should be based on the characteristics of the patient's dental arches, as well as the orthodontist's personal preference and experience [47].

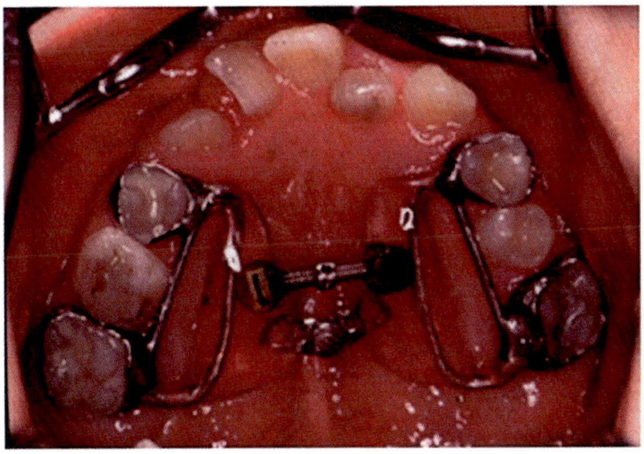

Figure 4: A fan type expander generates differential expansion of the transverse diameters of the upper arch. It is usually indicated for anteriorly constricted CLP patients.

Lateral expansion of the constricted maxillary arch may be indicated for physiological reasons. When the maxillary segments are displaced medially, the tongue cannot be accommodated in its normal position in the palate. Tongue position is critical for normal development of the maxilla as well as the mandible. If nasal respiration is impeded, the tongue may assume a low posture in order to facilitate oral respiration, which results in a posterior rotation of the mandible and opening of the Gonial angle [48].

Orthodontic tooth movement before bone grafting should be minimal, and movement of the teeth proximal to the cleft must be done with caution to avoid tipping the root into the cleft space [5]. The most important issue in orthodontics prior to bone grafting is to avoid perforating the thin lamina of the alveolar bone, covering the roots of teeth adjacent to the cleft site [49-51]. It is preferable to ensure that the incisor roots remain in the bone at the pre-grafting stage. Correction of tooth angulation can be achieved after a successful graft is achieved [5]. As a rule, the best outcomes for major orthodontic correction are accomplished after a bone graft has been completed [5].

The timing of secondary bone grafts in the mixed dentition is routinely between 9 and 11 years of age, when the canine roots have reached between one-quarter and two-thirds of their final length [52-55]. However, if the tooth germ of the lateral incisor tooth is present, earlier grafting may be considered [56, 57]. In such cases, bone grafting is performed before the eruption of the lateral incisor adjacent to the alveolar cleft [41, 57-60].

Approximately 1 to 3 months after bone grafting, it is usually possible to proceed with orthodontic movement of the teeth in the grafted area. A periapical radiograph is the best method to determine the quality and quantity of the bone around the teeth proximal to the cleft. The long-term treatment plan should be coordinated with the patient's growth and the degree of anteroposterior discrepancy [5, 47].

If oronasal fistulas are present, expansion may increase the size of the oronasal fistulas, complicating the surgical repair [47]. In the absence of a midpalatal suture, palatal expansion might enlarge the palatal fistula, leading to a requirement for more bone and the rotation of more soft tissue, especially in bilateral clefts [61]. Oronasal fistulas often occur in the labial vestibule. Defects in the alveolus, the hard palate, and at the junction between the hard and soft palate, are common complication of cleft palate repair [46]. The symptoms of these fistulas include nasality in speech, the leakage of fluids into the nose, and food lodging in the defect. The symptoms depend to some extent on the site of the fistula [62]. In addition, creating a cleft, whose width exceeds the coverage capabilities of the soft tissue, could negatively impact bone graft outcomes [61]. Covert oronasal fistulas can be repaired simultaneously with bone graft placement [61], so orthodontists should discuss this option with surgeons before the bone grafting procedure.

Maxillary Protraction

In growing CLP patients, sagittal discrepancies caused by the primary surgery may be corrected orthopedically with a protraction facemask [63]. Orthopedic force is applied to intraoral devices, such as a labiolingual arch, quad helix, or rapid maxillary expansion (RME). Such orthopedic force is transmitted to the circum-maxillary sutures and stimulates downward and forward movement of the maxillary complex. However, excessive scar tissue, adjacent to the pterygopalatine-tuberosity sutures and lip, can inhibit the forward growth of the maxilla [36].

Several clinical studies have shown that early maxillary protraction brings about short-term favorable effects on maxillary forward growth, when the treatment is started during the deciduous or early mixed dentition stage [32, 64, 65]. It is likely that circum-maxillary sutural growth is active during the early juvenile period, so it advantageous to facilitate the forward growth of the maxilla during these stages [66]. It is important to note that there was a lot of variation in the treatment response, and some populations displayed a poor response; *i.e.*, only 0-1 mm of advancement over the same time period.

Numerous papers report that facemask protraction improves the Class III skeletal patterns of CLP patients [66-73]. However, early orthopedic treatment in CLP cases is still controversial. Actually, there have also been reports of cases showing a poor treatment response in the basal maxilla [64, 65, 69, 74]. Ngan *et al.* [75] and MacDonald *et al.* [76] report that facemask therapy does not normalize the forward growth of the maxilla, and patients resume a Class III growth pattern, due to deficient maxillary growth, during the follow-up period. Ranta [77] showed that maxillary protraction was not effective when it was applied in older patients (9-15 yrs old). In addition, there are limitations to the degree of maxillary advancement in CLP patients, and they display a high relapse tendency due to scar tissue formation [78]. Variations in the amount of maxillary protraction may be associated with the degree of scar tissue formation [71].

RME is used to activate the circum-maxillary sutural system to possibly enhance the effect of the orthopedic facemask in CLP patients, as well as non-cleft class III patients. Palatal expansion before or during protraction of the maxilla is performed to facilitate protraction by disarticulating the circum-maxillary sutures. Baik [79] reported that more forward movement of the maxilla was achieved, when protraction was performed in conjunction with RME, compared to protraction without RME. One protocol is to perform alternating rapid maxillary expansions and constrictions, at weekly intervals, to disarticulate the circum-maxillary sutures without over expanding the maxilla [80]. Recent study demonstrated that such maxillary suture loosening with protraction therapy is effective in improving the skeletal discrepancy in cleft lip and palate patients [81].

When a rapid palatal expander is used as anchorage for protraction, the orthodontist should guard against unwanted side effects such as labioversion of the upper incisors, extrusion of the upper molars, counterclockwise rotation of the upper occlusal plane, and clockwise rotation of the mandible [82, 83]. Cleft patients display a more vertical growth pattern than non-cleft patients [11], and excessive clockwise rotation of the mandible during facemask therapy can worsen their facial profile.

To allow the direct transmission of orthopedic force to the circum-maxillary sutures, unique approaches had been developed, such as intentionally ankylosed primary canines and osseointegrated implants [84, 85]. Recently, orthodontic miniscrews have been used to provide skeletal anchorage for protraction facemasks [86-89]. This method is available for older patients (11-13 years) and produces minimal dentoalveolar side effects [89]. Facemask protraction with miniscrews succeeded in achieving more maxillary protraction compared to conventional protraction [90].

Surgical Treatment in Cleft Patients

Maxillary hypoplasia is a common deformity in CLP. Approximately 25-30% of these patients require orthognathic surgery to achieve adequate functional jaw relationships, harmonious facial aesthetics, or both [21, 91-93]. Improvement of the facial profile is achieved by surgical advancement of the maxilla to normalize the relationships between the jaws, teeth, lips, and tongue [12, 94]. Le Fort I osteotomy is widely employed for this purpose. However, poor maxillary and alveolar growth in the transverse and sagittal planes, as well as palatal scarring, render maxillary advancement of more than 6 mm difficult to achieve [95]. Improvement of the occlusal relationships by LeFort I osteotomy might also improve speech articulation and favor nasal breathing. However, Le Fort I osteotomy has many disadvantages when used for correcting a hypoplastic maxilla in CLP patients, such as limited advancement, a requirement for bone grafting, a negative effect on velopharyngeal closure, and a high risk of bone necrosis and relapse [96]. Actually, a high recurrence rate has been documented with conventional Le Fort I maxillary osteotomy in cleft lip and palate patients [97]. In addition, maxillary advancement changes the velopharyngeal configuration, enhancing the potential to adversely affect the velopharyngeal function of cleft patients, postoperatively [98].

Incomplete closure of the velum during speech, as seen in patients with velopharyngeal insufficiency (VPI), results in nasal air escape and difficulties establishing intraoral pressure. Moreover, increasing nasal resonance (hypernasality) becomes more pronounced as velopharyngeal function worsens [96, 98]. The increased risk of developing hypernasality and VPI in CLP patients could be due to their greatcr nasopharyngeal depth dimensions. An additional contributing factor is the decreased amount of velar tissue that is characteristic of repaired clefts [99]. It has also been pointed out that maxillary advancement results in (or aggravates) velopharyngeal incompetence and hypernasal speech in CLP patients, particularly if there is borderline incompetence before surgery [100] (Fig. **5**).

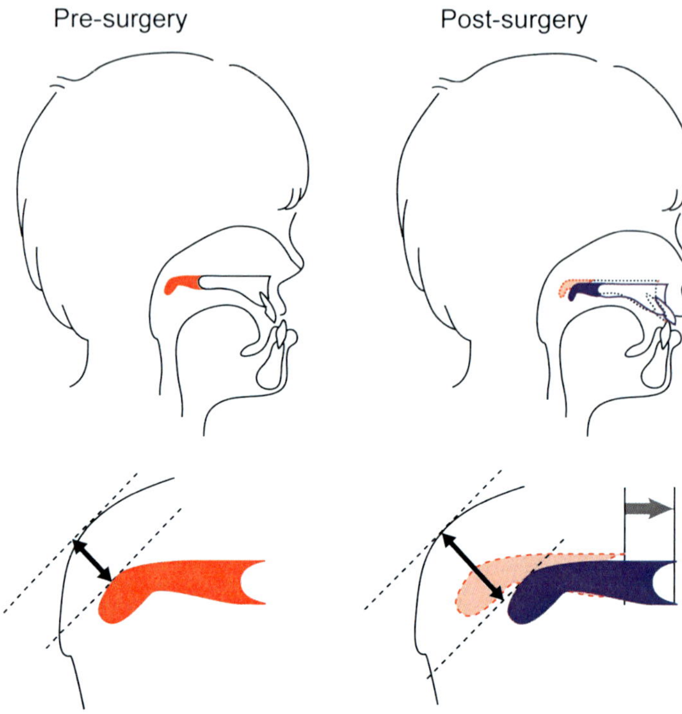

Figure 5: With advancement of the maxilla, the velum is also being pulled forward, raising the concern that velopharyngeal incompetence (VPI) may develop.

The precise effect of maxillary advancement on the velar mechanism is undefined, and previous studies have failed to find any correlation between the amount of maxillary advancement and velopharyngeal function in cleft patients [94, 101, 102]. Thus, appropriate surgical treatment planning can be individualized, based on a baseline speech assessment. If speech and velopharyngeal function deteriorate, after maxillary advancement, a pharyngeal flap can be harvested after orthognathic surgery to correct VPI in most patients [96, 103].

Maxillary advancement with distraction osteogenesis (DO) has become a standard treatment for patients with cleft lip and palate [104]. DO is more reliable than surgical advancement and the slow movement of the maxilla, due to the gradual distraction, seems to allow for easier adaptation of soft tissue structures and a reduction in skeletal relapse [103, 104]. Maxillary distraction, following a Le Fort I osteotomy, has many advantages, including greater advancement potential. Furthermore, this method produces more stable and reliable long-term results, less bone grafting is required, and there is less negative effects on velopharyngeal competence [105-111] (Fig. **6**). The gradual advancement of the maxilla is achieved *via* a cranially attached external distractor or an internal distractor; both devices are effective at distraction mediated maxillary advancement. External devices offer easier implantation and better control of the vectors of distraction, assuring a more predictable and effective outcome. In contrast, external devices are relatively difficult to utilize if the patient is uncooperative due to the bulkiness of the external frame [112]. Because of simultaneous elongation of the soft tissue, near the distraction segment, the relapse rate for maxillary distraction osteogenesis is greatly decreased, compared with traditional orthognathic surgical procedures [113].

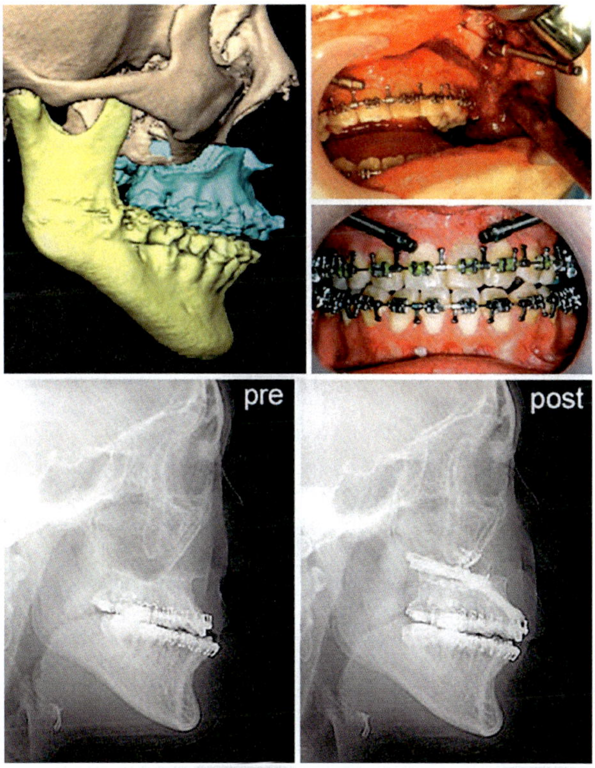

Figure 6: Maxillary distraction following Le Fort I osteotomy.

Whether distraction osteogenesis results in better velopharyngeal (VP) outcomes than traditional maxillary osteotomy remains a very important question. There has been a limited attempt to develop differential diagnostic and treatment planning criteria, to identify those maxillary deficient patients who would be most suited to routine orthognathic surgery, rather than distraction osteogenesis. Several subsequent studies have examined the effect of distraction osteogenesis on VP function and speech. No significant differences in speech or velopharyngeal function were noted [114-116].

Another approach to maxillary distraction osteogenesis is anterior segmental distraction osteogenesis, which allows forward advancement of the anterior maxillary segments without affecting the patient's velopharyngeal function. The advantage of this approach is that it does not affect the morphology of the posterior part of the oral cavity including the nasopharynx [117-119] (Fig. **7**). Recent results have shown that anterior segmental distraction osteogenesis can effectively correct the hypoplastic maxilla and severe dental crowding, associated with CLP, by increasing midfacial convexity and dental arch length, while preserving velopharyngeal function. Furthermore, dental crowding can be corrected without tooth extraction [118, 120-122].

Although no significant correlation was found between the degree of advancement and the outcome measures [112], Nohara described clinical indices that predict the postsurgical deterioration of velopharyngeal function [42]. The deterioration of velopharyngeal function associated with maxillary advancement was demonstrated in subjects whose levator activity was higher during speech than during blowing, regardless of the amount of maxillary advancement. Preoperative levator muscle electromyography could be used as a predictor, to identify patients who are at higher risk of postsurgical velopharyngeal insufficiency [42].

Eurocleft Project

The treatment of cleft lip and palate requires a comprehensive plan from birth to adulthood. Surgery is the primary treatment for cleft palate, resulting in subsequent problems with facial and dental development, speech, and hearing. Multiple procedures and a large number of specialist services are needed for years to fully correct the deficiencies. Major progress had been made towards the effective treatment of these complications. However, the diversity of approaches

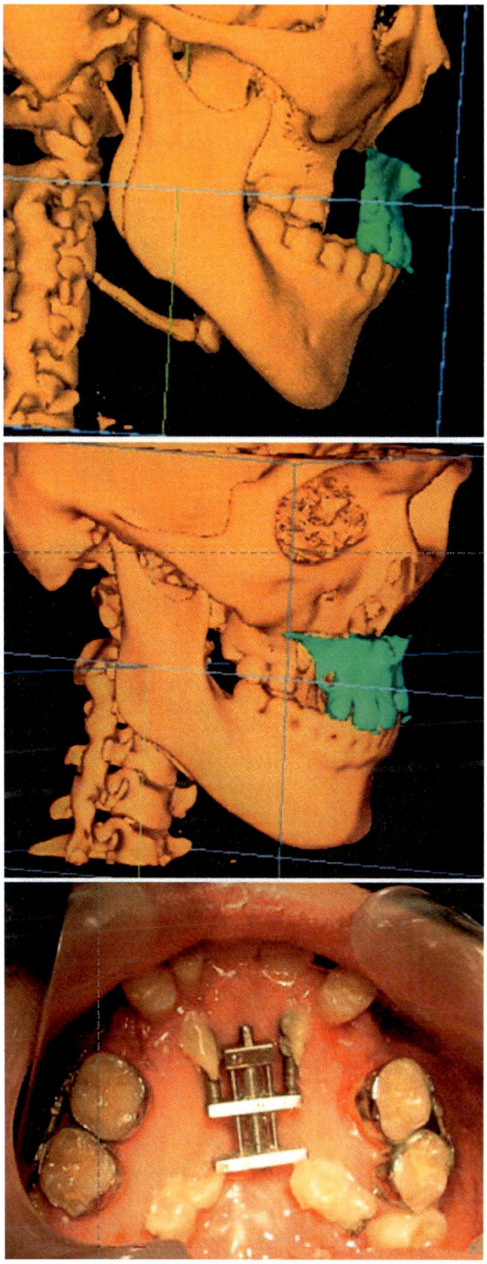

Figure 7: Anterior segmental distraction osteogenesis provides forward advancement of the anterior maxillary segments without affecting the patient's velopharyngeal function.

to cleft treatment remains great, and studies involving large samples are rare because of the relatively low frequency and numerous anatomical subtypes of cleft lip and palate. Thus, there is insufficient clinical data to establish evidence-based medical treatments for cleft palate [123]. To improve the standard of care for cleft palate patients, data about variables such as facial and dental appearance, speech outcome, and cost-effectiveness, should be efficiently collected in large studies.

In 1992, a European intercenter comparative study of treatment outcomes in CLP patients was published [6-10]. The study confirmed that a great diversity of clinical approaches and treatment protocols existed among the six centers examined, and also found dramatic differences in treatment outcomes. The study developed a preliminary methodology for comparing practices, and demonstrated the potential for wider European collaboration, including opportunities for promoting clinical trials. In addition, the study recognized the importance of intercenter comparisons [123]. Thereafter, the next "Eurocleft" project ran between 1996 and 2000 and aimed to discriminate between the favorable and unfavorable effects of various primary infant management protocols [123-128]. The recent published Americleft study [12-16] is expanding outcomes research into surgery, speech, and psychology [16].

These intercenter comparative studies suggest that providing decentralized care by low volume operators is associated with inferior outcomes. It was noteworthy that the necessity of maxillary osteotomy differed between the best and worst services [10]. Furthermore, care in the worst service was much more complex and expensive [10]. Rigorously managed intercenter evaluations force clinicians to compare outcomes for different protocols and identify harmful practices. Thus, significant improvements can be achieved at no extra cost assuming the underperforming teams recognize the need to change practice protocols [123].

A previous study indicated that different primary surgical procedures resulted in different levels of maxillary growth deficiency; Push-back closure of the palate impaired maxillary development, more than the von Langenbeck method, or for patients who had not yet had their hard palate closed [129]. Transverse maxillary growth disturbance was also more evident after the pushback method [43, 130, 131]. However, the Eurocleft study did not confirm whether the von Langenbeck method resulted in better development of the maxilla than the Wardill pushback method [125]. Regarding growth retardation, earlier studies indicated that primary bone grafting is associated with poor maxillary growth [132-134], and the Eurocleft study supported these findings [128].

It is noteworthy that the most favorable outcomes for dental arch relationships were obtained in centers with the simplest surgical protocols that avoided both presurgical orthopedics, and primary alveolar repair. The Eurocleft study confirmed that systematic differences in dental arch relationships can occur between different cleft centers, but did not identify specific causal factors [127].

SUMMARY POINTS

- Class III malocclusion and midfacial retrusion are major problems in patients with cleft lip and palate because postsurgical scar contraction results in maxillary growth deficiency.

- Velopharyngeal function is an important component of speech, and patients with CLP are at risk of speech difficulties due to impaired velopharyngeal function.

- In growing CLP patients, sagittal discrepancies caused by primary surgery can be corrected by orthopedic treatment, using a protraction facemask like in non-cleft patients.

- Maxillary advancement procedures in CLP patients can aggravate or result in velopharyngeal incompetence and hypernasality, especially if the patient shows signs of borderline incompetence before surgery.

- Maxillary distraction following Le Fort I osteotomy has many advantages, including allowing greater advancement potential, producing a more stable and reliable long-term result, and reducing the requirement for bone grafting.

- The diverse approach to cleft treatment remains great, and there is insufficient clinical evidence to establish an evidence-based protocol for CLP. Intercenter comparative studies, such as the Eurocleft project, confirmed that systematic differences in treatment outcomes can occur between different cleft centers.

ACKNOWLEDGEMENTS

Declared none.

CONFLICT OF INTEREST

The authors confirm that this chapter contents have no conflict of interest.

REFERENCES

[1] Bergland O and Sidhu SS. Occlusal changes from the deciduous to the early mixed dentition in unilateral complete clefts. Cleft Palate J 1974;11:317-326.

[2] Schwarz C and Gruner E. Logopaedic findings following advancement of the maxilla. J Maxillofac Surg 1976;4:40-55.

[3] Dahl E and Hanusardottir B. [prevalence of malocclusion in the primary and early mixed dentition in Danish children with complete cleft lip and palate]. Eur J Orthod 1979;1:81-88.

[4] Vargervik K. Growth characteristics of the premaxilla and orthodontic treatment principles in bilateral cleft lip and palate. Cleft Palate J 1983;20:289-302.

[5] Vlachos CC. Orthodontic treatment for the cleft palate patient. Semin Orthod 1996;2:197-204.

[6] Asher-McDade C, Brattstrom V, Dahl E, *et al.* A six-center international study of treatment outcome in patients with clefts of the lip and palate: Part 4. Assessment of nasolabial appearance. Cleft Palate Craniofac J 1992;29:409-412.

[7] Mars M, Asher-McDade C, Brattstrom V, *et al.* A six-center international study of treatment outcome in patients with clefts of the lip and palate: Part 3. Dental arch relationships. Cleft Palate Craniofac J 1992;29:405-408.

[8] Molsted K, Asher-McDade C, Brattstrom V, *et al.* A six-center international study of treatment outcome in patients with clefts of the lip and palate: Part 2. Craniofacial form and soft tissue profile. Cleft Palate Craniofac J 1992;29:398-404.

[9] Shaw WC, Asher-McDade C, Brattstrom V, *et al.* A six-center international study of treatment outcome in patients with clefts of the lip and palate: Part 1. Principles and study design. Cleft Palate Craniofac J 1992;29:393-397.

[10] Shaw WC, Dahl E, Asher-McDade C, *et al.* A six-center international study of treatment outcome in patients with clefts of the lip and palate: Part 5. General discussion and conclusions. Cleft Palate Craniofac J 1992;29:413-418.

[11] Van den Dungen GM, Ongkosuwito EM, Aartman IH, *et al.* Craniofacial morphology of dutch patients with bilateral cleft lip and palate and noncleft controls at the age of 15 years. Cleft Palate Craniofac J 2008;45:661-666.

[12] Daskalogiannakis J and Mehta M. The need for orthognathic surgery in patients with repaired complete unilateral and complete bilateral cleft lip and palate. Cleft Palate Craniofac J 2009;46:498-502.

[13] Long RE, Hathaway R, Daskalogiannakis J, *et al.* The Americleft study: An inter-center study of treatment outcomes for patients with unilateral cleft lip and palate part 1. Principles and study design. Cleft Palate Craniofac J 2011;48:239-243.

[14] Hathaway R, Daskalogiannakis J, Mercado A, *et al.* The Americleft study: An inter-center study of treatment outcomes for patients with unilateral cleft lip and palate part 2. Dental arch relationships. Cleft Palate Craniofac J 2011;48:244-251.

[15] Mercado A, Russell K, Hathaway R, *et al.* The Americleft study: An inter-center study of treatment outcomes for patients with unilateral cleft lip and palate part 4. Nasolabial aesthetics. Cleft Palate Craniofac J 2011;48:259-264.

[16] Russell K, Long RE, Hathaway R, *et al.* The Americleft study: An inter-center study of treatment outcomes for patients with unilateral cleft lip and palate part 5. General discussion and conclusions. Cleft Palate Craniofac J 2011;48:265-270.

[17] Graber TM. The congenital cleft palate deformity. J Am Dent Assoc 1954;48:375-395.

[18] Semb G and Shaw WC. Facial growth after different methods of surgical intervention in patients with cleft lip and palate. Acta Odontol Scand 1998;56:352-355.

[19] Yen SL. Protocols for late maxillary protraction in cleft lip and palate patients at childrens hospital Los Angeles. Semin Orthod 2011;17:138-148.

[20] Friede H and Pruzansky S. Long-term effects of premaxillary setback on facial skeletal profile in complete bilateral cleft lip and palate. Cleft Palate J 1985;22:97-105.

[21] Ross RB. Treatment variables affecting facial growth in complete unilateral cleft lip and palate. Cleft Palate J 1987;24:5-77.

[22] Trotman CA and Ross RB. Craniofacial growth in bilateral cleft lip and palate: Ages six years to adulthood. Cleft Palate Craniofac J 1993;30:261-273.

[23] Da Silva Filho OG, Normando AD and Capelozza Filho L. Mandibular growth in patients with cleft lip and/or cleft palate--the influence of cleft type. Am J Orthod Dentofacial Orthop 1993;104:269-275.

[24] Linder-Aronson S. Adenoids: their effect on mode of breathing and nasal airflow and their relationship to characteristics of the facial skeleton and the denition. A biometric, rhino-manometric and cephalometro-radiographic study on children with and without adenoids. Acta Otolaryngol Suppl 1970;265:1-132.

[25] Warren DW, Hairfield WM and Dalston ET. The relationship between nasal airway size and nasal-oral breathing in cleft lip and palate. Cleft Palate J 1990;27:46-51; discussion 51-42.

[26] Long RE, Jr. and McNamara JA, Jr. Facial growth following pharyngeal flap surgery: Skeletal assessment on serial lateral cephalometric radiographs. Am J Orthod 1985;87:187-196.

[27] Trotman CA, Long RE, Jr., Rosenstein SW, *et al.* Comparison of facial form in primary alveolar bone-grafted and nongrafted unilateral cleft lip and palate patients: Intercenter retrospective study. Cleft Palate Craniofac J 1996;33:91-95.

[28] Prydso U, Holm PC, Dahl E, *et al.* Bone formation in palatal clefts subsequent to palato-vomer plasty. Influence on transverse maxillary growth. Scand J Plast Reconstr Surg 1974;8:73-78.

[29] Heidbuchel KL, Kuijpers-Jagtman AM, Kramer GJ, *et al.* Maxillary arch dimensions in bilateral cleft lip and palate from birth until four years of age in boys. Cleft Palate Craniofac J 1998;35:233-239.

[30] Heidbuchel KL, Kuijpers-Jagtman AM, Van't Hof MA, *et al.* Effects of early treatment on maxillary arch development in bclp. A study on dental casts between 0 and 4 years of age. J Craniomaxillofac Surg 1998;26:140-147.

[31] Ross RB. The management of dental arch deformity in cleft lip and palate. Clin Plast Surg 1975;2:325-342.

[32] Rygh P and Tindlund R. Orthopedic expansion and protraction of the maxilla in cleft palate patients--a new treatment rationale. Cleft Palate J 1982;19:104-112.

[33] Kremenak CR, Jr. Dental exfoliation and eruption chronology in beagles. J Dent Res 1967;46:686-693.

[34] Kremenak CR, Huffman WC and Olin WH. Growth of maxillae in dogs after palatal surgery. I. Cleft Palate J 1967;4:6-17.

[35] Kremenak CR, Jr. and Kremenak CR, Sr. Influence of occlusion on amount of jaw growth inhibition induced by palate surgery in beagles. J Dent Res 1970;49:893.

[36] Ross RB. The clinical implications of facial growth in cleft lip and palate. Cleft Palate J 1970;7:37-47.

[37] Ross RB and Johnston MC. The effect of early orthodontic treatment on facial growth in cleft lip and palate. Cleft Palate J 1967;4:157-164.

[38] Ishikawa H, Nakamura S, Misaki K, *et al.* Scar tissue distribution on palates and its relation to maxillary dental arch form. Cleft Palate Craniofac J 1998;35:313-319.

[39] Shprintzen RJ and Golding-Kushner KJ. Evaluation of velopharyngeal insufficiency. Otolaryngol Clin North Am 1989;22:519-536.

[40] Smith B and Guyette TW. Evaluation of cleft palate speech. Clin Plast Surg 2004;31:251-260.

[41] Bergland O, Semb G and Abyholm FE. Elimination of the residual alveolar cleft by secondary bone grafting and subsequent orthodontic treatment. Cleft Palate J 1986;23:175-205.

[42] Nohara K, Tachimura T and Wada T. Prediction of deterioration of velopharyngeal function associated with maxillary advancement using electromyography of levator veli palatini muscle. Cleft Palate Craniofac J 2006;43:174-178.

[43] Nishio J, Yamanishi T, Kohara H, *et al.* Early two-stage palatoplasty using modified furlow's veloplasty. Cleft Palate Craniofac J 2010;47:73-81.

[44] Wong LP and Weiss CE. A clinical assessment of obturator-wearing cleft palate patients. J Prosthet Dent 1972;27:632-639.

[45] Nohara K, Kotani Y, Sasao Y, *et al.* Effect of a speech aid prosthesis on reducing muscle fatigue. J Dent Res 2010;89:478-481.

[46] Waite PD and Waite DE. Bone grafting for the alveolar cleft defect. Semin Orthod 1996;2:192-196.

[47] Santiago PE and Grayson BH. Role of the craniofacial orthodontist on the craniofacial and cleft lip and palate team. Semin Orthod 2009;15:225-243.

[48] Vargervik K. Orthodontic management of unilateral cleft lip and palate. Cleft Palate J 1981;18:256-270.

[49] Turvey TA, Vig K, Moriarty J, *et al.* Delayed bone grafting in the cleft maxilla and palate: a retrospective multidisciplinary analysis. Am J Orthod 1984;86:244-256.

[50] Vig KW and Turvey TA. Orthodontic-surgical interaction in the management of cleft lip and palate. Clin Plast Surg 1985;12:735-748.

[51] Vig KW. Alveolar bone grafts: the surgical/orthodontic management of the cleft maxilla. Ann Acad Med Singapore 1999;28:721-727.

[52] Boyne PJ and Sands NR. Secondary bone grafting of residual alveolar and palatal clefts. J Oral Surg 1972;30:87-92.

[53] Boyne PJ and Sands NR. Combined orthodontic-surgical management of residual palato-alveolar cleft defects. Am J Orthod 1976;70:20-37.

[54] Lilja J, Kalaaji A, Friede H, *et al.* Combined bone grafting and delayed closure of the hard palate in patients with unilateral cleft lip and palate: Facilitation of lateral incisor eruption and evaluation of indicators for timing of the procedure. Cleft Palate Craniofac J 2000;37:98-105.

[55] Rosenstein SW, Grasseschi M and Dado DV. A long-term retrospective outcome assessment of facial growth, secondary surgical need, and maxillary lateral incisor status in a surgical-orthodontic protocol for complete clefts. Plast Reconstr Surg 2003;111:1-13; discussion 14-16.

[56] Ozawa T, Omura S, Fukuyama E, *et al.* Factors influencing secondary alveolar bone grafting in cleft lip and palate patients: Prospective analysis using ct image analyzer. Cleft Palate Craniofac J 2007;44:286-291.

[57] El Deeb M, Messer LB, Lehnert MW, *et al.* Canine eruption into grafted bone in maxillary alveolar cleft defects. Cleft Palate J 1982;19:9-16.

[58] Sindet-Pedersen S and Enemark H. Comparative study of secondary and late secondary bone-grafting in patients with residual cleft defects. Short-term evaluation. Int J Oral Surg 1985;14:389-398.

[59] Paulin G, Astrand P, Rosenquist JB, *et al.* Intermediate bone grafting of alveolar clefts. J Craniomaxillofac Surg 1988;16:2-7.

[60] Witherow H, Cox S, Jones E, *et al.* A new scale to assess radiographic success of secondary alveolar bone grafts. Cleft Palate Craniofac J 2002;39:255-260.

[61] Long RE, Jr., Spangler BE and Yow M. Cleft width and secondary alveolar bone graft success. Cleft Palate Craniofac J 1995;32:420-427.

[62] Amaratunga NA. Occurrence of oronasal fistulas in operated cleft palate patients. J Oral Maxillofac Surg 1988;46:834-838.

[63] Delaire J. Maxillary development revisited: Relevance to the orthopaedic treatment of class iii malocclusions. Eur J Orthod 1997;19:289-311.

[64] Friede H and Lennartsson B. Forward traction of the maxilla in cleft lip and palate patients. Eur J Orthod 1981;3:21-39.

[65] Ranta R. Protraction of the cleft maxilla. Eur J Orthod 1988;10:215-222.

[66] Ishikawa H, Kitazawa S, Iwasaki H, *et al.* Effects of maxillary protraction combined with chin-cap therapy in unilateral cleft lip and palate patients. Cleft Palate Craniofac J 2000;37:92-97.

[67] Tindlund RS and Rygh P. Maxillary protraction: Different effects on facial morphology in unilateral and bilateral cleft lip and palate patients. Cleft Palate Craniofac J 1993;30:208-221.

[68] Tindlund RS, Rygh P and Boe OE. Orthopedic protraction of the upper jaw in cleft lip and palate patients during the deciduous and mixed dentition periods in comparison with normal growth and development. Cleft Palate Craniofac J 1993;30:182-194.

[69] Tindlund RS. Skeletal response to maxillary protraction in patients with cleft lip and palate before age 10 years. Cleft Palate Craniofac J 1994;31:295-308.

[70] Bhatia S and Nanda RS. Role of protraction headgear in correction of a skeletal midface deficiency in a unilateral cleft lip and palate--an interim case report. Am J Orthod Dentofacial Orthop 1994;105:529-535.

[71] Buschang PH, Porter C, Genecov E, *et al.* Face mask therapy of preadolescents with unilateral cleft lip and palate. Angle Orthod 1994;64:145-150.

[72] Chen KF and So LL. Sagittal skeletal and dental changes of reverse headgear treatment in chinese boys with complete unilateral cleft lip and palate. Angle Orthod 1996;66:363-372.

[73] Kawakami M, Yagi T and Takada K. Maxillary expansion and protraction in correction of midface retrusion in a complete unilateral cleft lip and palate patient. Angle Orthod 2002;72:355-361.

[74] Sarnas KV and Rune B. Extraoral traction to the maxilla with face mask: A follow-up of 17 consecutively treated patients with and without cleft lip and palate. Cleft Palate J 1987;24:95-103.

[75] Ngan PW, Hagg U, Yiu C, *et al.* Treatment response and long-term dentofacial adaptations to maxillary expansion and protraction. Semin Orthod 1997;3:255-264.

[76] Macdonald KE, Kapust AJ and Turley PK. Cephalometric changes after the correction of class iii malocclusion with maxillary expansion/facemask therapy. Am J Orthod Dentofacial Orthop 1999;116:13-24.

[77] Ranta R. Forward traction of the maxilla with cleft lip and palate in mixed and permanent dentitions. J Craniomaxillofac Surg 1989;17 Suppl 1:20-22.

[78] Baek SH, Lee JK, Lee JH, *et al.* Comparison of treatment outcome and stability between distraction osteogenesis and lefort i osteotomy in cleft patients with maxillary hypoplasia. J Craniofac Surg 2007;18:1209-1215.

[79] Baik HS. Clinical results of the maxillary protraction in korean children. Am J Orthod Dentofacial Orthop 1995;108:583-592.

[80] Liou EJ and Tsai WC. A new protocol for maxillary protraction in cleft patients: Repetitive weekly protocol of alternate rapid maxillary expansions and constrictions. Cleft Palate Craniofac J 2005;42:121-127.

[81] Borzabadi-Farahani A, Lane CJ, Yen SL. Late Maxillary Protraction in patients with unilateral cleft Lip and palate: A preliminary study. Cleft Palate Craniofac J. 2013 *in press.*

[82] Nartallo-Turley PE and Turley PK. Cephalometric effects of combined palatal expansion and facemask therapy on class iii malocclusion. Angle Orthod 1998;68:217-224.

[83] Kapust AJ, Sinclair PM and Turley PK. Cephalometric effects of face mask/expansion therapy in class iii children: A comparison of three age groups. Am J Orthod Dentofacial Orthop 1998;113:204-212.

[84] Kokich VG, Shapiro PA, Oswald R, *et al.* Ankylosed teeth as abutments for maxillary protraction: A case report. Am J Orthod 1985;88:303-307.

[85] Enacar A, Giray B, Pehlivanoglu M, *et al.* Facemask therapy with rigid anchorage in a patient with maxillary hypoplasia and severe oligodontia. Am J Orthod Dentofacial Orthop 2003;123:571-577.

[86] Hong H, Ngan P, Han G, *et al.* Use of onplants as stable anchorage for facemask treatment: A case report. Angle Orthod 2005;75:453-460.

[87] Vachiramon A, Urata M, Kyung HM, *et al.* Clinical applications of orthodontic microimplant anchorage in craniofacial patients. Cleft Palate Craniofac J 2009;46:136-146.

[88] Kircelli BH, Pektas ZO and Uckan S. Orthopedic protraction with skeletal anchorage in a patient with maxillary hypoplasia and hypodontia. Angle Orthod 2006;76:156-163.

[89] Kircelli BH and Pektas ZO. Midfacial protraction with skeletally anchored face mask therapy: A novel approach and preliminary results. Am J Orthod Dentofacial Orthop 2008;133:440-449.

[90] Baek SH, Kim KW and Choi JY. New treatment modality for maxillary hypoplasia in cleft patients. Protraction facemask with miniplate anchorage. Angle Orthod 2010;80:595-603.

[91] DeLuke DM, Marchand A, Robles EC, *et al.* Facial growth and the need for orthognathic surgery after cleft palate repair: Literature review and report of 28 cases. J Oral Maxillofac Surg 1997;55:694-697; discussion 697-698.

[92] Cohen SR, Corrigan M, Wilmot J, *et al.* Cumulative operative procedures in patients aged 14 years and older with unilateral or bilateral cleft lip and palate. Plast Reconstr Surg 1995;96:267-271.

[93] Schnitt DE, Agir H and David DJ. From birth to maturity: A group of patients who have completed their protocol management. Part i. Unilateral cleft lip and palate. Plast Reconstr Surg 2004;113:805-817.

[94] Chanchareonsook N, Samman N and Whitehill TL. The effect of ranio-maxillofacial osteotomies and distraction osteogenesis on speech and velopharyngeal status: A critical review. Cleft Palate Craniofac J 2006;43:477-487.

[95] Wang XX, Wang X, Li ZL, *et al.* Anterior maxillary segmental distraction for correction of maxillary hypoplasia and dental crowding in cleft palate patients: A preliminary report. Int J Oral Maxillofac Surg 2009;38:1237-1243.

[96] Janulewicz J, Costello BJ, Buckley MJ, *et al.* The effects of le fort i osteotomies on velopharyngeal and speech functions in cleft patients. J Oral Maxillofac Surg 2004;62:308-314.

[97] Posnick JC and Dagys AP. Skeletal stability and relapse patterns after le fort i maxillary osteotomy fixed with miniplates: The unilateral cleft lip and palate deformity. Plast Reconstr Surg 1994;94:924-932.

[98] Maegawa J, Sells RK and David DJ. Pharyngoplasty in patients with cleft lip and palate after maxillary advancement. J Craniofac Surg 1998;9:330-335; discussion 336-337.

[99] Mason R, Turvey TA and Warren DW. Speech considerations with maxillary advancement procedures. J Oral Surg 1980;38:752-758.

[100] Witzel MA and Munro IR. Velopharyngeal insufficiency after maxillary advancement. Cleft Palate J 1977;14:176-180.

[101] Watzke I, Turvey TA, Warren DW, *et al.* Alterations in velopharyngeal function after maxillary advancement in cleft palate patients. J Oral Maxillofac Surg 1990;48:685-689.

[102] Trindade IE, Yamashita RP, Suguimoto RM, *et al.* Effects of orthognathic surgery on speech and breathing of subjects with cleft lip and palate: Acoustic and aerodynamic assessment. Cleft Palate Craniofac J 2003;40:54-64.

[103] Maegawa J, Sells RK and David DJ. Speech changes after maxillary advancement in 40 cleft lip and palate patients. J Craniofac Surg 1998;9:177-182; discussion 183-174.

[104] Scolozzi P. Distraction osteogenesis in the management of severe maxillary hypoplasia in cleft lip and palate patients. J Craniofac Surg 2008;19:1199-1214.

[105] Molina F, Ortiz Monasterio F, de la Paz Aguilar M, *et al.* Maxillary distraction: Aesthetic and functional benefits in cleft lip-palate and prognathic patients during mixed dentition. Plast Reconstr Surg 1998;101:951-963.

[106] Cohen SR, Burstein FD, Stewart MB, *et al.* Maxillary-midface distraction in children with cleft lip and palate: A preliminary report. Plast Reconstr Surg 1997;99:1421-1428.

[107] Polley JW and Figueroa AA. Rigid external distraction: Its application in cleft maxillary deformities. Plast Reconstr Surg 1998;102:1360-1372; discussion 1373-1364.

[108] Figueroa AA, Polley JW, Friede H, *et al.* Long-term skeletal stability after maxillary advancement with distraction osteogenesis using a rigid external distraction device in cleft maxillary deformities. Plast Reconstr Surg 2004;114:1382-1392; discussion 1393-1384.

[109] Wang XX, Wang X, Yi B, *et al.* Internal midface distraction in correction of severe maxillary hypoplasia secondary to cleft lip and palate. Plast Reconstr Surg 2005;116:51-60.

[110] Nout E, Wolvius EB, Van Adrichem LN, *et al.* Complications in maxillary distraction using the red ii device: A retrospective analysis of 21 patients. Int J Oral Maxillofac Surg 2006;35:897-902.

[111] Rachmiel A. Treatment of maxillary cleft palate: Distraction osteogenesis *vs.* orthognathic surgery--part one: Maxillary distraction. J Oral Maxillofac Surg 2007;65:753-757.

[112] Pelo S, Gasparini G, Di Petrillo A, *et al.* Distraction osteogenesis in the surgical treatment of craniostenosis: A comparison of internal and external craniofacial distractor devices. Childs Nerv Syst 2007;23:1447-1453.

[113] Chua HD, Whitehill TL, Samman N, *et al.* Maxillary distraction *vs.* orthognathic surgery in cleft lip and palate patients: Effects on speech and velopharyngeal function. Int J Oral Maxillofac Surg 2010 39:633-640.

[114] Cedars MG, Linck DL, 2nd, Chin M. *et al.* Advancement of the midface using distraction techniques. Plast Reconstr Surg 1999;103:429-441.

[115] Scheuerle J and Habal MB. Functional impact of distraction osteogenesis of the midface on expressive language development. J Craniofac Surg 2001;12:69-72.

[116] Harada K, Ishii Y, Ishii M, *et al.* Effect of maxillary distraction osteogenesis on velopharyngeal function: A pilot study. Oral Surg Oral Med Oral Pathol Oral Radiol Endod 2002;93:538-543.

[117] Iida S, Kogo M, Aikawa T, *et al.* Maxillary distraction osteogenesis using the intraoral distractors and the full-covered tooth-supported maxillary splint. J Oral Maxillofac Surg 2007;65:813-817.

[118] Iida S, Yagi T, Yamashiro T, *et al.* Maxillary anterior segmental distraction osteogenesis with the dynaform system for severe maxillary retrusion in cleft lip and palate. Plast Reconstr Surg 2007;120:508-516.

[119] Iida S, Haraguchi S, Aikawa T, *et al.* Conventional bone-anchored palatal distractor using an orthodontic palatal expander for the transverse maxillary distraction osteogenesis: Technical note. Oral Surg Oral Med Oral Pathol Oral Radiol Endod 2008;105:e8-11.

[120] Karakasis D and Hadjipetrou L. Advancement of the anterior maxilla by distraction (case report). J Craniomaxillofac Surg 2004;32:150-154.

[121] Gunaseelan R, Cheung LK, Krishnaswamy R, *et al.* Anterior maxillary distraction by tooth-borne palatal distractor. J Oral Maxillofac Surg 2007;65:1044-1049.

[122] Alkan A, Bas B, Ozer M, *et al.* Maxillary anterior segmental advancement of hypoplastic maxilla in cleft patients by distraction osteogenesis: Report of 2 cases. J Oral Maxillofac Surg 2008;66:126-132.

[123] Shaw WC, Semb G, Nelson P, *et al.* The eurocleft project 1996-2000: Overview. J Craniomaxillofac Surg 2001;29:131-140; discussion 141-132.

[124] Semb G, Brattstrom V, Molsted K, *et al.* The eurocleft study: Intercenter study of treatment outcome in patients with complete cleft lip and palate. Part 1: Introduction and treatment experience. Cleft Palate Craniofac J 2005;42:64-68.

[125] Semb G, Brattstrom V, Molsted K, *et al.* The eurocleft study: Intercenter study of treatment outcome in patients with complete cleft lip and palate. Part 4: Relationship among treatment outcome, patient/parent satisfaction, and the burden of care. Cleft Palate Craniofac J 2005;42:83-92.

[126] Brattstrom V, Molsted K, Prahl-Andersen B, *et al.* The eurocleft study: Intercenter study of treatment outcome in patients with complete cleft lip and palate. Part 2: Craniofacial form and nasolabial appearance. Cleft Palate Craniofac J 2005;42:69-77.

[127] Molsted K, Brattstrom V, Prahl-Andersen B, *et al.* The eurocleft study: Intercenter study of treatment outcome in patients with complete cleft lip and palate. Part 3: Dental arch relationships. Cleft Palate Craniofac J 2005;42:78-82.

[128] Shaw WC, Brattstrom V, Molsted K, *et al.* The eurocleft study: Intercenter study of treatment outcome in patients with complete cleft lip and palate. Part 5: Discussion and conclusions. Cleft Palate Craniofac J 2005;42:93-98.

[129] Friede H, Enemark H, Semb G, *et al.* Craniofacial and occlusal characteristics in unilateral cleft lip and palate patients from four scandinavian centres. Scand J Plast Reconstr Surg Hand Surg 1991;25:269-276.

[130] Palmer CR, Hamlen M, Ross RB, *et al.* Cleft palate repair: Comparison of the results of two surgical techniques. Can J Surg 1969;12:32-39.

[131] Friede H and Lilja J. Dentofacial morphology in adolescent or early adult patients with cleft lip and palate after a treatment regimen that included vomer flap surgery and pushback palatal repair. Scand J Plast Reconstr Surg Hand Surg 1994;28:113-121.

[132] Friede H and Johanson B. A follow-up study of cleft children treated with primary bone grafting. 1. Orthodontic aspects. Scand J Plast Reconstr Surg 1974;8:88-103.

[133] Friede H and Johanson B. Adolescent facial morphology of early bone-grafted cleft lip and palate patients. Scand J Plast Reconstr Surg 1982;16:41-53.

[134] Brattstrom V, McWilliam J, Larson O, *et al.* Craniofacial development in children with unilateral clefts of the lip, alveolus, and palate treated according to four different regimes. I. Maxillary development. Scand J Plast Reconstr Surg Hand Surg 1991;25:259-267.

Index

A

Peter W. Ngan, ToshiDeguchi and Eugene Roberts (Eds)

B

C

D

E

P

R

V

Y

Made in United States
North Haven, CT
04 November 2026

21719566R00263